PDR®-for all of your drug info...

2004 Physicians' D...

Physicians have turned to th... scription drugs for 58 years... standard prescription drug reference and can be found in virtually every physician's office, hospital and pharmacy in the United States. You can search more than 4,000 drugs by using one of many indices and look at more than 2,100 full-color photos of drugs cross-referenced to the label information.

2004 PDR® Companion Guide

This unique 1,900-page all-in-one clinical companion to the PDR ensures safe, appropriate drug selection with eight critical checkpoint indices including *Indications, Side Effects, Interactions,* and much more.

PDR® Pharmacopoeia Pocket Dosing Guide – Fourth Ed 2004

This pocket dosing guide brings important dispensing information to the practitioner's fingertips. Organized in tabular format, this small, 300-page quick reference is easy to navigate and gives important FDA-approved dosing information, black box warning summaries and much more.

PDR® for Nutritional Supplements – 1st Ed

The definitive information source for more than 300 nutritional supplements. This unique, comprehensive, unbiased source of solid, evidence-based information about nutritional supplements provides practitioners with more than 700 pages of the most current and reliable information available.

2004 PDR® for Nonprescription Drugs and Dietary Supplements

This acknowledged authority offers full FDA-approved descriptions of the most commonly used OTC medicines in four separate indices within more than 400 pages. Plus, it includes a section on supplements, vitamins and herbal remedies.

...cines – 2nd Ed

The ... comprehensive reference on herbal remedies, is based upon the work of Germany's Commission E and Joe... Gruenwald, Ph.D., a renowned expert on herbal medicines. This detailed guide provides more than 1,100 pages of thorough descriptions on over 600 botanical remedies.

2004 PDR® for Ophthalmic Medicines

The definitive reference for the eye-care professional offers 230 pages of detailed information on drugs and equipment used in the fields of ophthalmology and optometry. With five full indices and information on specialized instruments, lenses and much more, this guide is the most comprehensive of its kind.

PDR® Medical Dictionary – 2nd Ed

The second edition reflects the thorough revision performed by 44 medical consultants as well as a team of skilled editors and lexicographers. This fully updated edition, with more than 2,100 pages, includes 1,000 images, numerous tables, an innovative Genus Finder to help you find the genus of organisms, and much more!

PDR® Drug Guide for Mental Health Professionals – 1st Ed

The growing use of psychotropic drugs has brought new opportunities and fresh challenges to the mental health care professional. That's why *PDR® Drug Guide for Mental Health Professionals* was created. It will help you understand the beneficial effects—and the dangerous side effects—of today's potent psychotherapeutic medications. Over 70 common psychotropic drugs are profiled by brand name. All this vital information is presented in a easy-to-read format, written in nontechnical language, and drawn from the FDA-approved PDR database.

Complete Your 2004 PDR® Library NOW! Enclose payment and save shipping costs.

250001	____ copies **2004 Physicians' Desk Reference®**	$92.95 ea.	$_____
250019	____ copies **2004 PDR® Companion Guide**	$68.95 ea.	$_____
250100	____ copies **PDR® Pharmacopoeia Pocket Dosing Guide***	$8.95 ea.	$_____
250068	____ copies **PDR® for Nutritional Supplements, 1st EDITION!**	$59.95 ea.	$_____
250027	____ copies **2004 PDR® for Nonprescription Drugs and Dietary Supplements**	$59.95 ea.	$_____
250050	____ copies **PDR® for Herbal Medicines, 2nd EDITION!**	$59.95 ea.	$_____
250035	____ copies **2004 PDR® for Ophthalmic Medicines**	$65.95 ea.	$_____
250043	____ copies **PDR® Medical Dictionary, 2nd EDITION!**	$49.95 ea.	$_____
250076	____ copies **2004 PDR® Drug Guide for Mental Health Professionals 1st EDITION!**	$39.95 ea.	$_____
	____ copies **PDR® Montly Prescribing Guide™** (yearly subscription)	$49.00 ea.	$_____

Shipping & Handling (Add $9.95 S&H per book if paying later*) $_____
Sales Tax (FL, IA, & NJ) $_____
(*Shipping and handling is $1.95 for PDR Pharmacopoeia) Total Amount of Order $_____

Mail this order form to: **PDR**, P.O. Box 10689, Des Moines, IA 50336-0689
e-mail: customer.service@medec.com

For Faster Service—FAX YOUR ORDER (515) 284-6714 or CALL TOLL-FREE (888) 859-8053
Do not mail a confirmation order in addition to this fax.
Valid for 2004 editions only, prices and shipping & handling higher outside U.S.

SAVE TIME AND MONEY EVERY YEAR AS A STANDING ORDER SUBSCRIBER

☐ Check here to enter your standing order for future editions of publications ordered. They will be shipped to you automatically, after advance notice. As a standing order subscriber, you are **guaranteed** our lowest price offer, earliest delivery and FREE shipping and handling.

PLEASE INDICATE METHOD OF PAYMENT:
Payment Enclosed (shipping & handling FREE)
☐ Check payable to PDR
☐ VISA   ☐ MasterCard
☐ Discover   ☐ American Express

_____
Account No.

_____
Exp. Date

_____
Telephone No.

_____
Signature

_____
Name

_____
Address

_____
City

_____
State/Zip

☐ **Bill me later** (Add $9.95 per book for shipping and handling*)

KEY 768838

PDR
25
EDITION
2004

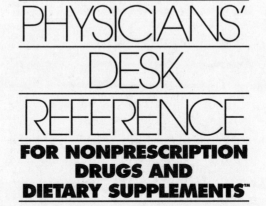

PHYSICIANS' DESK REFERENCE

FOR NONPRESCRIPTION DRUGS AND DIETARY SUPPLEMENTS™

Executive Vice President, PDR: David Duplay

Vice President, Sales and Marketing:
Dikran N. Barsamian

Senior Director, Sales: Anthony Sorce

Senior Account Manager: Frank Karkowsky

Account Managers: Denise Kelley, Eileen Sullivan

Director of Trade Sales: Bill Gaffney

Senior Director, Marketing and Product Management:
Valerie E. Berger

Senior Product Manager: Jeffrey D. Dubin

Finance Director: Mark S. Ritchin

Senior Director, Publishing Sales and Marketing:
Michael Bennett

Senior Marketing Manager: Jennifer M. Fronzaglia

Direct Mail Manager: Lorraine M. Loening

Manager of Marketing Analysis: Dina A. Maeder

Promotion Manager: Linda Levine

Vice President, Regulatory Affairs: Mukesh Mehta, RPh

Vice President, PDR Services: Brian Holland

Manager, Professional Data Services:
Thomas Fleming, PharmD

Manager, Editorial Services: Bette LaGow

Manager, Concise Data Content: Tammy Chernin, RPh

Drug Information Specialists: Min Ko, PharmD;
Sheila Talatala, PharmD; Greg Tallis, RPh

Project Editor: Harris Fleming

Senior Editor: Lori Murray

Production Editor: Gwynned L. Kelly

Director of PDR Operations: Jeffrey D. Schaefer

Manager of Production Operations: Thomas Westburgh

PDR Production Manager: Joseph F. Rizzo

Senior Production Coordinators: Gianna Caradonna,
Christina Klinger

Production Coordinator: Yasmin Hernández

Senior Index Editor: Shannon Reilly

Index Editor: Noel Deloughery

Format Editor: Michelle S. Guzman

Production Associate: Joan K. Akerlind

Production Design Supervisor: Adeline Rich

Electronic Publishing Designers: Bryan C. Dix,
Rosalia Sberna, Livio Udina

Digital Imaging Coordinator: Michael Labruyere

Director of Client Services: Stephanie Struble

THOMSON
PDR

Copyright © 2004 and published by Thomson PDR at Montvale, NJ 07645-1742. All rights reserved. None of the content of this publication may be reproduced, stored in a retrieval system, resold, redistributed, or transmitted in any form or by any means (electronic, mechanical, photocopying, recording, or otherwise) without the prior written permission of the publisher. Physicians' Desk Reference®, PDR®, Pocket PDR®, PDR Family Guide to Prescription Drugs®, PDR Family Guide to Women's Health and Prescription Drugs®, and PDR Family Guide to Nutrition and Health® are registered trademarks used herein under license. PDR® for Ophthalmic Medicines, PDR® for Nonprescription Drugs and Dietary Supplements, PDR® Companion Guide, PDR® Pharmacopoeia, PDR® for Herbal Medicines, PDR® for Nutritional Supplements, PDR® Medical Dictionary, PDR® Nurse's Drug Handbook, PDR® Nurse's Dictionary, PDR® Family Guide Encyclopedia of Medical Care, PDR® Family Guide to Natural Medicines and Healing Therapies, PDR® Family Guide to Common Ailments, PDR® Family Guide to Over-the-Counter Drugs, PDR® Family Guide to Nutritional Supplements, and PDR® Electronic Library are trademarks used herein under license.

Officers of Thomson Healthcare, Inc.: *President and Chief Executive Officer:* Richard Noble; *Chief Financial Officer:* Paul Hilger; *Executive Vice President, Clinical Trials:* Tom Kelly; *Executive Vice President, Medical Education:* Jeff MacDonald; *Executive Vice President, Clinical Solutions:* Jeff Reihl; *Executive Vice President, PDR:* David Duplay; *Senior Vice President, Business Development:* Robert Christopher; *Vice President, Human Resources:* Pamela M. Bilash; *President, Physician's World:* Marty Cearnal

ISBN: 1-56363-478-3

FOREWORD

Physicians' Desk Reference® has been providing unparalleled drug information to doctors and other healthcare professionals for 58 years. A wider variety of pharmaceutical reference options than ever before is now available and in more formats—in print, on CD, on the Internet, and for PDA.

About This Book

Physicians' Desk Reference® for Nonprescription Drugs and Dietary Supplements comprises five color-coded indices and a full-color Product Identification Guide followed by two distinct sections of product information. The first of these, entitled *Nonprescription Drug Information*, presents descriptions of conventional remedies marketed in compliance with the Code of Federal Regulations labeling requirements for over-the-counter drugs. The second section, entitled *Dietary Supplement Information*, contains information on herbal remedies and nutritional supplements marketed under the Dietary Supplement Health and Education Act of 1994. For your convenience, products in both sections are listed in the consolidated indices at the front of the book.

Physicians' Desk Reference for Nonprescription Drugs and Dietary Supplements is published annually by Thomson PDR in cooperation with participating manufacturers. The function of the publisher is the compilation, organization, and distribution of product information obtained from manufacturers. Each product description has been prepared by the manufacturer, and edited and approved by the manufacturer's medical department, medical director, and/or medical consultant. During compilation of this information, the publisher has emphasized the necessity of describing products comprehensively in order to provide all the facts necessary for sound and intelligent decision-making. Descriptions seen here include all information made available by the manufacturer. Please note that descriptions of OTC products marketed under the Dietary Supplement Health and Education Act of 1994 have not been evaluated by the Food and Drug Administration, and that such products are not intended to diagnose, treat, cure, or prevent any disease.

In organizing and presenting the material in *Physicians' Desk Reference for Nonprescription Drugs and Dietary Supplements*, the publisher does not warrant or guarantee any of the products described, or perform any independent analysis in connection with any of the product information contained herein. *Physicians' Desk Reference* does not assume, and expressly disclaims, any obligation to obtain and include any information other than that provided to it by the manufacturer. It should be understood that by making this material available, the publisher is not advocating the use of any product described herein, nor is the publisher responsible for misuse of a product due to typographical error. Additional information on any product may be obtained from the manufacturer.

Other Clinical Information Products from PDR®

For complicated cases and special patient problems, there is no substitute for the in-depth data contained in *Physicians' Desk Reference*. But on other occasions, you may find that the *PDR® Monthly Prescribing Guide™* provides a handy alternative. With concise summaries of the FDA-approved and other manufacturer-supplied labeling found in *PDR*, this 350-page digest-sized reference presents certain key facts on more than 1,000 drugs, including the form, strength, and route; therapeutic class; approved indications; dosage; contraindications; warnings; precautions; pregnancy rating; drug interactions; and adverse reactions. Each entry alerts you to significant precautions you need to take, spells out the most common or dangerous adverse effects, summarizes the recommended adult and pediatric dosages, and supplies you with the *PDR* page number to turn to for further information. A full-color insert of pill images allows you to correctly identify each product. Issued monthly, the guide is regularly updated, with detailed descriptions of the new drugs to receive FDA approval, as well as providing FDA-approved revisions to existing product information. In addition, you'll receive bulletins about major new developments on the pharmaceutical scene, an overview of important new agents nearing approval, and recent medical abstracts on commonly used herbs and nutritional supplements. In fact, in one neat package you'll find the critical information you need to make a prescribing decision—with confidence that you're acting on the latest information available. To order your personal subscription to this important free monthly publication, simply call 1-800-232-7379.

If you prefer to carry drug information with you on a handheld device like a Palm® or Pocket PC, you will want to know about *mobilePDR®*. This easy-to-use software allows you to retrieve in an instant concise summaries of the FDA-approved and other manufacturer-supplied labeling for 1,500 of the most frequently prescribed drugs, lets you run automatic interaction checks on multidrug regimens, and even alerts you to significant changes in drug labeling, usually within 24 to 48 hours of announcements. You can look up drugs by brand or generic name, by indication, and by therapeutic class. The drug interaction checker allows you to screen for interactions between as many as 32 drugs. The *What's New* feature provides daily alerts about drug recalls, labeling changes, new drug introductions, and so on. This portable electronic reference is updated daily with the latest available FDA-approved revisions to existing product information, plus the essential facts you need to make prescribing decisions for newly approved agents. Sync anytime, day or night, at your convenience, to be sure you have the most recent information available. Our auto-update feature updates the content and the software, so upgrades are easy to manage. *mobilePDR* works with both the Palm and Windows CE operating systems, and it's free to U.S.-based MDs, DOs, NPs, and PAs in full-time patient practice and to medical students and residents. Check it out today at www.PDR.net.

For those who prefer to view drug information on the Internet, **PDR.net** is the best online source for comprehensive FDA-approved and other manufacturer-supplied labeling information, as found in *PDR*. Updated monthly, this incredible resource allows you to look up drugs by brand or generic name, by key word, or by indication, side effect, contraindication, or manufacturer. The drug interaction checker allows you to screen for interactions between as many as 20 different drugs. The site provides an index that can be searched to find comparable drugs. As a terrific extra benefit, images of all products are included for easy identification. Finally, as an added benefit, *PDR.net* hosts the download for *mobilePDR*. At this one website, you get two great *PDR* products in one. In addition to all this, *PDR.net* provides links to such useful information as *Stedman's Medical Dictionary*, MEDLINE, online CME programs, clinical trials registries, evidence-based treatment decision tools, medical newsletters, Internet directories, online formularies, and the FDA's Medwatch. A wealth of information all in one place! Registration for *PDR.net* is free for U.S.-based MDs, DOs, NPs, and PAs in full-time patient practice as well as for medical students and residents. Visit www.PDR.net today to register.

For those times when all you need is quick confirmation of a particular dosage, you will want to have a copy of the **2004 PDR® Pharmacopoeia Pocket Dosing Guide**. This handy little book can accompany you wherever you need to go, around the office or on hospital rounds. Only slightly larger than an index card and a half inch thick, it fits easily into any pocket, while providing you with FDA-approved dosing recommendations for more than 1,500 drugs. Unlike other condensed drug references, the information is drawn almost exclusively from the FDA-approved drug labeling published in *Physicians' Desk Reference*. And its tabular presentation makes lookups a breeze. The *2004 PDR Pharmacopoeia Pocket Dosing Guide* is a tool you really can't afford to be without.

The use of over-the-counter nutritional supplements has skyrocketed, and *PDR* can help you to learn more about this unfamiliar—even exotic—set of agents. **PDR® for Nutritional Supplements** offers the latest scientific consensus on hundreds of popular supplement products, including an array of amino acids, cofactors, fatty acids, probiotics, phytoestrogens, phytosterols, over-the-counter hormones, hormonal

precursors, and much more. Focused on the scientific evidence for each supplement's claims, this unique reference offers you today's most detailed, informed, and objective overview of a burgeoning new area in the field of self-treatment. To protect your patients and ensure that they use only truly beneficial products, this book is a must.

For counseling patients who favor herbal remedies, another PDR reference may prove equally valuable. The very popular **PDR® for Herbal Medicines** provides you with the latest science-based assessment of some 700 botanicals. Indexed by scientific, common, and brand names (as well as Western, Asian, and homeopathic indications), this volume also includes a Side Effects Index, a Drug/Herb Interactions Guide, an Herb Identification Guide with nearly 400 color photos, and a Safety Guide that lists herbs to be avoided during pregnancy and herbs to be used only under professional supervision. Although botanical products are not officially regulated or monitored in the United States, *PDR for Herbal Medicines* provides you with authoritative information—the findings of the German Medicines Agency's expert committee on herbal medicines, Commission E.

To maximize the value of *PDR* itself, you'll also need a copy of the 2004 edition of the **PDR® Companion Guide**, a 1,700-page reference that augments *PDR* with nine unique decision-making tools: Interactions Index; Food Interactions Cross-Reference; Side Effects Index; Indications Index; Contraindications Index; International Drug Name Index; Generic Availability Guide; Imprint Identification Guide. The *2004 PDR Companion Guide* includes all drugs described in *PDR*, *PDR for Nonprescription Drugs and Dietary Supplements*, and *PDR® for Ophthalmic Medicines*. It will assist you in making safe, appropriate selection of drugs faster and more easily than ever before.

PDR and its major companion volumes are also found in the **PDR® Electronic Library** on CD-ROM, now used in more than 100,000 practices. This Windows-compatible disc provides users with a complete database of *PDR* prescribing information, electronically searchable for instant retrieval. A standard subscription includes *PDR's* sophisticated search software and an extensive file of chemical structures, illustrations, and full-color product photographs. Optional enhancements include the complete contents of *The Merck Manual Seventeenth Edition*, *Stedman's Medical Dictionary*, and *Stedman's Spellchecker*. For anyone who wants to run a fast double check on a proposed prescription, there's also the *PDR® Drug Interactions and Side Effects System* — sophisticated software capable of automatically screening a 20-drug regimen for conflicts, then proposing alternatives for any problematic medication. This unique decision-making tool now comes free with the *PDR Electronic Library*. For more information on these or any other members of the growing family of *PDR* products, please call, toll-free, 1-800-232-7379 or fax 201-722-2680.

CONTENTS

SECTION 1

MANUFACTURERS' INDEX

This index lists manufacturers that have supplied information for this edition. Each company's entry includes the address, phone, and fax number of its headquarters and regional offices, as well as company contacts for inquiries, orders, and emergency information.

Products with entries in the Nonprescription Drug Information section are listed with their page numbers under the heading "OTC Products Described." Products with entries in the Dietary Supplement Information section are listed with their page numbers under the

heading "Dietary Supplements Described." Other OTC products and dietary supplements available from the manufacturer follow these two sections.

If an entry in the index lists multiple page numbers, the first one shown refers to the photograph of the product, the last one to its prescribing information.

- The ◆ symbol marks drugs shown in the Product Identification Guide.

- *Italic page numbers* signify partial information.

A & Z PHARMACEUTICAL INC.   503, 784

180 Oser Avenue, Suite 300
Hauppauge, NY 11788
Direct Inquiries to:
Customer Service
(631) 952-3800
FAX: (631) 952-3900

Dietary Supplements Described:
◆ D-Cal Chewable Caplets **503, 784**

A. C. GRACE COMPANY   602

1100 Quitman Rd.
P.O. Box 570
Big Sandy, TX 75755
Direct Inquiries to:
(903) 636-4368
Orders Only:
(800) 833-4368

OTC Products Described:
Unique E Vitamin E Concentrate
    Capsules...........................**602**

ADAMS LABORATORIES, INC.   602

14801 Sovereign Road
Fort Worth, TX 76155
Direct Inquiries to:
Medical Affairs
(817) 786-1200

OTC Products Described:
Mucinex 600mg
    Extended-Release Tablets **602**
Mucinex 1200mg
    Extended-Release Tablets **602**

AK PHARMA INC.   503, 784

P.O. Box 111
Pleasantville, NJ 08232-0111
Direct Inquiries to:
Elizabeth Klein
(609) 645-5100
FAX: (609) 645-0767
For Medical Emergencies Contact:
Alan E. Kligerman
(609) 645-5100

Dietary Supplements Described:
◆ Prelief Tablets and Powder **503, 784**

ALPHARMA   602

U.S. Pharmaceuticals Division
7205 Windsor Boulevard
Baltimore, MD 21244
Direct Inquiries to:
Customer Service
(800) 432-8534

OTC Products Described:
Permethrin Lotion......................**602**

AMERICAN LONGEVITY   785

2400 Boswell Road
Chula Vista, CA 91914
Direct Inquiries to:
Customer Service
(800) 982-3189
FAX: (619) 934-3205
www.americanlongevity.net

Dietary Supplements Described:
Majestic Earth Ultimate Osteo-FX *785*
Plant Derived Minerals Liquid *785*

AMERIFIT NUTRITION, INC.   503, 785

166 Highland Park Drive
Bloomfield, CT 06002
Direct Inquiries to:
Consumer Resources
(800) 722-3476
FAX: (860) 243-9400
www.amerifit.com

Dietary Supplements Described:
◆ Estroven Caplets **503, 785**
Estroven Gelcaps......................**785**
◆ Extra Strength Estroven
    Caplets **503, 785**
◆ Vitaball Vitamin Gumballs *503, 786*

AWARENESS CORPORATION/dba AWARENESSLIFE   503, 786

25 South Arizona Place, Suite 500
Chandler, AZ 85225
Direct Inquiries to:
(800) 69AWARE
www.awarecorp.com
www.awarenesslife.com

Dietary Supplements Described:
Awareness Clear Capsules **786**
◆ Awareness Female Balance
    Capsules.....................**503, 786**
◆ Daily Complete Liquid............**503, 786**
◆ Experience Capsules **503, 787**
◆ Pure Gardens Cream **787**
◆ PureTrim Capsules................**503, 787**

AWARENESS CORPORATION/dba AWARENESSLIFE—cont.

◆ PureTrim Whole Food Wellness
   Shake............................**503, 787**
◆ SynergyDefense Capsules.......**503, 787**

BAUSCH & LOMB   503, 603

1400 North Goodman Street
Rochester, NY 14609
Direct Inquiries to:
Main Office
(585) 338-6000
Consumer Affairs
(800) 553-5340

OTC Products Described:
◆ Bausch & Lomb PreserVision
   Eye Vitamin and Mineral
   Supplement.....................**503, 604**
◆ Ocuvite Antioxidant Vitamin
   and Mineral Supplement.....**503, 603**
◆ Ocuvite Extra Vitamin and
   Mineral Supplement **503, 603**
◆ Ocuvite Lutein Vitamin and
   Mineral Supplement **503, 604**

BAYER HEALTHCARE LLC   503, 605
CONSUMER CARE
DIVISION

36 Columbia Road
P.O. Box 1910
Morristown, NJ 07962-1910
Direct Inquiries to:
Consumer Relations
(800) 331-4536
www.bayercare.com
For Medical Emergencies Contact:
Bayer Healthcare LLC Consumer Care
Division
(800) 331-4536

OTC Products Described:
◆ Aleve Tablets, Caplets and
   Gelcaps **503, 605**
◆ Aleve Cold & Sinus Caplets......**503, 605**
◆ Aleve Sinus & Headache
   Caplets **503, 606**
   Alka-Seltzer Original Antacid and
   Pain Reliever Effervescent
   Tablets **607**
◆ Alka-Seltzer Lemon Lime
   Antacid and Pain Reliever
   Effervescent Tablets.........**503, 607**
   Alka-Seltzer Extra Strength
   Antacid and Pain Reliever
   Effervescent Tablets...............**607**
◆ Alka-Seltzer Morning Relief
   Tablets **503, 608**
◆ Alka-Seltzer Plus Cold
   Medicine Liqui-Gels **504, 609**
◆ Alka-Seltzer Plus Cold Medicine
   Effervescent Tablets (Original &
   Cherry).............................*503*
◆ Alka-Seltzer Plus Cold
   Medicine Ready Relief
   Tablets **504, 609**
◆ Alka-Seltzer Plus Night-Time
   Cold Medicine Liqui-Gels **504, 609**
◆ Alka-Seltzer Plus Cold &
   Cough Medicine Liqui-Gels...**504, 609**
◆ Alka-Seltzer Heartburn Relief
   Tablets **503, 607**
◆ Alka-Seltzer PM Tablets..........**504, 610**
   Bactine First Aid Liquid **612**
◆ Genuine Bayer Tablets and
   Caplets **504, 612**
   Extra Strength Bayer Caplets..........**615**
   Aspirin Regimen Bayer Adult 81
   mg Mint Chewable Tablets **613**

◆ Aspirin Regimen Bayer Adult
   Low Strength 81 mg
   Tablets **504, 612**
◆ Aspirin Regimen Bayer Regular
   Strength 325 mg Caplets....**504, 612**
◆ Aspirin Regimen Bayer
   Children's Chewable
   Tablets (Orange or Cherry
   Flavored)....................**504, 613**
   Genuine Bayer Professional
   Labeling (Aspirin Regimen
   Bayer).............................**614**
   Extra Strength Bayer Plus Caplets....**616**
   Bayer Nighttime Relief Caplets **617**
   Bayer Extra Strength Back & Body
   Pain Caplets.......................**616**
   Bayer Muscle & Joint Cream **617**
◆ Bayer Women's Aspirin Plus
   Calcium Caplets **504, 617**
   Domeboro Powder Packets............**618**
   Domeboro Tablets....................**618**
◆ Maximum Strength Midol
   Menstrual Caplets and
   Gelcaps **504, 619**
◆ Maximum Strength Midol PMS
   Caplets and Gelcaps.........**504, 619**
◆ Neo-Synephrine Nasal Drops,
   Regular Strength.............**504, 620**
◆ Neo-Synephrine 12 Hour Nasal
   Spray *504*
   Neo-Synephrine 12 Hour Extra
   Moisturizing Nasal Spray **504, 620**
   Neo-Synephrine Nasal Sprays, Extra
   Strength *504*
   Neo-Synephrine Nasal Sprays, Mild
   Strength *504*
   Neo-Synephrine Nasal Sprays,
   Regular Strength.................**620**
◆ Phillips' Chewable Tablets............**621**
◆ Phillips' Liqui-Gels **505, 621**
◆ Phillips' Milk of Magnesia
   Liquid (Original, Cherry, &
   Mint) **505, 621**
◆ Phillips' M-O Original Formula ...**505, 622**
◆ Phillips' M-O Refreshing Mint
   Formula **505, 622**
   Maximum Strength Rid Mousse **623**
   Maximum Strength Rid
   Shampoo & Conditioner in
   One **505, 622**
   Vanquish Caplets **623**

Dietary Supplements Described:
◆ Fergon Iron Tablets.............**504, 787**
◆ Flintstones Bone Building
   Calcium Chews **504, 788**
◆ Flintstones Complete
   Children's Mutivitamin/
   Multimineral Chewable
   Tablets **504, 788**
◆ My First Flintstones
   Multivitamin Tablets **504, 788**
   One-A-Day Kids Complete Scooby
   Doo Multivitamin/Multimineral
   Tablets **789**
   One-A-Day Kids Bugs Bunny and
   Friends Complete Sugar Free
   Tablets **789**
   One-A-Day Kids Scooby Doo Plus
   Calcium Multivitamin Tablets **790**
◆ One-A-Day Men's Health
   Formula Tablets **505, 790**
◆ One-A-Day Weight Smart
   Tablets **505, 791**
◆ One-A-Day Women's Tablets **505, 791**
◆ Phillips' Soft Chews Laxative
   Dietary Supplement **505, 792**

Other Products Available:
Alka-Mints
Bactine Cleansing Spray
Bactine Cleansing Wipes
Bactine Protective Antibiotic
Bronkaid Caplets

Campho-Phenique Antiseptic Gel
Campho-Phenique Cold Sore Gel
Campho-Phenique Maximum Strength First
   Aid Antibiotic Plus Pain Reliever
   Ointment
Campho-Phenique Liquid
Concentrated Phillips' Milk of Magnesia
   (Strawberry)

BEACH PHARMACEUTICALS   792

Division of Beach Products, Inc.
EXECUTIVE OFFICE:
5220 South Manhattan Avenue
Tampa, FL 33611
(813) 839-6565
Direct Inquiries to:
Richard Stephen Jenkins, Exec. V.P.:
(813) 839-6565
Clete Harmon, Vice President Q.A.:
(864) 277-7282
Manufacturing and Distribution:
201 Delaware Street
Greenville, SC 29605
(800) 845-8210

Dietary Supplements Described:
Beelith Tablets.........................**792**

BEUTLICH LP   624
PHARMACEUTICALS

1541 Shields Drive
Waukegan, IL 60085-8304
Direct Inquiries to:
(847) 473-1100
(800) 238-8542 in the U.S. and Canada
FAX: (847) 473-1122
www.beutlich.com
E-mail: beutlich@beutlich.com

OTC Products Described:
Ceo-Two Evacuant Suppository........**624**
Hurricaine Topical Anesthetic Gel,
   1 oz. Fresh Mint, Wild Cherry,
   Pina Colada, Watermelon,
   1/6 oz. Wild Cherry **624**
Hurricaine Topical Anesthetic
   Liquid, 1 oz. Wild Cherry, Pina
   Colada, .25 ml Swab
   Applicator Wild Cherry.............**624**
Hurricaine Topical Anesthetic
   Spray Extension Tubes (200)......**624**
Hurricaine Topical Anesthetic
   Spray Kit, 2 oz. Wild Cherry **624**
Hurricaine Topical Anesthetic
   Spray, 2 oz. Wild Cherry...........**624**

Dietary Supplements Described:
Peridin-C Tablets......................**793**

BOEHRINGER INGELHEIM   505, 625
CONSUMER
HEALTHCARE
PRODUCTS

Division of Boehringer Ingelheim
Pharmaceuticals, Inc.
900 Ridgebury Road
P.O. Box 368
Ridgefield, CT 06877
Direct Inquiries to:
(888) 285-9159

OTC Products Described:
◆ Dulcolax Bowel Cleansing Kit....**505, 625**
◆ Dulcolax Bowel Prep Kit **505, 625**
◆ Dulcolax Milk of Magnesia.......**505, 627**
◆ Dulcolax Stool Softener **505, 626**
◆ Dulcolax Suppositories **505, 626**
◆ Dulcolax Tablets **505, 625**

(◆) **Shown in Product Identification Guide**   *Italic Page Number* **Indicates Brief Listing**

UAS LABORATORIES　**759**
9953 Valley View Road
Eden Prairie, MN 55344
Direct Inquiries to:
Dr. S.K. Dash
(952) 935-1707
FAX: (952) 935-1650
For Medical Emergencies Contact:
Dr. S.K. Dash
(952) 935-1707
FAX: (952) 935-1650

UPSHER-SMITH　**760**
LABORATORIES, INC.
6701 Evenstad Drive
Maple Grove, MN 55369
Direct Inquiries to:
Professional Services
(800) 654-2299
FAX: (763) 315-2001
For Medical Emergencies Contact:
Professional Services
(800) 654-2299
FAX: (763) 315-2001
Branch Offices:
14905 23rd Avenue N.
Plymouth, MN 55447
(763) 473-4412
FAX: (800) 328-3344
301 South Cherokee Street
Denver, CO 80223
(800) 445-8091
(303) 607-4500
FAX (303) 607-4503

WARNER-LAMBERT
CONSUMER HEALTHCARE
(See PFIZER CONSUMER HEALTHCARE,
PFIZER INC.)

WELLNESS INTERNATIONAL　**760**
NETWORK, LTD.
5800 Democracy Drive
Plano, TX 75024
Direct Inquiries to:
Product Coordinator
(972) 312-1100
FAX: (972) 943-5250

WHITEHALL-ROBINS
HEALTHCARE
(See WYETH CONSUMER HEALTHCARE)

WHITEHALL-ROBINS
HEALTHCARE AMERICAN
HOME PRODUCTS
CORPORATION
(See WYETH CONSUMER HEALTHCARE)

WYETH CONSUMER　**762**
HEALTHCARE
Wyeth
Five Giralda Farms
Madison, NJ 07940-0871
Direct Inquiries to:
Wyeth Consumer Healthcare
(800) 322-3129 (9-5 E.S.T.)

Centrum Performance Complete
  Multivitamin Tablets **820**
Centrum Silver Tablets **821**
Robitussin Sunny Orange and
  Raspberry Vitamin C
  Supplement Drops **780**

Other Products Available:
Regular Strength Anbesol Gel
Regular Strength Anbesol Liquid
Axid AR
Caltrate 600 Plus Chewable
Caltrate 600 Tablets
Centrum Liquid
Centrum Chewable Tablets
Centrum Kids Extra C Children's
  Chewables

Centrum Kids Rugrats Extra C Children's
  Chewables
Centrum Kids Rugrats Extra Calcium
  Children's Chewables
ChapStick All Natural
ChapStick Cold Sore Therapy
ChapStick Flava-Craze
ChapStick Lip Balm
ChapStick Lip Moisturizer
ChapStick LipSations
ChapStick Medicated
ChapStick OverNight Lip Treatment
ChapStick Ultra SPF 30
Dimetapp Cold & Allergy Tablets
Dimetapp Cold & Congestion Caplets

Dimetapp Maximum Strength 12 Hour
  Non-Drowsy Extentabs
Children's Dimetapp Nighttime Flu Syrup
Children's Dimetapp Non-Drowsy Flu
  Syrup
Dristan 12 Hour Nasal Spray
Dristan Cold Multi-Symptom Tablets
Dristan Maximum Strength Cold
  Non-Drowsiness Caplets
Dristan Sinus Caplets
Orudis KT Tablets
Riopan Plus Suspension
Riopan Plus Double Strength Suspension
Robitussin Cough & Congestion Liquid
Robitussin Night Relief Liquid
Robitussin Pediatric Night Relief Liquid

SECTION 2

PRODUCT NAME INDEX

This index includes all entries in the Product Information sections. Products are listed alphabetically by brand name.

If an entry in the index lists multiple page numbers, the first one shown refers to the photograph of the product, the last one to its prescribing information.

- **Bold page numbers** indicate that the entry contains full product information.

- *Italic page numbers* signify partial information.

Italic Page Number **Indicates Brief Listing**

Italic Page Number **Indicates Brief Listing**

Italic Page Number **Indicates Brief Listing**

SECTION 3

PRODUCT CATEGORY INDEX

This index cross-references each brand by pharmaceutical category. All fully described products in the Product Information sections are included.

If an entry in the index lists multiple page numbers, the first one shown refers to the photograph of the product,

the last one to its prescribing information.

The classification of each product is determined by the publisher in cooperation with the product's manufacturer or, when necessary, by the publisher alone.

E

EAR WAX REMOVAL
(see under:
OTIC PREPARATIONS
CERUMENOLYTICS)

ELECTROLYTES
(see under:
DIETARY SUPPLEMENTS
MINERALS & ELECTROLYTES)

EXPECTORANTS
(see under:
RESPIRATORY AGENTS
DECONGESTANTS, EXPECTORANTS & COMBINATIONS
EXPECTORANTS & COMBINATIONS)

F

FEVER PREPARATIONS
(see under:
ANALGESICS
ACETAMINOPHEN & COMBINATIONS
NONSTEROIDAL ANTI-INFLAMMATORY DRUGS (NSAIDS)
SALICYLATES)

FUNGAL MEDICATIONS
(see under:
SKIN & MUCOUS MEMBRANE AGENTS
ANTI-INFECTIVES
ANTIFUNGALS & COMBINATIONS)

G

GASTROINTESTINAL AGENTS

ANTACIDS

SECTION 4

ACTIVE INGREDIENTS INDEX

This index cross-references each brand by its generic ingredients. All entries in the Product Information sections are included. Under each generic heading, all fully described products are listed first, followed by those with only partial descriptions.

If an entry in the index lists multiple page numbers, the first one shown refers to the photograph of the product, the last one to its prescribing information.

- **Bold page numbers** indicate full product information.

- *Italic page numbers* signify partial information.

Classification of products under these headings has been determined in cooperation with the products' manufacturers or, if necessary, by the publisher alone.

Italic Page Number **Indicates Brief Listing**

SECTION 5

COMPANION DRUG INDEX

This index is a quick-reference guide to OTC products that may be used in conjunction with prescription drug therapy to reverse drug-induced side effects, relieve symptoms of the illness itself, or treat sequelae of the initial disease. All entries are derived from the FDA-approved prescribing information published by *PDR*.

The products listed are generally considered effective for temporary symptomatic relief. They may not, however, be appropriate for sustained therapy, and each case must be approached on an individual basis. Certain common side effects may be harbingers of more serious reactions. When making a recommendation, be sure to adjust for the patient's age, concurrent medical conditions, and complete drug regimen.

Consider timing as well, since simultaneous ingestion may not be recommended in all instances.

Please note that only products fully described in *Physicians' Desk Reference* and its companion volumes are included in this index. The publisher therefore cannot guarantee that all entries are totally accurate or complete. Keep in mind, too, that although a given OTC product is usually an appropriate companion for an entire class of prescription medications, certain drugs within the class may be exceptions. If you have any doubt about the suitability of a particular OTC product in a given situation, be sure to check the underlying *PDR* prescribing information and the relevant medical literature.

ANCYLOSTOMIASIS, IRON-DEFICIENCY ANEMIA SECONDARY TO

Ancylostomiasis may be treated with mebendazole or thiabendazole. The following products may be recommended for relief of iron-deficiency anemia:

ANEMIA, IRON-DEFICIENCY

May result from the use of chronic salicylate therapy or nonsteroidal anti-inflammatory drugs. The following products may be recommended:

ANGINA, UNSTABLE

May be treated with beta blockers, calcium channel blockers or nitrates. The following products may be recommended for relief of symptoms:

ARTHRITIS

May be treated with corticosteroids or nonsteroidal anti-inflammatory drugs. The following products may be recommended for relief of symptoms:

BRONCHITIS, CHRONIC, ACUTE EXACERBATION OF

May be treated with quinolones, sulfamethoxazole-trimethoprim, cefixime, cefpodoxime proxetil, cefprozil, ceftibuten dihydrate, cefuroxime axetil, cilastatin, clarithromycin, imipenem or loracarbef. The following products may be recommended for relief of symptoms:

BURN INFECTIONS, SEVERE, NUTRIENTS DEFICIENCY SECONDARY TO

Severe burn infections may be treated with anti-infectives. The following products may be recommended for relief of nutrients deficiency:

CANCER, NUTRIENTS DEFICIENCY SECONDARY TO

Cancer may be treated with chemotherapeutic agents. The following products may be recommended for relief of nutrients deficiency:

CANDIDIASIS, VAGINAL

May be treated with antifungal agents The following products may be recommended for relief of symptoms:

CONGESTIVE HEART FAILURE, NUTRIENTS DEFICIENCY SECONDARY TO

Congestive heart failure may be treated with ace inhibitors, cardiac glycosides or diuretics. The following products may be recommended for relief of nutrients deficiency:

CONSTIPATION

May result from the use of ace inhibitors, hmg-coa reductase inhibitors, anticholinergics, anticonvulsants, antidepressants, beta blockers, bile acid sequestrants, butyrophenones, calcium and aluminum-containing antacids, calcium channel blockers, ganglionic blockers, hematinics, monoamine oxidase inhibitors, narcotic analgesics, nonsteroidal anti-inflammatory drugs or phenothiazines.The following products may be recommended:

CYSTIC FIBROSIS, NUTRIENTS DEFICIENCY SECONDARY TO

Cystic fibrosis may be treated with dornase alfa. The following products may be recommended for relief of nutrients deficiency:

DENTAL CARIES

May be treated with fluoride preparations or vitamin and fluoride supplements. The following products may be recommended for relief of symptoms:

DIABETES MELLITUS, CONSTIPATION SECONDARY TO

Diabetes mellitus may be treated with insulins or oral hypoglycemic agents. The following products may be recommended for relief of constipation:

DIABETES MELLITUS, POORLY CONTROLLED, GINGIVITIS SECONDARY TO

Diabetes mellitus may be treated with insulins or oral hypoglycemic agents. The following products may be recommended for relief of gingivitis:

DIABETES MELLITUS, POORLY CONTROLLED, VITAMINS AND MINERALS DEFICIENCY SECONDARY TO

Diabetes mellitus may be treated with insulins or oral hypoglycemic agents. The following products may be recommended for relief of vitamins and minerals deficiency:

DIABETES MELLITUS, PRURITUS SECONDARY TO

Diabetes mellitus may be treated with insulins or oral hypoglycemic agents. The following products may be recommended for relief of pruritus:

DIAPER DERMATITIS

May result from the use of cefpodoxime proxetil, cefprozil, cefuroxime axetil or varicella virus vaccine, live. The following products may be recommended:

DIARRHEA

May result from the use of ace inhibitors, beta blockers, cardiac glycosides, chemotherapeutic agents, diuretics, magnesium-containing antacids, nonsteroidal anti-inflammatory drugs, potassium supplements, acarbose, alprazolam, colchicine, divalproex sodium, ethosuximide, fluoxetine hydrochloride, guanethidine monosulfate, hydralazine hydrochloride, levodopa, lithium carbonate, lithium citrate, mesna, metformin hydrochloride, misoprostol, olsalazine sodium, pancrelipase, procainamide hydrochloride, reserpine, succimer, ticlopidine hydrochloride or valproic acid. The following products may be recommended:

FLUSHING EPISODES
May result from the use of lipid lowering doses of niacin. The following products may be recommended:

GASTRITIS, IRON-DEFICIENCY SECONDARY TO
Gastritis may be treated with histamine h2 receptor antagonists, proton pump inhibitors or sucralfate. The following products may be recommended for relief of iron deficiency:

GASTROESOPHAGEAL REFLUX DISEASE
May be treated with histamine h2 receptor antagonists, proton pump inhibitors or sucralfate. The following products may be recommended for relief of symptoms:

GINGIVAL HYPERPLASIA
May result from the use of calcium channel blockers, cyclosporine, fosphenytoin sodium or phenytoin. The following products may be recommended:

HUMAN IMMUNODEFICIENCY VIRUS (HIV) INFECTIONS, NUTRIENTS DEFICIENCY SECONDARY TO
HIV infections may be treated with non-nucleo-side reverse transcriptase inhibitors, nucleo-side reverse transcriptase inhibitors or pro-tease inhibitors. The following products may be recommended for relief of nutrients deficiency:

PHOTOSENSITIVITY REACTIONS

May result from the use of antidepressants, antihistamines, estrogens, nonsteroidal anti-inflammatory drugs, phenothiazines, quinolones, sulfonamides, sulfonylurea hypoglycemic agents, tetracyclines, thiazides, topical retinoids, captopril, diltiazem hydrochloride, enalapril maleate, fluorouracil, griseofulvin, labetalol hydrochloride, lisinopril, methoxsalen, methyldopa, minoxidil, nalidixic acid or nifedipine. The following products may be recommended:

PRURITUS, PERIANAL

May result from the use of broad-spectrum antibiotics. The following products may be recommended:

PSORALEN WITH UV-A LIGHT (PUVA) THERAPY

May be treated with methoxsalen. The following products may be recommended for relief of symptoms:

RENAL OSTEODYSTROPHY, HYPOCALCEMIA SECONDARY TO

Renal osteodystrophy may be treated with vitamin d sterols. The following products may be recommended for relief of hypocalcemia:

RESPIRATORY TRACT ILLNESS, INFLUENZA A VIRUS-INDUCED

May be treated with amantadine hydrochloride or rimantadine hydrochloride. The following products may be recommended for relief of symptoms:

SINUSITIS, HALITOSIS SECONDARY TO
Sinusitis may be treated with amoxicillin,
amoxicillin-clavulanate, cefprozil, cefuroxime
axetil, clarithromycin or loracarbef. The
following products may be recommended for
relief of halitosis:

SKIN IRRITATION
May result from the use of transdermal drug
delivery systems. The following products may
be recommended:

STOMATITIS, APHTHOUS
May result from the use of selective serotonin
reuptake inhibitors, aldesleukin, clomipramine
hydrochloride, didanosine, foscarnet sodium,
indinavir sulfate, indomethacin, interferon alfa-2b,
recombinant, methotrexate sodium, naproxen,
naproxen sodium, nicotine polacrilex or stavudine.
The following products may be recommended:

TASTE DISTURBANCES
May result from the use of biguanides, acetazolamide, butorphanol tartrate, captopril, cefuroxime axetil, clarithromycin, etidronate disodium,
felbamate, flunisolide, gemfibrozil, griseofulvin,
interferon alfa-2b, recombinant, lithium carbonate, lithium citrate, mesna, metronidazole,
nedocromil sodium, penicillamine, rifampin or
succimer. The following products may be
recommended:

TONSILITIS, HALITOSIS SECONDARY TO
Tonsilitis may be treated with erythromycin,
macrolide antibiotics, cefaclor, cefadroxil,
cefixime, cefpodoxime proxetil, cefprozil,
ceftibuten dihydrate or cefuroxime axetil. The
following products may be recommended for
relief of halitosis:

TUBERCULOSIS, NUTRIENTS DEFICIENCY SECONDARY TO

Tuberculosis may be treated with capreomycin sulfate, ethambutol hydrochloride, ethionamide, isoniazid, pyrazinamide, rifampin or strepto-mycin sulfate. The following products may be recommended for relief of nutrients deficiency:

VAGINOSIS, BACTERIAL

May be treated with sulfabenzamide/sulfac-etamide/sulfathiozole or metronidazole. The following products may be recommended for relief of symptoms:

XERODERMA

May result from the use of aldesleukin, protease inhibitors, retinoids, topical acne preparations, topical corticosteroids, topical retinoids, benzoyl peroxide, clofazimine, inter-feron alfa-2a, recombinant, interferon alfa-2b, recombinant or pentostatin. The following products may be recommended:

XEROMYCTERIA

May result from the use of anticholinergics, antihistamines, retinoids, apraclonidine hydrochloride, clonidine, etretinate, ipratropium bromide, isotretinoin or lodoxamide tromethamine. The following products may be recommended:

XEROSTOMIA

May result from the use of anticholinergics, antidepressants, diuretics, phenothiazines, alprazolam, bromocriptine mesylate, buspirone hydrochloride, butorphanol tartrate, clomipramine hydrochloride, clonidine, clozap-ine, dexfenfluramine hydrochloride, didanosine, disopyramide phosphate, etretinate, flumazenil, fluvoxamine maleate, guanfacine hydrochloride, isotretinoin, leuprolide acetate, pergolide mesy-late, selegiline hydrochloride, tramadol hydrochloride or zolpidem tartrate. The follow-ing products may be recommended:

VERIFIED HERBAL INDICATIONS

Claims made for herbs in the popular press often outdistance their actual benefits. Which indications should be taken seriously and which dismissed? The most authoritative answers come from Germany, where the efficacy of medicinal herbs undergoes official scrutiny by the German Regulatory Authority's "Commission E." This agency has conducted an intensive analysis of the peer-reviewed literature on some 300 common botanicals, weighing the quality of the clinical evidence and identifying the uses for which the herb can reasonably be considered effective. The results of this effort are summarized in the table below.

Herb	Indications	Herb	Indications
Adonis (Adonis vernalis)	Arrhythmias Anxiety disorders, management of	**Asparagus** (Asparagus officinalis)	Infections, urinary tract Renal calculi
Agrimony (Agrimonia eupatoria)	Diarrhea, symptomatic relief of Skin, inflammatory conditions Stomatitis	**Bean Pod** (Phaseolus vulgaris)	Infections, urinary tract Renal calculi
Aloe Vera (Aloe barbadensis)	Constipation	**Belladonna** (Atropa belladonna)	Liver and gallbladder complaints
Angelica (Angelica archangelica)	Appetite, stimulation of Digestive disorders, symptomatic relief of Cold, common, symptomatic relief of Fever associated with common cold Infections, urinary tract	**Bilberry** (Vaccinium myrtillus)	Diarrhea, symptomatic relief of Stomatitis
		Birch (Betula species)	Infections, urinary tract Renal calculi Rheumatic disorders, unspecified
Anise (Pimpinella anisum)	Appetite, stimulation of Bronchitis, acute Cold, common, symptomatic relief of Cough, symptomatic relief of Digestive disorders, symptomatic relief of Fever associated with common cold Stomatitis	**Bitter Orange** (Citrus aurantium)	Appetite, stimulation of Digestive disorders, symptomatic relief of
		Bittersweet Nightshade (Solanum dulcamara)	Acne, unspecified Furunculosis Dermatitis, eczematoid Warts
		Black Cohosh (Cimicifuga racemosa)	Menopause, climacteric complaints Premenstrual syndrome, management of
Arnica (Arnica montana)	Bronchitis, acute Cold, common, symptomatic relief of Cough, symptomatic relief of Fever associated with common cold Infection, tendency to Rheumatic disorders, unspecified Skin, inflammatory conditions Stomatitis Trauma, blunt	**Blackberry** (Rubus fruticosus)	Diarrhea, symptomatic relief of Stomatitis
		Blessed Thistle (Cnicus benedictus)	Appetite, stimulation of Digestive disorders, symptomatic relief of
		Bog Bean (Menyanthes trifoliata)	Appetite, stimulation of Digestive disorders, symptomatic relief of
Artichoke (Cynara scolymus)	Appetite, stimulation of Liver and gallbladder complaints	**Boldo** (Peumus boldus)	Digestive disorders, symptomatic relief of

Herb	Indications	Herb	Indications
Brewer's Yeast (*Saccharomyces cerevisiae*)	Acne vulgaris Appetite, stimulation of Digestive disorders, symptomatic relief of Furunculosis Skin, inflammatory conditions	**Chaste Tree** (*Vitex agnus-castus*)	Premenstrual syndrome, management of Menopause, climacteric complaints
Buckthorn (*Rhamnus catharticus*)	Constipation	**Chicory** (*Cichorium intybus*)	Appetite, stimulation of Digestive disorders, symptomatic relief of
Bugleweed (*Lycopus virginicus*)	Anxiety disorders, management of Premenstrual syndrome, management of Sleep, induction of	**Chinese Cinnamon** (*Cinnamomum aromaticum*)	Appetite, stimulation of Digestive disorders, symptomatic relief of
Butcher's Broom (*Ruscus aculeatus*)	Hemorrhoids, symptomatic relief of Venous conditions	**Chinese Rhubarb** (*Rheum palmatum*)	Constipation
Cajuput (*Melaleuca leucadendra*)	Rheumatic disorders, unspecified Infection, tendency to Pain, muscular, temporary relief of Pain, neurogenic Wound care, adjunctive therapy in	**Cinnamon** (*Cinnamomum verum*)	Appetite, stimulation of Digestive disorders, symptomatic relief of
		Cinquefoil (*Potentilla erecta*)	Diarrhea, symptomatic relief of Stomatitis
Camphor Tree (*Cinnamomum camphora*)	Anxiety disorders, management of Arrhythmias Bronchitis, acute Cough, symptomatic relief of Hypotension Rheumatic disorders, unspecified	**Clove** (*Syzygium aromaticum*)	Pain, dental Stomatitis
		Coffee (*Coffea arabica*)	Diarrhea, symptomatic relief of Stomatitis
		Cola (*Cola acuminata*)	Lack of stamina
Canadian Golden Rod (*Solidago canadensis*)	Infections, urinary tract Renal calculi	**Colchicum** (*Colchicum autumnale*)	Brucellosis Gout, management of signs and symptoms
Caraway (*Carum carvi*)	Digestive disorders, symptomatic relief of	**Colt's Foot** (*Tussilago farfara*)	Bronchitis, acute Cough, symptomatic relief of Stomatitis
Cardamom (*Elettaria cardamomum*)	Digestive disorders, symptomatic relief of		
Cascara Sagrada (*Rhamnus purshianus*)	Constipation	**Comfrey** (*Symphytum officinale*)	Trauma, blunt
Cayenne (*Capsicum annuum*)	Muscle tension Rheumatic disorders, unspecified	**Condurango** (*Marsdenia condurango*)	Appetite, stimulation of Digestive disorders, symptomatic relief of
Celandine (*Chelidonium majus*)	Liver and gallbladder complaints	**Coriander** (*Coriandrum sativum*)	Appetite, stimulation of Digestive disorders, symptomatic relief of
Centaury (*Centaurium erythraea*)	Appetite, stimulation of Digestive disorders, symptomatic relief of	**Cowslip** (*Primula veris*)	Bronchitis, acute Cough, symptomatic relief of

Herb	Indications	Herb	Indications
Curcuma *(Curcuma xanthorrhizia)*	Appetite, stimulation of Digestive disorders, symptomatic relief of	**Eucalyptus** *(Eucalyptus globulus)*	Bronchitis, acute Cough, symptomatic relief of Rheumatic disorders, unspecified
Dandelion *(Taraxacum officinale)*	Appetite, stimulation of Digestive disorders, symptomatic relief of Infections, urinary tract Liver and gallbladder complaints	**European Elder** *(Sambucus nigra)*	Bronchitis, acute Cold, common, symptomatic relief of Cough, symptomatic relief of Fever associated with common cold
Devil's Claw *(Harpagophytum procumbens)*	Appetite, stimulation of Digestive disorders, symptomatic relief of Rheumatic disorders, unspecified	**European Mistletoe** *(Viscum album)*	Rheumatic disorders, unspecified Tumor therapy adjuvant
Dill *(Anethum graveolens)*	Digestive disorders, symptomatic relief of	**European Sanicle** *(Sanicula europaea)*	Bronchitis, acute Cough, symptomatic relief of
Echinacea Pallida *(Echinacea pallida)*	Cold, common, symptomatic relief of Fever associated with common cold	**Fennel** *(Foeniculum vulgare)*	Bronchitis, acute Cough, symptomatic relief of Digestive disorders, symptomatic relief of
Echinacea Purpurea *(Echinacea purpurea)*	Bronchitis, acute Cold, common, symptomatic relief of Cough, symptomatic relief of Fever associated with common cold Infections, tendency to Infections, urinary tract Stomatitis Wound care, adjunctive therapy in	**Fenugreek** *(Trigonella foenum-graecum)*	Appetite, stimulation of Skin, inflammatory conditions
		Flax *(Linum usitatissimum)*	Constipation Skin, inflammatory conditions
English Hawthorn *(Crataegus laevigata)*	Cardiac output, low	**Frangula** *(Rhamnus frangula)*	Constipation
		Fumitory *(Fumaria officinalis)*	Liver and gallbladder complaints
English Ivy *(Hedera helix)*	Bronchitis, acute Cough, symptomatic relief of	**Garlic** *(Allium sativum)*	Arteriosclerosis Hypercholesterolemia Hypertension
English Lavender *(Lavandula angustifolia)*	Anxiety disorders, management of Appetite, stimulation of Circulatory disorders Digestive disorders, symptomatic relief of Sleep, induction of	**German Chamomile** *(Matricaria recutita)*	Bronchitis, acute Cold, common, symptomatic relief of Cough, symptomatic relief of Fever associated with common cold Infection, tendency to Skin, inflammatory conditions Stomatitis Wound care, adjunctive therapy in
English Plantain *(Plantago lanceolata)*	Bronchitis, acute Cold, common, symptomatic relief of Cough, symptomatic relief of Fever associated with common cold Skin, inflammatory conditions Stomatitis	**Ginger** *(Zingiber officinale)*	Appetite, stimulation of Digestive disorders, symptomatic relief of Motion sickness

Herb	Indications	Herb	Indications
Ginkgo (*Ginkgo biloba*)	Claudication, intermittent Organic brain dysfunction, symptomatic relief of Tinnitus Vertigo	**Iceland Moss** (*Cetraria islandica*)	Appetite, stimulation of Bronchitis, acute Cough, symptomatic relief of Digestive disorders, symptomatic relief of Stomatitis
Ginseng (*Panax ginseng*)	Lack of stamina	**Immortelle** (*Helichrysum arenarium*)	Digestive disorders, symptomatic relief of
Guaiac (*Guaiacum officinale*)	Rheumatic disorders, unspecified	**Jambolan** (*Syzygium cumini*)	Diarrhea, symptomatic relief of Skin, inflammatory conditions Stomatitis
Gumweed (*Grindelia* species)	Bronchitis, acute Cough, symptomatic relief of	**Japanese Mint** (*Mentha arvensis piperascens*)	Bronchitis, acute Cold, common, symptomatic relief of Cough, symptomatic relief of Fever associated with common cold Infection, tendency to Liver and gallbladder complaints Pain, unspecified Stomatitis
Haronga (*Haronga madagascariensis*)	Digestive disorders, symptomatic relief of		
Heartsease (*Viola tricolor*)	Skin, inflammatory conditions		
Hempnettle (*Galeopsis segetum*)	Bronchitis, acute Cough, symptomatic relief of	**Java Tea** (*Orthosiphon spicatus*)	Infections, urinary tract Renal calculi
Henbane (*Hyoscyamus niger*)	Digestive disorders, symptomatic relief of	**Juniper** (*Juniperus communis*)	Appetite, stimulation of Digestive disorders, symptomatic relief of
High Mallow (*Malva sylvestris*)	Bronchitis, acute Cough, symptomatic relief of Stomatitis	**Kava-Kava** (*Piper methysticum*)	Anxiety disorders, management of Sleep, induction of
Hops (*Humulus lupulus*)	Anxiety disorders, management of Sleep, induction of	**Knotweed** (*Polygonum aviculare*)	Bronchitis, acute Cough, symptomatic relief of Stomatitis
Horehound (*Marrubium vulgare*)	Appetite, stimulation of Digestive disorders, symptomatic relief of	**Lady's Mantle** (*Alchemilla vulgaris*)	Diarrhea, symptomatic relief of
Horse Chestnut (*Aesculus hippocastanum*)	Venous conditions	**Larch** (*Larix decidua*)	Blood pressure problems Bronchitis, acute Cold, common, symptomatic relief of Cough, symptomatic relief of Fever associated with common cold Infection, tendency to Rheumatic disorders, unspecified Stomatitis
Horseradish (*Armoracia rusticana*)	Bronchitis, acute Cough, symptomatic relief of Infections, urinary tract		
Horsetail (*Equisetum arvense*)	Infections, urinary tract Renal calculi Wound care, adjunctive therapy in	**Lemon Balm** (*Melissa officinalis*)	Anxiety disorders, management of Sleep, induction of

Herb	Indications	Herb	Indications
Lesser Galangal (*Alpinia officinarum*)	Appetite, stimulation of Digestive disorders, symptomatic relief of Stomatitis	**Mullein** (*Verbascum densiflorum*)	Bronchitis, acute Cough, symptomatic relief of
Licorice (*Glycyrrhiza glabra*)	Bronchitis, acute Cough, symptomatic relief of Gastritis	**Myrrh** (*Commiphora molmol*)	Stomatitis
Lily-of-the-Valley (*Convallaria majalis*)	Anxiety disorders, management of Arrhythmias Cardiac output, low	**Nasturtium** (*Tropaeolum majus*)	Bronchitis, acute Cough, symptomatic relief of Infections, urinary tract
Linden (*Tilia* species)	Bronchitis, acute Cough, symptomatic relief of	**Niauli** (*Melaleucea viridiflora*)	Bronchitis, acute Cough, symptomatic relief of
Lovage (*Levisticum officinale*)	Infections, urinary tract Renal calculi	**Oak** (*Quercus robur*)	Bronchitis, acute Cough, symptomatic relief of Diarrhea, symptomatic relief of Skin, inflammatory conditions Stomatitis
Ma-Huang (*Ephedra sinica*)	Bronchitis (acute), cough **Note:** The FDA banned ephedra products in Feb. 2004.	**Oats** (*Avena sativa*)	Skin, inflammatory conditions Warts
Manna (*Fraxinus ornus*)	Constipation	**Onion** (*Allium cepa*)	Appetite, stimulation of Arteriosclerosis Bronchitis, acute Cold, common, symptomatic relief of Cough, symptomatic relief of Digestive disorders, symptomatic relief of Fever associated with common cold Hypertension Infection, tendency to Stomatitis
Marigold (*Calendula officinalis*)	Stomatitis Wound care, adjunctive therapy in		
Marshmallow (*Althaea officinalis*)	Bronchitis, acute Cough, symptomatic relief of		
Maté (*Ilex paraguariensis*)	Lack of stamina		
Mayapple (*Podophyllum peltatum*)	Warts	**Parsley** (*Petroselinum crispum*)	Infections, urinary tract Renal calculi
Meadowsweet (*Filipendula ulmaria*)	Bronchitis, acute Cold, common, symptomatic relief of Cough, symptomatic relief of Fever associated with common cold	**Passion Flower** (*Passiflora incarnata*)	Anxiety disorders, management of Sleep, induction of
Milk Thistle (*Silybum marianum*)	Digestive disorders, symptomatic relief of Liver and gallbladder complaints	**Peppermint** (*Mentha piperita*)	Bronchitis, acute Cold, common, symptomatic relief of Cough, symptomatic relief of Digestive disorders, symptomatic relief of Fever associated with common cold Infection, tendency to Liver and gallbladder complaints Stomatitis
Motherwort (*Leonurus cardiaca*)	Anxiety disorders, management of		

Herb	Indications	Herb	Indications
Petasites (*Petasites hybridus*)	Renal calculi	**Rosemary** (*Rosmarinus officinalis*)	Appetite, stimulation of Blood pressure problems Digestive disorders, symptomatic relief of Rheumatic disorders, unspecified
Pimpinella (*Pimpinella major*)	Cough, symptomatic relief of Bronchitis, acute		
Pineapple (*Ananas comosus*)	Wound care, adjunctive therapy in	**Sage** (*Salvia officinalis*)	Appetite, stimulation of Hyperhidrosis Stomatitis
Poplar (*Populus* species)	Hemorrhoids, symptomatic relief of Wound care, adjunctive therapy in	**Sandalwood** (*Santalum album*)	Infections, urinary tract
Potentilla (*Potentilla anserina*)	Diarrhea, symptomatic relief of Premenstrual syndrome, management of Stomatitis	**Saw Palmetto** (*Serenoa repens*)	Urinary frequency, symptomatic relief of Prostatic hyperplasia, benign, symptomatic treatment of
Psyllium (*Plantago ovata*)	Constipation Diarrhea, symptomatic relief of Hemorrhoids Hypercholesterolemia, primary, adjunct to diet	**Scopolia** (*Scopolia carniolica*)	Liver and gallbladder complaints
		Scotch Broom (*Cytisus scoparius*)	Hypertension Circulatory disorders
Psyllium Seed (*Plantago afra*)	Constipation Diarrhea, symptomatic relief of	**Scotch Pine** (*Pinus* species)	Blood pressure problems Bronchitis, acute Cold, common, symptomatic relief of Cough, symptomatic relief of Fever associated with common cold Infection, tendency to Pain, neurogenic Rheumatic disorders, unspecified Stomatitis
Pumpkin (*Cucurbita pepo*)	Urinary frequency, symptomatic relief of Prostatic hyperplasia, benign, symptomatic treatment of		
Quinine (*Cinchona pubescens*)	Appetite, stimulation of Digestive disorders, symptomatic relief of		
Radish (*Raphanus sativus*)	Bronchitis, acute Cough, symptomatic relief of Digestive disorders, symptomatic relief of	**Seneca Snakeroot** (*Polygala senega*)	Bronchitis, acute Cough, symptomatic relief of
		Senna (*Cassia senna*)	Constipation
Rauwolfia (*Rauwolfia serpentina*)	Anxiety disorders, management of Hypertension Sleep, induction of	**Shepherd's Purse** (*Capsella bursa-pastoris*)	Hemorrhage, nasal Premenstrual syndrome, management of Wound care, adjunctive therapy in
Rhatany (*Krameria triandra*)	Stomatitis	**Siberian Ginseng** (*Eleutherococcus senticosus*)	Infection, tendency to Lack of stamina
Rose (*Rosa centifolia*)	Stomatitis	**Sloe** (*Prunus spinosa*)	Stomatitis

Herb	Indications	Herb	Indications
Soapwort (*Saponaria officinalis*)	Bronchitis, acute Cough, symptomatic relief of	**Tolu Balsam** (*Myroxylon balsamum*)	Bronchitis, acute Cough, symptomatic relief of Hemorrhoids, symptomatic relief of Wound care, adjunctive therapy in
Soybean (*Glycine soja*)	Hypercholesterolemia, primary, adjunct to diet	**Triticum** (*Agropyron repens*)	Infections, urinary tract Renal calculi
Spiny Rest Harrow (*Ononis spinosa*)	Infections, urinary tract Renal calculi	**Turmeric** (*Curcuma domestica*)	Appetite, stimulation of Digestive disorders, symptomatic relief of
Spruce (*Picea* species)	Bronchitis, acute Cold, common, symptomatic relief of Cough, symptomatic relief of Fever associated with common cold Infection, tendency to Pain, neurogenic Rheumatic disorders, unspecified Stomatitis	**Usnea** (*Usnea* species) **Uva-Ursi** (*Arctostaphylos uva-ursi*)	Stomatitis Infections, urinary tract
Squill (*Drimia maritima*)	Anxiety disorders, management of Arrhythmias Cardiac output, low	**Uzara** (*Xysmalobium undulatum*)	Diarrhea, symptomatic relief of
St. John's Wort (*Hypericum perforatum*)	Anxiety disorders, management of Depression, relief of symptoms Skin, inflammatory conditions Trauma, blunt Wound care, adjunctive therapy in	**Valerian** (*Valeriana officinalis*)	Anxiety disorders, management of Sleep, induction of
Star Anise (*Illicium verum*)	Appetite, stimulation of Bronchitis, acute Cough, symptomatic relief of	**Walnut** (*Juglans regia*)	Hyperhidrosis Skin, inflammatory conditions
Stinging Nettle (*Urtica dioica*)	Infections, urinary tract Renal calculi Rheumatic disorders, unspecified Prostatic hyperplasia, benign, symptomatic treatment of Urinary frequency, symptomatic relief of	**Watercress** (*Nasturtium officinale*) **White Fir** (*Abies alba*)	Bronchitis, acute Cough, symptomatic relief of Pain, neurogenic Rheumatic disorders, unspecified
Sundew (*Drosera rotundifolia*)	Bronchitis, acute Cough, symptomatic relief of	**White Mustard** (*Sinapis alba*)	Bronchitis, acute Cold, common, symptomatic relief of Cough, symptomatic relief of Rheumatic disorders, unspecified
Sweet Clover (*Melilotus officinalis*)	Hemorrhoids, symptomatic relief of Trauma, blunt Venous conditions	**White Nettle** (*Lamium album*)	Bronchitis, acute Cough, symptomatic relief of Skin, inflammatory conditions Stomatitis
Sweet Orange (*Citrus sinensis*)	Appetite, stimulation of Digestive disorders, symptomatic relief of	**White Willow** (*Salix* species)	Pain, unspecified Rheumatic disorders, unspecified
Thyme (*Thymus vulgaris*)	Bronchitis, acute Cough, symptomatic relief of	**Wild Thyme** (*Thymus serpyllum*)	Bronchitis, acute Cough, symptomatic relief of

Herb	Indications	Herb	Indications
Witch Hazel (Hamamelis virginiana)	Hemorrhoids, symptomatic relief of Skin disorders Skin, inflammatory conditions Venous conditions Wound care, adjunctive therapy in	**Yarrow** (Achillea millefolium)	Appetite, stimulation of Digestive disorders, symptomatic relief of Liver and gallbladder complaints
Wormwood (Artemisia absinthium)	Appetite, stimulation of Digestive disorders, symptomatic relief of Liver and gallbladder complaints	**Yellow Gentian** (Gentiana lutea)	Appetite, stimulation of Digestive disorders, symptomatic relief of

HERBS THAT REQUIRE SUPERVISION

Although herbal remedies enjoy a benign, "natural" image among consumers, some pose the danger of significant adverse reactions. Indeed, in some instances, overdosage can lead to fatalities. Listed below are herbs that should be used only under direct supervision of a medical expert.

Omission from this list does not necessarily imply that an herb presents no possibility of adverse effects. For detailed information on overdosage and side effects of more than 700 botanicals, please consult the *PDR® for Herbal Medicines*.

Almond *(Prunus dulcis)*

American Hellebore *(Veratrum viride)*

Belladonna *(Atropa belladonna)*

Birthwort *(Aristolochia clematitis)*

Boxwood *(Buxus sempervirens)*

Digitalis *(Digitalis purpurea)*

Germander *(Teucrium chamaedrys)*

Indian-Hemp *(Apocynum cannabinum)*

Jaborandi *(Pilocarpus microphyllus)*

Lily-of-the-Valley *(Convallaria majalis)*

Ma-Huang *(Ephedra sinica)**

Mandrake *(Mandragora officinarum)*

Mayapple *(Podophyllum peltatum)*

Monkshood *(Aconitum napellus)*

Nutmeg *(Myristica fragrans)*

Poke *(Phytolacca americana)*

Scopolia *(Scopolia carniolica)*

Scotch Broom *(Cytisus scoparius)*

Tonka Beans *(Dipteryx odorata)*

Wahoo *(Euonymus atropurpurea)*

Yohimbe Bark *(Pausinystalia yohimbe)*

*The FDA banned dietary supplements containing ephedra in February 2004.

PRODUCT IDENTIFICATION GUIDE

For quick identification, this section provides full-color reproductions of product packaging, as well as some actual-sized photographs of tablets and capsules. In all, the section contains some 600 photos.

Products in this section are arranged alphabetically by manufacturer. In some instances, not all dosage forms and sizes are pictured. For more information on any of the products in this section, please turn to the page indicated above the product's photo or check directly with the product's manufacturer.

While every effort has been made to guarantee faithful reproduction of the photos in this section, changes in size, color, and design are always a possibility. Be sure to confirm a product's identity with the manufacturer or your pharmacist.

MANUFACTURER'S INDEX

A & Z PHARMACEUTICAL INC.

A & Z Pharmaceutical Inc.
P. 784

Calcium supplement with fruit flavor in packages of 30 and 60 caplets.

D-Cal™

AKPHARMA INC.

AkPharma Inc.
P. 784

Dietary Supplement Granulate and Tablets

Prelief®

AMERIFIT NUTRITION

Amerifit Nutrition
P. 785

Dietary Supplement
Also available in 40 ct easy-to-swallow gelcaps.

Estroven®

Amerifit Nutrition
P. 786

Multivitamin Supplement

**Vitaball®
Vitamin Gumballs**

AWARENESS CORPORATION

Awareness Corporation/AwarenessLife
P. 786

Experience®
Regularity/Colon Cleanse

Daily Complete®
Liquid Vitamins/
Minerals

Female Balance®
Menopause/PMS

SynergyDefense®
Enzyme/Probiotic/
Antioxidant

**Awareness Natural
Dietary Supplements**

Awareness Corporation/AwarenessLife
P. 787

PureTrim®
Capsules

PureTrim®
Wholefood
Wellness Shake

Dietary Supplement

**PureTrim® Weight
Management System**

BAUSCH & LOMB

Bausch & Lomb Incorporated
P. 603

Vitamin and Mineral Supplement

Ocuvite®

Bausch & Lomb Incorporated
P. 604

Vitamin and Mineral Supplement

Ocuvite® Lutein

Bausch & Lomb Incorporated
P. 604

Eye Vitamin and Mineral Supplement

Ocuvite® PreserVision™

BAYER HEALTHCARE LLC

Bayer Healthcare LLC
P. 605

Tablets and Caplets available in 24, 50, 100, 150 and 200 count.
Caplets also available in 200 count.
Gelcaps available in 20, 40 and 80 count.
Easy-open Arthritis cap available.

Aleve®

Bayer Healthcare LLC
P. 605

Aleve® Cold & Sinus

Bayer Healthcare LLC
P. 606

Aleve® Sinus & Headache

Bayer Healthcare LLC
P. 607

Lemon Lime Effervescent Antacid and Pain Reliever.
Also available in Original flavor and Extra Strength.

Alka-Seltzer®

Bayer Healthcare LLC
P. 607

**Alka-Seltzer®
Heartburn Relief**

Bayer Healthcare LLC
P. 608

**Alka-Seltzer® Morning
Relief™**

Bayer Healthcare LLC
P. 609

Also available in
Orange Zest flavor.

**Alka-Seltzer Plus®
Cold Medicine**

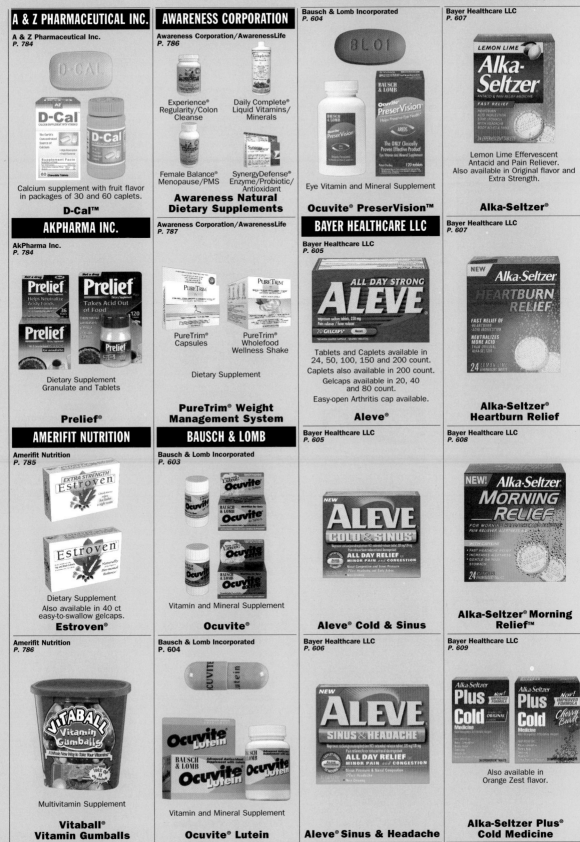

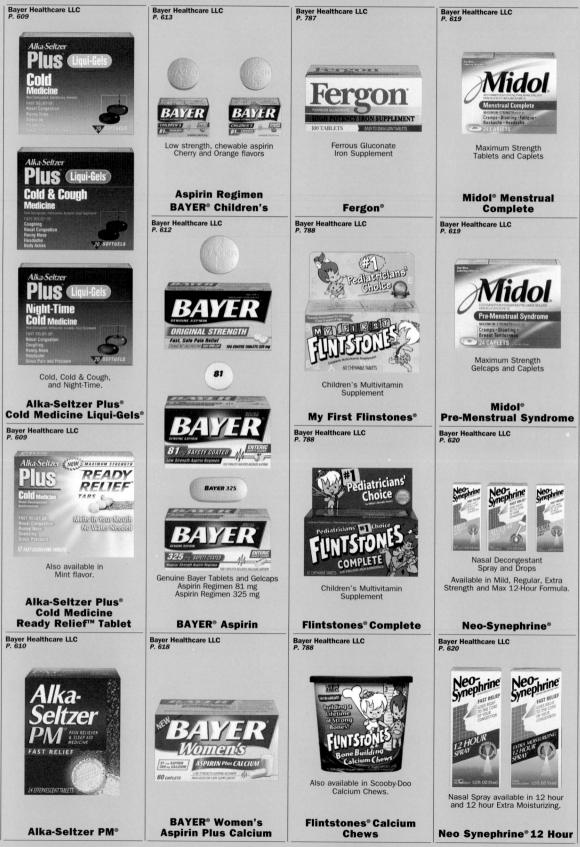

Bayer Healthcare LLC
P. 609

Bayer Healthcare LLC
P. 613

Low strength, chewable aspirin
Cherry and Orange flavors

**Aspirin Regimen
BAYER® Children's**

Bayer Healthcare LLC
P. 787

Ferrous Gluconate
Iron Supplement

Fergon®

Bayer Healthcare LLC
P. 619

Maximum Strength
Tablets and Caplets

**Midol® Menstrual
Complete**

Cold, Cold & Cough,
and Night-Time.

**Alka-Seltzer Plus®
Cold Medicine Liqui-Gels®**

Bayer Healthcare LLC
P. 612

Bayer Healthcare LLC
P. 788

Children's Multivitamin
Supplement

My First Flinstones®

Bayer Healthcare LLC
P. 619

Maximum Strength
Gelcaps and Caplets

**Midol®
Pre-Menstrual Syndrome**

Bayer Healthcare LLC
P. 609

Also available in
Mint flavor.

**Alka-Seltzer Plus®
Cold Medicine
Ready Relief™ Tablet**

Genuine Bayer Tablets and Gelcaps
Aspirin Regimen 81 mg
Aspirin Regimen 325 mg

BAYER® Aspirin

Bayer Healthcare LLC
P. 788

Children's Multivitamin
Supplement

Flintstones® Complete

Bayer Healthcare LLC
P. 620

Nasal Decongestant
Spray and Drops

Available in Mild, Regular, Extra
Strength and Max 12-Hour Formula.

Neo-Synephrine®

Bayer Healthcare LLC
P. 610

Alka-Seltzer PM®

Bayer Healthcare LLC
P. 618

**BAYER® Women's
Aspirin Plus Calcium**

Bayer Healthcare LLC
P. 788

Also available in Scooby-Doo
Calcium Chews.

**Flintstones® Calcium
Chews**

Bayer Healthcare LLC
P. 620

Nasal Spray available in 12 hour
and 12 hour Extra Moisturizing.

Neo Synephrine® 12 Hour

Bayer Healthcare LLC
P. 790

One-A-Day® Men's Health

Bayer Healthcare LLC
P. 791

Dietary Supplement

**One-A-Day®
Weight Smart®**

Bayer Healthcare LLC
P. 792

One-A-Day® Women's

Bayer Healthcare LLC
P. 621

Stool Softener Laxative

Phillips'® Liqui-Gels

Bayer Healthcare LLC
P. 622

Original Flavor
Also available in
Fresh Mint, Wild Cherry and
French Vanilla flavors.

**Phillips'®
Milk of Magnesia**

Bayer Healthcare LLC
P. 622

Lubricant Laxative in Mint Formula.

Phillips'® M-O

Bayer Healthcare LLC
P. 622

Chocolate Creme
Laxative Dietary Supplement

**Phillips'®
Soft Chews**

Bayer Healthcare LLC
P. 622

Also available in mousse form.

**Rid® Lice Killing
Shampoo**

SEEKING AN
ALTERNATIVE?

Check the
Product Category Index,
where you'll find
alphabetical listings of
all the products in each
therapeutic class.

BOEHRINGER INGELHEIM

Boehringer Ingelheim Consumer H.C.
P. 625

Dulcolax® Bowel Prep Kit
(bisacodyl USP)

Boehringer Ingelheim Consumer H.C.
P. 625

(4) Dulcolax® 5 mg tablets

(1) Dulcolax® 10 mg suppository

(1) Dulcolax® 10 fl. oz. bottle of
Magnesium Citrate

**Dulcolax® Bowel
Cleansing Kit**

Boehringer Ingelheim Consumer H.C.
P. 626

4 Comfort Shaped Suppositories
Also available in boxes of 8, 16
and 28 suppositories.

Dulcolax® Laxative

Boehringer Ingelheim Consumer H.C.
P. 626

25 Comfort Coated Tablets
Also available in 10, 50 and 100 ct.

Dulcolax® Laxative

Boehringer Ingelheim Consumer H.C.
P. 626

25 Liquid Gels
Blister pack of 10 and bottles of
25, 50 or 100 liquid gels

Dulcolax® Stool Softener

Boehringer Ingelheim Consumer H.C.
P. 627

12 fl. oz.
Original and Mint Flavor
Also available in 26 fl. oz.

**Dulcolax®
Milk of Magnesia
Laxative & Antacid**

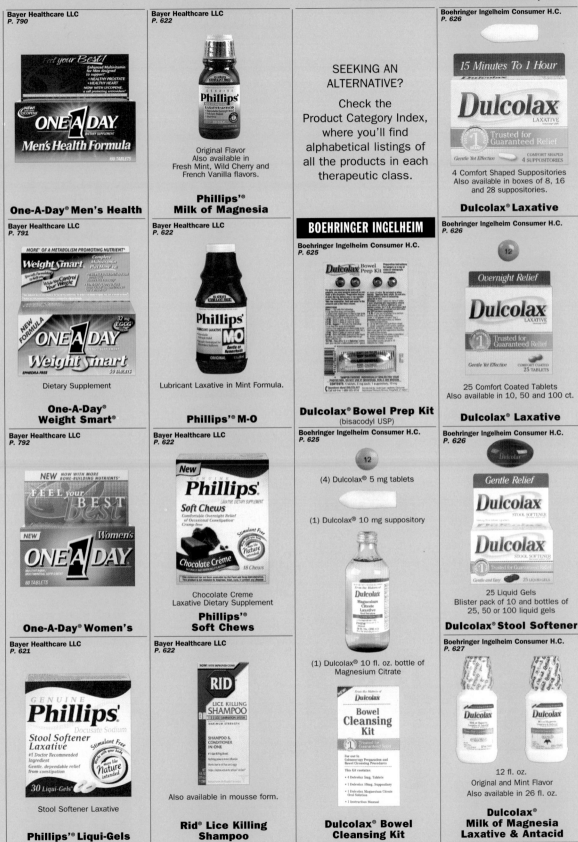

BRISTOL-MYERS SQUIBB

Bristol-Myers Squibb Products
P. 628

Bottles of 24, 50, 100
and 250 tablets, and pocket size
container of 10 tablets.
Bottles of 24, 50, 100, 250 caplets
and 24, 50 and 100 geltabs.

Excedrin® Extra Strength

Bristol-Myers Squibb Products
P. 629

Bottles of 24, 50, 100
and 250 tablets.
Bottles of 24, 50 and 100 caplets.
Bottles of 24, 50 and 100 geltabs.

Excedrin® Migraine

Bristol-Myers Squibb Products
P. 629

Tablets, Caplets and Geltabs in
bottles of 24, 50 and 100.

Excedrin PM®

Bristol-Myers Squibb Products
P. 628

Caplets, Geltabs and Tablets
in bottles of 24, 50 and 100.
Also available in bottles of
250 caplets and tablets.

Excedrin® Tension
Headache

CADBURY ADAMS USA LLC

Cadbury Adams USA LLC
P. 632

Supplement Drops. 100% Daily Value
Vitamin C in each drop. Available in
Watermelon, Assorted Citrus and
Strawberry flavors.

Halls Defense®

Cadbury Adams USA LLC
P. 631

Supplement Drops
Available in Harvest Cherry.

Halls Defense®
Multi-Blend

Cadbury Adams USA LLC
P. 630

Pectin Throat Drops

Halls Fruit Breezers®

Cadbury Adams USA LLC
P. 631

Cough Suppressant/Oral Anesthetic
Throat Drops with Medicine Center
Available in Honey-Lemon,
Mentho-Lyptus® & Cherry.

Halls® Plus

Cadbury Adams USA LLC
P. 630

Cough Suppressant/
Oral Anesthetic Drops
Available in Spearmint,
Mentho-Lyptus®,
Ice Blue™, Honey-Lemon,
Cherry, Strawberry and
Tropical Fruit flavors.

Halls® Mentho-Lyptus®

Cadbury Adams USA LLC
P. 631

Cough Suppressant/
Oral Anesthetic Drops
Available in Black Cherry,
Citrus Blend™, Honey-Lemon and
Mountain Menthol™ flavors.

Halls® Sugar Free
Squares Mentho-Lyptus®

Cadbury Adams USA LLC
P. 632

Sugarless Dental Gum available in
Berry Bubble Gum flavor in an
8-stick pack.

Trident for Kids™
with Recaldent™

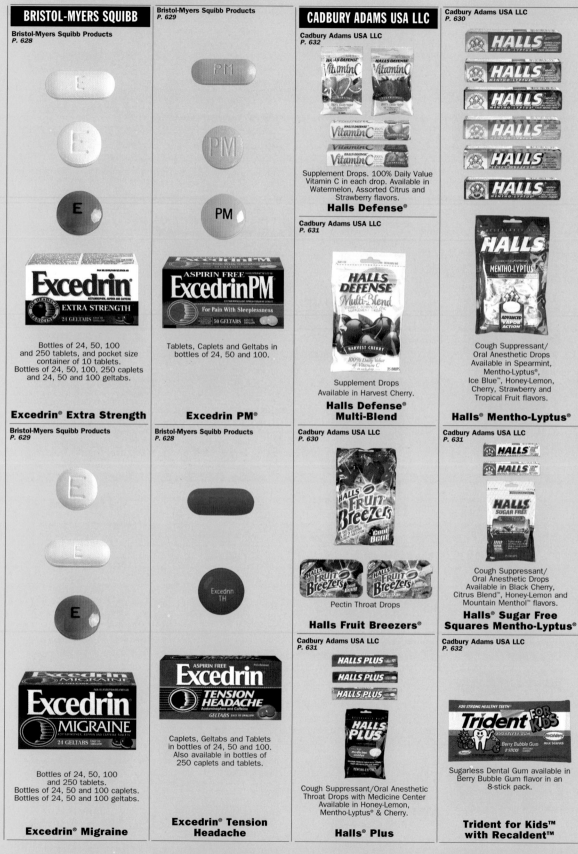

Cadbury Adams USA LLC
P. 632

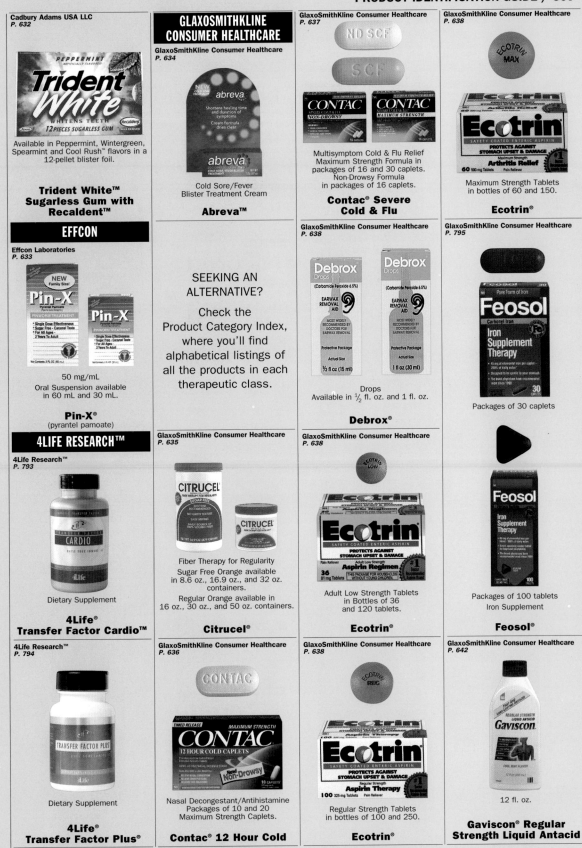

Available in Peppermint, Wintergreen, Spearmint and Cool Rush™ flavors in a 12-pellet blister foil.

Trident White™ Sugarless Gum with Recaldent™

EFFCON

Effcon Laboratories
P. 633

NEW Family Size!

50 mg/mL
Oral Suspension available in 60 mL and 30 mL.

Pin-X®
(pyrantel pamoate)

4LIFE RESEARCH™

4Life Research™
P. 793

Dietary Supplement

4Life® Transfer Factor Cardio™

4Life Research™
P. 794

Dietary Supplement

4Life® Transfer Factor Plus®

GLAXOSMITHKLINE CONSUMER HEALTHCARE

GlaxoSmithKline Consumer Healthcare
P. 634

Cold Sore/Fever Blister Treatment Cream

Abreva™

SEEKING AN ALTERNATIVE?

Check the Product Category Index, where you'll find alphabetical listings of all the products in each therapeutic class.

GlaxoSmithKline Consumer Healthcare
P. 635

Fiber Therapy for Regularity
Sugar Free Orange available in 8.6 oz., 16.9 oz., and 32 oz. containers.
Regular Orange available in 16 oz., 30 oz., and 50 oz. containers.

Citrucel®

GlaxoSmithKline Consumer Healthcare
P. 636

Nasal Decongestant/Antihistamine Packages of 10 and 20 Maximum Strength Caplets.

Contac® 12 Hour Cold

GlaxoSmithKline Consumer Healthcare
P. 637

Multisymptom Cold & Flu Relief Maximum Strength Formula in packages of 16 and 30 caplets.
Non-Drowsy Formula in packages of 16 caplets.

Contac® Severe Cold & Flu

GlaxoSmithKline Consumer Healthcare
P. 638

Drops
Available in ½ fl. oz. and 1 fl. oz.

Debrox®

GlaxoSmithKline Consumer Healthcare
P. 638

Adult Low Strength Tablets in Bottles of 36 and 120 tablets.

Ecotrin®

GlaxoSmithKline Consumer Healthcare
P. 638

Regular Strength Tablets in bottles of 100 and 250.

Ecotrin®

GlaxoSmithKline Consumer Healthcare
P. 638

Maximum Strength Tablets in bottles of 60 and 150.

Ecotrin®

GlaxoSmithKline Consumer Healthcare
P. 795

Packages of 30 caplets

Packages of 100 tablets
Iron Supplement

Feosol®

GlaxoSmithKline Consumer Healthcare
P. 642

12 fl. oz.

Gaviscon® Regular Strength Liquid Antacid

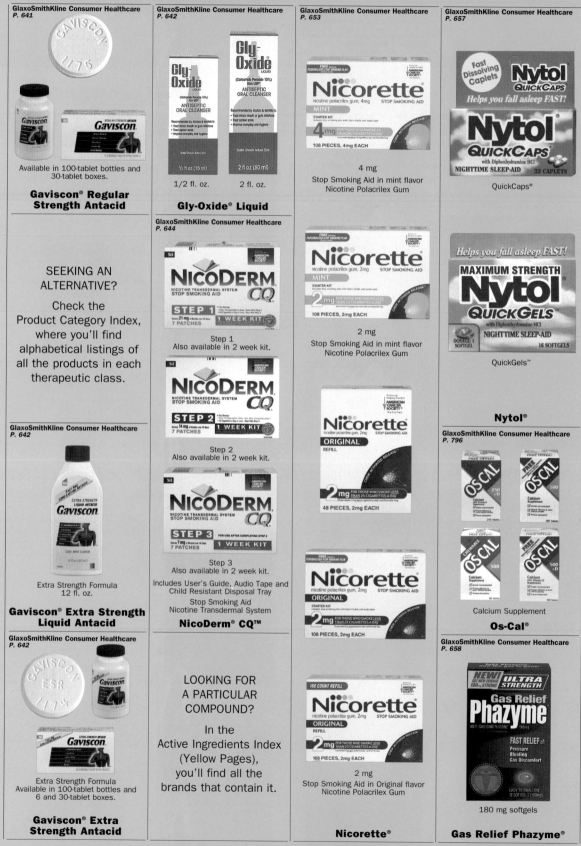

GlaxoSmithKline Consumer Healthcare
P. 641

Available in 100-tablet bottles and 30-tablet boxes.

Gaviscon® Regular Strength Antacid

SEEKING AN ALTERNATIVE?

Check the Product Category Index, where you'll find alphabetical listings of all the products in each therapeutic class.

GlaxoSmithKline Consumer Healthcare
P. 642

Extra Strength Formula
12 fl. oz.

Gaviscon® Extra Strength Liquid Antacid

GlaxoSmithKline Consumer Healthcare
P. 642

Extra Strength Formula
Available in 100-tablet bottles and 6 and 30-tablet boxes.

Gaviscon® Extra Strength Antacid

GlaxoSmithKline Consumer Healthcare
P. 642

1/2 fl. oz.   2 fl. oz.

Gly-Oxide® Liquid

GlaxoSmithKline Consumer Healthcare
P. 644

Step 1
Also available in 2 week kit.

Step 2
Also available in 2 week kit.

Step 3
Also available in 2 week kit.
Includes User's Guide, Audio Tape and Child Resistant Disposal Tray
Stop Smoking Aid
Nicotine Transdermal System

NicoDerm® CQ™

LOOKING FOR A PARTICULAR COMPOUND?

In the Active Ingredients Index (Yellow Pages), you'll find all the brands that contain it.

GlaxoSmithKline Consumer Healthcare
P. 653

4 mg
Stop Smoking Aid in mint flavor
Nicotine Polacrilex Gum

2 mg
Stop Smoking Aid in mint flavor
Nicotine Polacrilex Gum

2 mg
Stop Smoking Aid in Original flavor
Nicotine Polacrilex Gum

Nicorette®

GlaxoSmithKline Consumer Healthcare
P. 657

QuickCaps®

QuickGels™

Nytol®

GlaxoSmithKline Consumer Healthcare
P. 796

Calcium Supplement

Os-Cal®

GlaxoSmithKline Consumer Healthcare
P. 658

180 mg softgels

Gas Relief Phazyme®

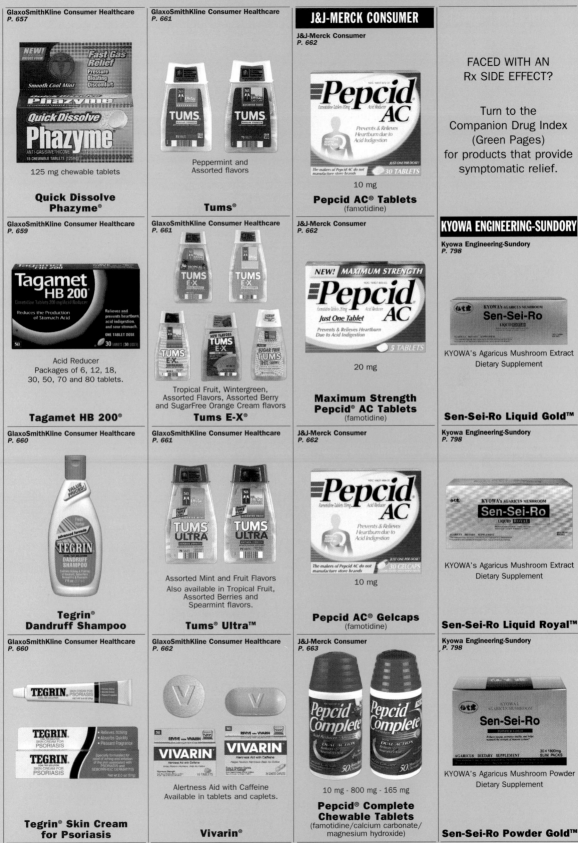

GlaxoSmithKline Consumer Healthcare
P. 657

NEW!
Fast Gas Relief
Pressure Bloating Discomfort
Smooth Cool Mint
Phazyme
Quick Dissolve
Phazyme
ANTI-GAS/SIMETHICONE
18 CHEWABLE TABLETS (125mg)

125 mg chewable tablets

Quick Dissolve Phazyme®

GlaxoSmithKline Consumer Healthcare
P. 659

Tagamet
HB 200
Cimetidine Tablets 200 mg/Acid Reducer
Reduces and prevents heartburn, acid indigestion, and sour stomach.
Reduces the Production of Stomach Acid
ONE TABLET DOSE
30 TABLETS (30 DOSES)

Acid Reducer
Packages of 6, 12, 18,
30, 50, 70 and 80 tablets.

Tagamet HB 200®

GlaxoSmithKline Consumer Healthcare
P. 660

VALUE PRICED!
advanced formula
TEGRIN
DANDRUFF SHAMPOO

**Tegrin®
Dandruff Shampoo**

GlaxoSmithKline Consumer Healthcare
P. 660

TEGRIN
SKIN CREAM FOR PSORIASIS

TEGRIN
SKIN CREAM FOR PSORIASIS
Relieves itching
Absorbs Quickly
Pleasant Fragrance
Specially formulated for relief of itching and scaling of the skin associated with PSORIASIS and SEBORRHEIC DERMATITIS
Net wt 2.0 oz (57g)

**Tegrin® Skin Cream
for Psoriasis**

GlaxoSmithKline Consumer Healthcare
P. 661

TUMS
TUMS

Peppermint and
Assorted flavors

Tums®

GlaxoSmithKline Consumer Healthcare
P. 661

TROPICAL FRUIT
TUMS
E·X
TUMS
E·X
TUMS
E·X
TUMS
E·X
NEW FLAVORS
SUGAR FREE
TUMS
E·X

Tropical Fruit, Wintergreen,
Assorted Flavors, Assorted Berry
and SugarFree Orange Cream flavors

Tums E-X®

GlaxoSmithKline Consumer Healthcare
P. 661

TUMS
ULTRA
TUMS
ULTRA

Assorted Mint and Fruit Flavors
Also available in Tropical Fruit,
Assorted Berries and
Spearmint flavors.

Tums® Ultra™

GlaxoSmithKline Consumer Healthcare
P. 662

V
V

REVIVE with VIVARIN
VIVARIN
Alertness Aid with Caffeine
REVIVE with VIVARIN
VIVARIN
Alertness Aid with Caffeine

Alertness Aid with Caffeine
Available in tablets and caplets.

Vivarin®

J&J-MERCK CONSUMER

J&J-Merck Consumer
P. 662

Pepcid
AC
Famotidine Tablets 10mg   Acid Reducer
Prevents & Relieves
Heartburn due to
Acid Indigestion
JUST ONE PER DOSE!
The makers of Pepcid AC do not manufacture store brands
30 TABLETS

10 mg

Pepcid AC® Tablets
(famotidine)

J&J-Merck Consumer
P. 662

NEW! MAXIMUM STRENGTH
Pepcid
AC
Famotidine Tablets 20mg   Acid Reducer
Just One Tablet
Prevents & Relieves Heartburn
Due to Acid Indigestion
5 TABLETS

20 mg

**Maximum Strength
Pepcid® AC Tablets**
(famotidine)

J&J-Merck Consumer
P. 662

Pepcid
AC
Famotidine Tablets 10mg   Acid Reducer
Prevents & Relieves
Heartburn due to
Acid Indigestion
JUST ONE PER DOSE!
The makers of Pepcid AC do not manufacture store brands
30 GELCAPS

10 mg

Pepcid AC® Gelcaps
(famotidine)

J&J-Merck Consumer
P. 663

Pepcid
Complete
Acid Reducer + Antacid
DUAL ACTION
50
Pepcid
Complete
Acid Reducer + Antacid
DUAL ACTION
50

10 mg - 800 mg - 165 mg

**Pepcid® Complete
Chewable Tablets**
(famotidine/calcium carbonate/
magnesium hydroxide)

FACED WITH AN
Rx SIDE EFFECT?

Turn to the
Companion Drug Index
(Green Pages)
for products that provide
symptomatic relief.

KYOWA ENGINEERING-SUNDORY

Kyowa Engineering-Sundory
P. 798

KYOWA's AGARICUS MUSHROOM
Sen-Sei-Ro
LIQUID GOLD

KYOWA's Agaricus Mushroom Extract
Dietary Supplement

Sen-Sei-Ro Liquid Gold™

Kyowa Engineering-Sundory
P. 798

KYOWA's AGARICUS MUSHROOM
Sen-Sei-Ro
LIQUID ROYAL

KYOWA's Agaricus Mushroom Extract
Dietary Supplement

Sen-Sei-Ro Liquid Royal™

Kyowa Engineering-Sundory
P. 798

KYOWA
AGARICUS MUSHROOM
Sen-Sei-Ro
POWDER GOLD
AGARICUS DIETARY SUPPLEMENT
30 x 1800mg
SLIM PACKS

KYOWA's Agaricus Mushroom Powder
Dietary Supplement

Sen-Sei-Ro Powder Gold™

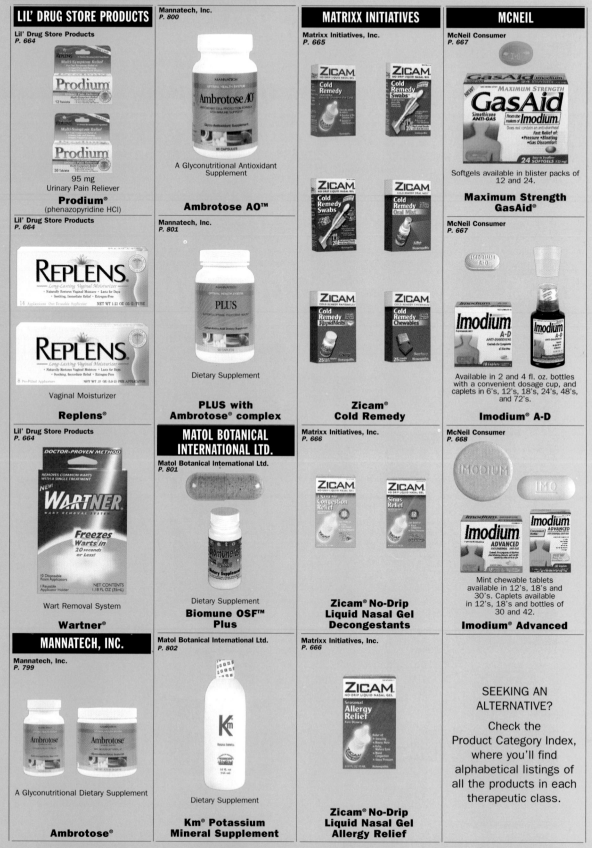

LIL' DRUG STORE PRODUCTS

Lil' Drug Store Products
P. 664

95 mg
Urinary Pain Reliever
Prodium®
(phenazopyridine HCI)

Lil' Drug Store Products
P. 664

Vaginal Moisturizer
Replens®

Lil' Drug Store Products
P. 664

Wart Removal System
Wartner®

MANNATECH, INC.

Mannatech, Inc.
P. 799

A Glyconutritional Dietary Supplement

Ambrotose®

Mannatech, Inc.
P. 800

A Glyconutritional Antioxidant
Supplement

Ambrotose AO™

Mannatech, Inc.
P. 801

Dietary Supplement

**PLUS with
Ambrotose® complex**

MATOL BOTANICAL INTERNATIONAL LTD.

Matol Botanical International Ltd.
P. 801

Dietary Supplement
**Biomune OSF™
Plus**

Matol Botanical International Ltd.
P. 802

Dietary Supplement

**Km® Potassium
Mineral Supplement**

MATRIXX INITIATIVES

Matrixx Initiatives, Inc.
P. 665

**Zicam®
Cold Remedy**

Matrixx Initiatives, Inc.
P. 666

**Zicam® No-Drip
Liquid Nasal Gel
Decongestants**

Matrixx Initiatives, Inc.
P. 666

**Zicam® No-Drip
Liquid Nasal Gel
Allergy Relief**

MCNEIL

McNeil Consumer
P. 667

Softgels available in blister packs of
12 and 24.

**Maximum Strength
GasAid®**

McNeil Consumer
P. 667

Available in 2 and 4 fl. oz. bottles
with a convenient dosage cup, and
caplets in 6's, 12's, 18's, 24's, 48's,
and 72's.

Imodium® A-D

McNeil Consumer
P. 668

Mint chewable tablets
available in 12's, 18's and
30's. Caplets available
in 12's, 18's and bottles of
30 and 42.

Imodium® Advanced

SEEKING AN
ALTERNATIVE?

Check the
Product Category Index,
where you'll find
alphabetical listings of
all the products in each
therapeutic class.

Lactaid Inc. Marketed By
McNeil Consumer
P. 803

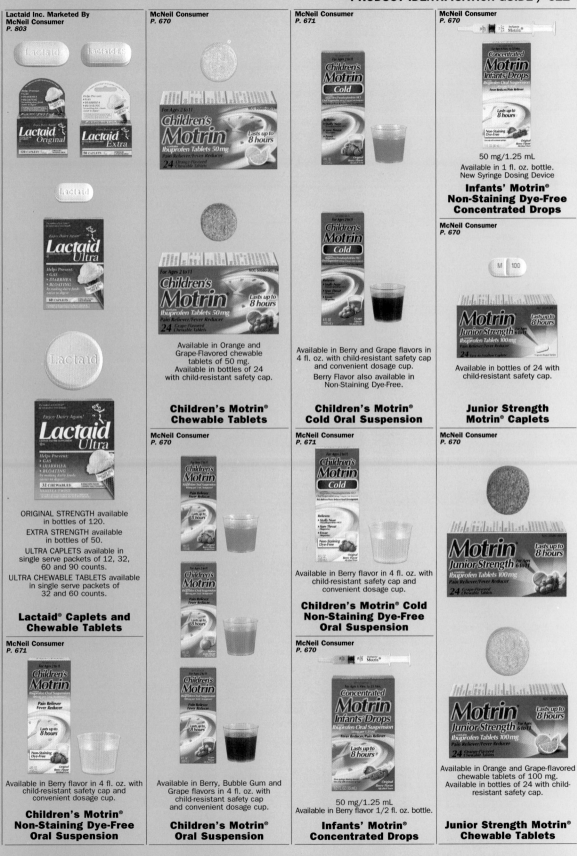

ORIGINAL STRENGTH available
in bottles of 120.

EXTRA STRENGTH available
in bottles of 50.

ULTRA CAPLETS available in
single serve packets of 12, 32,
60 and 90 counts.

ULTRA CHEWABLE TABLETS available
in single serve packets of
32 and 60 counts.

**Lactaid® Caplets and
Chewable Tablets**

McNeil Consumer
P. 671

Available in Berry flavor in 4 fl. oz. with
child-resistant safety cap and
convenient dosage cup.

**Children's Motrin®
Non-Staining Dye-Free
Oral Suspension**

McNeil Consumer
P. 670

Available in Orange and
Grape-Flavored chewable
tablets of 50 mg.
Available in bottles of 24
with child-resistant safety cap.

**Children's Motrin®
Chewable Tablets**

McNeil Consumer
P. 670

Available in Berry, Bubble Gum and
Grape flavors in 4 fl. oz. with
child-resistant safety cap
and convenient dosage cup.

**Children's Motrin®
Oral Suspension**

McNeil Consumer
P. 671

Available in Berry and Grape flavors in
4 fl. oz. with child-resistant safety cap
and convenient dosage cup.

Berry Flavor also available in
Non-Staining Dye-Free.

**Children's Motrin®
Cold Oral Suspension**

McNeil Consumer
P. 671

Available in Berry flavor in 4 fl. oz. with
child-resistant safety cap and
convenient dosage cup.

**Children's Motrin® Cold
Non-Staining Dye-Free
Oral Suspension**

McNeil Consumer
P. 670

50 mg/1.25 mL
Available in Berry flavor 1/2 fl. oz. bottle.

**Infants' Motrin®
Concentrated Drops**

McNeil Consumer
P. 670

50 mg/1.25 mL
Available in 1 fl. oz. bottle.
New Syringe Dosing Device

**Infants' Motrin®
Non-Staining Dye-Free
Concentrated Drops**

McNeil Consumer
P. 670

Available in bottles of 24 with
child-resistant safety cap.

**Junior Strength
Motrin® Caplets**

McNeil Consumer
P. 670

Available in Orange and Grape-flavored
chewable tablets of 100 mg.
Available in bottles of 24 with child-
resistant safety cap.

**Junior Strength Motrin®
Chewable Tablets**

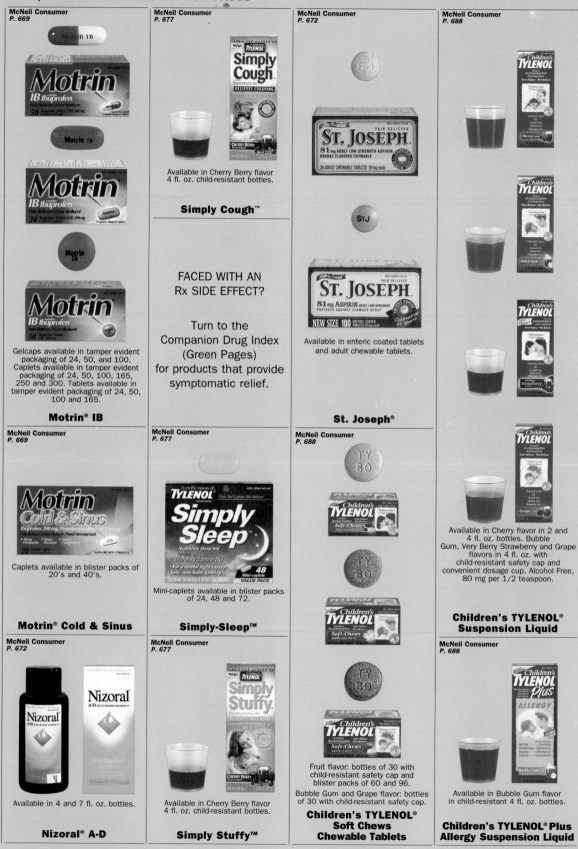

McNeil Consumer
P. 669

Gelcaps available in tamper evident packaging of 24, 50, and 100. Caplets available in tamper evident packaging of 24, 50, 100, 165, 250 and 300. Tablets available in tamper evident packaging of 24, 50, 100 and 165.

Motrin® IB

McNeil Consumer
P. 669

Caplets available in blister packs of 20's and 40's.

Motrin® Cold & Sinus

McNeil Consumer
P. 672

Available in 4 and 7 fl. oz. bottles.

Nizoral® A-D

McNeil Consumer
P. 677

Available in Cherry Berry flavor 4 fl. oz. child-resistant bottles.

Simply Cough™

FACED WITH AN
Rx SIDE EFFECT?

Turn to the
Companion Drug Index
(Green Pages)
for products that provide
symptomatic relief.

McNeil Consumer
P. 677

Mini-caplets available in blister packs of 24, 48 and 72.

Simply-Sleep™

McNeil Consumer
P. 677

Available in Cherry Berry flavor 4 fl. oz. child-resistant bottles.

Simply Stuffy™

McNeil Consumer
P. 672

Available in enteric coated tablets and adult chewable tablets.

St. Joseph®

McNeil Consumer
P. 688

Fruit flavor: bottles of 30 with child-resistant safety cap and blister packs of 60 and 96.
Bubble Gum and Grape flavor: bottles of 30 with child-resistant safety cap.

**Children's TYLENOL®
Soft Chews
Chewable Tablets**

McNeil Consumer
P. 688

Available in Cherry flavor in 2 and 4 fl. oz. bottles. Bubble Gum, Very Berry Strawberry and Grape flavors in 4 fl. oz. with child-resistant safety cap and convenient dosage cup. Alcohol Free, 80 mg per 1/2 teaspoon.

**Children's TYLENOL®
Suspension Liquid**

McNeil Consumer
P. 688

Available in Bubble Gum flavor in child-resistant 4 fl. oz. bottles.

**Children's TYLENOL® Plus
Allergy Suspension Liquid**

McNeil Consumer
P. 690

Available in 4 fl. oz. bottle with child-resistant safety cap and convenient dosage cup. Great Grape flavor.

Children's TYLENOL® Plus Cold Suspension Liquid

McNeil Consumer
P. 691

Available in Bubble Gum flavor in child-resistant 4 fl. oz. bottles.

Children's TYLENOL® Plus Flu Suspension Liquid

McNeil Consumer
P. 688

Available in 1/2 fl. oz. bottle with child-resistant safety cap and calibrated dropper. Cherry flavor, Alcohol-free.

Concentrated TYLENOL® Infants' Drops Plus Cold & Cough

McNeil Consumer
P. 678

Tablets available in tamper resistant bottles of 50's and 100's.

Regular Strength TYLENOL®

McNeil Consumer
P. 690

Available in blister pack of 24 chewable tablets. Great Grape flavor.

Children's TYLENOL® Plus Cold Chewable Tablets

McNeil Consumer
P. 695

Available in Fruit flavor in child-resistant 4 fl. oz. bottles.

Children's TYLENOL® Plus Sinus Suspension Liquid

McNeil Consumer
P. 688

Available in blister pack of 24 chewable tablets. Fruit flavor and Grape flavor.

Junior Strength TYLENOL® Soft Chews Chewable Tablets

McNeil Consumer
P. 678

McNeil Consumer
P. 690

Available in 4 fl. oz. bottle with child-resistant safety cap and convenient dosage cup. Cherry flavor.

Children's TYLENOL® Plus Cold & Cough Suspension Liquid

McNeil Consumer
P. 688

Available in Cherry and Grape flavor 1/2 fl. oz. and 1 fl. oz. bottles with child-resistant safety cap and calibrated droppers. Alcohol Free, 80 mg per 0.8 mL.

Concentrated TYLENOL® Infants' Drops

McNeil Consumer
P. 678

Geltabs available in tamper-evident bottles of 20's, 40's and 80's. Caplets available in bottles of 24's, 50's, 100's, 150's and 200's.

TYLENOL® 8 Hour Extended Release

McNeil Consumer
P. 690

Available in blister pack of 24 chewable tablets. Cherry flavor.

Children's TYLENOL® Plus Cold & Cough Chewable Tablets

McNeil Consumer
P. 690

Available in 1/2 fl. oz. bottle with child-resistant safety cap and calibrated dropper. Bubble Gum flavor, Alcohol-free.

Concentrated TYLENOL® Infants' Drops Plus Cold

Caplets: tamper-resistant vials of 10 and bottles of 8's, 16's, 24's, 50's, 100's, 150's, 250's and 325's.
Tablets: tamper-resistant vials of 10 and bottles of 30's, 60's, 100's and 200's.
Liquid: tamper-evident 8 fl. oz. bottles.

Extra Strength TYLENOL®

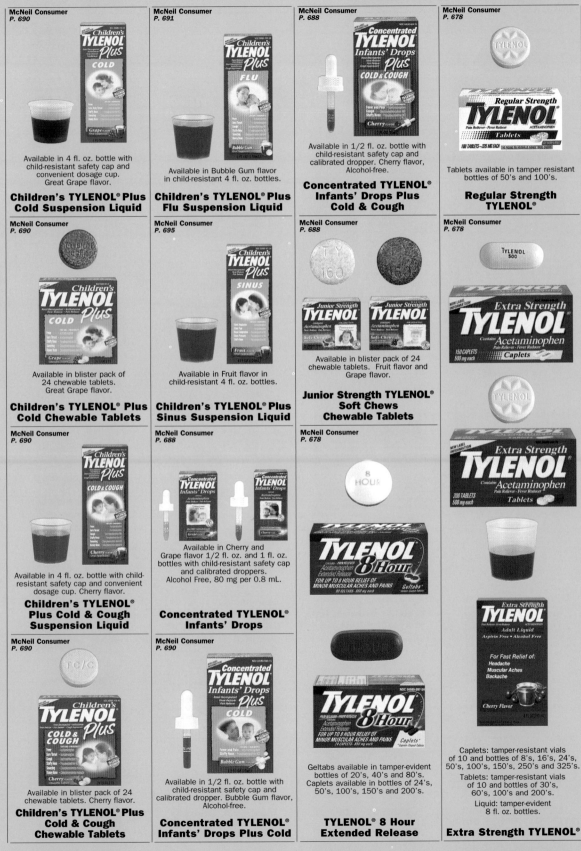

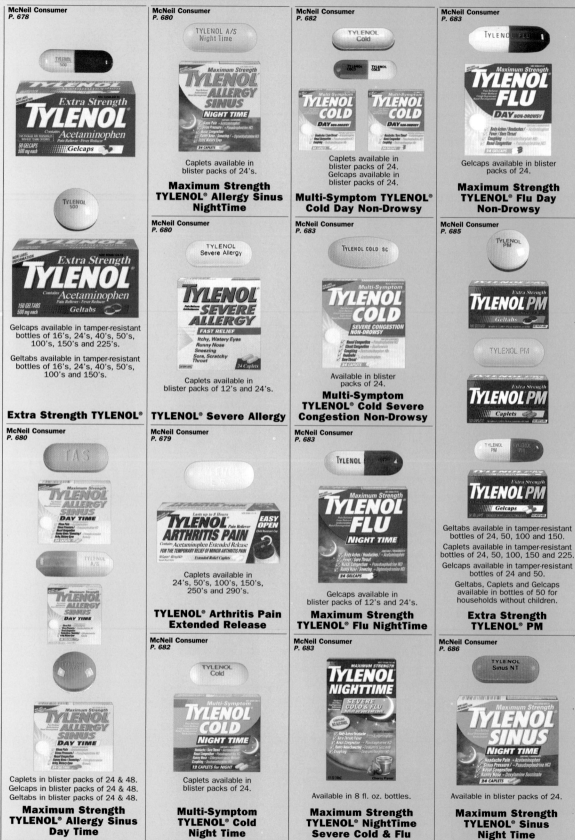

McNeil Consumer
P. 678

Gelcaps available in tamper-resistant bottles of 16's, 24's, 40's, 50's, 100's, 150's and 225's.

Geltabs available in tamper-resistant bottles of 16's, 24's, 40's, 50's, 100's and 150's.

Extra Strength TYLENOL®

McNeil Consumer
P. 680

Caplets in blister packs of 24 & 48.
Gelcaps in blister packs of 24 & 48.
Geltabs in blister packs of 24 & 48.

Maximum Strength TYLENOL® Allergy Sinus Day Time

McNeil Consumer
P. 680

Caplets available in blister packs of 24's.

Maximum Strength TYLENOL® Allergy Sinus NightTime

McNeil Consumer
P. 680

Caplets available in blister packs of 12's and 24's.

TYLENOL® Severe Allergy

McNeil Consumer
P. 679

Caplets available in 24's, 50's, 100's, 150's, 250's and 290's.

TYLENOL® Arthritis Pain Extended Release

McNeil Consumer
P. 682

Caplets available in blister packs of 24.

Multi-Symptom TYLENOL® Cold Night Time

McNeil Consumer
P. 682

Caplets available in blister packs of 24.
Gelcaps available in blister packs of 24.

Multi-Symptom TYLENOL® Cold Day Non-Drowsy

McNeil Consumer
P. 683

Available in blister packs of 24.

Multi-Symptom TYLENOL® Cold Severe Congestion Non-Drowsy

McNeil Consumer
P. 683

Gelcaps available in blister packs of 12's and 24's.

Maximum Strength TYLENOL® Flu NightTime

McNeil Consumer
P. 683

Available in 8 fl. oz. bottles.

Maximum Strength TYLENOL® NightTime Severe Cold & Flu

McNeil Consumer
P. 683

Gelcaps available in blister packs of 24.

Maximum Strength TYLENOL® Flu Day Non-Drowsy

McNeil Consumer
P. 685

Geltabs available in tamper-resistant bottles of 24, 50, 100 and 150.

Caplets available in tamper-resistant bottles of 24, 50, 100, 150 and 225.

Gelcaps available in tamper-resistant bottles of 24 and 50.

Geltabs, Caplets and Gelcaps available in bottles of 50 for households without children.

Extra Strength TYLENOL® PM

McNeil Consumer
P. 686

Available in blister packs of 24.

Maximum Strength TYLENOL® Sinus Night Time

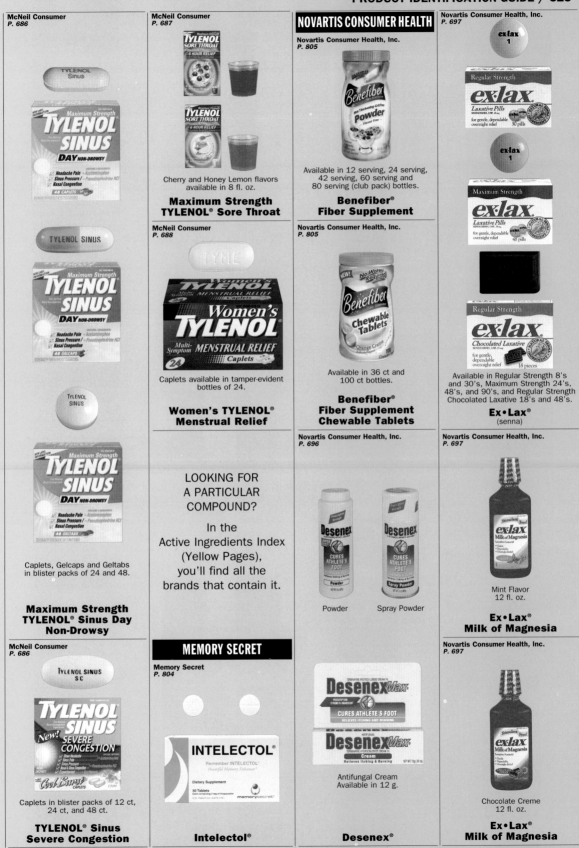

McNeil Consumer
P. 686

**Maximum Strength
TYLENOL® Sinus Day
Non-Drowsy**

Caplets, Gelcaps and Geltabs
in blister packs of 24 and 48.

McNeil Consumer
P. 686

Caplets in blister packs of 12 ct,
24 ct, and 48 ct.

**TYLENOL® Sinus
Severe Congestion**

McNeil Consumer
P. 687

Cherry and Honey Lemon flavors
available in 8 fl. oz.

**Maximum Strength
TYLENOL® Sore Throat**

McNeil Consumer
P. 688

Caplets available in tamper-evident
bottles of 24.

**Women's TYLENOL®
Menstrual Relief**

LOOKING FOR
A PARTICULAR
COMPOUND?

In the
Active Ingredients Index
(Yellow Pages),
you'll find all the
brands that contain it.

MEMORY SECRET

Memory Secret
P. 804

Intelectol®

NOVARTIS CONSUMER HEALTH

Novartis Consumer Health, Inc.
P. 805

Available in 12 serving, 24 serving,
42 serving, 60 serving and
80 serving (club pack) bottles.

**Benefiber®
Fiber Supplement**

Novartis Consumer Health, Inc.
P. 805

Available in 36 ct and
100 ct bottles.

**Benefiber®
Fiber Supplement
Chewable Tablets**

Novartis Consumer Health, Inc.
P. 696

Powder   Spray Powder

Antifungal Cream
Available in 12 g.

Desenex®

Novartis Consumer Health, Inc.
P. 697

Available in Regular Strength 8's
and 30's, Maximum Strength 24's,
48's, and 90's, and Regular Strength
Chocolated Laxative 18's and 48's.

Ex•Lax®
(senna)

Novartis Consumer Health, Inc.
P. 697

Mint Flavor
12 fl. oz.

**Ex•Lax®
Milk of Magnesia**

Novartis Consumer Health, Inc.
P. 697

Chocolate Creme
12 fl. oz.

**Ex•Lax®
Milk of Magnesia**

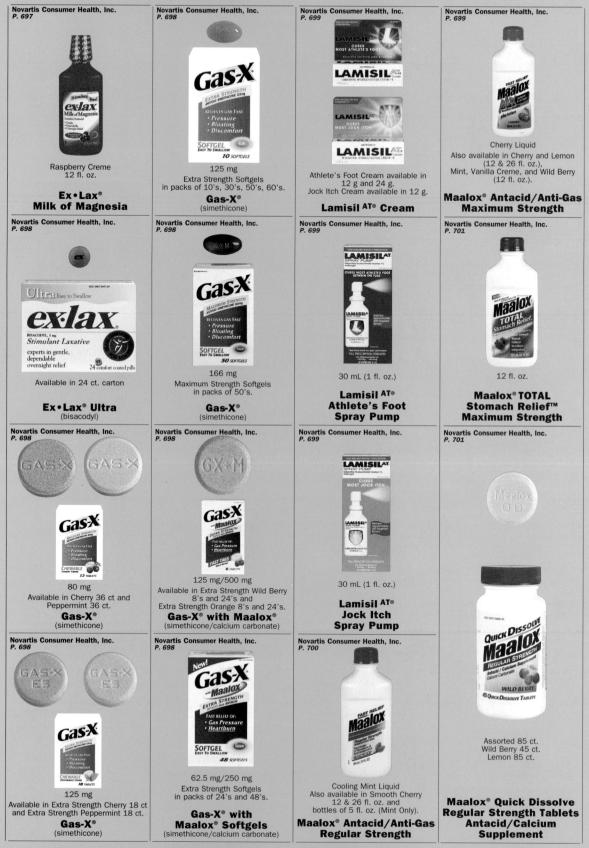

Novartis Consumer Health, Inc.
P. 697

Raspberry Creme
12 fl. oz.

**Ex•Lax®
Milk of Magnesia**

Novartis Consumer Health, Inc.
P. 698

Available in 24 ct. carton

Ex•Lax® Ultra
(bisacodyl)

Novartis Consumer Health, Inc.
P. 698

80 mg
Available in Cherry 36 ct and
Peppermint 36 ct.

Gas-X®
(simethicone)

Novartis Consumer Health, Inc.
P. 698

125 mg
Available in Extra Strength Cherry 18 ct
and Extra Strength Peppermint 18 ct.

Gas-X®
(simethicone)

Novartis Consumer Health, Inc.
P. 698

125 mg
Extra Strength Softgels
in packs of 10's, 30's, 50's, 60's.

Gas-X®
(simethicone)

Novartis Consumer Health, Inc.
P. 698

166 mg
Maximum Strength Softgels
in packs of 50's.

Gas-X®
(simethicone)

Novartis Consumer Health, Inc.
P. 698

125 mg/500 mg
Available in Extra Strength Wild Berry
8's and 24's and
Extra Strength Orange 8's and 24's.

Gas-X® with Maalox®
(simethicone/calcium carbonate)

Novartis Consumer Health, Inc.
P. 698

62.5 mg/250 mg
Extra Strength Softgels
in packs of 24's and 48's.

**Gas-X® with
Maalox® Softgels**
(simethicone/calcium carbonate)

Novartis Consumer Health, Inc.
P. 699

Athlete's Foot Cream available in
12 g and 24 g.
Jock Itch Cream available in 12 g.

Lamisil AT® Cream

Novartis Consumer Health, Inc.
P. 699

30 mL (1 fl. oz.)

**Lamisil AT®
Athlete's Foot
Spray Pump**

Novartis Consumer Health, Inc.
P. 699

30 mL (1 fl. oz.)

**Lamisil AT®
Jock Itch
Spray Pump**

Novartis Consumer Health, Inc.
P. 700

Cooling Mint Liquid
Also available in Smooth Cherry
12 & 26 fl. oz. and
bottles of 5 fl. oz. (Mint Only).

**Maalox® Antacid/Anti-Gas
Regular Strength**

Novartis Consumer Health, Inc.
P. 699

Cherry Liquid
Also available in Cherry and Lemon
(12 & 26 fl. oz.),
Mint, Vanilla Creme, and Wild Berry
(12 fl. oz.).

**Maalox® Antacid/Anti-Gas
Maximum Strength**

Novartis Consumer Health, Inc.
P. 701

12 fl. oz.

**Maalox® TOTAL
Stomach Relief™
Maximum Strength**

Novartis Consumer Health, Inc.
P. 701

Assorted 85 ct.
Wild Berry 45 ct.
Lemon 85 ct.

**Maalox® Quick Dissolve
Regular Strength Tablets
Antacid/Calcium
Supplement**

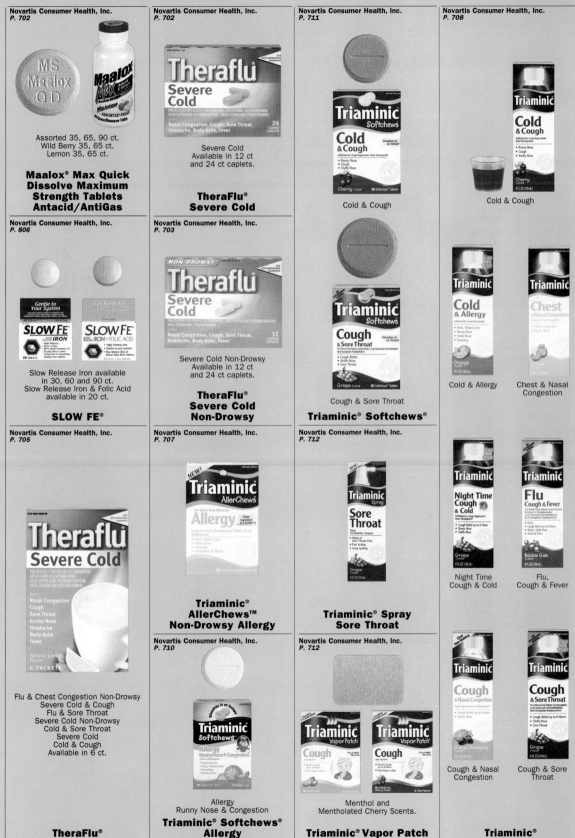

Novartis Consumer Health, Inc.
P. 702

Assorted 35, 65, 90 ct.
Wild Berry 35, 65 ct.
Lemon 35, 65 ct.

**Maalox® Max Quick
Dissolve Maximum
Strength Tablets
Antacid/AntiGas**

Novartis Consumer Health, Inc.
P. 806

Slow Release Iron available
in 30, 60 and 90 ct.
Slow Release Iron & Folic Acid
available in 20 ct.

SLOW FE®

Novartis Consumer Health, Inc.
P. 705

Flu & Chest Congestion Non-Drowsy
Severe Cold & Cough
Flu & Sore Throat
Severe Cold Non-Drowsy
Cold & Sore Throat
Severe Cold
Cold & Cough
Available in 6 ct.

TheraFlu®

Novartis Consumer Health, Inc.
P. 702

Severe Cold
Available in 12 ct
and 24 ct caplets.

**TheraFlu®
Severe Cold**

Novartis Consumer Health, Inc.
P. 703

Severe Cold Non-Drowsy
Available in 12 ct
and 24 ct caplets.

**TheraFlu®
Severe Cold
Non-Drowsy**

Novartis Consumer Health, Inc.
P. 707

**Triaminic®
AllerChews™
Non-Drowsy Allergy**

Novartis Consumer Health, Inc.
P. 710

Allergy
Runny Nose & Congestion

**Triaminic® Softchews®
Allergy**

Novartis Consumer Health, Inc.
P. 711

Cold & Cough

Cough & Sore Throat

Triaminic® Softchews®

Novartis Consumer Health, Inc.
P. 712

**Triaminic® Spray
Sore Throat**

Novartis Consumer Health, Inc.
P. 712

Menthol and
Mentholated Cherry Scents.

Triaminic® Vapor Patch

Novartis Consumer Health, Inc.
P. 708

Cold & Cough

Cold & Allergy   Chest & Nasal
                        Congestion

Night Time   Flu,
Cough & Cold   Cough & Fever

Cough & Nasal   Cough & Sore
Congestion   Throat

Triaminic®

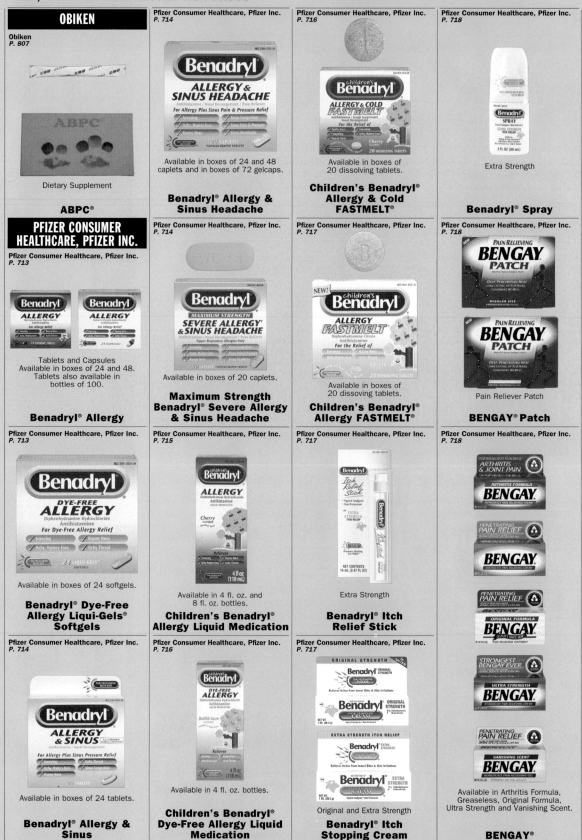

OBIKEN

Obiken
P. 807

Dietary Supplement

ABPC®

PFIZER CONSUMER HEALTHCARE, PFIZER INC.

Pfizer Consumer Healthcare, Pfizer Inc.
P. 713

Tablets and Capsules
Available in boxes of 24 and 48.
Tablets also available in
bottles of 100.

Benadryl® Allergy

Pfizer Consumer Healthcare, Pfizer Inc.
P. 713

Available in boxes of 24 softgels.

Benadryl® Dye-Free Allergy Liqui-Gels® Softgels

Pfizer Consumer Healthcare, Pfizer Inc.
P. 714

Available in boxes of 24 tablets.

Benadryl® Allergy & Sinus

Pfizer Consumer Healthcare, Pfizer Inc.
P. 714

Available in boxes of 24 and 48
caplets and in boxes of 72 gelcaps.

Benadryl® Allergy & Sinus Headache

Pfizer Consumer Healthcare, Pfizer Inc.
P. 714

Available in boxes of 20 caplets.

Maximum Strength Benadryl® Severe Allergy & Sinus Headache

Pfizer Consumer Healthcare, Pfizer Inc.
P. 715

Available in 4 fl. oz. and
8 fl. oz. bottles.

Children's Benadryl® Allergy Liquid Medication

Pfizer Consumer Healthcare, Pfizer Inc.
P. 716

Available in 4 fl. oz. bottles.

Children's Benadryl® Dye-Free Allergy Liquid Medication

Pfizer Consumer Healthcare, Pfizer Inc.
P. 716

Available in boxes of
20 dissolving tablets.

Children's Benadryl® Allergy & Cold FASTMELT®

Pfizer Consumer Healthcare, Pfizer Inc.
P. 717

Available in boxes of
20 dissoving tablets.

Children's Benadryl® Allergy FASTMELT®

Pfizer Consumer Healthcare, Pfizer Inc.
P. 717

Extra Strength

Benadryl® Itch Relief Stick

Pfizer Consumer Healthcare, Pfizer Inc.
P. 717

Original and Extra Strength

Benadryl® Itch Stopping Cream

Pfizer Consumer Healthcare, Pfizer Inc.
P. 718

Extra Strength

Benadryl® Spray

Pfizer Consumer Healthcare, Pfizer Inc.
P. 718

Pain Reliever Patch

BENGAY® Patch

Pfizer Consumer Healthcare, Pfizer Inc.
P. 718

Available in Arthritis Formula,
Greaseless, Original Formula,
Ultra Strength and Vanishing Scent.

BENGAY®

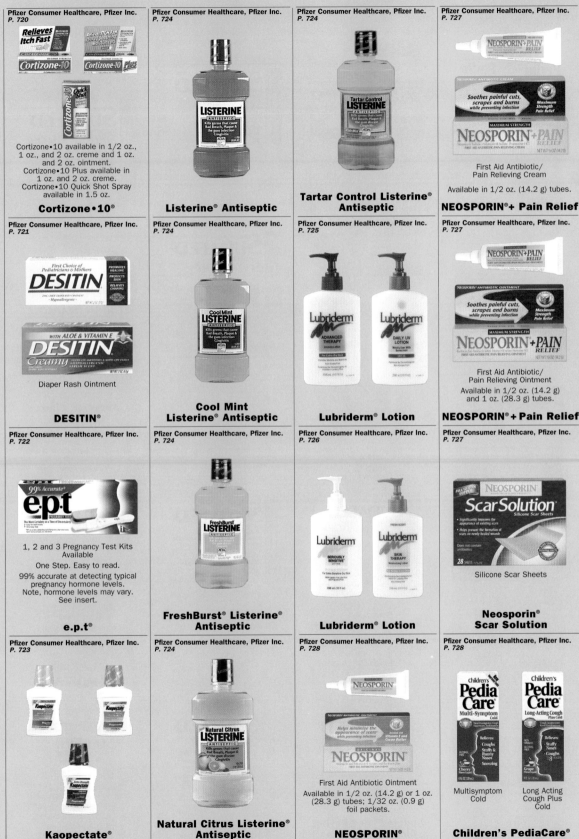

Pfizer Consumer Healthcare, Pfizer Inc.
P. 720

Cortizone•10 available in 1/2 oz.,
1 oz., and 2 oz. creme and 1 oz.
and 2 oz. ointment.
Cortizone•10 Plus available in
1 oz. and 2 oz. creme.
Cortizone•10 Quick Shot Spray
available in 1.5 oz.

Cortizone•10®

Pfizer Consumer Healthcare, Pfizer Inc.
P. 721

Diaper Rash Ointment

DESITIN®

Pfizer Consumer Healthcare, Pfizer Inc.
P. 722

1, 2 and 3 Pregnancy Test Kits
Available
One Step. Easy to read.
99% accurate at detecting typical
pregnancy hormone levels.
Note, hormone levels may vary.
See insert.

e.p.t®

Pfizer Consumer Healthcare, Pfizer Inc.
P. 723

Kaopectate®

Pfizer Consumer Healthcare, Pfizer Inc.
P. 724

Listerine® Antiseptic

Pfizer Consumer Healthcare, Pfizer Inc.
P. 724

**Cool Mint
Listerine® Antiseptic**

Pfizer Consumer Healthcare, Pfizer Inc.
P. 724

**FreshBurst® Listerine®
Antiseptic**

Pfizer Consumer Healthcare, Pfizer Inc.
P. 724

**Natural Citrus Listerine®
Antiseptic**

Pfizer Consumer Healthcare, Pfizer Inc.
P. 724

**Tartar Control Listerine®
Antiseptic**

Pfizer Consumer Healthcare, Pfizer Inc.
P. 725

Lubriderm® Lotion

Pfizer Consumer Healthcare, Pfizer Inc.
P. 726

Lubriderm® Lotion

Pfizer Consumer Healthcare, Pfizer Inc.
P. 728

First Aid Antibiotic Ointment
Available in 1/2 oz. (14.2 g) or 1 oz.
(28.3 g) tubes; 1/32 oz. (0.9 g)
foil packets.

NEOSPORIN®

Pfizer Consumer Healthcare, Pfizer Inc.
P. 727

First Aid Antibiotic/
Pain Relieving Cream

Available in 1/2 oz. (14.2 g) tubes.

NEOSPORIN®+ Pain Relief

Pfizer Consumer Healthcare, Pfizer Inc.
P. 727

First Aid Antibiotic/
Pain Relieving Ointment
Available in 1/2 oz. (14.2 g)
and 1 oz. (28.3 g) tubes.

NEOSPORIN®+ Pain Relief

Pfizer Consumer Healthcare, Pfizer Inc.
P. 727

Silicone Scar Sheets

**Neosporin®
Scar Solution**

Pfizer Consumer Healthcare, Pfizer Inc.
P. 728

Multisymptom
Cold

Long Acting
Cough Plus
Cold

Children's PediaCare®

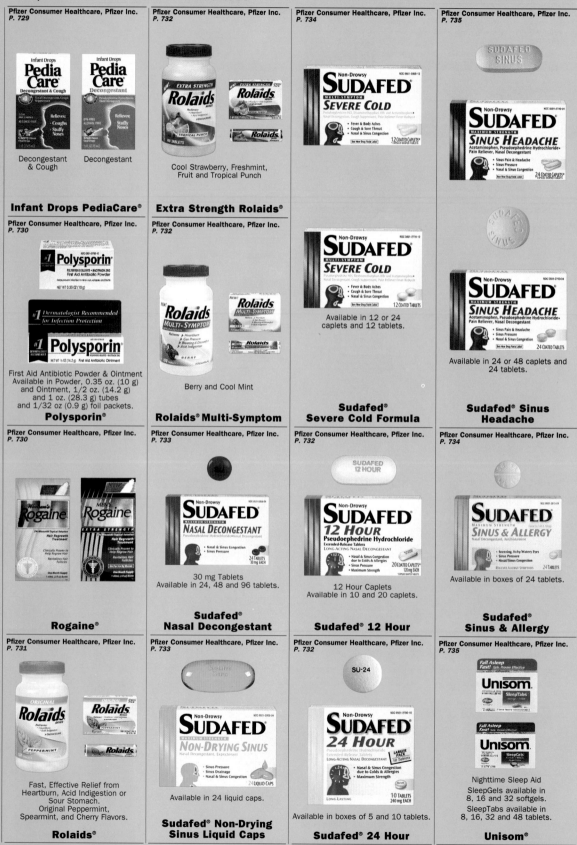

Pfizer Consumer Healthcare, Pfizer Inc.
P. 729

Decongestant & Cough

Decongestant

Infant Drops PediaCare®

Pfizer Consumer Healthcare, Pfizer Inc.
P. 730

First Aid Antibiotic Powder & Ointment
Available in Powder, 0.35 oz. (10 g)
and Ointment, 1/2 oz. (14.2 g)
and 1 oz. (28.3 g) tubes
and 1/32 oz (0.9 g) foil packets.

Polysporin®

Pfizer Consumer Healthcare, Pfizer Inc.
P. 730

Rogaine®

Pfizer Consumer Healthcare, Pfizer Inc.
P. 731

Fast, Effective Relief from
Heartburn, Acid Indigestion or
Sour Stomach.
Original Peppermint,
Spearmint, and Cherry Flavors.

Rolaids®

Pfizer Consumer Healthcare, Pfizer Inc.
P. 732

Cool Strawberry, Freshmint,
Fruit and Tropical Punch

Extra Strength Rolaids®

Pfizer Consumer Healthcare, Pfizer Inc.
P. 732

Berry and Cool Mint

Rolaids® Multi-Symptom

Pfizer Consumer Healthcare, Pfizer Inc.
P. 733

30 mg Tablets
Available in 24, 48 and 96 tablets.

**Sudafed®
Nasal Decongestant**

Pfizer Consumer Healthcare, Pfizer Inc.
P. 733

Available in 24 liquid caps.

**Sudafed® Non-Drying
Sinus Liquid Caps**

Pfizer Consumer Healthcare, Pfizer Inc.
P. 734

Available in 12 or 24
caplets and 12 tablets.

**Sudafed®
Severe Cold Formula**

Pfizer Consumer Healthcare, Pfizer Inc.
P. 732

12 Hour Caplets
Available in 10 and 20 caplets.

Sudafed® 12 Hour

Pfizer Consumer Healthcare, Pfizer Inc.
P. 732

Available in boxes of 5 and 10 tablets.

Sudafed® 24 Hour

Pfizer Consumer Healthcare, Pfizer Inc.
P. 735

Available in 24 or 48 caplets and
24 tablets.

**Sudafed® Sinus
Headache**

Pfizer Consumer Healthcare, Pfizer Inc.
P. 734

Available in boxes of 24 tablets.

**Sudafed®
Sinus & Allergy**

Pfizer Consumer Healthcare, Pfizer Inc.
P. 735

Nighttime Sleep Aid
SleepGels available in
8, 16 and 32 softgels.

SleepTabs available in
8, 16, 32 and 48 tablets.

Unisom®

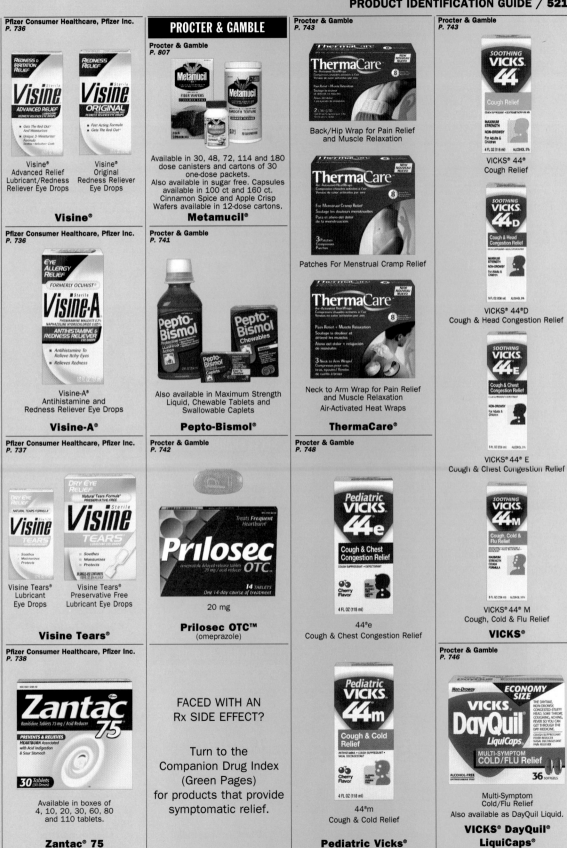

Pfizer Consumer Healthcare, Pfizer Inc.
P. 736

Visine®
Advanced Relief
Lubricant/Redness
Reliever Eye Drops

Visine®
Original
Redness Reliever
Eye Drops

Visine®

Pfizer Consumer Healthcare, Pfizer Inc.
P. 736

Visine-A®
Antihistamine and
Redness Reliever Eye Drops

Visine-A®

Pfizer Consumer Healthcare, Pfizer Inc.
P. 737

Visine Tears®
Lubricant
Eye Drops

Visine Tears®
Preservative Free
Lubricant Eye Drops

Visine Tears®

Pfizer Consumer Healthcare, Pfizer Inc.
P. 738

Available in boxes of
4, 10, 20, 30, 60, 80
and 110 tablets.

Zantac® 75

PROCTER & GAMBLE

Procter & Gamble
P. 807

Available in 30, 48, 72, 114 and 180
dose canisters and cartons of 30
one-dose packets.
Also available in sugar free. Capsules
available in 100 ct and 160 ct.
Cinnamon Spice and Apple Crisp
Wafers available in 12-dose cartons.

Metamucil®

Procter & Gamble
P. 741

Also available in Maximum Strength
Liquid, Chewable Tablets and
Swallowable Caplets

Pepto-Bismol®

Procter & Gamble
P. 742

20 mg

Prilosec OTC™
(omeprazole)

FACED WITH AN
Rx SIDE EFFECT?

Turn to the
Companion Drug Index
(Green Pages)
for products that provide
symptomatic relief.

Procter & Gamble
P. 743

Back/Hip Wrap for Pain Relief
and Muscle Relaxation

Patches For Menstrual Cramp Relief

Neck to Arm Wrap for Pain Relief
and Muscle Relaxation
Air-Activated Heat Wraps

ThermaCare®

Procter & Gamble
P. 748

44®e
Cough & Chest Congestion Relief

44®m
Cough & Cold Relief

Pediatric Vicks®

Procter & Gamble
P. 743

VICKS® 44®
Cough Relief

VICKS® 44®D
Cough & Head Congestion Relief

VICKS® 44® E
Cough & Chest Congestion Relief

VICKS® 44® M
Cough, Cold & Flu Relief

VICKS®

Procter & Gamble
P. 746

Multi-Symptom
Cold/Flu Relief
Also available as DayQuil Liquid.

**VICKS® DayQuil®
LiquiCaps®**

Procter & Gamble
P. 745

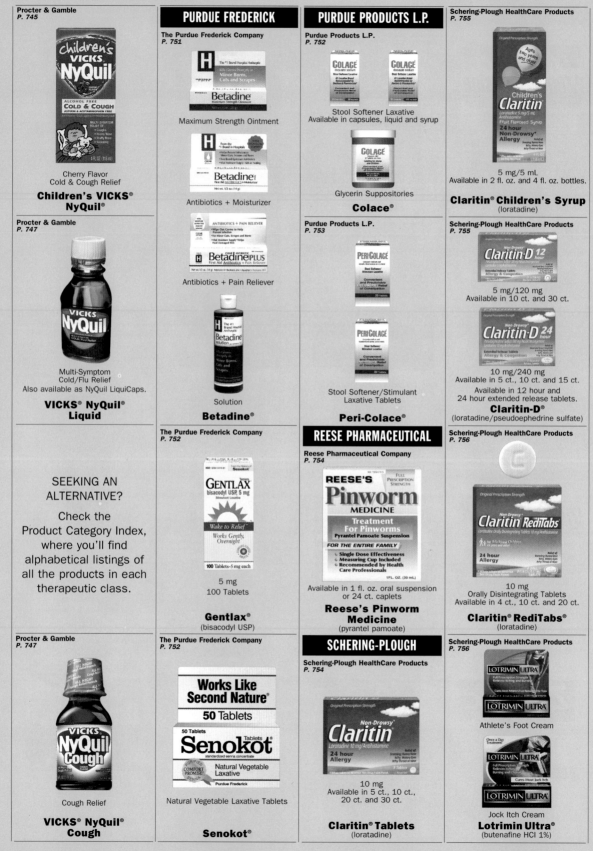

Cherry Flavor
Cold & Cough Relief
Children's VICKS®
NyQuil®

Procter & Gamble
P. 747

Multi-Symptom
Cold/Flu Relief
Also available as NyQuil LiquiCaps.

VICKS® NyQuil®
Liquid

SEEKING AN
ALTERNATIVE?

Check the
Product Category Index,
where you'll find
alphabetical listings of
all the products in each
therapeutic class.

Procter & Gamble
P. 747

Cough Relief
VICKS® NyQuil®
Cough

PURDUE FREDERICK

The Purdue Frederick Company
P. 751

Maximum Strength Ointment

Antibiotics + Moisturizer

Antibiotics + Pain Reliever

Solution
Betadine®

The Purdue Frederick Company
P. 752

5 mg
100 Tablets
Gentlax®
(bisacodyl USP)

The Purdue Frederick Company
P. 752

Natural Vegetable Laxative Tablets
Senokot®

PURDUE PRODUCTS L.P.

Purdue Products L.P.
P. 752

Stool Softener Laxative
Available in capsules, liquid and syrup

Glycerin Suppositories
Colace®

Purdue Products L.P.
P. 753

Stool Softener/Stimulant
Laxative Tablets
Peri-Colace®

REESE PHARMACEUTICAL

Reese Pharmaceutical Company
P. 754

Available in 1 fl. oz. oral suspension
or 24 ct. caplets
Reese's Pinworm
Medicine
(pyrantel pamoate)

SCHERING-PLOUGH

Schering-Plough HealthCare Products
P. 754

10 mg
Available in 5 ct., 10 ct.,
20 ct. and 30 ct.
Claritin® Tablets
(loratadine)

Schering-Plough HealthCare Products
P. 755

5 mg/5 mL
Available in 2 fl. oz. and 4 fl. oz. bottles.
Claritin® Children's Syrup
(loratadine)

Schering-Plough HealthCare Products
P. 755

5 mg/120 mg
Available in 10 ct. and 30 ct.

10 mg/240 mg
Available in 5 ct., 10 ct. and 15 ct.
Available in 12 hour and
24 hour extended release tablets.
Claritin-D®
(loratadine/pseudoephedrine sulfate)

Schering-Plough HealthCare Products
P. 756

10 mg
Orally Disintegrating Tablets
Available in 4 ct., 10 ct. and 20 ct.
Claritin® RediTabs®
(loratadine)

Schering-Plough HealthCare Products
P. 756

Athlete's Foot Cream

Jock Itch Cream
Lotrimin Ultra®
(butenafine HCl 1%)

SINOFRESH HEALTHCARE

SinoFresh Healthcare, Inc.
P. 757

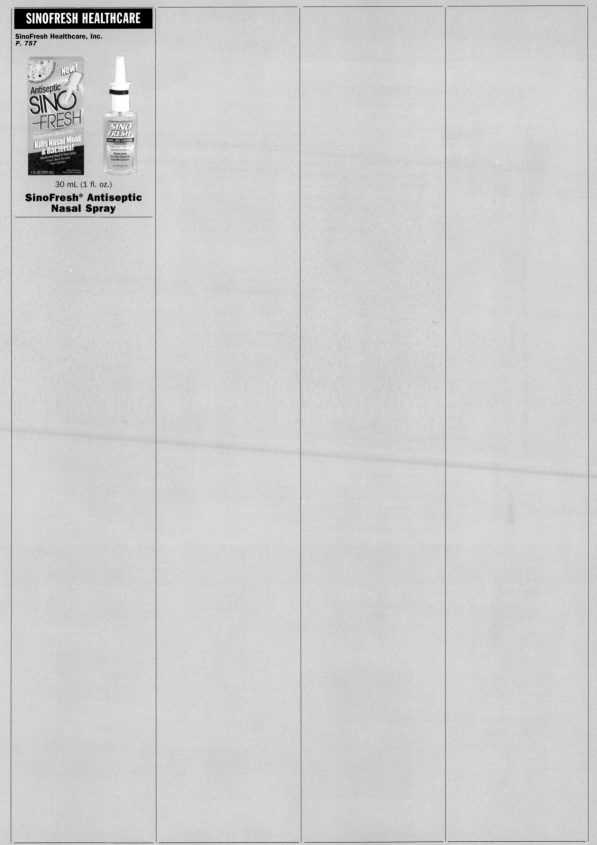

30 mL (1 fl. oz.)

**SinoFresh® Antiseptic
Nasal Spray**

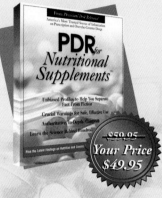
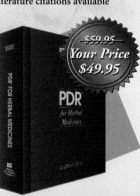
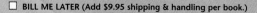

NONPRESCRIPTION DRUG INFORMATION

This section presents information on nonprescription drugs, self-testing kits, and other medical products marketed for home use by consumers. It is made possible through the courtesy of the manufacturers whose products appear on the following pages. The information concerning each product has been prepared, edited, and approved by the manufacturer's professional staff.

Pharmaceutical product descriptions in this section must be in compliance with the Code of Federal Regulations' labeling requirements for over-the-counter drugs. The descriptions are designed to provide all information necessary for informed use, including, when applicable, active ingredients, inactive ingredients, indications, actions, warnings, cau-tions, drug interactions, symptoms and treatment of oral overdosage, dosage and directions for use, professional labeling, and how supplied. In some cases, additional information has been supplied to complement the standard labeling.

In compiling this section, the publisher has emphasized the necessity of describing products comprehensively. The descriptions seen here include all information made available by the manufacturer. The publisher does not warrant or guarantee any product described here, and does not perform any independent analysis of the information provided. Inclusion of a product in this book does not represent an endorsement, and the publisher does not necessarily advocate the use of any product listed.

A.C. Grace Co.
1100 QUITMAN ROAD
P.O. BOX 570
BIG SANDY, TX 75755

Direct Inquiries to:
Inquiries:　(903) 636-4368
Orders Only:　800-833-4368
www.acgraceco.com

UNIQUE E®
NATURAL VITAMIN E COMPLEX
MIXED TOCOPHEROL CONCENTRATE

Description:
Established 1962... OUR ONLY PRODUCT.
WHY UNIQUE?
All NATURAL VITAMIN E COMPLEX.
NOT the *dl* SYNTHETIC CHEMICAL
form, *NOT ESTER*IFIED TOCOPH-
ERYL ACETATE (OR SUCCINATE),
NOT the ORDINARY SOY OIL
DILUTED MIXED TOCOPHEROLS OR
ADULTERATED FORMS.

Each soft easy-to-swallow high quality
GEL CAPSULE contains **ALL NATU-
RAL *UN*ESTERIFIED VITAMIN E
COMPLEX** providing **400 I.U. ANTI-
*THROMBIC*** function d-alpha tocoph-
erol with other naturally occuring **AN-
TIOXIDANT** tocopherols; **d-beta, d
GAMMA, d-delta** for maximum protec-
tion against <u>harmful</u> free radical dam-
age and inhibiting peroxynitrites dam-
aging to brain cells.

NO SOY or other OIL FILLER additives
which can turn rancid and cause harmful free radical damage even in sealed
gel capsules.

NO ALLERGY CAUSING PRESERVA-
TIVES, COLORS OR FLAVORINGS.

UNIQUE E® capsule potency is stabil-
ized and Certified by Assay.

Dosage: Up to 6 capsules daily as
directed by your physician according to
individual weight or need, usually 1
capsule per each 40 lbs. of total body
weight. Best results when <u>ENTIRE</u> daily
dose is taken just before or with the
morning meal.

How Supplied:
Bottles of 180 and 90 easy-to-swallow
high quality gel capsules in safety sealed
light protected bottles.

UNKNOWN DRUG?
Consult the
Product Identification Guide
(Gray Pages)
for full-color photos of
leading over-the-counter
medications

Adams Laboratories, Inc.
14801 SOVEREIGN ROAD
FORT WORTH, TX 76155

Direct Inquiries to:
Medical Affairs 817-786-1200

MUCINEX® 600 mg
(Guaifenesin) Extended-Release
Tablets
MUCINEX® 1200 mg
(Guaifenesin) Extended-Release
Tablets

Drug Facts
Active Ingredient:
(in each extended-release tablet)
　　　　　　　　　　　　　Purpose:
MUCINEX® 600 mg
Guaifenesin 600 mg .... Expectorant
MUCINEX® 1200 mg
Guaifenesin 1200 mg .... Expectorant
Uses: Helps loosen phlegm (mucus)
and thin bronchial secretions to rid the
bronchial passageways of bothersome
mucus and make coughs more productive

Warnings:
Do not use
• for children under 12 years of age
Ask a doctor before use if you have
• persistent or chronic cough such as occurs with smoking, asthma, chronic
bronchitis, or emphysema
• cough accompanied by too much
phlegm (mucus)
Stop use and ask a doctor if
• cough lasts more than 7 days, comes
back, or occurs with fever, rash, or persistent headache. These could be signs
of a serious illness.
If pregnant or breast-feeding, ask a
health professional before use.
Keep out of reach of children. In case of
overdose, get medical help or contact a
Poison Control Center right away.

Directions:
• do not crush, chew, or break tablet
• take with a full glass of water
• this product can be administered without regard for the timing of meals
MUCINEX® 600 mg
• adults and children 12 years of age
and over: one or two tablets every 12
hours. Do not exceed 4 tablets in 24
hours.
MUCINEX® 1200 mg
• adults and children 12 years of age
and over: 1 tablet every 12 hours. Do
not exceed 2 tablets in 24 hours.
• children under 12 years of age: do
not use
Other Information:
• tamper evident: do not use if seal on
bottle printed "SEALED for YOUR
PROTECTION" is broken or missing
• store between 20–25°C (68–77°F)
• see bottom of bottle for lot code and expiration date
Inactive Ingredients:　carbomer 934P,
NF; FD&C blue #1 aluminum lake
(600 mg) or green lake blend (1200 mg);
hypromellose, USP; magnesium stearate, NF; microcrystalline cellulose, NF;
sodium starch glycolate, NF

How Supplied:
MUCINEX® 600 mg
Bottles of 20 tablets, (NDC 63824-008-
20), 40 tablets (NDC 63824-008-40) and
sample bottles of 2 tablets (NDC 63824-
008-82). Round tablet debossed with "A"
on the light blue, marbled layer and
"600" on the white bi-layer. Each tablet
provides 600 mg guaifenesin.
MUCINEX® 1200 mg
Bottles of 10 tablets (NDC 63824-052-
01), bottles of 20 tablets (NDC 63824-
052-20) and sample bottles of 2 tablets
(NDC 63824-052-82). Modified oval tablet debossed with "Adams" on the light
green, marbled layer and "1200" on the
white bi-layer. Each tablet provides 1200
mg guaifenesin.
US Patent No. 6,372,252 B1
REV 0104

Alpharma
U.S. Pharmaceuticals Division
7205 WINDSOR BOULEVARD
BALTIMORE, MD 21244

For General Inquiries Contact:
Customer Service
800-432-8534

PERMETHRIN LOTION 1%
Lice Treatment

Description:
EACH FLUID OUNCE CONTAINS: Active Ingredient: Permethrin 280 mg (1%).
Inactive Ingredients: Balsam fir canada,
cetyl alcohol, citric acid, FD&C Yellow
No. 6, fragrance, hydrolyzed animal protein, hydroxyethylcellulose, polyoxyethylene 10 cetyl ether, propylene glycol,
stearalkonium chloride, water, isopropyl
alcohol 5.6 g (20%), methylparaben
56 mg (0.2%), and propylparaben 22 mg
(0.08%).
Permethrin Lotion 1% kills lice and their
unhatched eggs with usually only one
application. Permethrin Lotion 1% protects against head lice reinfestation for
14 days. The creme rinse formula leaves
hair manageable and easy to comb.

Indications: For the treatment of
head lice. For prophylactic use during
head lice epidemics.

Warnings: For external use only. Keep
out of eyes when rinsing hair. Adults and
children: Close eyes and do not open eyes
until product is rinsed out. If product
gets into the eyes, immediately flush
with water. Do not use near the eyes or
permit contact with mucous membranes,
such as inside the nose, mouth, or vagina, as irritation may occur. Children:

Also protect children's eyes with a washcloth, towel or other suitable material or method. This product should not be used on pediatric patients less than 2 months of age. Itching, redness, or swelling of the scalp may occur. If skin irritation persists or infection is present or develops, discontinue use and consult a doctor. Consult a doctor if infestation of eyebrows or eyelashes occurs. This product may cause breathing difficulty or an asthmatic episode in susceptible persons. As with any drug, if you are pregnant or nursing a baby, seek the advice of a health professional before using this product. Keep this and all drugs out of the reach of children. In case of accidental ingestion, seek professional assistance or contact a Poison Control Center immediately.

Dosage and Administration:

Treatment: Permethrin Lotion 1% should be used after hair has been washed with patient's regular shampoo, rinsed with water and towel dried. A sufficient amount should be applied to saturate hair and scalp (especially behind the ears and on the nape of the neck). Leave on hair for 10 minutes but not longer. Rinse with water. A single application is usually sufficient. If live lice are observed seven days or more after the first application of this product, a second treatment should be given. For proper head lice management, remove nits with the nit comb provided.

Head lice live on the scalp and lay small white eggs (nits) on the hair shaft close to the scalp. The nits are most easily found on the nape of the neck or behind the ears. All personal headgear, scarfs, coats, and bed linen should be disinfected by machine washing in hot water and drying, using the hot cycle of a dryer for at least 20 minutes. Personal articles of clothing or bedding that cannot be washed may be dry-cleaned, sealed in a plastic bag for a period of about 2 weeks, or sprayed with a product specifically designed for this purpose. Personal combs and brushes may be disinfected by soaking in hot water (above 130°F) for 5 to 10 minutes. Thorough vacuuming of rooms inhabited by infected patients is recommended.

Prophylaxis: Prophylactic use of Permethrin Lotion 1% is only recommended for individuals exposed to head lice epidemics in which at least 20% of the population at an institution are infested and for immediate household members of infested individuals. Casual use is strongly discouraged.

The method of application of Permethrin Lotion 1% for prophylaxis is identical to that described above for treatment of a lice infestation except nit removal is not required.

Directions For Use: One application of Permethrin Lotion 1% has been shown to protect greater than 95% of patients against reinfestation for at least two weeks. In epidemic settings, a second prophylactic application is recommended two weeks after the first because the life cycle of a head louse is approximately four weeks.

How Supplied: Bottles of 2 fl. oz. (59 mL) with nit removal comb and Family Pack of 2 bottles, 2 fl. oz. (59 mL) each, with 2 nit removal combs. Store at 15° to 25°C (59° to 77°F).

Manufactured by
Alpharma USPD Inc.
Baltimore, MD 21244
FORM NO. 5242   Rev. 9/99
                                VC1587

Bausch & Lomb
**1400 NORTH GOODMAN STREET
ROCHESTER, NY 14609**

Direct Inquiries to:
Main Office
(585) 338-6000
Consumer Affairs
1-800-553-5340

OCUVITE®
Antioxidant Vitamin and Mineral Supplement

Description: Each tablet contains:
[See table below]

Inactive Ingredients: Dibasic calcium phosphate, microcrystalline cellulose, calcium carbonate, crospovidone, hydroxypropyl methylcellulose, titanium dioxide, silicon dioxide, magnesium stearate, stearic acid, FD&C Yellow No. 6, triethyl citrate, polysorbate 80 and sodium lauryl sulfate.

Indications: OCUVITE is specifically formulated to provide nutritional support for the eye, and is recommended for those patients who are already taking a daily multi-vitamin supplement but would like to include Lutein. The Ocuvite formulation contains essential antioxidant vitamins and minerals plus 2 mg of Lutein.

Recommended Intake: Adults. One tablet, one or two times daily or as directed by their doctor.

Current and Former Smokers: Consult your eye care professional about the risks associated with smoking and using Beta-Carotene.

How Supplied: Peach, eye shaped, film coated tablet engraved LL on one side, 04 on the other side.
NDC 24208-387-60—Bottle of 60
NDC 24208-387-62—Bottle of 120
Store at Room Temperature.
MADE IN Germany
Marketed by
Bausch & Lomb
Rochester, NY 14609
Shown in Product Identification Guide, page 503

OCUVITE® EXTRA®
Vitamin and Mineral Supplement

Description: Each tablet contains:
[See first table at top of next page]

Inactive Ingredients: dibasic calcium phosphate, microcrystalline cellulose, calcium carbonate, crospovidone, hydroxypropyl methylcellulose, titanium dioxide, silicon dioxide, magnesium stearate, stearic acid, FD&C yellow No. 6, triethyl citrate, polysorbate 80 and sodium lauryl sulfate.

Indications: OCUVITE EXTRA is specifically formulated to provide nutritional support for the eye, and is recommended for those patients who are not taking a daily multi-vitamin supplement. The Ocuvite Extra formulation contains essential antioxidant vitamins and minerals, vitamins B-2 and B-3, plus 2 mg of Lutein.

Recommended Intake: Adults: One tablet, one or two times daily or as directed by their doctor.

Continued on next page

	Source	Amount	% Daily Value
Vitamin A	beta carotene	1000 IU	20%
Vitamin C	ascorbic acid	200 mg	330%
Vitamin E	dl-alpha tocopheryl acetate	60 IU	200%
Zinc	zinc oxide*	40 mg	270%
Selenium	sodium selenate	55 mcg	80%
Copper	cupric oxide	2 mg	100%
Lutein		2 mg	†

* Zinc oxide is the most concentrated form of zinc and contains more elemental zinc than any other zinc salt (ie: zinc sulfate or zinc acetate).
† Daily value not established.

Ocuvite Extra—Cont.

Current and Former Smokers: Consult your eye care professional about the risks associated with smoking and using Beta-Carotene.

How Supplied: Orange, eye shaped, film coated tablet engraved OCUVITE on one side, 05 on the other side.
NDC 24208-388-19—Bottle of 50
Store at Room Temperature
MADE IN Germany
Marketed by
Bausch & Lomb
Rochester, NY 14609
Shown in Product Identification Guide, page 503

OCUVITE® LUTEIN
[lu "teen]
Vitamin and Mineral Supplement

Description: Each capsule contains:
[See second table at right]

Inactive Ingredients: Lactose monohydrate, Crospovidone, Magnesium Stearate, Silicone dioxide.

- Lutein is a carotenoid found in dark leafy green vegetables such as spinach. Carotenoids are concentrated in the Macula, the part of the eye responsible for central vision. Clinical studies suggest that Lutein plays an essential role in maintaining healthy central vision by protecting against free radical damage and filtering blue light.*
- Lutein levels in your eye are related to the amount in your diet. Ocuvite Lutein contains 6 mg of Lutein per capsule. The leading multi-vitamin contains only a fraction of the amount of lutein used in clinical studies.
- Ocuvite® Lutein helps supplement your diet with antioxidant vitamins and essential minerals that can play an important role in your ocular health.*

Indications: Ocuvite Lutein is an advanced antioxidant supplement formulated to provide nutritional support for the eye. The Ocuvite Lutein formulation contains essential antioxidant vitamins, minerals and 6 mg of Lutein.

Recommended Intake: Adults: One capsule, one or two times daily or as directed by their physician.

> ***THESE STATEMENTS HAVE NOT BEEN EVALUATED BY THE FOOD AND DRUG ADMINISTRATION. THIS PRODUCT IS NOT INTENDED TO DIAGNOSE, TREAT, CURE OR PREVENT ANY DISEASE.**

How Supplied: Yellow capsule with Ocuvite Lutein printed in black.
NDC 24208-403-19—Bottle of 36
Store at Room Temperature
MADE IN U.S.A.

	Source	Amount	% Daily Value
Vitamin A	beta carotene	1000 IU	20%
Vitamin C	ascorbic acid	300 mg	500%
Vitamin E	dl-alpha tocopheryl acetate	100 IU	330%
Riboflavin		3 mg	180%
Niacinamide		40 mg	200%
Zinc	zinc oxide*	40 mg	270%
Selenium	sodium selenate	55 mcg	80%
Copper	cupric oxide	2 mg	100%
Manganese		5 mg	250%
L-Glutathione		5 mg	†
Lutein		2 mg	†

---

* Zinc oxide is the most concentrated form of zinc and contains more elemental zinc than any other zinc salt (ie: zinc sulfate or zinc acetate).
† Daily value not established.

	Source	Amount	% Daily Value
Vitamin C	ascorbic acid	**60 mg**	**100%**
Vitamin E	dl-alpha tocopheryl acetate	**30 IU**	**100%**
Zinc	zinc oxide*	**15 mg**	**100%**
Copper	cupric oxide	**2 mg**	**100%**
Lutein		**6 mg**	†

*Zinc oxide is the most concentrated form of zinc and contains more elemental zinc than any other zinc salt (ie:zinc sulfate or zinc acetate)
† Daily value not established

Contents	Two tablets		Daily Dosage (4 tablets)	
	Amount	% of Daily Value	Amount	% of Daily Value
Vitamin A (Beta-carotene)	14,320 IU	286%	28,640 IU	573%
Vitamin C (ascorbic acid)	226 mg	376%	452 mg	753%
Vitamin E (dl-alpha tocopheryl acetate)	200 IU	666%	400 IU	1333%
Zinc (zinc oxide)	34.8 mg	232%	89.5 mg	484%
Cooper (cupric oxide)	0.8 mg	40%	1.6 mg	80%

Marketed by
Bausch & Lomb
Rochester, NY 14609
Shown in Product Identification Guide, page 503

BAUSCH & LOMB PRESERVISION®
High Potency Eye Vitamin and Mineral Supplement†

Description: Each capsule contains
[See third table above]

Other Ingredients: Lactose Monohydrate, Microcrystalline Cellulose, Crospovidone, Stearic Acid, Magnesium Stearate, Silicon Dioxide, Polysorbate 80, Triethyl Citrate, FD&C Yellow #6, FD&C Red #40

- Age-related macular degeneration is the leading cause of vision loss and blindness in people over 55. The National Institutes of Health (NIH) Age Related Eye Disease Study (AREDS) proved that a unique high-potency vitamin and mineral supplement was effective in helping to preserve the sight of certain people most at risk.*
- †Bausch & Lomb **Ocuvite PreserVision** was the one and only eye vitamin and mineral supplement tested and clinically proven effective in the NIH AREDS Study.
- Bausch & Lomb **Ocuvite PreserVision** is a high-potency antioxidant and mineral supplement with the antioxidant vitamins A, C, E and select minerals in amounts well above those in ordinary multivitamins and generally cannot be attained through diet alone.

For a FREE 16-page brochure on Age-Related Macular Degeneration call toll-free 1-886-467-3263 Extension #81 (1-868-HOPE-AMD)

Recommended Intake: To get the high levels proven in the NIH AREDS Study it is important to take 4 tablets per day – 2 in the morning, 2 in the evening taken with meals.

Current and Former Smokers: Consult your eye care professional about the risks associated with smoking and using Beta-Carotene.
Bausch & Lomb Ocuvite PreserVision is the #1 recommended eye vitamin and mineral supplement brand among Retinal Specialists.[1]

Adults and children 12 years and older	• take 1 tablet (caplet, gelcap) every 8 to 12 hours while symptoms last • for the first dose you may take 2 tablets (caplets, gelcaps) within the first hour • the smallest effective dose should be used • do not exceed 2 tablets (caplets, gelcaps) in any 8- to 12-hour period • do not exceed 3 tablets (caplets, gelcaps) in a 24-hour period
Adults over 65 years	• do not take more than 1 tablet (caplet, gelcap) every 12 hours unless directed by a doctor
Children under 12 years	• ask a doctor

* This statement has not been evaluated by the Food and Drug Administration. This product is not intended to diagnose, treat, cure or prevent any disease.

How Supplied: Orange, eye shaped film coated tablet, engraved BL 01 on one side, scored on the other side.
Store at room temperature.
Made in USA
Marketed by
Bausch & Lomb
Rochester, NY 14609

References: 1. Data on file, Bausch & Lomb, Inc.
© Bausch & Lomb Incorporated. All Rights Reserved.
Bausch & Lomb, Ocuvite and PreserVision are trademarks of Bausch & Lomb Incorporated or its affiliates. Other brand names are trademarks of their respective owners.
Shown in Product Identification Guide, page 503

Bayer HealthCare LLC Consumer Care Division

36 COLUMBIA ROAD
P.O. BOX 1910
MORRISTOWN, NJ 07962-1910

Direct Inquiries to:
Consumer Relations
(800) 331-4536
www.bayercare.com

For Medical Emergency Contact:
Bayer HealthCare LLC
Consumer Care Division
(800) 331-4536

ALEVE®
All Day Strong
naproxen sodium tablets, 220 mg
Pain reliever/fever reducer

ALEVE® Caplets*, Gelcaps, or Tablets Naproxen Sodium Tablets, USP**

Active Ingredient: **Purpose:**
(in each tablet/caplet/gelcap)
Naproxen sodium 220 mg (naproxen 200 mg) .... Pain reliever/fever reducer

Uses: Temporarily relieves minor aches and pains due to:

• headache
• muscular aches
• minor pain of arthritis
• toothache
• backache
• common cold
• menstrual cramps
temporarily reduces fever

Warnings: Allergy alert: Naproxen sodium may cause a severe allergic reaction which may include:
• hives
• facial swelling
• asthma (wheezing)
• shock
Alcohol warning: If you consume 3 or more alcoholic drinks every day, ask your doctor whether you should take naproxen sodium or other pain relievers/fever reducers. Naproxen sodium may cause stomach bleeding.
Do not use if you have ever had an allergic reaction to any other pain reliever/fever reducer
Ask a doctor before use if you have had serious side effects from any pain reliever/fever reducer
Ask a doctor or pharmacist before use if you are
• under a doctor's care for any serious condition
• taking other drug
• taking any other product that contains naproxen sodium, or any other pain reliever/fever reducer
Stop use and ask a doctor if
• an allergic reaction occurs. Seek medical help right away.
• pain gets worse or lasts more than 10 days
• fever gets worse or lasts more than 3 days
• you have difficulty swallowing
• it feels like the pill is stuck in your throat
• you develop heartburn
• stomach pain occurs or lasts, even if symptoms are mild
• redness or swelling is present in the painful area
• any new symptoms appear
If pregnant or breast-feeding, ask a health professional before use. It is especially important not to use naproxen sodium during the last 3 months of pregnancy unless definitely directed to do so by a doctor because it may cause problems in the unborn child or complications during delivery.
Keep out of reach of children. In case of overdose, get medical help or contact a Poison Control Center right away.

Directions:
• **do not take more than directed**
• drink a full glass of water with each dose
[See table above]
Other Information:
• **each contains:** sodium 20 mg
• store at 20–25°C (68–77°F) avoid high humidity and excessive heat above 40°C (104°F)
Aleve tablets, caplets:

Inactive Ingredients: FD&C blue #2 lake, hypromellose, magnesium stearate, microcrystalline cellulose, polyethylene glycol, povidone, talc, titanium dioxide
Aleve gelcaps:

Inactive Ingredients: D&C yellow #10 aluminum lake, EDTA disodium, edible ink, FD&C blue #1, FD&C yellow #6 aluminum lake, gelatin, glycerin, hypromellose, magnesium stearate, microcrystalline cellulose, polyethylene glycol, povidone, stearic acid, talc, titanium dioxide

* capsule-shaped tablet(s)
** gelatin coated capsule-shaped tablet(s)

How Supplied:
ALEVE® Caplets in boxes of 24, 50, 100, 150, 200.
ALEVE® Gelcaps in boxes of 20, 40, 80.
ALEVE® Tablets in boxes of 24, 50, 100, 150. + 8 count vials
Questions or comments? call **1-800-395-0689** or www.aleve.com
Do not use if carton is open or if foil seal imprinted with "Safety *SQUEASE*®" on bottle opening is missing or broken.
Distributed by
Bayer HealthCare LLC
PO Box 1910
Morristown, NJ 07962-1910 USA
B-R LLC
Shown in Product Identification Guide, page 503

ALEVE® COLD & SINUS
Pain reliever/fever reducer/nasal decongestant

Active Ingredients:
(in each caplet):   **Purposes:**
Naproxen sodium 220 mg (naproxen 200 mg) ... Pain reliever/fever reducer

Continued on next page

Aleve Cold & Sinus—Cont.

Pseudoephedrine HCl 120 mg,
extended-release ..... Nasal decongestant
Uses: temporarily relieves these cold,
sinus, and flu symptoms:
- sinus pressure
- minor body aches and pains
- headache
- nasal and sinus congestion (promotes
  sinus drainage and restores freer
  breathing through the nose)
- fever

Warnings:
Allergy alert: Naproxen sodium may
cause a severe allergic reaction which
may include:
- hives
- facial swelling
- asthma (wheezing)
- shock

Alcohol warning: If you consume 3 or
more alcoholic drinks every day, ask your
doctor whether you should take
naproxen sodium or other pain relievers/
fever reducers. Naproxen sodium may
cause stomach bleeding.
Do not use
- if you have ever had an allergic reaction to any other pain reliever/fever reducer
- if you are now taking a prescription
  monoamine oxidase inhibitor (MAOI)
  (certain drugs for depression, psychiatric, or emotional conditions, or Parkinson's disease), or for 2 weeks after
  stopping the MAOI drug. If you do not
  know if your prescription drug contains an MAOI, ask a doctor or pharmacist before taking this product.
Ask a doctor before use if you have
- heart disease
- high blood pressure
- thyroid disease
- diabetes
- trouble urinating due to an enlarged
  prostate gland
- had serious side effects from any pain
  reliever/fever reducer
**Ask a doctor or pharmacist before use if
you are**
- using any other product containing
  naproxen or pseudoephedrine
- taking any other pain reliever/fever reducer or nasal decongestant
- under a doctor's care for any continuing medical condition
- taking other drugs on a regular basis
**When using this product do not use
more than directed.**
Stop use and ask a doctor if
- an allergic reaction occurs. Seek medical help right away.
- you get nervous, dizzy, or sleepless
- you develop heartburn
- nasal congestion lasts more than 7
  days
- symptoms continue or get worse
- you have trouble swallowing or the caplet feels stuck in your throat
- new or unexpected symptoms occur
- stomach pain occurs with use of this
  product or if even mild symptoms persist
- fever lasts for more than 3 days
If pregnant or breast-feeding, ask a
health professional before use.
It is especially important not to use
naproxen sodium during the last 3

months of pregnancy unless definitely
directed to do so by a doctor because it
may cause problems in the unborn child
or complications during delivery.
Keep out of reach of children. In case of
overdose, get medical help or contact a
Poison Control Center right away.

Directions:
- **swallow whole;** do not crush or chew
- **drink a full glass of water with each
  dose**
- adults and children 12 years and
  older: **1 caplet every 12 hours;** do not
  take more than 2 caplets in 24 hours
- children under 12 years: ask a doctor
Other Information:
- **each caplet contains:** sodium 20 mg
- store at 20 to 25° C (68–77°F)
- store in a dry place

Inactive Ingredients: colloidal silicon
dioxide, hypromellose, lactose, magnesium stearate, microcrystalline cellulose,
polyethylene glycol, povidone, talc, titanium dioxide
**Questions or comments? 1-800-395-
0689 or www.aleve.com**

How Supplied: Boxes of 10, 20, or 30
caplets (capsule-shaped tablets)
Distributed by: Bayer HealthCare, LLC
Consumer Care Division
Morristown, NJ 07962-1910 USA

B-R LLC

*Shown in Product Identification
Guide, page 503*

ALEVE® SINUS & HEADACHE
**Pain reliever/fever reducer/nasal
decongestant**

Active Ingredients
(in each caplet):   **Purposes:**
Naproxen sodium 220 mg
(naproxen 200 mg) ... Pain reliever/fever
reducer
Pseudoephedrine HCl 120 mg,
extended-release ..... Nasal decongestant

Uses: temporarily relieves these cold,
sinus, and flu symptoms:
- sinus pressure
- minor body aches and pains
- headache
- nasal and sinus congestion (promotes
  sinus drainage and restores freer
  breathing through the nose)
- fever

Warnings: Allergy alert: Naproxen
sodium may cause a severe allergic reaction which may include:
- hives
- facial swelling
- asthma (wheezing)
- shock
Alcohol warning: If you consume 3 or
more alcoholic drinks every day, ask your
doctor whether you should take
naproxen sodium or other pain relievers/
fever reducers. Naproxen sodium may
cause stomach bleeding.

Do not use
- if you have ever had an allergic reaction to any other pain reliever/fever reducer
- if you are now taking a prescription
  monoamine oxidase inhibitor (MAOI)
  (certain drugs for depression, psychiatric or emotional conditions, or Parkinson's disease), or for 2 weeks after
  stopping the MAOI drug. If you do not
  know if your prescription drug contains an MAOI, ask a doctor or pharmacist before taking this product.

Ask a doctor before use if you have
- heart disease
- high blood pressure
- thyroid disease
- diabetes
- trouble urinating due to an enlarged
  prostate gland
- had serious side effects from any pain
  reliever/fever reducer

**Ask a doctor or pharmacist before
use if you are**
- using any other product containing
  naproxen or pseudoephedrine
- taking any other pain reliever/fever reducer or nasal decongestant
- under a doctor's care for any continuing medical condition
- taking other drugs on a regular basis

**When using this product do not use
more than directed.**

Stop use and ask a doctor if:
- an allergic reaction occurs. Seek medical help right away.
- you get nervous, dizzy, or sleepless
- you develop heartburn
- nasal congestion lasts more than 7
  days
- symptoms continue or get worse
- you have trouble swallowing or the caplet feels stuck in your throat
- new or unexpected symptoms occur
- stomach pain occurs with use of this
  product or if even mild symptoms persist
- fever lasts for more than 3 days

If pregnant or breast-feeding, ask a
health professional before use. It is especially important not to use naproxen
sodium during the last 3 months of pregnancy unless definitely directed to do so
by a doctor because it may cause problems in the unborn child or complications during delivery.

Keep out of reach of children. If case of
overdose, get medical help or contact a
Poison Control Center right away.

Directions:
- **swallow whole;** do not crush or chew
- **drink a full glass of water with each
  dose**
- adults and children 12 years and
  older: **1 caplet every 12 hours;** do not
  take more than 2 caplets in 24 hours
- children under 12 years: ask a doctor

Other Information: • **each caplet
contains:** sodium 20 mg
- store at 20 to 25°C (68–77°F)
- store in a dry place

Inactive Ingredients: colloidal silicon
dioxide, hypromellose, lactose, magnesium stearate, microcrystalline cellulose,

polyethylene glycol, povidone, talc, titanium dioxide

Questions or comments? **1-800-395-0689**

How Supplied: Box of 10 or 20 Caplets
(Capsule-Shaped Tablets).

Visit our website at www.aleve.com

Distributed by:

Bayer HealthCare, LLC

Consumer Care Division

PO Box 1910

Morristown, NJ 07962-1910 USA

B-R LLC

154043

Shown in Product Identification Guide, page 503

ALKA-SELTZER® Original
ALKA-SELTZER® Extra Strength
ALKA-SELTZER® Lemon Lime
Effervescent Antacid Pain Reliever

Active Ingredients

(in each tablet):	Purposes:

ALKA-SELTZER® Original:

Aspirin 325 mg .... Analgesic

Citric acid
  1000 mg .... Antacid

Sodium bicarbonate (heat-treated)
  1916 mg .... Antacid

ALKA-SELTZER® Lemon-Lime:

Aspirin 325 mg .... Analgesic

Citric acid
  1000 mg .... Antacid

Sodium bicarbonate (heat-treated)
  1700 mg .... Antacid

ALKA-SELTZER® Extra Strength:

Aspirin 500 mg .... Analgesic

Citric acid
  1000 mg .... Antacid

Sodium bicarbonate (heat-treated)
  1985 mg .... Antacid

Uses: for the relief of:

ALKA-SELTZER® Original, Lemon-Lime, and Extra Strength:

- heartburn, acid indigestion, and sour stomach when accompanied with headache or body aches and pains
- upset stomach with headache from overindulgence in food or drink
- pain alone (headache or body and muscular aches and pains)

Warnings:

ALKA-SELTZER® Original, Lemon-Lime and Extra Strength:

Reye's syndrome: Children and teenagers should not use this medicine for chicken pox or flu symptoms before a doctor is consulted about Reye's syndrome, a rare but serious illness reported to be associated with aspirin.

- fully dissolve tablets in 4 ounces of water before taking

adults and children 12 years and over	2 tablets every 4 hours, or as directed by a doctor	do not exceed 8 tablets in 24 hours, or as directed by a doctor
adults 60 years and over	2 tablets every 4 hours, or as directed by a doctor	do not exceed 4 tablets in 24 hours, or as directed by a doctor

- fully dissolve tablets in 4 ounces of water before taking

adults and children 12 years and over	2 tablets every 6 hours, or as directed by a doctor	do not exceed 7 tablets in 24 hours
adults 60 years and over	2 tablets every 6 hours, or as directed by a doctor	do not exceed 4 tablets in 24 hours

Allergy alert: Aspirin may cause a severe allergic reaction which may include:
- hives • facial swelling • asthma (wheezing) • shock

Alcohol warning: If you consume 3 or more alcoholic drinks every day, ask your doctor whether you should take aspirin or other pain relievers/fever reducers. Aspirin may cause stomach bleeding.

Do not use if you are allergic to aspirin or any other pain reliever/fever reducer

Ask a doctor before use if you have
- asthma
- ulcers
- bleeding problems
- stomach problems that last or come back frequently, such as heartburn, upset stomach, or pain

Ask a doctor or pharmacist before use if you are
- presently taking a prescription drug. Antacids may interact with certain prescription drugs.
- on a sodium-restricted diet
- taking a prescription drug for anticoagulation (blood thinning), diabetes, gout, or arthritis

When using this product do not exceed recommended dosage

Stop use and ask a doctor if
- an allergic reaction occurs. Seek medical help right away.
- symptoms get worse or last more than 10 days
- new symptoms occur
- redness or swelling is present
- ringing in the ears or loss of hearing occurs

If pregnant or breast-feeding, ask a health professional before use. **It is especially important not to use aspirin during the last 3 months of pregnancy unless definitely directed to do so by a doctor because it may cause problems in the unborn child or complications during delivery.**

Keep out of reach of children. In case of overdose, get medical help or contact a Poison Control Center right away.

Directions:
Alka Seltzer® Original and Lemon-Lime:
[See first table above]
Alka Seltzer Extra Strength:
[See second table above]

Other Information:
- **each tablets contains:** sodium 567 mg (Original), sodium 503 mg (Lemon-Lime), sodium 588 mg (Extra Strength)
- **phenylketonurics:** contains phenylalaline 9 mg (Lemon-Lime) per tablet
- protect from excessive heat
- Alka-Seltzer in water contains principally the antacid sodium citrate and the analgesic sodium acetylsalicylate

Inactive Ingredients:

Original: None

Lemon-Lime: aspartame, dimethylpolysiloxane powder, docusate sodium, flavor, povidone, sodium benzoate

Extra Strength: Flavors

How Supplied: 2 effervescent tablets per foil pack

Original: Box of 12, 24, 36, 72, and 100 tablets

Lemon-Lime: Box of 12, 24, 36 tablets

Extra Strenth: Box of 12 and 24 tablets

Questions or comments? **1-800-800-4793** or www.alka-seltzer.com

Bayer HealthCare LLC

Consumer Care Division

P.O. Box 1910

Morristown, NJ 07962-1910

USA

Shown in Product Identification Guide, page 503

ALKA-SELTZER® HEARTBURN RELIEF
Antacid Medicine

Active Ingredients:	**Purposes:**
(in each tablet)	

Citric acid 1000 mg .... antacid

Sodium bicarbonate (heat-treated)
1940 mg .... antacid

Uses:

for the relief of:
- heartburn
- acid indigestion
- upset stomach associated with these conditions

Continued on next page

Alka-Seltzer Heartburn—Cont.

Warnings:

Do not use this product if you are on a sodium-restricted diet unless directed by a doctor.

Ask a doctor or pharmacist before use if you are presently taking a prescription drug. Antacids may interact with certain prescription drugs.

When using this product do not exceed recommended dosage.

Stop use and ask a doctor if symptoms last for more than 14 days.

If pregnant or breast-feeding, ask a health professional before use.

Keep out of reach of children.

Directions: Fully dissolve tablets in 4 ounces of water before taking.

[See first table at right]

Other Information:

- **each tablet contains:** sodium 578 mg.
- **phenylketonurics:** contains phenylalanine 5.6 mg per tablet
- protect from excessive heat
- Alka-Seltzer Heartburn Relief in water contains the antacid sodium citrate as the principal active ingredient.

Inactive Ingredients: acesulfame potassium, aspartame, flavor enhancer, flavors, magnesium stearate, mannitol

How Supplied: Alka-Seltzer Heartburn Relief is available in 12, 24 & 36 count packages in lemon lime flavor.

Questions or comments: 1-800-800-4793 or www.alka-seltzer.com

Made in Germany.

Bayer HealthCare LLC

Consumer Care Division

P.O. Box 1910

Morristown, NJ 07962-1910

USA

Shown in Product Identification Guide, page 503

ALKA-SELTZER® MORNING RELIEF

Pain Reliever, Alertness Aid
For Morning Headache and Fatigue
with Caffeine
- **Fast Headache Relief**
- **Increases Alertness**
- **Gentle on your stomach**

Active Ingredients: **Purposes:**
(in each tablet)

Aspirin 500 mg .... Analgesic

Caffeine 65 mg .... Alertness aid/
pain reliever aid

Uses:
- for the temporary relief of minor aches and pains with fatigue or drowsiness associated with a hangover
- also effective for headaches, body aches and pains alone

adults and children 12 years and over	2 tablets every 4 hours as needed, or as directed by a doctor	do not exceed 8 tablets in 24 hours, or as directed by a doctor
adult 60 years of age and over	2 tablets every 4 hours as needed, or as directed by a doctor	do not exceed 4 tablets in 24 hours, or as directed by a doctor
children under 12 years	Consult a doctor.	

adults and children 12 years and over	2 tablets every 6 hours, as needed, or as directed by a doctor	do not exceed 8 tablets in 24 hours
adults 60 years and over	2 tablets every 6 hours, as needed, or as directed by a doctor	do not exceed 4 tablets in 24 hours
children under 12 years	do not use	

Warnings:

Reye's syndrome: Children and teenagers should not use this medicine for chicken pox or flu symptoms before a doctor is consulted about Reye's syndrome, a rare but serious illness reported to be associated with aspirin.

Allergy alert: Aspirin may cause a severe allergic reaction which may include:

- hives • facial swelling • asthma (wheezing) • shock

Alcohol warning: If you consume 3 or more alcoholic drinks every day, ask your doctor whether you should take aspirin or other pain relievers/fever reducers. Aspirin may cause stomach bleeding.

Do not use
- if you are allergic to aspirin or any other pain reliever/fever reducer
- this product if you are on a sodium-restricted diet unless directed by a doctor
- in children under 12 years of age

Ask a doctor before use if you have
- asthma • ulcers • bleeding problems
- stomach problems that last or come back, such as heartburn, upset stomach, or pain

Ask a doctor or pharmacist before use if you are taking a prescription drug for

- anticoagulation (blood thinning) • gout
- diabetes • arthritis

When using this product
- limit the use of caffeine-containing medications, foods or beverages because too much caffeine may cause nervousness, irritability, sleeplessness, and occasionally, rapid heart beat. The recommended dose of this product contains about as much caffeine as a cup of coffee.
- if fatigue or drowsiness persists or continues to recur, consult a doctor. For occasional use only. Not intended for use as a substitute for sleep.

Stop use and ask a doctor if
- allergic reaction occurs. Seek medical help right away.

- pain gets worse or lasts more than 10 days
- new symptoms occur
- redness or swelling is present
- ringing in the ears or loss of hearing occurs

If pregnant or breast-feeding, ask a health professional before use. **It is especially important not to use aspirin during the last 3 months of pregnancy unless definitely directed to do so by a doctor because it may cause problems in the unborn child or complications during delivery.**

Keep out of reach of children. In case of overdose, get medical help or contact a Poison Control Center right away.

Directions:
- do not exceed recommended dosage
- do not use for more than 2 days for hangover
- fully dissolve tablets in 4 ounces of water before taking

[See second table above]

Other Information:
- **each tablet contains:** sodium 415 mg
- **phenylketonurics:** contains phenylalanine 9 mg per tablet
- protect from excessive heat

Inactive Ingredients: acesulfame potassium, aspartame, citric acid, dimethylpolysiloxane powder, docusate sodium, flavor, mannitol, povidone, sodium benzoate, sodium bicarbonate

How Supplied: 2 Citrus effervescent tablets per foil pack in boxes of 12 and 24 tablets

Questions or comments? 1-800-800-4793 or www.alka-seltzer.com

Made in U.S.A.

Bayer HealthCare LLC

Consumer Care Division

P.O. Box 1910

Morristown, NJ 07962-1910 USA

Shown in Product Identification Guide, page 503

ALKA-SELTZER PLUS® COLD MEDICINE LIQUI-GELS®
Analgesic, Antihistamine, Nasal Decongestant

ALKA-SELTZER PLUS® COLD& COUGH MEDICINE LIQUI-GELS®
Analgesic, Antihistamine, Cough Suppressant, Nasal Decongestant

ALKA-SELTZER PLUS® NIGHT-TIME COLD MEDICINE LIQUI-GELS®
Analgesic, Cough Suppressant, Antihistamine, Nasal Decongestant

[See first table at right]
[See second table at right]
[See third table at right]
[See first table at top of next page]

Alka-Seltzer Plus® Liqui-Gels®: Warnings and Other Information
1- Alka Seltzer Plus Cold Medicine Liqui-Gels
3- Alka Seltzer Plus Cold & Cough Medicine Liqui-Gels
4- Alka Seltzer Plus Night-Time Cold Medicine Liqui-Gels

Warnings:
(The numbers following the warnings correspond to the products listed above.)
[See second table on pages 610 and 611]

Other Information:
(The numbers following the warnings correspond to the products listed above.)
[See first table at top of page 611]

How Supplied: ALKA-SELTZER PLUS® Cold Medicine, ALKA-SELTZER PLUS® Cold & Cough Medicine, ALKA-SELTZER PLUS® Night-Time Cold Medicine: Carton of 20 softgels.

Questions or comments? 1-800-800-4793 or www.alka-seltzerplus.com
Distributed by:
Bayer HealthCare LLC
PO Box 1910
Morristown, NJ 07962-1910 USA
Liqui-Gels is a registered trademark of R.P. Scherer Corporation.

Shown in Product Identification Guide, page 504

ALKA-SELTZER PLUS®
[ăl-kă sĕlt-sər]
Cold Medicine
Maximum Strength Cool Mint and Orange Zest Flavors
Ready Relief™ Tabs
Nasal Decongestant, Antihistamine

Active Ingredients
(in each tablet):   **Purpose:**
Chlorpheniramine
  maleate 2 mg .... Antihistamine
Pseudoephedrine
  HCl 30 mg .... Nasal decongestant

Active Ingredients:

Per softgel	Cold	Cold & Cough	Night-Time
Acetaminophen 325 mg	√	√	√
Chlorpheniramine maleate 2 mg	√	√	
Dextromethorphan hydrobromide 10 mg		√	√
Doxylamine succinate 6.25 mg			√
Pseudophedrine HCl 30 mg	√	√	√

Inactive Ingredients:

per softgel	Cold	Cold & Cough	Night-Time
FD&C blue #1	√	√	√
FD&C red #40	√		
D&C red #33		√	
D&C yellow #10			√
gelatin	√	√	√
glycerin	√	√	√
polyethylene glycol	√	√	√
polyvinyl acetate phthalate	√	√	√
potassium acetate	√	√	√
povidone	√	√	√
propylene glycol	√	√	√
sorbitol	√	√	√
titanium dioxide	√	√	√
Water	√	√	√

Uses:

	Cold	Cold & Cough	Night-Time
body aches & pains	√	√	√
headache	√	√	√
coughing		√	√
fever	√	√	√
runny nose	√	√	√
sinus pain & pressure			
sneezing	√	√	√
nasal & sinus congestion	√	√	√
sore throat	√	√	√

Uses:
• provides temporary relief of these symptoms associated with a cold, hay fever, or other upper respiratory allergies:
  • runny nose • sneezing • nasal and sinus congestion

• provides temporary relief of these additional symptoms associated with hay fever or other upper respiratory allergies:

Continued on next page

Alka-Seltzer Plus—Cont.

- itching of the nose and throat
- itchy, watery eyes

Warnings:

Do not use if you are now taking a prescription monoamine oxidase inhibitor (MAOI) (certain drugs for depression, psychiatric, or emotional conditions, or Parkinson's disease), or for 2 weeks after stopping the MAOI drug. If you do not know if your prescription drug contains an MAOI, ask a doctor or pharmacist before taking this product.

Ask a doctor before use if you have
- heart disease • high blood pressure
- diabetes
- thyroid disease • glaucoma
- difficulty in urination due to enlargement of the prostate gland
- a breathing problem such as emphysema or chronic bronchitis

Ask a doctor or pharmacist before use if you are taking sedatives or tranquilizers

When using this product
- **do not exceed recommended dosage**
- you may get drowsy • avoid alcoholic drinks
- alcohol, sedatives, and tranquilizers may increase drowsiness
- be careful when driving a motor vehicle or operating machinery
- excitability may occur, especially in children

Stop use and ask a doctor if
- nervousness, dizziness, or sleeplessness occurs
- symptoms do not improve within 7 days or are accompanied by a fever

If pregnant or breast-feeding, ask a health professional before use.

Keep out of reach of children. In case of overdose, get medical help or contact a Poison Control Center right away.

Directions:
- do not take more than the recommended dose
- for best taste, do not chew tablets

[See table at bottom of next page]

Other Information:
- **phenylketonurics:** contains phenylalanine 0.1 mg per tablet
- this product does not contain phenylpropanolamine (PPA)
- store at room temperature and protect from excessive heat

Inactive Ingredients: Cool Mint: acesulfame potassium, aspartame, carnauba wax, citric acid, colloidal silicon dioxide, crospovidone, ethylcellulose, flavors, hypromellose, magnesium stearate, mannitol, mono- and di-glycerides, polyethylene, sorbitol, sucralose, sucrose

Orange Zest: acesulfame potassium ascorbic acid, aspartame, carnauba wax, citric acid, colloidal silicon dioxide, crospovidone, ethylcellulose, FD&C yellow #6 aluminum lake, flavors, hypromellose, magnesium stearate, mannitol, mono- and di-glycerides, polyethylene, sorbitol, sucralose, sucrose

Questions or comments? 1-800-800-4793 or www.alka-seltzerplus.com

Bayer HealthCare LLC

Shown in Product Identification Guide, page 504

Directions:

ALKA-SELTZER PLUS® NIGHT-TIME COLD MEDICINE LIQUI-GELS®

adults and children 12 years and over	swallow 2 softgels with water at bedtime (may be taken every 6 hours)	do not exceed 8 softgels in 24 hours or as directed by a doctor
children under 12 years	consult a doctor	

ALKA-SELTZER PLUS® COLD MEDICINE LIQUI-GELS®
ALKA-SELTZER PLUS® COLD & COUGH MEDICINE LIQUI-GELS®

adults and children 12 years and over	swallow 2 softgels with water every 4 hours	do not exceed 8 softgels in 24 hours or as directed by a doctor
children 6 to under 12 years	take 1 softgel with water every 4 hours	do not exceed 4 softgels in 24 hours or as directed by a doctor
children under 6 years	consult a doctor	

Alcohol warning: If you consume 3 or more alcoholic drinks every day, ask your doctor whether you should take acetaminophen or other pain relievers/fever reducers. Acetaminophen may cause liver damage.	**ALL**
Sore throat warning: If sore throat is severe, persists for more than 3 days, is accompanied or followed by fever, headache, rash nausea, or vomiting, consult a doctor promptly.	1,3,4
Do not use:	
• with any other products containing acetaminophen	**ALL**
• If you are now taking a prescription Monamine Oxidase Inhibitor (MAOI) (certain drugs for depression, psychiatric or emotional conditions, or Parkinson's disease), or for 2 weeks after stopping the MAOI drug. If you are uncertain whether your prescription drug contains an MAOI, ask a doctor or pharmacist before taking this product.	**ALL**
Ask a doctor before use if you have	
• heart disease, high blood pressure, diabetes, thyroid disease	**ALL**
• glaucoma	1,3,4
• difficulty in urination due to enlargement of the prostate gland	**ALL**
• a breathing problem such as emphysema or chronic bronchitis	1,3,4
• persistent or chronic cough such as occurs with smoking, asthma, or emphysema	3,4
• cough with excessive phlegm (mucus)	3,4
Ask a doctor or pharmacist before use if you are:	
• taking sedatives or tranquilizers	1,3,4

(Table continued on next page)

ALKA-SELTZER PM™
[əl-ka sĕl-sur]
Pain Reliever &
Sleep Aid Medicine

Active Ingredients: (in each tablet)	**Purposes:**
Aspirin 325 mg	Pain reliever
Diphenhydramine citrate 38 mg	Nighttime sleep aid

When using this product:	
• **do not exceed recommended dosage**	ALL
• you may get drowsy	1
• marked drowsiness may occur	3,4
• avoid alcoholic drinks	1,3,4
• excitability may occur, especially in children	1,3,4
• alcohol, sedatives, and tranquilizers may increase drowsiness	1,3,4
• be careful when driving a motor vehicle or operating machinery	1,3,4
Stop use and ask a doctor if:	
• nervousness, dizziness, or sleeplessness occurs	ALL
• new symptoms occur	ALL
• symptoms do not improve within 7 days (adults) or 5 days (children) or are accompanied by a fever	1,3
• symptoms do not improve within 7 days or are accompanied by a fever	4
• fever gets worse or lasts for more than 3 days	ALL
• redness or swelling is present	ALL
• cough persists for more than 7 days, tends to recur, or is accompanied by a fever, rash, or persistent headache. These may be signs of a serious condition.	3,4
If pregnant or breast-feeding, ask a health professional before use.	ALL
Keep out of reach of children	ALL
Overdose Warning: Taking more than the recommended dose can cause serious health problems. In case of overdose, get medical help or contact a Poison Control Center right away. Quick medical attention is critical for adults as well as for children even if you do not notice any signs or symptoms.	ALL

• this product does not contain phenylpropanolamine (PPA)	ALL
• store at room temperature and protect from excessive heat	ALL

Uses: temporarily relieves occasional headache and minor aches and pains with accompanying sleeplessness

Warnings: Reye's syndrome: Children and teenagers should not use this medicine for chicken pox or flu symptoms before a doctor is consulted about Reye's syndrome, a rare but serious illness reported to be associated with aspirin.
Allergy alert: Aspirin may cause a severe allergic reaction which may include: • hives • facial swelling • asthma (wheezing) • shock
Alcohol warning: If you consume 3 or more drinks every day, ask your doctor whether you should take aspirin or other pain relievers/fever reducers. Aspirin may cause stomach bleeding.

Do not use
• if you are allergic to aspirin or any other pain reliever/fever reducer
• in children under 12 years of age
• with any other product containing diphenhydramine, even one used on skin

Ask a doctor before use if you have:
• stomach problems (such as heartburn, upset stomach, or stomach pain) that continue or come back
• bleeding problems
• ulcers

• breathing problems such as emphysema, chronic bronchitis or asthma
• glaucoma
• trouble urinating due to an enlarged prostate gland
Ask a doctor or pharmacist before use if you are:
• taking a prescription drug for
  • anticoagulation (blood thinning)
  • diabetes
  • gout
  • arthritis
• taking tranquilizers or sedatives
• on a sodium-restricted diet
When using this product avoid alcoholic drinks
Stop use and ask a doctor if:
• an allergic reaction occurs. Seek medical help right away.
• pain gets worse or lasts for more than 10 days
• redness or swelling is present
• new symptoms occur
• ringing in the ears or loss of hearing occurs
• sleeplessness lasts for more than 2 weeks. Insomnia may be a symptom of a serious underlying medical illness.
If pregnant or breast-feeding, ask a health professional before use. **It is especially important not to use aspirin during the last 3 months of pregnancy unless definitely directed to do so by a doctor because it may cause problems in the unborn child or complications during delivery.**
Keep out of reach of children. In case of overdose, get medical help or contact a Poison Control Center right away.

Directions:
• **do not exceed recommended dosage**
• fully dissolve tablets in 4 ounces of water before taking

adults and children 12 years and over	take 2 tablets with water at bedtime, if needed, or as directed by a doctor
children under 12 years	do not use

Other Information:
• **each tablet contains:** sodium 503 mg
• **phenylketonurics:** contains phenylalanine 4.0 mg per tablet
• protect from excessive heat

Inactive Ingredients: acesulfame potassium, aspartame, citric acid, dimethylpolysiloxane powder, docusate sodium, flavors, mannitol, povidone, sodium benzoate, sodium bicarbonate

Place two (2) tablets in 4 oz of water. Dissolve tablets completely.

Drink Alka-Seltzer. You do not have to drink any of the residue that may be on the bottom of the glass. The medicines of Alka-Seltzer are in the water.

adults and children 12 years and over	allow 2 tablets to dissolve fully on the tongue every 4 to 6 hours	do not exceed 8 tablets in 24 hours or as directed by a doctor
children 6 to under 12 years	allow 1 tablet to dissolve fully on the tongue every 4 to 6 hours	do not exceed 4 tablets in 24 hours or as directed by a doctor
children under 6 years	consult a doctor	

Continued on next page

Alka-Seltzer PM—Cont.

How Supplied Foil Packs of 24 Effervescent Tablets.
FOIL SEALED FOR YOUR SAFETY. DO NOT USE IF FOIL PACKS ARE TORN OR BROKEN.
Questions or comments?
1-800-800-4793 or www.alka-seltzer.com
For more information, visit our website at www.alka-seltzer.com
Questions or comments?
Please call 1-800-800-4793.
Made in the U.S.A.
Bayer HealthCare LLC
Consumer Care Division
P.O. Box 1910
Morristown, NJ 07962-1910 USA
Shown in Product Identification Guide, page 504

BACTINE® Antiseptic-Anesthetic First Aid Liquid

Drug Facts

Active Ingredients: Purpose:
Benzalkonium chloride
0.13% w/w .... First aid antiseptic
Lidocaine hydrochloride
2.5% w/w .... Pain reliever

Uses: first aid to help prevent skin infection, and temporarily relieves pain and itching associated with minor: • cuts • scrapes • burns

Warnings:
For external use only
Ask a doctor before use if you have
• deep or puncture wounds
• animal bites
• serious burns
When using this product:
• do not use in or near the eyes
• do not apply over large areas of the body or in large quantities
• do not apply over raw surfaces or blistered areas
Stop use and ask a doctor if:
• condition worsens
• symptoms persist for more than 7 days, or clear up and occur again within a few days
Keep out of reach of children. If swallowed, get medical help or contact a Poison Control Center right away

Directions: • children under 2 years ask a doctor • adults and children 2 years and older: clean affected area; apply small amount on area 1–3 times daily; may be covered with a sterile bandage (let dry first)
Other Information:
• protect from excessive heat

Inactive ingredients: Disodium EDTA, fragrances, octoxynol 9, propylene glycol, water.
Questions: 1-800-800-4793 or www-.bayercare.com
CHILD RESISTANT CAP

How Supplied: Bactine Antiseptic-Anesthetic First Aid Liquid is available in 2, 4 and 5 oz sizes.
Bayer HealthCare LLC
Consumer Care Division

Genuine BAYER® Aspirin Caplets and Tablets

Active Ingredient: Purposes:
(in each caplet, gelcap, tablet)
Aspirin
325 mg ..... pain reliever/fever reducer

Uses: Temporarily relieves:
• headache
• muscle pain
• toothache
• menstrual pain
• pain and fever of colds
• minor pain of arthritis

Warnings: Reye's syndrome: Children and teenagers should not use this medicine for chicken pox or flu symptoms before a doctor is consulted about Reye's syndrome, a rare but serious illness reported to be associated with aspirin.

Allergy alert: Aspirin may cause a severe allergic reaction which may include:
• hives
• facial swelling
• asthma (wheezing)
• shock
Alcohol warning: If you consume 3 or more alcoholic drinks every day, ask your doctor whether you should take aspirin or other pain relievers/fever reducers. Aspirin may cause stomach bleeding.
Do not use if you are allergic to aspirin or any other pain reliever/fever reducer.
Ask a doctor before use if you have:
• stomach problems (such as heartburn, upset stomach, or stomach pain) that continue or come back
• bleeding problems
• ulcers
• asthma
Ask a doctor or pharmacist before use if you are taking a prescription drug for
• anticoagulation (blood thinning)
• gout
• diabetes
• arthritis
Stop use and ask a doctor if:
• an allergic reaction occurs. Seek medical help right away.
• pain gets worse or lasts for more than 10 days
• fever lasts for more than 3 days
• new symptoms occur
• ringing in the ears or loss of hearing occurs
• redness or swelling is present
If pregnant or breast-feeding, ask a health professional before use. **It is especially important not to use aspirin during the last 3 months of pregnancy unless definitely directed to do so by a doctor because it may cause problems in the unborn child or complications during delivery.**
Keep out of reach of children. In case of overdose, get medical help or contact a Poison Control Center right away.

Directions:
• drink a full glass of water with each dose
• adults and children 12 years and over: take 1 or 2 caplets every 4 hours not to exceed 12 caplets in 24 hours

• children under 12 years: consult a doctor
Other Information:
• save carton for full directions and warnings
• store at room temperature

Inactive Ingredients:
BAYER® Genuine Aspirin Caplets: Cellulose, hypromellose, starch, triacetin
BAYER® Genuine Aspirin Tablets: Cellulose, Hypromellose, Starch, Triacetin

How Supplied: BAYER® Genuine Aspirin Original Strength 325 mg is available in bottles of 100 coated caplets, and in bottles of 100 coated tablets.
Questions or comments?
1-800-331-4536 or
www.bayeraspirin.com
Bayer HealthCare LLC
PO Box 1910
Morristown, NJ 07962-1910 USA
Shown in Product Identification Guide, page 504

ASPIRIN REGIMEN BAYER® 81 mg ASPIRIN REGIMEN BAYER® 325 mg
Delayed Release Enteric Aspirin Adult Low Strength 81 mg Tablets and Regular Strength 325 mg Caplets

Active Ingredient:
(in each tablet)   Purpose:
Aspirin 81 mg .... Pain reliever
Aspirin 325 mg .... Pain reliever

Uses: For the temporary relief of minor aches and pains or as recommended by your doctor. **Because of its delayed action, this product will not provide fast relief of headaches or other symptoms needing immediate relief.**

Warnings: Reye's syndrome: Children and teenagers should not use this medicine for chicken pox or flu symptoms before a doctor is consulted about Reye's syndrome, a rare but serious illness reported to be associated with aspirin.
Allergy alert: Aspirin may cause a severe allergic reaction which may include: • hives • facial swelling • asthma (wheezing) • shock
Alcohol warning: If you consume 3 or more alcoholic drinks every day, ask your doctor whether you should take aspirin or other pain relievers/fever reducers. Aspirin may cause stomach bleeding.
Do not use if you are allergic to aspirin or any other pain reliever/fever reducer.
Ask a doctor before use if you have:
• stomach problems (such as heartburn, upset stomach, or stomach pain) that continue or come back
• bleeding problems
• ulcers
• asthma
Ask a doctor or pharmacist before use if you are taking a prescription drug for
• anticoagulation (blood thinning)
• gout

- diabetes
- arthritis

Stop use and ask a doctor if

- an allergic reaction occurs. Seek medical help right away.
- pain gets worse or lasts for more than 10 days
- new symptoms occur
- ringing in the ears or loss of hearing occurs
- redness or swelling is present

If pregnant or breast-feeding, ask a health professional before use. **It is especially important not to use aspirin during the last 3 months of pregnancy unless definitely directed to do so by a doctor because it may cause problems in the unborn child or complications during delivery.**

Keep out of reach of children. In case of overdose, get medical help or contact a Poison Control Center right away.

Directions:

ASPIRIN REGIMEN BAYER® 81 mg:

- drink a full glass of water with each dose
- adults and children 12 years and over: take 4 to 8 tablets every 4 hours not to exceed 48 tablets in 24 hours unless directed by a doctor
- children under 12 years: consult a doctor

ASPIRIN REGIMEN BAYER® 325 mg:

- drink a full glass of water with each dose
- adults and children 12 years and over: take 1 or 2 caplets every 4 hours not to exceed 12 caplets in 24 hours unless directed by a doctor
- children under 12 years: consult a doctor

Other Information:

- save carton for full directions and warnings
- store at room temperature

Inactive Ingredients:

ASPIRIN REGIMEN BAYER® 81 mg: Carnauba wax, cellulose, croscarmellose sodium, D&C yellow #10 aluminum lake, FD&C yellow #6 aluminum lake, hypromellose, iron oxides, lactose, methacrylic acid copolymer, microcrystalline cellulose, polysorbate 80, propylene glycol, shellac, sodium lauryl sulfate, starch, titanium dioxide, triacetin

ASPIRIN REGIMEN BAYER® 325 mg: Carnauba wax, cellulose, D&C yellow #10 aluminum lake, FD&C yellow #6 aluminum lake, hypromellose, iron oxides, methacrylic acid copolymer, polysorbate 80, propylene gylcol, shellac, sodium lauryl sulfate, starch, titanium dioxide, triacetin

How Supplied:

ASPIRIN REGIMEN BAYER® 81 mg: Bottle of 120 tablets delayed release enteric safety coated aspirin.

ASPIRIN REGIMEN BAYER® 325 mg: Bottle of 100 caplets delayed release enteric safety coated aspirin.

Questions or comments?
1-800-331-4536 or
www.bayeraspirin.com

Bayer HealthCare LLC
PO Box 1910
Morristown, NJ 07962-1910 USA
*Shown in Product Identification
Guide, page 504*

BAYER® Children's Chewable Tablets
Genuine Aspirin
Cherry & Orange Flavored
Adult Regimen Chewable Mint
81 mg

Active Ingredient:
(in each tablet)   **Purposes:**
Aspirin
 81 mg .... Pain reliever/fever reducer

Uses: For the temporary relief of:
- minor aches, pains, and headaches
- to reduce fever associated with colds, sore throats, and teething

Warnings: Reye's syndrome: Children and teenagers should not use this medicine for chicken pox or flu symptoms before a doctor is consulted about Reye's syndrome, a rare but serious illness reported to be associated with aspirin.

Allergy alert: Aspirin may cause a severe allergic reaction which may include:
- hives
- facial swelling
- asthma (wheezing)
- shock

Alcohol warning: If you consume 3 or more alcoholic drinks every day, ask your doctor whether you should take aspirin or other pain relievers/fever reducers. Aspirin may cause stomach bleeding.

Sore throat warning: If sore throat is severe, persists for more than 2 days, is accompanied or followed by fever, headache, rash, nausea, or vomiting, consult a doctor promptly.

Do not use:
- if you are allergic to aspirin or any other pain reliever/fever reducer
- for at least 7 days after tonsillectomy or oral surgery

Ask a doctor before use if you have:
- stomach problems (such as heartburn, upset stomach, or stomach pain) that continue or come back
- bleeding problems
- ulcers
- asthma
- a child experiencing arthritis pain

Ask a doctor or pharmacist before use if you are taking a prescription drug for

- anticoagulation (blood thinning)
- gout
- diabetes
- arthritis

Stop use and ask a doctor if:

- an allergic reaction occurs. Seek medical help right away.
- pain gets worse or lasts more than 10 days (for adults) or 5 days (for children)
- fever gets worse or lasts more than 3 days
- new symptoms occur
- ringing in the ears or loss of hearing occurs
- redness or swelling is present

If pregnant or breast-feeding, ask a health professional before use. **It is especially important not to use aspirin during the last 3 months of pregnancy unless definitely directed to do so by a doctor because it may cause problems in the unborn child or complications during delivery.**

Keep out of reach of children. In case of overdose, get medical help or contact a Poison Control Center right away.

Directions:

- drink a full glass of water with each dose
- to be administered only under adult supervision
- if possible use weight to dose. Otherwise use age.
[See table below]

Other Information:

- save carton for full directions and warnings.
- store at room temperature.

Inactive Ingredients:
BAYER® Children's Chewable: Cherry Flavored: D&C Red #27 Aluminum Lake, Dextrose, FD&C Red #40 Aluminum Lake, Flavor, Sodium, Saccharin, Starch
BAYER Children's Chewable: Orange Flavored: Dextrose, FD&C Yellow #6 Aluminum Lake, Flavor, Sodium Saccharin, starch

How Supplied: Bottle of 36 chewable tablets.

USE ONLY IF SEAL UNDER BOTTLE CAP WITH WHITE "Bayer Corporation" PRINT IS INTACT.

Questions or comments?
1-800-331-4536 or
www.bayeraspirin.com

Continued on next page

Weight (lb)	Age (years)	Dosage	Maximum Dosage
under 32	children under 3	consult a doctor	
32 to 35	3 to under 4	2 tablets	
36 to 45	4 to under 6	3 tablets	
46 to 65	6 to under 9	4 tablets	repeat every 4 hours while symptoms persist up to a maximum of 5 doses in 24 hours or as directed by a doctor
66 to 76	9 to under 11	4 to 5 tablets	
77 to 83	11 to under 12	4 to 6 tablets	
	adults and children 12 years and over	5 to 8 tablets	

Bayer Children's—Cont.

Bayer HealthCare LLC
PO Box 1910
Morristown, NJ 07962-1910 USA
*Shown in Product Identification
Guide, page 504*

PROFESSIONAL LABELING

Genuine Bayer Aspirin
Aspirin Regimen Bayer 325 mg
Aspirin Regimen Bayer 81 mg
Bayer Women's Aspirin with Calcium
Aspirin Regimen Bayer Childrens
Chewable Orange/Cherry 81 mg
Adult Regimen Chewable Mint

Professional Labeling:

Indications And Usage: Vascular Indications (Ischemic Stroke, TIA, Acute MI, Prevention of Recurrent MI, Unstable Angina Pectoris, and Chronic Stable Angina Pectoris): Aspirin is indicated to: (1) Reduce the combined risk of death and nonfatal stroke in patients who have had ischemic stroke or transient ischemia of the brain due to fibrin platelet emboli, (2) reduce the risk of vascular mortality in patients with a suspected acute MI, (3) reduce the combined risk of death and nonfatal MI in patients with a previous MI or unstable angina pectoris, and (4) reduce the combined risk of MI and sudden death in patients with chronic stable angina pectoris.
Revascularization Procedures (Coronary Artery Bypass Graft (CABG), Percutaneous Transluminal Coronary Angioplasty (PTCA), and Carotid Endarterectomy): Aspirin is indicated in patients who have undergone revascularization procedures (i.e., CABG, PTCA, or carotid endarterectomy) when there is a pre-existing condition for which aspirin is already indicated.
Rheumatologic Disease Indications (Rheumatoid Arthritis, Juvenile Rheumatoid Arthritis, Spondyloarthropathies, Osteoarthritis, and the Arthritis and Pleurisy of Systemic Lupus Erythematosus (SLE)): Aspirin is indicated for the relief of the signs and symptoms of rheumatoid arthritis, juvenile rheumatoid arthritis, osteoarthritis, spondyloarthropathies, and arthritis and pleurisy associated with SLE.

Contraindications: Allergy: Aspirin is contraindicated in patients with known allergy to nonsteroidal anti-inflammatory drug products and in patients with the syndrome of asthma, rhinitis, and nasal polyps. Aspirin may cause severe urticaria, angioedema, or bronchospasm (asthma).
Reye's syndrome: Aspirin should not be used in children or teenagers for viral infections, with or without fever, because of the risk of Reye's syndrome with concomitant use of aspirin in certain viral illnesses.

Warnings: Alcohol Warning: Patients who consume three or more alcoholic drinks every day should be counseled about the bleeding risks involved with chronic, heavy alcohol use while taking aspirin.
Coagulation Abnormalities: Even low doses of aspirin can inhibit platelet function leading to an increase in bleeding time. This can adversely affect patients with inherited (hemophilia) or acquired (liver disease or vitamin K deficiency) bleeding disorders.
GI Side Effects: GI side effects include stomach pain, heartburn, nausea, vomiting, and gross GI bleeding. Although minor upper GI symptoms, such as dyspepsia, are common and can occur anytime during therapy, physicians should remain alert for signs of ulceration and bleeding, even in the absence of previous GI symptoms. Physicians should inform patients about the signs and symptoms of GI side effects and what steps to take if they occur.
Peptic Ulcer Disease: Patients with a history of active peptic ulcer disease should avoid using aspirin, which can cause gastric mucosal irritation and bleeding.

Precautions:

General: Renal Failure: Avoid aspirin in patients with severe renal failure (glomerular filtration rate less than 10 mL/minute).
Hepatic Insufficiency: Avoid aspirin in patients with severe hepatic insufficiency.
Sodium Restricted Diets: Patients with sodium-retaining states, such as congestive heart failure or renal failure, should avoid sodium-containing buffered aspirin preparations because of their high sodium content.
Laboratory Tests: Aspirin has been associated with elevated hepatic enzymes, blood urea nitrogen and serum creatinine, hyperkalemia, proteinuria, and prolonged bleeding time.

Drug Interactions: Angiotensin Converting Enzyme (ACE) Inhibitors: The hyponatremic and hypotensive effects of ACE inhibitors may be diminished by the concomitant administration of aspirin due to its indirect effect on the renin-angiotensin conversion pathway.
Acetazolamide: Concurrent use of aspirin and acetazolamide can lead to high serum concentrations of acetazolamide (and toxicity) due to competition at the renal tubule for secretion.
Anticoagulant Therapy (Heparin and Warfarin): Patients on anticoagulation therapy are at increased risk for bleeding because of drug-drug interactions and the effect on platelets. Aspirin can displace warfarin from protein binding sites, leading to prolongation of both the prothrombin time and the bleeding time. Aspirin can increase the anticoagulant activity of heparin, increasing bleeding risk.
Anticonvulsants: Salicylate can displace protein-bound phenytoin and valproic acid, leading to a decrease in the total concentration of phenytoin and an increase in serum valproic acid levels.
Beta Blockers: The hypotensive effects of beta blockers may be diminished by the concomitant administration of aspirin due to inhibition of renal prostaglandins, leading to decreased renal blood flow, and salt and fluid retention.
Diuretics: The effectiveness of diuretics in patients with underlying renal or cardiovascular disease may be diminished by the concomitant administration of aspirin due to inhibition of renal prostaglandins, leading to decreased renal blood flow and salt and fluid retention.
Methotrexate: Salicylate can inhibit renal clearance of methotrexate, leading to bone marrow toxicity, especially in the elderly or renal impaired.
Nonsteroidal Anti-inflammatory Drugs (NSAID's): The concurrent use of aspirin with other NSAID's should be avoided because this may increase bleeding or lead to decreased renal function.
Oral Hypoglycemics: Moderate doses of aspirin may increase the effectiveness of oral hypoglycemic drugs, leading to hypoglycemia.
Uricosuric Agents (Probenecid and Sulfinpyrazone): Salicylates antagonize the uricosuric action of uricosuric agents.
Carcinogenesis, Mutagenesis, Impairment of Fertility: Administration of aspirin for 68 weeks at 0.5 percent in the feed of rats was not carcinogenic. In the Ames Salmonella assay, aspirin was not mutagenic; however, aspirin did induce chromosome aberrations in cultured human fibroblasts. Aspirin inhibits ovulation in rats. (See Pregnancy.)
Pregnancy: Pregnant women should only take aspirin if clearly needed. Because of the known effects of NSAID's on the fetal cardiovascular system (closure of the ductus arteriosus), use during the third trimester of pregnancy should be avoided. Salicylate products have also been associated with alterations in maternal and neonatal hemostasis mechanisms, decreased birth weight, and with perinatal mortality.
Labor and Delivery: Aspirin should be avoided 1 week prior to and during labor and delivery because it can result in excessive blood loss at delivery. Prolonged gestation and prolonged labor due to prostaglandin inhibition have been reported.
Nursing Mothers: Nursing mothers should avoid using aspirin because salicylate is excreted in breast milk. Use of high doses may lead to rashes, platelet abnormalities, and bleeding in nursing infants.
Pediatric Use: Pediatric dosing recommendations for juvenile rheumatoid arthritis are based on well-controlled clinical studies. An initial dose of 90–130 mg/kg/day in divided doses, with an increase as needed for anti-inflammatory efficacy (target plasma salicylate levels of 150–300 mcg/mL) are effective.

At high doses (i.e., plasma levels of greater than 200 mcg/mL), the incidence of toxicity increases.

Adverse Reactions: Many adverse reactions due to aspirin ingestion are dose-related. The following is a list of adverse reactions that have been reported in the literature. (See **Warnings**.)

Body as a Whole: Fever, hypothermia, thirst.

Cardiovascular: Dysrhythmias, hypotension, tachycardia.

Central Nervous System: Agitation, cerebral edema, coma, confusion, dizziness, headache, subdural or intracranial hemorrhage, lethargy, seizures.

Fluid and Electrolyte: Dehydration, hyperkalemia, metabolic acidosis, respiratory alkalosis.

Gastrointestinal: Dyspepsia, GI bleeding, ulceration and perforation, nausea, vomiting, transient elevations of hepatic enzymes, hepatitis, Reye's Syndrome, pancreatitis.

Hematologic: Prolongation of the prothrombin time, disseminated intravascular coagulation, coagulopathy, thrombocytopenia.

Hypersensitivity: Acute anaphylaxis, angioedema, asthma, bronchospasm, laryngeal edema, urticaria.

Musculoskeletal: Rhabdomyolysis.

Metabolism: Hypoglycemia (in children), hyperglycemia.

Reproductive: Prolonged pregnancy and labor, stillbirths, lower birth weight infants, antepartum and postpartum bleeding.

Respiratory: Hyperpnea, pulmonary edema, tachypnea.

Special Senses: Hearing loss, tinnitus. Patients with high frequency hearing loss may have difficulty perceiving tinnitus. In these patients, tinnitus cannot be used as a clinical indicator of salicylism.

Urogenital: Interstitial nephritis, papillary necrosis, proteinuria, renal insufficiency and failure.

Drug Abuse and Dependence: Aspirin is nonnarcotic. There is no known potential for addiction associated with the use of aspirin.

Overdosage: Salicylate toxicity may result from acute ingestion (overdose) or chronic intoxication. The early signs of salicylic overdose (salicylism), including tinnitus (ringing in the ears), occur at plasma concentrations approaching 200 mcg/mL. Plasma concentrations of aspirin above 300 mcg/mL are clearly toxic. Severe toxic effects are associated with levels above 400 mcg/mL. (See **Clinical Pharmacology**.) A single lethal dose of aspirin in adults is not known with certainty but death may be expected at 30 g. For real or suspected overdose, a Poison Control Center should be contacted immediately. Careful medical management is essential.

Signs and Symptoms: In acute overdose, severe acid-base and electrolyte disturbances may occur and are complicated by hyperthermia and dehydration. Respiratory alkalosis occurs early while hyperventilation is present, but is quickly followed by metabolic acidosis.

Treatment: Treatment consists primarily of supporting vital functions, increasing salicylate elimination, and correcting the acid-base disturbance. Gastric emptying and/or lavage is recommended as soon as possible after ingestion, even if the patient has vomited spontaneously. After lavage and/or emesis, administration of activated charcoal, as a slurry, is beneficial, if less than 3 hours have passed since ingestion. Charcoal adsorption should not be employed prior to emesis and lavage.

Severity of aspirin intoxication is determined by measuring the blood salicylate level. Acid-base status should be closely followed with serial blood gas and serum pH measurements. Fluid and electrolyte balance should aslo be maintained.

In severe cases, hyperthermia and hypovolemia are the major immediate threats to life. Children should be sponged with tepid water. Replacement fluid should be administered intravenously and augmented with correction of acidosis. Plasma electrolytes and pH should be monitored to promote alkaline diuresis of salicylate if renal function is normal. Infusion of glucose may be required to control hypoglycemia.

Hemodialysis and peritoneal dialysis can be performed to reduce the body drug content. In patients with renal insufficiency or in cases of life-threatening intoxication, dialysis is usually required. Exchange transfusion may be indicated in infants and young children.

Dosage and Administration: Each dose of aspirin should be taken with a full glass of water unless patient is fluid restricted. Anti-inflammatory and analgesic dosages should be individualized. When aspirin is used in high doses, the development of tinnitus may be used as a clinical sign of elevated plasma salicylate levels except in patients with high frequency hearing loss.

Ischemic Stroke and TIA: 50–325 mg once a day. Continue therapy indefinitely.

Suspected Acute MI: The initial dose of 160–162.5 mg is administered as soon as an MI is suspected. The maintenance dose of 160–162.5 mg a day is continued for 30 days post-infaction. After 30 days, consider further therapy based on dosage and administration for prevention of recurrent MI.

Prevention of Recurrent MI: 75–325 mg once a day. Continue therapy indefinitely.

Unstable Angina Pectoris: 75–325 mg once a day. Continue therapy indefinitely.

Chronic Stable Angina Pectoris: 75–325 mg once a day. Continue therapy indefinitely.

CABG: 325 mg daily starting 6 hours post-procedure. Continue therapy for 1 year post-procedure.

PTCA: The initial dose of 325 mg should be given 2 hours presurgery. Maintenance dose is 160–325 mg daily. Continue therapy indefinitely.

Carotid Endarterectomy: Doses of 80 mg once daily to 650 mg twice daily, started presurgery, are recommended. Continue therapy indefinitely.

Rheumatoid Arthritis: The initial dose is 3 g a day in divided doses. Increase as needed for anti-inflammatory efficacy with target plasma salicylate levels of 150–300 mcg/mL. At high doses (i.e., plasma levels of greater than 200 mcg/mL), the incidence of toxicity increases.

Juvenile Rheumatoid Arthritis: Initial dose is 90–130 mg/kg/day in divided doses. Increase as needed for anti-inflammatory efficacy with target plasma salicylate levels of 150–300 mcg/mL. At high doses (i.e., plasma levels of greater than 200 mcg/mL), the incidence of toxicity increases.

Spondyloarthropathies: Up to 4 g per day in divided doses.

Osteoarthritis: Up to 3 g per day in divided doses.

Arthritis and Pleurisy of SLE: The initial dose is 3 g a day in divided doses. Increase as needed for anti-inflammatory efficacy with target plasma salicylate levels of 150–300 mcg/mL. At high doses (i.e., plasma levels of greater than 200 mcg/mL, the incidence of toxicity increases.

Extra Strength BAYER® Aspirin Caplets

Active Ingredient: **Purposes:**
(in each caplet)
Aspirin
500 mg ...... Pain reliever/fever reducer

Uses: For the temporary relief of
- headache
- pain and fever of colds
- muscle pain
- menstrual pain
- toothache
- minor pain of arthritis

Warnings: Reye's syndrome: Children and teenagers should not use this medicine for chicken pox or flu symptoms before a doctor is consulted about Reye's syndrome, a rare but serious illness reported to be associated with aspirin.

Allergy alert: Aspirin may cause a severe allergic reaction which may include:
- hives • facial swelling • asthma (wheezing) • shock

Alcohol warning: If you consume 3 or more alcoholic drinks every day, ask your doctor whether you should take aspirin or other pain relievers/fever reducers. Aspirin may cause stomach bleeding.

Do not use if you are allergic to aspirin or any other pain reliever/fever reducer.

Ask a doctor before use if you have:
- stomach problems (such as heartburn, upset stomach, or stomach pain) that last or come back

Continued on next page

Bayer Extra Strength—Cont.

- bleeding problems
- ulcers
- asthma

Ask a doctor or pharmacist before use if you are taking a prescription drug for
- anticoagulation (blood thinning)
- gout
- diabetes
- arthritis

Stop use and ask a doctor if:
- an allergic reaction occurs. Seek medical help right away.
- pain gets worse or lasts for more than 10 days
- fever lasts for more than 3 days
- new symptoms occur
- ringing in the ears or loss of hearing occurs
- redness or swelling is present

If pregnant or breast-feeding, ask a health professional before use. **It is especially important not to use aspirin during the last 3 months of pregnancy unless definitely directed to do so by a doctor because it may cause problems in the unborn child or complications during delivery.**

Keep out of reach of children. In case of overdose, get medical help or contact a Poison Control Center right away.

Directions:
- drink a full glass of water with each dose
- adults and children 12 years and over: take 1 or 2 caplets every 4 to 6 hours not to exceed 8 caplets in 24 hours
- children under 12 years: consult a doctor

Other Information:
- save carton for full directions and warnings
- store at room temperature

Inactive Ingredients: Extra Strength BAYER® Aspirin Caplets: Carnauba Wax, Cellulose, D&C Red #7 Calcium Lake, FD&C Blue #2 Aluminum Lake, FD&C Red #40 Aluminum Lake, Hypromellose, Propylene Glycol, Shellac, Starch, Titanium Dioxide, Triacetin

How Supplied:
Extra Strength BAYER® Aspirin Caplets: Bottle of 50 coated caplets (500 mg).

Questions or comments?
1-800-331-4536 or
www.bayeraspirin.com
Bayer HealthCare LLC
PO Box 1910
Morristown, NJ 07962-1910 USA

BAYER® Extra Strength
back & body pain

Drug Facts

Active Ingredients: **Purpose:**
(in each caplet)
Aspirin 500 mg .... Pain reliever
Caffeine 32.5 mg .... Pain reliever aid

Uses: for the temporary relief of
- backache pain • muscle aches and pains
- minor aches and pains of arthritis

Warnings:
Reye's syndrome: Children and teenagers should not use this medicine for chicken pox or flu symptoms before a doctor is consulted about Reye's syndrome, a rare but serious illness reported to be associated with aspirin.

Allergy alert: Aspirin may cause a severe allergic reaction which may include:
- hives • facial swelling • asthma (wheezing) • shock

Alcohol warning: If you consume 3 or more alcoholic drinks every day, ask your doctor whether you should take aspirin or other pain relievers/fever reducers. Aspirin may cause stomach bleeding.

Do not use if you are allergic to aspirin or any other pain reliever/fever reducer

Ask a doctor before use if you have
- stomach problems (such as heartburn, upset stomach, or stomach pain) that continue or come back
- bleeding problems • ulcers • asthma

Ask a doctor or pharmacist before use if you are taking a prescription drug for
- anticoagulation (blood thinning)
- gout • diabetes • arthritis

Stop use and ask a doctor if
- an allergic reaction occurs. Seek medical help right away.
- pain gets worse or lasts more than 10 days
- redness or swelling is present
- new symptoms occur
- ringing in the ears or loss of hearing occurs

If pregnant or breast-feeding, ask a health professional before use. **It is especially important not to use aspirin during the last 3 months of pregnancy unless definitely directed to do so by a doctor because it may cause problems in the unborn child or complications during delivery.**

Keep out of reach of children. In case of overdose, get medical help or contact a Poison Control Center right away.

Directions: • drink a full glass of water with each dose
- adults and children 12 years and over: take 2 caplets every 6 hours not to exceed 8 caplets in 24 hours
- children under 12 years: consult a doctor

Other Information: • save carton for full directions and warnings
- store at room temperature

Inactive Ingredients: carnauba wax, cellulose, D&C red #30 aluminum lake, D&C yellow #10 aluminum lake, hypromellose, propylene glycol, shellac, starch, titanium dioxide, triacetin

How Supplied: 50 Coated Caplets
Questions or comments?
1-800-331-4536 or
www.bayeraspirin.com
Bayer
Bayer HealthCare LLC
Consumer Care Division
P.O. Box 1910
Morristown, NJ 07962-1910 USA

Extra Strength BAYER® PLUS
Buffered Aspirin Caplets

Active Ingredient:
(in each caplet)   **Purposes:**
Aspirin
500 mg .... Pain reliever/fever reducer

Uses: For the temporary relief of
- headache
- pain and fever of colds
- muscle pain
- menstrual pain
- toothache
- minor pain of arthritis

Warnings: Reye's syndrome: Children and teenagers should not use this medicine for chicken pox or flu symptoms before a doctor is consulted about Reye's syndrome, a rare but serious illness reported to be associated with aspirin.

Allergy alert: Aspirin may cause a severe allergic reaction which may include
- hives
- facial swelling
- asthma (wheezing)
- shock

Alcohol warning: If you consume 3 or more alcoholic drinks every day, ask your doctor whether you should take aspirin or other pain relievers/fever reducers. Aspirin may cause stomach bleeding.

Do not use if you are allergic to aspirin or any other pain reliever/fever reducer.

Ask a doctor before use if you have
- stomach problems (such as heartburn, upset stomach, or stomach pain) that continue or come back
- bleeding problems
- ulcers
- asthma

Ask a doctor or pharmacist before use if you are taking a prescription drug for
- anticoagulation (blood thinning)
- gout
- diabetes
- arthritis

Stop use and ask a doctor if
- an allergic reaction occurs. Seek medical help right away.
- pain gets worse or lasts more than 10 days
- fever lasts more than 3 days
- new symptoms occur
- ringing in the ears or loss of hearing occurs
- redness or swelling is present

If pregnant or breast-feeding, ask a health professional before use. **It is especially important not to use aspirin during the last 3 months of pregnancy unless definitely directed to do so by a doctor because it may cause problems in the unborn child or complications during delivery.**

Keep out of reach of children. In case of overdose, get medical help or contact a Poison Control Center right away.

Directions:
- drink a full glass of water with each dose
- adults and children 12 years and over: take 1 or 2 caplets every 4 to 6 hours as needed, not to exceed 8 caplets in 24 hours
- children under 12 years: consult a doctor

Other Information:
- contains calcium carbonate (350 mg = 140 mg elemental calcium)

- save carton for full directions and warnings
- store at room temperature

Inactive Ingredients: Calcium carbonate, carnauba wax, colloidal silicon dioxide, D&C red #7 calcium lake, FD&C blue #2 aluminum lake, FD&C red #40 aluminum lake, hypromellose, microcrystalline cellulose, propylene glycol, shellac, sodium starch glycolate, starch, titanium dioxide, zinc stearate

How Supplied: Bottle of 50 buffered caplets (500 mg).
Questions or comments?
1-800-331-4536 or
www.bayeraspirin.com
USE ONLY IF SEAL UNDER BOTTLE CAP WITH GREEN "Bayer Corporation" PRINT IS INTACT.
Bayer HealthCare LLC
PO Box 1910
Morristown, NJ 07962-1910 USA

BAYER® NIGHTTIME RELIEF
For Pain with Sleeplessness
Caplets

Drug Facts

Active Ingredients: **Purpose:**
(in each caplet)
Aspirin 500 mg .... Pain reliever
Diphenhydramine citrate
  38.3 mg .... Nighttime sleep-aid

Uses: for the temporary relief of occasional headache and minor aches and pains with accompanying sleeplessness

Warnings:
Reye's syndrome: Children and teenagers should not use this medicine for chicken pox or flu symptoms before a doctor is consulted about Reye's syndrome, a rare but serious illness reported to be associated with aspirin.
Allergy alert: Aspirin may cause a severe allergic reaction which may include:
• hives • facial swelling • asthma (wheezing) • shock
Alcohol warning: If you consume 3 or more alcoholic drinks every day, ask your doctor whether you should take aspirin or other pain relievers/fever reducers. Aspirin may cause stomach bleeding.
Do not use
- if you are allergic to aspirin or any other pain reliever/fever reducer
- in children under 12 years of age
- with any other product containing diphenhydramine, even one used on the skin

Ask a doctor before use if you have
- stomach problems (such as heartburn, upset stomach, or stomach pain) that last or come back
- bleeding problems • ulcers
- a breathing problem such as emphysema, chronic bronchitis, or asthma
- glaucoma
- trouble urinating due to an enlarged prostate gland

Ask a doctor or pharmacist before use if you are
- taking a prescription drug for
  • anticoagulation (blood thinning) • diabetes • gout • arthritis

- taking tranquilizers or sedatives
When using this product avoid alcoholic drinks
Stop use and ask a doctor if
- an allergic reaction occurs. Seek medical help right away.
- pain gets worse or lasts more than 10 days
- redness or swelling is present
- new symptoms occur
- ringing in the ears or loss of hearing occurs
- sleeplessness lasts for more than 2 weeks. Insomnia may be a symptom of a serious underlying medical illness.
If pregnant or breast-feeding, ask a health professional before use. **It is especially important not to use aspirin during the last 3 months of pregnancy unless definitely directed to do so by a doctor because it may cause problems in the unborn child or complications during delivery.**
Keep out of reach of children. In case of overdose, get medical help or contact a Poison Control Center right away.

Directions:
- do not exceed recommended dosage
- drink a full glass of water with each dose
- adults and children 12 years and over: take 2 caplets at bedtime, if needed, or as directed by a doctor.
- children under 12 years: do not use
Other Information:
- save carton for full directions and warnings
- store at room temperature

Inactive Ingredients: carnauba wax, citric acid, colloidal silicon dioxide, FD&C blue #1 aluminum lake, FD&C blue #2 aluminum lake, hypromellose, microcrystalline cellulose, pregelatinized starch, propylene glycol, shellac, titanium dioxide, zinc stearate
Questions or comments?
1-800-331-4536 or
www.bayeraspirin.com

BAYER®
Muscle & Joint Cream
Non-Greasy Pain Relieving Cream

Drug Facts
Active Ingredients: **Purpose:**
Camphor 4% .... Topical analgesic
Menthol 10% .... Topical analgesic
Methyl
  salicylate 30% .... Topical analgesic

Uses: for temporary relief of minor aches and pains of muscles and joints associated with
- arthritis • simple backache • strains
- sprains

Warnings:
For external use only
Do not use
- for arthritis-like conditions in children under 12. Consult a physician.
- with a heating pad
- on wounds, damaged, broken or irritated skin
When using this product
- use only as directed
- do not swallow

- do not bandage tightly
- avoid contact with the eyes and mucous membranes
Stop use and ask a doctor if
- skin redness or irritation develops
- condition worsens or pain lasts for more than 7 days or clears up and occurs again within a few days
Keep out of reach of children. If swallowed, get medical help or contact a Poison Control Center right away.

Directions: Adults and children 12 years of age and older:
- apply generously to affected area
- massage gently until absorbed in the skin
- repeat 3 to 4 times a day
Children under 12 years of age, consult a doctor.
Other Information: store at room temperature

Inactive Ingredients: carbomer 940, edetate disodium, glyceryl stearate SE, isopropyl myristate, lanolin, polysorbate 60, purified water, sorbitan monostearate, stearyl alcohol, trolamine
Questions or comments?

How Supplied: 2 oz. tube, 4 oz tube
1-800-331-4536 or www.bayercare.com
Made in U.S.A.
Distributed by:
Bayer Healthcare LLC
Consumer Care Division
P.O. Box 1910
Morristown, NJ 07962-1910 USA
    30000091-00

BAYER® WOMEN'S ASPIRIN PLUS CALCIUM
Low Strength Aspirin Regimen
Analgesic/Dietary Supplement
81 mg Aspirin-300 mg Calcium

Directions: For calcium, take up to 4 caplets per day.

Serving Size: One Caplet

	Amount Per Serving	% Daily Value
Calcium (elemental)	300 mg	30%

Ingredients: Calcium Carbonate, Microcrystalline Cellulose, Aspirin, Lactose, Cellulose, Maltodextrin, Starch, Carnauba Wax, Hypromellose, Polydextrose, Titanium Dioxide, Triacetin, Sodium Starch Glycolate, Colloidal Silicon Dioxide, Zinc Stearate, Mineral Oil, Crospovidone, Magnesium Stearate, Stearic Acid.
What you should know about Osteoporosis
Menopausal women and women with a family history of the disease are groups at risk for developing osteoporosis. Adequate calcium intake throughout life, along with a healthy diet and regular exercise, builds and maintains good bone

Continued on next page

Bayer Women's—Cont.

health and may reduce the risk of osteoporosis. While adequate calcium intake is important, daily intakes above 2,000 mg may not provide additional benefits.

Active Ingredient:

(in each caplet)   **Purpose**
Aspirin 81 mg .... Pain reliever

Uses: For the temporary relief of minor aches and pains or as recommended by your doctor

Warnings: Reye's syndrome: Children and teenagers should not use this medicine for chicken pox or flu symptoms before a doctor is consulted about Reye's syndrome, a rare but serious illness reported to be associated with aspirin.

Alcohol warning: If you consume 3 or more alcoholic drinks every day, ask your doctor whether you should take aspirin or other pain relievers/fever reducers. Aspirin may cause stomach bleeding.

Allergy alert: Aspirin may cause a severe allergic reaction which may include:
• hives
• facial swelling
• asthma (wheezing)
• shock

Do not use if you are allergic to aspirin or any other pain reliever/fever reducer.

Ask a doctor before use if you have
• stomach problems (such as heartburn, upset stomach, or stomach pain) that continue or come back
• bleeding problems
• ulcers
• asthma

Ask a doctor or pharmacist before use if you are taking a prescription drug for
• anticoagulation (blood thinning)
• gout
• diabetes
• arthritis

Stop use and ask a doctor if
• an allergic reaction occurs. Seek medical help right away.
• pain gets worse or lasts more than 10 days
• new symptoms occur
• ringing in the ears or loss of hearing occurs
• redness or swelling is present

If pregnant or breast-feeding, ask a health professional before use. **It is especially important not to use aspirin during the last 3 months of pregnancy unless definitely directed to do so by a doctor because it may cause problems in the unborn child or complications during delivery.**

Keep out of reach of children. In case of overdose, get medical help or contact a Poison Control Center right away.

Directions:
• talk to your doctor about regimen use of aspirin
• drink a full glass of water with each dose
• for pain, adults and children 12 years and over: take 4 caplets not to exceed 4 caplets in 24 hours
• children under 12 years: consult a doctor

Other Information:
• save carton for full directions and warnings
• store at room temperature

Inactive Ingredients: Calcium carbonate, carnauba wax, cellulose, colloidal silicon dioxide, crospovidone, hypromellose, lactose, magnesium stearate, maltodextrin, microcrystalline cellulose, mineral oil, polydextrose, sodium starch glycolate, starch, stearic acid, titanium dioxide, triacetin, zinc stearate.

How Supplied: Bottle of 90 Caplets
Aspirin is not appropriate for everyone, so be sure to talk to your doctor before you begin an aspirin regimen.
Ideal for women on an aspirin regimen, as directed by a doctor, who need a head start on their daily calcium requirements to help fight Osteoporosis. *For more information on how to fight heart disease and stroke, visit the American Heart Association Web Site at www.americanheart.org.*
USE ONLY IF SEAL UNDER BOTTLE CAP WITH GREEN "Bayer Corporation" PRINT IS INTACT.
Questions or comments?
1-800-331-4536 or
www.bayeraspirin.com
Bayer HealthCare LLC
Consumer Care Division
PO Box 1910
Morristown, NJ 07962-1910 USA
Shown in Product Identification Guide, page 504

DOMEBORO® POWDER PACKETS
DOMEBORO® TABLETS
DOMEBORO® Astringent Solution

Drug Facts
Active Ingredient   **Purpose:**
(in each packet):
Aluminum acetate .... Astringent
(Each powder packet, when mixed in water and ready for use, provides the active ingredient aluminum acetate resulting from the reaction of calcium acetate 839 mg and aluminum sulfate 1191 mg.)
DOMEBORO® Tablets
Active Ingredient   **Purpose:**
(in each tablet):
Aluminum acetate
   467 mg .... Astringent
(Each tablet, when dissolved in water and ready for use, provides the active ingredient aluminum acetate resulting from the reaction of hydrated calcium acetate 605 mg and aluminum sulfate 879 mg.)

Uses: temporarily relieves minor skin irritations due to:
• poison ivy
• poison oak
• poison sumac
• insect bites
• athlete's foot
• rashes caused by soaps, detergents, cosmetics, or jewelry

Warnings:
For external use only
When using this product
• avoid contact with the eyes
• do not cover compress or wet dressing with plastic to prevent evaporation

Stop use and ask a doctor if condition worsens or symptoms persist more than 7 days.

Keep out of reach of children. If swallowed, get medical help or contact a Poison Control Center right away.

Directions:
DOMEBORO® Astringent Solution
• mix one, two, or three packets in 16 oz of water to obtain the following modified Burow's Solution

Number of Packets	Dilution	% Aluminum acetate
one packet	1:40 dilution	0.14%
two packets	1:20 dilution	0.28%
three packets	1:13 dilution	0.42%

• do not strain or filter the solution
• can be used as a compress, wet dressing, or a soak.

DOMEBORO® Tablets
• dissolve one, two, or three tablets in 12 oz of water and stir the solution until fully dissolved to obtain the following modified Burow's Solution

Number of Tablets	Dilution	% Aluminum acetate
one tablet	1:40 dilution	0.13%
two tablets	1:20 dilution	0.26%
three tablets	1:13 dilution	0.39%

• do not strain or filter the solution
• can be used as a compress, wet dressing, or a soak

AS A COMPRESS OR WET DRESSING:
• saturate a clean, soft, white cloth (such as a diaper or torn sheet) in the solution
• gently squeeze and apply loosely to the affected area
• saturate the cloth in the solution every 15 to 30 minutes and apply to the affected area
• discard the solution after each use
• repeat as often as necessary

AS A SOAK:
• soak affected area in the solution for 15 to 30 minutes
• discard solution after each use
• repeat 3 times a day

Other Information: • protect from excessive heat

Inactive Ingredients:
DOMEBORO® Powder Packets
dextrin
DOMEBORO® Tablets:
dextrin, polyethylene glycol, sodium bicarbonate

How Supplied:
Tablets and Packets available in 12 and 100 count sizes
Questions or comments? 1-800-800-4793 or www.bayercare.com
Bayer HealthCare LLC

**Maximum Strength
MIDOL® Menstrual
Pain & Multi-Symptom Menstrual Relief
Aspirin Free
Caplets and Gelcaps**

Active Ingredients:
(in each caplet and gelcap)   Purpose:
Acetaminophen 500 mg .... Pain reliever
Caffeine 60 mg .... Stimulant
Pyrilamine maleate 15 mg .... Diuretic

Uses: For the temporary relief of these symptoms associated with menstrual periods:
• cramps
• bloating
• water-weight gain
• breast tenderness
• headache
• backache
• muscle aches
• fatigue

Warnings: Alcohol warning: If you consume 3 or more alcoholic drinks every day, ask your doctor whether you should take acetaminophen or other pain relievers/fever reducers. Acetaminophen may cause liver damage.
Do not use with any other product containing acetaminophen.
Ask a doctor before use if you have:
• glaucoma
• difficulty in urination due to enlargement of the prostate gland
• a breathing problem such as emphysema or chronic bronchitis
Ask a doctor or pharmacist before use if you are taking sedatives or tranquilizers.
When using this product:
• you may get drowsy
• avoid alcoholic drinks
• excitability may occur, especially in children
• alcohol, sedatives, and tranquilizers may increase drowsiness
• be careful when driving a motor vehicle or operating machinery
• limit the use of caffeine-containing medications, foods, or beverages. Too much caffeine may cause nervousness, irritability, sleeplessness, and occasionally, rapid heartbeat. The recommended dose of this product contains about as much caffeine as a cup of coffee.
Stop use and ask a doctor if:
• new symptoms occur
• redness or swelling is present
• pain gets worse or lasts for more than 10 days
If pregnant or breast-feeding, ask a health professional before use.

Keep out of reach of children.
Overdose warning: Taking more than the recommended dose can cause serious health problems. In case of overdose, get medical help or contact a Poison Control Center right away. Quick medical attention is critical for adults as well as children even if you do not notice any signs or symptoms.

Directions:
MIDOL® Extra Strength Caplets:
Do not take more than the recommended dose. (see **Overdose Warning**)
• adults and children 12 years and older
   • take 2 caplets with water
   • repeat every 4 hours, as needed
   • do not exceed 8 caplets per day
• children under 12 years, consult a doctor

Other Information:
• store at room temperature
MIDOL® Extra Strength Gelcaps:
Do not take more than the recommended dose. (see **Overdose Warning**)
• adults and children 12 years and older
   • take 2 gelcaps with water
   • repeat every 6 hours, as needed
   • do not exceed 8 gelcaps per day
• children under 12 years, consult a doctor

Other Information:
• store at room temperature
• avoid excessive heat 104°F (40°C)

Inactive Ingredients:
MIDOL® Extra Strength Caplets:
Croscarmellose Sodium, FD&C Blue #2, Hypromellose, Magnesium Stearate, Microcrystalline Cellulose, Pregelatinized Starch, Triacetin.

MIDOL® Extra Strength Gelcaps:
Carnauba Wax, Croscarmellose Sodium, D&C Red #33 Lake, Disodium EDTA, FD&C Blue #1 Lake, Gelatin, Glycerin, Hypromellose, Iron Oxide, Lecithin, Magnesium Stearate, Microcrystalline Cellulose, Pharmaceutical Glaze, Simethicone, Starch, Stearic Acid, Titanium Dioxide, Triacetin

How Supplied:
MIDOL® Extra Strength Caplets:
Capsule-shaped caplets available in packages of 24 caplets containing 3 blisters of 8 capsules each.

MIDOL® Extra Strength Gelcaps:
Capsule-shaped gelcaps available in packages of 24 gelcaps containing 3 blisters of 8 gelcaps each.

Use only if blister unit is unbroken.

Store at room temperature; avoid excessive heat 40°C (104°F).

Questions? Comments?
Please call 1-800-331-4536.
Visit our website at www.midol.com
ASPIRIN-FREE
B-R LLC
Distributed by:
Bayer HealthCare LLC
Consumer Care Division
Morristown, NJ 07960 USA
Shown in Product Identification Guide, page 504

**Maximum Strength
MIDOL® PMS
Pain & Premenstrual Symptom Relief
Aspirin Free/Caffeine Free
Caplets and Gelcaps**

Active Ingredients:
(in each caplet and in each gelcap)   Purpose:
Acetaminophen 500 mg .... Pain reliever
Pamabrom 25 mg .... Diuretic
Pyrilamine maleate 15 mg .... Diuretic

Uses: For the temporary relief of these symptoms associated with menstrual periods:
• bloating
• water-weight gain
• cramps
• breast tenderness
• headache
• backache

Warnings: Alcohol warning: If you consume 3 or more alcoholic drinks every day, ask your doctor whether you should take acetaminophen or other pain relievers/fever reducers. Acetaminophen may cause liver damage.
Do not use with any other product containing acetaminophen.
Ask a doctor before use if you have:
• glaucoma
• difficulty in urination due to enlargement of the prostate gland
• a breathing problem such as emphysema or chronic bronchitis
Ask a doctor or pharmacist before use if you are taking sedatives or tranquilizers.
When using this product:
• you may get drowsy
• excitability may occur, especially in children
• alcohol, sedatives, and tranquilizers may increase drowsiness
• avoid alcoholic drinks
• be careful when driving a motor vehicle or operating machinery
Stop use and ask a doctor if:
• new symptoms occur
• redness or swelling is present
• pain gets worse or lasts for more than 10 days
If pregnant or breast-feeding, ask a health professional before use.
Keep out of reach of children.
Overdose warning: Taking more than the recommended dose can cause serious health problems. In case of overdose, get medical help or contact a Poison Control Center right away. Quick medical attention is critical for adults as well as children even if you do not notice any signs or symptoms.

Directions:
MIDOL® Maximum Strength PMS Caplets:
Do not take more than the recommended dose. (see Overdose Warning)
• adults and children 12 years and older
   • take 2 caplets with water
   • repeat every 6 hours, as needed
   • do not exceed 8 caplets per day
• children under 12 years, consult a doctor

Continued on next page

Midol PMS—Cont.

Other Information: Store at room temperature. Avoid excessive heat 104° F (40° C)

MIDOL® Maximum Strength PMS Gelcaps:

Do not take more than the recommended dose. (see Overdose Warning)
- adults and children 12 years and older
  - take 2 gelcaps with water
  - repeat every 6 hours, as needed
  - do not exceed 8 gelcaps per day
- children under 12 years, consult a doctor

Other Information: Store at room temperature. Avoid excessive heat 104° F (40° C)

Inactive Ingredients:
MIDOL® Maximum Strength PMS: Carnauba Wax, Croscarmellose Sodium, D&C Red #30 Aluminum Lake, D&C Yellow #10 Aluminum Lake, Hypromellose, Magnesium Stearate, Microcrystalline Cellulose, Propylene Glycol, Shellac, Starch, Titanium Dioxide, Triacetin
MIDOL® Maximum Strength PMS Gelcaps: Croscarmellose Sodium, D&C Red #27 Lake, EDTA Disodium, FD&C Blue #1, FD&C Red #40 Lake, Gelatin, Glycerin, Hypromellose, Iron Oxide, Magnesium Stearate, Microcrystalline Cellulose, Starch, Stearic Acid, Titanium Dioxide, Triacetin.

How Supplied:
MIDOL® Maximum Strength PMS Caplets: Capsule-shaped caplets available in packages of 24 caplets containing 3 blisters of 8 caplets each.
MIDOL® Maximum Strength PMS Gelcaps: Capsule-shaped gelcaps available in packages of 24 gelcaps containing 3 blisters of 8 gelcaps each.
Use only if blister unit is unbroken.
Store at room temperature; avoid excessive heat 40°C (104°F).
Questions? Comments?
Please call 1-800-331-4536.
Visit our website at
www.midol.com
ASPIRIN-FREE CAFFEINE-FREE
B-R LLC
Distributed by:
Bayer HealthCare LLC
Consumer Care Division
Morristown, NJ 07960 USA
Shown in Product Identification Guide, page 504

NEO-SYNEPHRINE®
Regular Strength

Neo-Synephrine® Regular Strength Drops
Neo-Synephrine® Regular Strength Spray
Active Ingredient: **Purpose:**
Phenylephrine
Hydrochloride 0.5% .... Nasal
decongestant

Uses:
- temporarily relieves nasal congestion:
  — due to common cold
  — due to hay fever or other upper respiratory allergies (allergic rhinitis)
  — associated with sinusitis
- temporarily relieves stuffy nose
- helps clear nasal passages; shrinks swollen membranes
- temporarily restores freer breathing through the nose
- helps decongest sinus openings and passages; temporarily relieves sinus congestion and pressure

Warnings:
Ask a doctor before use if you have
- heart disease
- high blood pressure
- thyroid disease
- diabetes
- difficulty in urination due to enlargement of the prostate gland

When using this product
- **do not exceed recommended dosage**
- do not use more than 3 days. Use only as directed. Frequent or prolonged use may cause nasal congestion to recur or worsen.
- temporary discomfort may occur such as burning, stinging, sneezing, and an increase in nasal discharge
- use by more than one person may spread infection

Stop use and ask a doctor if symptoms persist more than 3 days.

If pregnant or breast-feeding, ask a health professional before use.

Keep out of reach of children. If swallowed, get medical help or contact a Poison Control Center right away.

Directions: use only as directed

adults and children 12 years and older	2 or 3 drops in each nostril not more often than every 4 hours
children under 12 years	ask a doctor

Neo-Synephrine® Regular Strength Spray
To spray, squeeze bottle quickly and firmly.

adults and children 12 years and older	2 or 3 sprays in each nostril not more often than every 4 hours
children under 12 years	ask a doctor

Other Information:
- store at room temperature
- protect from light

Inactive Ingredients: benzalkonium chloride, citric acid, sodium chloride, sodium citrate, purified water

How Supplied:
Neo-Synephrine Regular Strength Drops: 15ml (0.5%)
DO NOT USE IF IMPRINTED BOTTLE OVERWRAP IS BROKEN OR MISSING.

Neo-Synephrine Regular Strength Spray: 15ml (0.5%)
USE ONLY IF NECKBAND PRINTED WITH "Bayer" IS INTACT.

Questions or comments? 1-800-331-4536 or www.bayercare.com

Bayer HealthCare LLC
Consumer Care Division
P.O. Box 1910
Morristown, NJ 07962-1910 USA
Shown in Product Identification Guide, page 504

NEO-SYNEPHRINE®
12 Hour Extra Moisturizing
(nasal spray)

Active Ingredients: **Purpose:**
Oxymetazoline
hydrochloride 0.05% .... Nasal
decongestant

Uses:
- temporarily relieves nasal congestion:
  — due to common cold
  — due to hay fever or other upper respiratory allergies (allergic rhinitis)
  — associated with sinusitis
- temporarily relieves stuffy nose
- helps clear nasal passages; shrinks swollen membranes
- temporarily restores freer breathing through the nose
- helps decongest sinus openings and passages; temporarily relieves sinus congestion and pressure

Warnings:
Ask a doctor before use if you have
- heart disease
- high blood pressure
- thyroid disease
- diabetes
- difficulty in urination due to enlargement of the prostate gland

When using this product
- **do not exceed recommended dosage**
- do not use more than 3 days. Frequent or prolonged use may cause nasal congestion to recur or worsen.
- temporary discomfort may occur such as burning, stinging, sneezing, and an increase in nasal discharge
- use by more than one person may spread infection

Stop use and ask a doctor if symptoms persist for more than 3 days.

If pregnant or breast-feeding, ask a health professional before use.

Keep out of reach of children. If swallowed, get medical help or contact a Poison Control Center right away.

Directions:
- use only as directed
- to spray, squeeze bottle quickly and firmly

adults and children 6 to under 12 years (with adult supervision)	2 to 3 sprays in each nostril not more often than every 10 to 12 hours. Do not exceed 2 doses in 24 hours.
children under 6 years	ask a doctor

Other Information:
- store at room temperature
- protect from light

Inactive Ingredients:
NEO-SYNEPHRINE® 12 Hour Extra Moisturizing Spray: benzalkonium chlo-

ride, dibasic sodium phosphate, edetate disodium, monobasic sodium phosphate, purified water, sodium chloride

How Supplied: Plastic squeeze bottle of 15 ml (½ Fl oz).
USE ONLY IF NECKBAND PRINTED WITH "Bayer" IS INTACT.
Questions or comments? 1-800-331-4536 or www.bayercare.com
Bayer HealthCare LLC
Consumer Care Division
P.O. Box 1910
Morristown, NJ 07962-1910 USA
Shown in Product Identification Guide, page 504

PHILLIPS'® CHEWABLE TABLETS ANTACID-LAXATIVE STIMULANT FREE
Mint Flavor

Drug Facts

Active Ingredient
(in each tablet):   **Purposes:**
Magnesium hydroxide
 311 mg .... Saline laxative/antacid

Uses:
Laxative
• relieves occasional constipation (irregularity)
• this product usually causes bowel movement in ½ to 6 hours
Antacid
• relieves:
 • heartburn
 • acid indigestion
 • sour stomach
 • upset stomach associated with these symptoms

Warnings:
Ask a doctor before use if you have
• kidney disease
• stomach pain, nausea, or vomiting
• a sudden change in bowel habits that lasts over 14 days
Ask a doctor or pharmacist before use if you are taking a prescription drug. Antacids may interact with certain prescription drugs.
When using this product as an antacid, it may have a laxative effect.

Stop use and ask a doctor if
Laxative
• you have rectal bleeding or no bowel movement after using this product. These could be signs of a serious condition.
• you need to use a laxative for more than 1 week
Antacid
• you have taken the maximum dose for 2 weeks
If pregnant or breast-feeding, ask a health professional before use.
Keep out of reach of children. In case of overdose, get medical help or contact a Poison Control Center right away.

Directions:
• do not exceed the maximum recommended daily dose in a 24 hour period [See table below]

Other Information:
• each tablet contains: sodium 1 mg
• store at room temperature

Inactive Ingredients: colloidal silicon dioxide, corn starch, dextrates, flavor, magnesium stearate, maltodextrin, sucrose
Questions? call **1-800-331-4536** or www.bayercare.com

How Supplied: Bottles of 100 Tablets and 200 Tablets
Bayer HealthCare LLC

PHILLIP'S® LIQUI-GELS®

Active Ingredient
(in each softgel):   **Purpose:**
Docusate sodium
 100 mg .... Stool softener laxative

Uses:
• for the relief of occasional constipation (irregularity)
• this product generally produces a bowel movement in 12 to 72 hours

Phillips' Liqui-Gels are a very low sodium product. Each softgel contains 5 mg of sodium.

Warnings:
Ask a doctor before use if you have
• stomach pain, nausea or vomiting
• a sudden change in bowel habits that lasts over 14 days

Laxative		Antacid	
• dose may be taken once in a 24 hour period preferably at bedtime, in divided doses, or as directed by a doctor • drink a full glass (8 oz) of liquid with each laxative dose		• take every 4 hours up to 4 times in a 24 hour period or as directed by a doctor	
adults and children 12 years and older	chew 8 tablets	adults and children 12 years and older	chew 2 to 4 tablets
children 6 to 11 years	chew 4 tablets	children under 12 years	ask a doctor
children 3 to 5 years	chew 2 tablets		
children under 3 years	ask a doctor		

Ask a doctor or pharmacist before use if you are presently taking mineral oil.
Stop use and ask a doctor if
• you have rectal bleeding or no bowel movement after using this product. These could be signs of a serious condition.
• you need to use a laxative for more than 1 week
If pregnant or breast-feeding, ask a health professional before use.
Keep out of reach of children. In case or overdose, get medical help or contact a Poison Control Center right away.

Directions:
• take softgels with a full glass (8 oz) of water

adults and children 12 years and older	take 1 to 3 softgels daily or as directed by a doctor. This dose may be taken as a single daily dose or in divided doses.
children 6 to under 12 years	take 1 softgel daily or as directed by a doctor
children under 6 years of age	ask a doctor

Other Information:
• store at room temperature
• avoid excessive heat 104°F (40°C)
Inactive Ingredients: FD&C blue #2 lake, gelatin, glycerin, methylparaben, polyethylene glycol, propylene glycol, propylparaben, shellac, sorbitol, titanium dioxide
Questions? 1-800-331-4536 or www.bayercare.com
Bayer HealthCare
Consumer Care Division
P.O. Box 1910
Morristown, NJ 07962-1910
USA

How Supplied: Blister packs of 10, 30 & 50 Liqui-Gels.

Liqui-Gels is a registered trademark of R.P. Scherer Corp.
Bayer HealthCare LLC
Shown in Product Identification Guide, page 505

PHILLIPS'® MILK OF MAGNESIA
Original Formula
Cherry Formula
Mint Formula

Active Ingredient
(in each 5 mL tsp):   **Purposes:**
Magnesium hydroxide
 400 mg .... Saline laxative
Uses:
Laxative • relieves occasional constipation (irregularity)
 • this product usually causes bowel movement in ½ to 6 hours

Continued on next page

Phillips' MoM—Cont.

Warnings:
Ask a doctor before use if you have
• kidney disease • stomach pain, nausea, or vomiting
• a sudden change in bowel habits that lasts over 14 days
Ask a doctor or pharmacist before use if you are taking a prescription drug. This product may interact with certain prescription drugs.
Stop use and ask a doctor if
• you have rectal bleeding or no bowel movement after using this product. These could be signs of a serious condition.
• you need to use a laxative for more than 1 week
If pregnant or breast-feeding, ask a health professional before use.
Keep out of reach of children. In case of overdose, get medical help or contact a Poison Control Center right away.

Directions: • do not exceed the maximum recommended daily dose in a 24 hour period
• shake well before use
• dose may be taken once a day preferably at bedtime, in divided doses, or as directed by a doctor. Drink a full glass (8 oz) of liquid with each laxative dose.

adults and children 12 years and older	2 to 4 tablespoonsful
children 6 to 11 years	1 to 2 tablespoonsful
children under 6 years	ask a doctor

Other Information:
• **each teaspoon (5 mL) contains:** sodium 2 mg
• store at room temperature and avoid freezing • keep tightly closed

Inactive Ingredients:
Phillips' Milk of Magnesia Original Flavor
purified water, sodium hypochlorite
Phillips' Milk of Magnesia Cherry Flavor
carboxymethylcellulose sodium, citric acid, D&C red #28, flavor, glycerin, microcrystalline cellulose, purified water, sodium citrate, sodium hypochlorite, sucrose, xanthan gum
Phillips' Milk of Magnesia Fresh Mint
flavor, mineral oil, purified water, sodium hypochlorite, sodium saccharin

How Supplied:
Original, Fresh Mint and Wild Cherry are available in 4 fl. oz., 12 fl. oz. and 26 fl. oz. bottle. French Vanilla is available in a 12 fl. oz. bottle.
Questions:
1-800-331-4536 or www.bayercare.com
Bayer HealthCare LLC
Consumer Care Division
P.O. Box 1910
Morristown, NJ 07962-1910
USA

Shown in Product Identification Guide, page 505

PHILLIPS' MO
Lubricant Laxative
Original Formula
Refreshing Mint Formula

Active Ingredients:
(in each 5 mL tsp)   **Purpose:**
Magnesium hydroxide
300 mg .... Saline laxative
Mineral oil
1.25 mL .... Lubricant laxative

Uses:
• relieves occasional constipation (irregularity)
• this product usually causes bowel movement in ½ to 6 hours

Warnings:
Do not use
• in children under 6 years, or if pregnant, bedridden, or have difficulty swallowing
• if you are presently taking a stool softener laxative
Ask a doctor before use if you have
• kidney disease
• stomach pain, nausea, or vomiting
• a sudden change in bowel habits that lasts over 14 days
Ask a doctor or pharmacist before use if you are taking a prescription drug. This product may interact with certain prescription drugs.
When using this product
• take only at bedtime. Do not use at any other time or administer to infants, except upon the advice of a physician.
• do not take with meals
Stop use and ask a doctor if
• you have rectal bleeding or no bowel movement after using this product. These could be signs of a serious condition.
• you need to use a laxative for more than 1 week
If breast-feeding, ask a health professional before use.
Keep out of reach of children. In case of overdose, get medical help or contact a Poison Control Center right away.

Directions:
• shake well before use
• drink a full glass (8 oz) of liquid with each dose
• do not use dosage cup for children
• dose may be taken as a single dose, or in divided doses, or as directed by a doctor
• do not exceed the maximum recommended daily dose in a 24 hour period

adults and children 12 years and older	3 to 4 tablespoonsful
children 6 to 11 years	4 to 6 teaspoonsful
children under 6 years	ask a doctor

Other Information: • **each teaspoon (5 mL) contains:** sodium 3 mg • store at room temperature and avoid freezing • keep tightly closed

Inactive Ingredients:
Phillips' MO Original
purified water, sodium citrate, sodium hypochlorite

Phillips' MO Mint Flavor
carboxymethylcellulose sodium, flavor, glycerin, microcrystalline cellulose, purified water, saccharin sodium, sodium citrate, sodium hypochlorite

How Supplied:
Original Flavor available in 12 fl. oz. bottle
Mint Flavor available in 12 and 26 fl. oz. bottles
Questions?   1-800-331-4536   or
www.bayercare.com
Bayer HealthCare LLC
Consumer Care Division
P.O. Box 1910
Morristown, NJ 07962-1910
USA

Shown in Product Identification Guide, page 505

RID®
LICE KILLING SHAMPOO
LICE TREATMENT
MAXIMUM STRENGTH
SHAMPOO & CONDITIONER IN ONE

• Kills lice and eggs
• Leaves no chemical residue
• Use on **DRY** hair
• Includes patented comb

Active Ingredients: **Purpose:**
Piperonyl butoxide
(4%) .... Lice treatment
Pyrethrum extract (equivalent to 0.33% pyrethrins) .... Lice treatment

Uses: treats head, pubic (crab), and body lice

Warnings:
For external use only
Do not use near the eyes or permit contact with mucous membranes, such as inside of the nose, mouth, or vagina. Irritation may occur.
Ask a doctor before use if you have an allergy to ragweed.
When using this product:
• keep out of eyes when rinsing hair
• close eyes tightly and do not open eyes until product is rinsed out
• protect eyes with washcloth, towel, or other suitable method
• if product gets into the eyes, immediately flush with water
Stop use and ask a doctor if:
• skin irritation or infection is present or develops
• infestation of eyebrows or eyelashes occurs
Keep out of reach of children. If swallowed, get medical help or contact a Poison Control Center right away.

Directions:
• **important: Read warnings and complete directions in the Consumer Information Insert before using.**
• apply to **DRY HAIR** only. Massage until hair and scalp are thoroughly wet with product (see insert)
• after completing application, allow product to remain on hair for 10 minutes but no longer.
• add sufficient warm water to form a lather and shampoo as usual. Rinse thoroughly.

- a fine-toothed comb or a special lice/nit removing comb (included) must be used to help remove dead lice, eggs, and nits from hair.
- **a second treatment must be done in 10 days to kill any newly hatched lice.**

Other Information:
- it is important to wash in hot water (130°F) all clothing, bedding, towels, and hair products (combs, brushes) used by infested persons.
- dry clean non-washable fabrics.
- to eliminate infestation of furniture and bedding that cannot be washed or dry cleaned, a multi-use lice spray may be used.

Inactive Ingredients: ammonium laureth sulfate, fragrance, PEG-25 hydrogenated castor oil, polyquaternium-10, purified water, SD alcohol

RID® Lice Killing Shampoo will kill lice completely without leaving a chemical residue. To help prevent reinfestation, use it twice (Day 1 and Day 10). Amount of shampoo needed will vary by hair length. See below for guidelines:

Hair Length	Approximate Dosage for 1 Adult/Child:
Short (ear length or shorter)	Day 1: 1 oz - 2 oz Day 10: 1 oz - 2 oz **Total: 2 oz - 4 oz**
Medium (shoulder length)	Day 1: 2 oz - 3 oz Day 10: 2 oz - 3 oz **Total: 4 oz - 6 oz**
Long (past shoulder length)	Day 1: 3 oz - 4 oz Day 10: 3 oz - 4 oz **Total: 6 oz - 8 oz**

The patented RID® comb is proven 100% effective as demonstrated in laboratory studies performed by trained testers. Individual results may vary.

RID® 1-2-3 LICE Elimination System
Completely eliminate lice from your family and home.
Step 1—Kill Lice
- apply RID® **Lice Killing Shampoo** according to label directions.
- repeat this step 10 days later to help prevent reinfestation.
Step 2—Comb-Out Eggs & Nits
- after Step 1, apply RID® **Egg & Nit Comb-Out Gel** on damp hair to make removal faster and easier. *(Purchase separately)*
- comb out the eggs and nits in the hair with a fine-toothed comb or with the RID® patented comb (included).
Step 3—Clean Home
- use RID® **Home Lice Control Spray** to kill lice and their eggs on mattresses, furniture, car interiors, and other non-washable items. *(Purchase separately)*
- wash bed linens, clothing, and other items in hot water and dry in high heat.

How Supplied: 6 FL OZ (177 ml), 1 Comb.

Questions or comments?
1-800-RID-LICE (1-800-743-5423) or www.ridlice.com

Distributed by: Bayer HealthCare LLC
Consumer Care Division
P.O. Box 1910
Morristown, NJ 07962-1910 USA
Shown in Product Identification Guide, page 505

RID® MOUSSE
MAXIMUM STRENGTH
LICE KILLING NO-DRIP MOUSSE
pyrethrum extract*/piperonyl butoxide aerosolized foam   Lice Treatment

- Kills lice
- Use on **DRY** hair
- Includes patented comb

Active Ingredients: (calculated without propellant)	Purpose:
Piperonyl butoxide (4%)	Lice treatment
Pyrethrum extract* (equivalent to 0.33% pyrethrins)	Lice treatment

Uses: treats head, pubic (crab), and body lice

Warnings:
For external use only
Flammable: Keep away from fire or flame
Do not use near the eyes or permit contact with the inside of the nose, mouth, or vagina. Irritation may occur.
Ask a doctor before use if you have an allergy to ragweed
When using this product:
- keep out of eyes when rinsing hair
- close eyes tightly and do not open eyes until product is rinsed out of hair
- protect eyes with washcloth, towel, or other suitable method
- if product gets into the eyes, immediately flush with water
- do not inhale; use in a well ventilated area
- do not puncture or incinerate. Contents under pressure.
Stop use and ask a doctor if:
- skin irritation or infection is present or develops
- infestation of eyebrows or eyelashes occurs
Keep out of reach of children. If swallowed, get medical help or contact a Poison Control Center right away.

Directions:
- **important: Read warnings and complete directions in the Consumer Information Insert before using.**
- shake well before using.
- holding the can upside down, apply RID® No-Drip Mousse to **DRY HAIR** or other affected area. Massage until hair and scalp are thoroughly wet with product.
- after completing application, allow product to remain on the hair for 10 minutes but no longer.
- rinse thoroughly with warm water and wash hair with soap or regular shampoo.
- a fine-toothed comb or a special lice/nit removing comb (included) must be used to help remove dead lice or their eggs (nits) from hair.
- a second treatment must be done in 7 to 10 days to kill any newly hatched lice.

Other Information:
- it is important to wash in hot water (130°F) all clothing, bedding, towels, and hair products (combs, brushes) used by infested persons.
- dry clean non-washable fabrics.
- to eliminate infestation of furniture and bedding that cannot be washed or dry cleaned, a multi use lice spray may be used.
- store at 20°–25°C (68°–77°F).
- do not store at temperature above 43°C (110°F).
- keep in a cool place out of the sun.

Inactive Ingredients: cetearyl alcohol, isobutane, PEG-20 stearate, propane, propylene glycol, purified water, quaternium-52, SD Alcohol 3-C (26.5% w/w)

Questions or comments? 1-800-RID-LICE (1-800-743-5423) or www.ridlice.com
To help prevent reinfestation, use it **twice** (Day 1 and Day 10)†.

---

†While you must apply the 2nd application within 7–10 days of the 1st treatment, it is strongly recommended to wait until Day 10 for maximum effectiveness. The patented RID® comb is proven 100% effective as demonstrated in laboratory studies performed by trained testers. Individual results may vary.

How Supplied: 5.5 oz (156 g), 1 Comb.

*50% extract (not USP)
Distributed by:
Bayer HealthCare LLC
P.O. Box 1910
Morristown, NJ 07962-1910 USA

VANQUISH®
Extra Strength Pain Reliever
Analgesic Caplets

Active Ingredients: (in each caplet)	Purpose:
Acetaminophen 194 mg	Pain reliever
Aspirin 227 mg	Pain reliever
Caffeine 33 mg	Pain reliever aid

Uses: Temporarily relieves minor pain due to
- headache
- backache
- menstrual cramps
- arthritis
- colds and flu
- muscle aches

Warnings: Reye's syndrome: Children and teenagers should not use this medicine for chicken pox or flu symptoms before a doctor is consulted about Reye's syndrome, a rare but serious illness reported to be associated with aspirin.

Alcohol warning: If you consume 3 or more alcoholic drinks every day, ask your doctor whether you should take acetaminophen and aspirin or other pain relievers/fever reducers. Acetaminophen and aspirin may cause liver damage and stomach bleeding.

Continued on next page

Vanquish—Cont.

Do not use
- if you have had an allergic reaction to any other pain reliever/fever reducer
- with any other product containing acetaminophen

Ask a doctor before use if you have
- stomach problems (such as heartburn, upset stomach or stomach pain) that last or come back
- bleeding problems
- ulcers
- asthma

Ask a doctor or pharmacist before use if you are taking a prescription drug for
- anticoagulation (blood thinning)
- gout
- diabetes
- arthritis

Stop use and ask doctor if
- an allergic reaction occurs. Seek medical help right away.
- pain gets worse or lasts more than 10 days
- redness or swelling is present
- new symptoms occur
- ringing in the ears or loss of hearing occurs

If pregnant or breast-feeding, ask a health professional before use. It is especially important not to use aspirin during the last 3 months of pregnancy unless definitely directed to do so by a doctor because it may cause problems in the unborn child or complications during delivery.

Keep out of reach of children.

Overdose warning: Taking more than the recommended dose can cause serious health problems. In case of overdose, get medical help or contact a Poison Control Center right away. Prompt medical attention is critical for adults as well as children even if you do not notice any signs or symptoms.

Directions
- adults and children 12 years and over: take 2 caplets with water every 6 hours, not to exceed 8 caplets in 24 hours unless directed by a doctor
- children under 12 years: consult a doctor

Other Information
- save carton for full directions and warnings
- store at room temperature
- buffered with aluminum hydroxide and magnesium hydroxide

Inactive Ingredients: Aluminum hydroxide, colloidal silicon dioxide, hypromellose, magnesium hydroxide, microcrystalline cellulose, propylene glycol, starch, titanium dioxide, zinc stearate

How Supplied: Bottle of 100 analgesic caplets.

USE ONLY IF SEAL UNDER BOTTLE CAP WITH GREEN "Bayer Corporation" PRINT IS INTACT.

Questions or comments?
1-800-331-4536 or www.bayeraspirin.com
Distributed by:
Bayer HealthCare LLC
PO Box 1910
Morristown, NJ 07962-1910

Beutlich LP Pharmaceuticals
1541 SHIELDS DRIVE
WAUKEGAN, IL 60085-8304

Direct Inquiries to:
847-473-1100
800-238-8542 in US & Canada
FAX 847–473-1122
www.beutlich.com
e-mail beutlich@beutlich.com

CEO–TWO® Evacuant Laxative Adult Rectal Suppository

NDC #0283-0763-09

Composition: Each suppository contains sodium bicarbonate and potassium bitartrate in a special blend of water-soluble polyethylene glycols.

Indications: For relief of occasional constipation, irregularity or for bowel training programs. CEO-TWO generally produces a bowel movement in 5–30 minutes. The lubrication provided by the emollient base combined with the gentle pressure of the released carbon dioxide slowly distends the rectal ampulla stimulating peristalsis. CEO-TWO does not interfere with normal digestion, is not habit forming, won't cause cramping or irritation or alter the normal peristaltic reflex, and it leaves no residue.

Administration and Dosage: Adults and children over 12 years of age. Rectal dosage is one suppository containing 0.6 gram of sodium bicarbonate and 0.9 gram potassium bitartrate in a single daily dose. For children under 12 years of age: consult a doctor. For most effective results and ease of insertion, moisten a CEO-TWO suppository by placing it under a warm water tap for 30 seconds or in a cup of water for 10 seconds before insertion. Insert rectally past the largest diameter of the suppository. Patient should retain in the rectum as long as possible (usually about 5–30 minutes).

Warnings: For rectal use only. Do not use this product if you are on a low salt diet unless directed by a doctor. (172 milligrams of sodium per suppository) Do not lubricate with mineral oil or petrolatum prior to use. Do not use when abdominal pain, nausea or vomiting are present unless directed by a doctor. Laxative products should not be used for longer than one week unless directed by a doctor. If you have noticed a sudden change of bowel habits that persists over a period of 2 weeks, consult a doctor before using a laxative. Rectal bleeding or failure to have a bowel movement after use of a laxative may indicate a serious problem. Discontinue use and consult your doctor.

How Supplied: In box of 10 individually foil wrapped white opaque suppositories. Keep in cool dry place. DO NOT REFRIGERATE

HURRICAINE® TOPICAL ANESTHETIC

Composition: HURRICAINE contains 20% benzocaine in a flavored, water soluble polyethylene glycol base.

Action and Indications: HURRICAINE is a topical anesthetic that provides rapid anesthesia on all accessible mucous membrane in 15 to 30 seconds, short duration of 15 minutes, has virtually no systemic absorption, and tastes good. Hurricaine is used as a lubricant and topical anesthetic to facilitate passage of fiberoptic gastroscopes, laryngoscopes, proctoscopes and sigmoidoscopes. In addition, Hurricaine is effective in suppressing the pharyngeal and tracheal gag reflex during the placement of nasogastric tubes. Hurricaine is used to control pain and discomfort during certain gynecological procedures such as IUD insertion, vaginal speculum placement, and as a preinjection anesthesia prior to LEEP procedures and paracervical blocks. Hurricaine is also effective for the temporary relief of pain due to sore throat, stomatitis and mucositis. It is also effective in controlling various types of pain associated with dental procedures and the temporary relief of minor mouth irritations, canker sores and irritation to the mouth and gums caused by dentures or orthodontic appliances.

Contraindications: Patients with a known hypersensitivity to benzocaine should not use HURRICAINE. True allergic reactions are rare.

Adverse Reactions: Methemoglobinemia has been reported following the use of benzocaine on extremely rare occasions. Intravenous methylene blue is the specific therapy for this condition.

**Cautions: DO NOT USE IN THE EYES.
NOT FOR INJECTION.
KEEP THIS AND ALL DRUGS OUT OF THE REACH OF CHILDREN.**

Packaging Available
GEL
1 oz. Jar Fresh Mint NDC #0283-0998-31
1 oz. Jar Wild Cherry NDC #0283-0871-31
1 oz. Jar Pina Colada NDC #0283-0886-31
1 oz. Jar Watermelon NDC #0283-0293-31
1/6 oz. Tube Wild Cherry NDC #0283-0871-75
LIQUID
1 fl. oz. Jar Wild Cherry NDC #0283-0569-31
1 fl. oz. Jar Pina Colada NDC #0283-1886-31

.25 ml Dry Handle Swab Wild Cherry 100 Each Per Box NDC #0283-0569-01
.25 ml Dry Handle Swab Wild Cherry 6 Each Per Travel Pack NDC #0283-0569-36

SPRAY
2 oz. Aerosol Wild Cherry NDC #0283-0679-02

SPRAY KIT
2 oz. Aerosol Wild Cherry NDC #0283-0679-60 with 200 Disposable Extension Tubes

---

Boehringer Ingelheim Consumer Healthcare Products Division of Boehringer Ingelheim Pharmceuticals Inc.

900 RIDGEBURY ROAD
P.O. BOX 368
RIDGEFIELD, CT 06877

For Direct Inquiries Contact:
1-888-285-9159

DULCOLAX® Bowel Cleansing Kit
For use in Colonoscopy Preparation and Bowel Cleansing Procedures

Drug Facts:

Active Ingredient:	Purpose:
Bisacodyl USP 5 mg (in each tablet)	Laxative
Bisacodyl USP 10 mg (in each suppository)	Laxative
Magnesium Citrate, 17.45 g per dose	Laxative

Uses: For use as part of a bowel cleansing regimen in preparing patients for surgery or for preparing the colon for x-ray or endoscopic examination.

Warnings:
Do note use:
- Unless directed by a doctor.
- If you cannot swallow tablets without chewing.
- In children under 6 years of age.
- Within one hour after taking an antacid or milk.
- If you are on a low salt diet.

Ask a doctor or pharmacist before use if you have:
- Kidney disease.
- Abdominal pain, nausea or vomiting.
- Noticed sudden change in bowel habits that persists over a period of 2 weeks.
- Already used a laxative for a period longer than 1 week.

When using this product:
- Do not chew or crush tablets.
- You may have stomach discomfort, faintness, rectal burning or cramps.

Stop use and ask a doctor if:
- You have rectal bleeding or failure to have a bowel movement after use. These could be signs of a serious condition.

If pregnant or breast-feeding, ask a doctor before use.

Keep out of reach of children. In case of overdose, get medical help or contact a Poison Control Center right away.

Directions:
- Read the entire label and enclosed directions at least 24 hours in advance of examination.
- Follow each step and complete all instructions or the entire x-ray or the endoscopic examination may have to be repeated.
- Use as directed by your doctor.

Other Information:
- Store at controlled room temperature 20–25°C (68–77°F). Avoid excessive humidity.
- Sodium content of liquid 500 mg per dose.

Inactive Ingredients: Tablets: Acacia, acetylated monoglyceride, carnauba wax, cellulose acetate phthalate, corn starch, dibutyl phthalate, docusate sodium, gelatin, glycerin, iron oxides, kaolin, lactose, magnesium stearate, methylparaben, pharmaceutical glaze, polyethylene glycol, povidone, propylparaben, Red No. 30 lake, sodium benzoate, sorbitan monooleate, sucrose, talc, titanium dioxide, white wax, Yellow No. 10 lake.

Oral Solution: Citric acid, lemon oil, polyethylene glycol, sodium bicarbonate, sodium saccharin, sucrose, water purified.

Suppository: Hydrogenated vegetable oil.

How Supplied:
4 Dulcolax 5 mg Tablets
1 Dulcolax 10 mg Suppository
1 Dulcolax 10oz Magnesium Citrate Oral Solution
1 Instruction Manual

Questions about Dulcolax?
Call toll-free 1-888-285-9159.
Distributed by:
Boehringer Ingelheim Consumer Healthcare Products
Division of Boehringer Ingelheim Pharmaceuticals, Inc.
Ridgefield, CT 06877
©Boehringer Ingelheim Pharmaceuticals, Inc. 2003

Shown in Product Identification Guide, page 505

DULCOLAX® Bowel Prep Kit
brand of bisacodyl USP

Drug Facts

Active Ingredient:	Purpose:
Bisacodyl USP 5 mg (in each tablet)	Laxative
Bisacodyl USP 10 mg (in each suppository)	Laxative

Use: For use as part of a bowel cleansing regimen in preparing patients for surgery or for preparing the colon for x-ray or endoscopic examination.

Warnings:
Do not use:
- unless directed by a doctor.
- if you cannot swallow without chewing.
- in children under 6 years of age.
- within one hour after taking an antacid or milk.

When using this product:
- Do not chew or crush tablets.
- You may have stomach discomfort, faintness, rectal burning or cramps.

If pregnant or breast-feeding, ask a doctor before use. **Keep out of reach of children.** In case of overdose, get medical help or contact a Poison Control Center right away.

Directions:
- Read the entire label and directions at least 24 hours in advance of examination.
- Follow each step and complete all instructions or the entire x-ray or the endoscopic examination may have to be repeated.

Other Information:
- Store at controlled room temperature 20–25°C (68–77°F). Avoid excessive humidity.

Inactive Ingredients:
Tablets
Acacia, acetylated monoglyceride, carnauba wax, cellulose acetate phthalate, corn starch, dibutyl phthalate, docusate sodium, gelatin, glycerin, iron oxides, kaolin, lactose, magnesium stearate, methylparaben, pharmaceutical glaze, polyethylene glycol, povidone, propylparaben, Red No. 30 lake, sodium benzoate, sorbitan monooleate, sucrose, talc, titanium dioxide, white wax, Yellow No. 10 lake.

Suppository
Hydrogenated vegetable oil.

How Supplied: 4 tablets, 5 mg each and 1 suppository, 10 mg
Questions about Dulcolax
Call toll-free 1-888-285-9159
Distributed by:
Boehringer Ingelheim Consumer Healthcare Products
Division of Boehringer Ingelheim Pharmaceuticals, Inc. Ridgefield, CT 06877
©Boehringer Ingelheim Pharmaceuticals, Inc.

Shown in Product Identification Guide, page 505

DULCOLAX®
[dul 'cō-Lax]
brand of bisacodyl USP
Tablets of 5 mg
Laxative

Drug Facts
Active Ingredient:

(in each tablet)	Purpose:
Bisacodyl USP, 5 mg	Laxative

Continued on next page

Dulcolax—Cont.

Uses:
- Relieves occasional constipation and irregularity.
- This product usually causes bowel movement in 6 to 12 hours.

Warnings:

Do not use • If you cannot swallow without chewing.

Ask a doctor before use if you have:
- Stomach pain, nausea or vomiting.
- A sudden change in bowel habits that lasts more than 2 weeks.

When using this product:
- Do not chew or crush tablet.
- Do not use within 1 hour after taking an antacid or milk.
- You may have stomach discomfort, faintness or cramps.

Stop use and ask a doctor if:
- You do not have a bowel movement within 12 hours or if rectal bleeding occurs. These could be signs of a serious condition.
- You need to use a laxative for more than 1 week.

If pregnant or breast-feeding, ask a doctor before use. **Keep out of reach of children.** In case of overdose, get medical help or contact a Poison Control Center right away.

Directions:

Adults and children 12 years and over	Take 1 to 3 tablets (usually 2) daily.
Children 6 to under 12 years	Take 1 tablet daily.
Children under 6 years	Ask a doctor.

Other Information • Store at 20–25°C (68–77°F). Avoid excessive humidity.

Inactive Ingredients: Acacia, acetylated monoglyceride, carnauba wax, cellulose acetate phthalate, corn starch, dibutyl phthalate, docusate sodium, gelatin, glycerin, iron oxides, kaolin, lactose, magnesium stearate, methylparaben, pharmaceutical glaze, polyethylene glycol, povidone, propylparaben, Red No. 30 lake, sodium benzoate, sorbitan monooleate, sucrose, talc, titanium dioxide, white wax, Yellow No. 10 lake.

How Supplied: Boxes of 25 Tablets.
Boehringer Ingelheim Consumer Healthcare Products.
Division of Boehringer Ingelheim Pharmaceuticals, Inc., Ridgefield, CT 06877
Made in Mexico ©Boehringer Ingelheim Pharmaceuticals, Inc. 2002

Questions about DULCOLAX?

Call toll-free 1-888-285-9159

Shown in Product Identification Guide, page 505

DULCOLAX®

[dul' co-lax]
brand of bisacodyl USP
Suppositories of 10 mg
Laxative

Drug Facts:

Active Ingredient:
(in each suppository)   Purpose:
Bisacodyl USP, 10 mg .... Laxative

Uses:
- Relieves occasional constipation and irregularity.
- This product usually causes bowel movement in 15 minutes to 1 hour.

Warnings:

For rectal use only.

Do not use • When abdominal pain, nausea, or vomiting are present.

Ask a doctor before use if you have:
- Stomach pain, nausea or vomiting.
- A sudden change in bowel habits that lasts more than 2 weeks.

When using this product:
You may have abdominal discomfort, faintness, rectal burning and mild cramps.

Stop use and ask a doctor if:
- Rectal bleeding occurs or you fail to have a bowel movement after using a laxative. This may indicate a serious condition.
- You need to use a laxative for more than 1 week.

If pregnant or breast-feeding, ask a doctor before use. **Keep out of reach of children.** If swallowed, get medical help or contact a Poison Control Center right away.

Directions:

Adults and children 12 years and over	1 suppository once daily. Remove foil. Insert suppository well into rectum, pointed end first. Retain about 15 to 20 minutes.
Children 6 to under 12 years	1/2 suppository once daily.
Children under 6 years	Ask a doctor.

Other Information • Store at controlled room temperature 20–25°C (68–77°F)

Inactive Ingredients: Hydrogenated vegetable oil.

How Supplied: Boxes of 4 Comfort Shaped Suppositories
Boehringer Ingelheim Consumer Healthcare Products.
Division of Boehringer Ingelheim Pharmaceuticals, Inc., Ridgefield, CT 06877   Made in Italy.
©Boehringer Ingelheim Pharmaceuticals, Inc. 2002
Questions? 1-888-285-9159

Shown in Product Identification Guide, page 505

DULCOLAX®

Drug Facts:

Active Ingredient:
(in each softgel)   Purpose:
Docusate sodium USP,
100 mg .... Stool Softener

Uses:
- Temporary relief of occasional constipation.
- This product generally produces bowel movement within 12 to 72 hours.

Warnings:

Do not use:
- If abdominal pain, nausea or vomiting are present.

Ask a doctor before use if:
- You have noticed a sudden change in bowel habits that persists over a period of 2 weeks.
- You are presently taking mineral oil.

Stop use and ask a doctor if:
- Rectal bleeding or failure to have a bowel movement occur after use, which may indicate a serious condition.
- You need to use a laxative for more than 1 week.

If pregnant or breast-feeding, ask a health professional before use.

Keep out of reach of children. In case of overdose, get medical help or contact a Poison Control Center immediately.

Directions:

Adults and children 12 years and over.	Take 1 to 3 softgels daily.
Children 2 to under 12 years.	Take 1 softgel daily.
Children under 2 years.	Ask a doctor.

Other Information
- Each softgel contains: sodium, 5 mg
- Store at 15–30°C (59–86°F).
- Protect from excessive moisture.

Inactive Ingredients FD&C Red #40, FD&C Yellow #6, gelatin, glycerin, polyethylene glycol, propylene glycol, purified water and sorbitol special.

How Supplied: Blister Pack of 10, and bottles of 25, 50, or 100 liquid gels.
Boehringer Ingelheim Consumer Healthcare Products.
Division of Boehringer Ingelheim Pharmaceuticals, Inc., Ridgefield, CT 06877
©Boehringer Ingelheim Pharmaceuticals, Inc. 2002

Questions about DULCOLAX?

Call toll-free 1-888-285-9159

*Among Stool Softener ingredients

Shown in Product Identification Guide, page 505

DULCOLAX® MILK OF MAGNESIA
Laxative & Antacid:
Original Flavor & Mint Flavor

Drug Facts:

Active Ingredient: **Purpose:**
Magnesium hydroxide – 400mg
per teaspoon (5mL) .... Laxative
& Antacid

Uses: As a Laxative: to relieve occasional constipation (irregularity). This saline laxative product generally produces a bowel movement in ½ to 6 hours. As an Antacid: to relieve acid indigestion, sour stomach and heartburn.

Warnings:

Ask a doctor before use if you have:
• Kidney disease • Stomach pain, nausea or vomiting • Noticed a sudden change in bowel habits that lasts more than 2 weeks

Ask a doctor or pharmacist before use if you are presently taking a prescription drug.
Antacids may interact with certain prescription drugs.

When using this product it may have a laxative effect. Do not exceed the maximum recommended daily dosage in a 24-hour period.

Stop use and ask a doctor if:
Laxative
• You have rectal bleeding or failure to have a bowel movement after use. This may indicate a serious condition.
• You need to use a laxative for more than one week.
Antacid
• Symptoms last for more than 2 weeks
If pregnant or breast-feeding, ask a health professional before use.

Keep out of reach of children. In case of overdose, get medical help or contact a Poison Control Center right away.

Directions: Shake well before using.
[See table below]

Other Information:
• Do not freeze. Store at room temperature tightly closed.

Inactive Ingredients:
Original Flavor: purified water
Mint Flavor: flavor, mineral oil, purified water, saccharin sodium

How Supplied:
Original and Mint Flavors in 12 fl. oz. (355mL) and 26 fl. oz. (769mL) bottles

Questions about Dulcolax?
Call toll-free 1-888-285-9159.
Distributed by:
Boehringer Ingelheim Consumer Healthcare Products
Division of Boehringer Ingelheim Pharmaceuticals, Inc.
Ridgefield, CT 06877
©Boehringer Ingelheim Pharmaceuticals, Inc. 2003
Shown in Product Identification Guide, page 505

Bristol-Myers Squibb Company
345 PARK AVENUE
NEW YORK, NY 10154

Direct Inquiries to:
Products Division
Consumer Affairs Department
1350 Liberty Avenue
Hillside, NJ 07205
(800) 468-7746

OVERDOSE PROFESSIONAL INFORMATION FOR EXCEDRIN® PRODUCTS

All of the following listed Excedrin drug products contain acetaminophen. In case of overdose, please read the following Acetylcysteine information:

Overdose Information:
Acetylcysteine As An Antidote For Acetaminophen Overdose
Acetaminophen is rapidly absorbed from the upper gastrointestinal tract with peak plasma levels occurring between 30 and 60 minutes after therapeutic doses and usually within 4 hours following an overdose. The parent compound, which is nontoxic, is extensively metabolized in the liver to form principally the sulfate and glucuronide conjugates which are also nontoxic and are rapidly excreted in the urine. A small fraction of an ingested dose is metabolized in the liver by the cytochrome P-450 mixed function oxidase enzyme system to form a reactive, potentially toxic, intermediate metabolite which preferentially conjugates with hepatic glutathione to form the nontoxic cysteine and mercapturic acid derivatives which are then excreted by the kidney. Therapeutic doses of acetaminophen do not saturate the glucuronide and sulfate conjugation pathways and do not result in the formation of sufficient reactive metabolite to deplete glutathione stores. However, following ingestion of a large overdose (150 mg/kg or greater) the glucuronide and sulfate conjugation pathways are saturated resulting in a larger fraction of the drug being metabolized via the P-450 pathway. The increased formation of reactive metabolite may deplete the hepatic stores of glutathione with subsequent binding of the metabolite to protein molecules within the hepatocyte resulting in cellular necrosis. Acetylcysteine has been shown to reduce the extent of liver injury following acetaminophen overdose.

Early symptoms following a potentially hepatotoxic overdose may include: nausea, vomiting, diaphoresis and general malaise. Clinical and laboratory evidence of hepatic toxicity may not be apparent until 48 to 72 hours postingestion. In most adults and adolescents, regardless of the quantity of acetaminophen reported to have been ingested, administer acetylcysteine immediately. Acetylcysteine therapy should be initiated and continued for a full course of therapy. Its effectiveness depends on early administration, with benefit seen principally in patients treated within 16 hours of the overdose.

If acetaminophen plasma assay capability is not available, and the estimated acetaminophen ingestion exceeds 150 mg/kg, acetylcysteine therapy should be initiated and continued for a full course of therapy.

For full prescribing information, refer to the acetylcysteine package insert. Do not await the results of assays for acetaminophen level before initiating treatment with acetylcysteine. The following additional procedures are recommended: the stomach should be emptied promptly by lavage or by induction of emesis with syrup of ipecac.

A serum acetaminophen assay should be obtained as early as possible, but no sooner than four hours following ingestion. Liver function studies should be obtained initially and repeated at 24-hour intervals.

For additional emergency information call your regional poison center or toll-free (1-800-525-6115) to the Rocky Mountain Poison Center for assistance in diagnosis and for directions in the use of acetylcysteine as an antidote.

Aspirin Free
EXCEDRIN® TENSION HEADACHE
[ĕx″ cĕd′ rin]
Pain Reliever

Active Ingredients: Each tablet, caplet or geltab contains Acetaminophen 500 mg (formulated with 65 mg caffeine).

Age	Laxative use: Do not use dosage cup for ages under 12 years. Follow each dose with a full glass (8oz) of liquid.	Antacid use: Do not use dosage cup. Follow each dose with a little water.
adults and children 12 years and older	2 – 4 tablespoonfuls (30 – 60 mL) once a day	1 – 3 teaspoonfuls (5 – 15 mL) up to 4 times a day
6 to 11 years	1 – 2 tablespoonfuls (15 – 30 mL) once a day	ask a doctor
2 to 5 years	1 – 3 teaspoonfuls (5 – 15 mL) once a day	ask a doctor
Under 2 years	ask a doctor	ask a doctor

Continued on next page

Excedrin Aspirin Free—Cont.

Inactive Ingredients: (tablet, caplet) benzoic acid, carnauba wax, corn starch, croscarmellose sodium, D&C red #27 lake, D&C yellow #10 lake, FD&C blue #1 lake, FD&C red #40, hypromellose, magnesium stearate, methylparaben*, microcrystalline cellulose, mineral oil, polysorbate 20, povidone, propylene glycol, propylparaben*, simethicone emulsion, sorbitan monolaurate, stearic acid, titanium dioxide

_____

*may contain these ingredients

Inactive Ingredients: (geltab) benzoic acid, corn starch, croscarmellose sodium, FD&C blue #1, FD&C red #40, FD&C yellow #6, gelatin, glycerin, hypromellose, magnesium stearate, methylparaben*, microcrystalline cellulose, mineral oil, polysorbate 20, povidone, propylene glycol, propylparaben*, simethicone emulsion, sorbitan monolaurate, stearic acid, titanium dioxide

_____

*may contain these ingredients

Uses:
• temporarily relieves minor aches and pains due to:
　• headache • muscular aches

Warnings:

Alcohol warning: If you consume 3 or more alcoholic drinks every day, ask your doctor whether you should take acetaminophen or other pain relievers/fever reducers. Acetaminophen may cause liver damage.

Caffeine warning: The recommended dose of this product contains about as much caffeine as a cup of coffee. Limit the use of caffeine-containing medications, foods, or beverages while taking this product because too much caffeine may cause nervousness, irritability, sleeplessness, and, occasionally, rapid heart beat.

Do not use • with any other products containing acetaminophen. Taking more than directed may cause liver damage.

Stop use and ask a doctor if
• new symptoms occur
• symptoms do not get better or worsen
• painful area is red or swollen
• pain gets worse or lasts for more than 10 days
• fever gets worse or lasts for more than 3 days

If pregnant or breast-feeding, ask a health professional before use.

Keep out of reach of children.

Overdose warning: Taking more than the recommended dose can cause serious health problems. In case of overdose, get medical help or contact a Poison Control Center right away. Quick medical attention is critical for adults as well as for children even if you do not notice any signs or symptoms.

Directions:
• do not use more than directed (see overdose warning)
• adults and children 12 years of age and over: take 2 (tablets, caplets or geltabs) every 6 hours; not more than 8 (tablets, caplets or geltabs) in 24 hours
• children under 12 years of age: ask a doctor

Overdose: Acetylcysteine as an antidote for acetaminophen overdose. See OVERDOSE PROFESSIONAL INFORMATION FOR EXCEDRIN PRODUCTS section at the beginning of the Bristol-Myers Squibb Co. listing.

How Supplied: EXCEDRIN® Tension Headache is supplied as: Coated red tablets and caplets with "ETH" debossed on one side in bottles of 24, 50, 100, and 250. Easy to swallow red geltabs with "Excedrin TH" printed in white on one side supplied in bottles of 24, 50, and 100. Store at room temperature.

Shown in Product Identification Guide, page 506

_____

EXCEDRIN® Extra-Strength Pain Reliever/Pain Reliever Aid
[ĕx "cĕd 'rin]

Active Ingredients: Each tablet, caplet, or geltab contains Acetaminophen 250 mg, Aspirin 250 mg, and Caffeine 65 mg.

Inactive Ingredients: (tablet, caplet) benzoic acid, carnauba wax, FD&C blue #1*, hydroxypropylcellulose, hypromellose, microcrystalline cellulose, mineral oil, polysorbate 20, povidone, propylene glycol, simethicone emulsion, sorbitan monolaurate, stearic acid, titanium dioxide*

_____

*may contain these ingredients

Inactive Ingredients: (geltab) benzoic acid, D&C yellow #10 lake, disodium EDTA, FD&C blue #1 lake, FD&C red #40 lake, ferric oxide, gelatin, glycerin, hydroxypropylcellulose, hypromellose, maltitol solution, microcrystalline cellulose, mineral oil, pepsin, polysorbate 20, povidone, propylene glycol, propyl gallate, simethicone emulsion, sorbitan monolaurate, stearic acid, titanium dioxide

Uses: Temporarily relieves minor aches and pains due to: • headache • a cold • arthritis • muscular aches • sinusitis • toothache • premenstrual & menstrual cramps

Warnings:

Reye's syndrome: Children and teenagers who have or are recovering from chicken pox or flu-like symptoms should not use this product. When using this product, if changes in behavior with nausea and vomiting occur, consult a doctor because these symptoms could be an early sign of Reye's syndrome, a rare but serious illness.

Allergy alert: Aspirin may cause a severe allergic reaction which may include:
• hives • facial swelling • asthma (wheezing) • shock

Alcohol Warning: If you consume 3 or more alcoholic drinks every day, ask your doctor whether you should take acetaminophen and aspirin or other pain relievers/fever reducers. Acetaminophen and aspirin may cause liver damage and stomach bleeding.

Caffeine warning: The recommended dose of this product contains about as much caffeine as a cup of coffee. Limit the use of caffeine-containing medications, foods, or beverages while taking this product because too much caffeine may cause nervousness, irritability, sleeplessness, and, occasionally, rapid heart beat.

Do not use
• if you have ever had an allergic reaction to any other pain reliever/fever reducer
• with any other products containing acetaminophen. Taking more than directed may cause liver damage.

Ask a doctor before use if you have
• asthma
• ulcers
• bleeding problems
• stomach problems such as heartburn, upset stomach, or stomach pain that do not go away or return

Ask a doctor or pharmacist before use if you are taking a prescription drug for:
• anticoagulation (thinning of the blood)
• diabetes
• gout
• arthritis

Stop use and ask a doctor if
• an allergic reaction occurs. Seek medical help right away.
• new symptoms occur
• symptoms do not get better or worsen
• ringing in the ears or loss of hearing occurs
• painful area is red or swollen
• pain gets worse or lasts for more than 10 days
• fever gets worse or lasts for more than 3 days

If pregnant or breast-feeding, ask a health professional before use. It is especially important not to use aspirin during the last 3 months of pregnancy unless definitely directed to do so by a doctor because it may cause problems in the unborn child or complications during delivery.

Keep out of reach of children.

Overdose warning: Taking more than the recommended dose can cause serious health problems. In case of overdose, get medical help or contact a Poison Control Center right away. Quick medical attention is critical for adults as well as for children even if you do not notice any signs or symptoms.

Directions:
• do not use more than directed (see overdose warning) • drink a full glass of water with each dose • adults and children 12 years and over: take 2 (tablets, caplets or geltabs) every 6 hours; not more than 8 (tablets, caplets, or geltabs) in 24 hours • children under 12 years: ask a doctor.

Overdose: Acetylcysteine as an antidote for acetaminophen overdose. See OVERDOSE PROFESSIONAL INFORMATION FOR COMTREX AND

EXCEDRIN PRODUCTS section at the beginning of the Bristol-Myers Products listing.

How Supplied: Excedrin Extra Strength is supplied as:

Coated white circular tablet with letter "E" debossed on one side. Supplied in bottles of 24, 50, 100, 250. Tablets also available in vials of 10 tablets.

Coated white caplets with "E" debossed on one side. Supplied in bottles of 24, 50, 100, 175, 275.

Gel-coated round geltabs–green on one side, white on the other, printed with black "E" on one side. Supplied in bottles of 24, 50, 100 (2 bottles of 50 each).

Store at room temperature.

Shown in Product Identification Guide, page 506

EXCEDRIN® MIGRAINE

[ĕx" cĕd' rin]

Pain Reliever/Pain Reliever Aid

Active Ingredients: Each tablet, caplet or geltab contains Acetaminophen 250 mg, Aspirin 250 mg and Caffeine 65 mg.

Inactive Ingredients: (tablet and caplet) benzoic acid, carnauba wax, FD&C blue #1* hydroxypropylcellulose, hypromellose, microcrystalline cellulose, mineral oil, polysorbate 20, povidone, propylene glycol, simethicone emulsion, sorbitan monolaurate, stearic acid, titanium dioxide.*

---

*may contain these ingredients

Inactive Ingredients: (geltab) benzoic acid, D&C yellow #10 lake, disodium EDTA, FD&C blue #1 lake, FD&C red #40 lake, ferric oxide, gelatin, glycerin, hydroxypropylcellulose, hypromellose, maltitol solution, microcrystalline cellulose, mineral oil, pepsin, polysorbate 20, povidone, propylene glycol, propyl gallate, simethicone emulsion, sorbitan monolaurate, stearic acid, titanium dioxide.

Use: Treats migraine.

Warnings:

Reye's Syndrome: Children and teenagers who have or are recovering from chicken pox or flu-like symptoms should not use this product. When using this product, if changes in behavior with nausea and vomiting occur, consult a doctor because these symptoms could be an early sign of Reye's syndrome, a rare but serious illness.

Allergy alert: Aspirin may cause a severe allergic reaction which may include: • hives • facial swelling • asthma (wheezing) • shock

Alcohol warning: If you consume 3 or more alcoholic drinks every day, ask your doctor whether you should take acetaminophen and aspirin or other pain relievers/fever reducers. Acetaminophen and aspirin may cause liver damage and stomach bleeding.

Caffeine warning: The recommended dose of this product contains about as much caffeine as a cup of coffee. Limit the use of caffeine-containing medications, foods, or beverages while taking this product because too much caffeine may cause nervousness, irritability, sleeplessness, and, occasionally, rapid heart beat.

Do not use • if you have ever had an allergic reaction to any other pain reliever/fever reducer • with any other products containing acetaminophen. Taking more than directed may cause liver damage.

Ask a doctor before use if you have

- never had migraines diagnosed by a health professional
- a headache that is different from your usual migraines
- the worst headache of your life
- fever and stiff neck
- headaches beginning after or caused by head injury, exertion, coughing or bending
- experienced your first headache after the age of 50
- daily headaches
- asthma
- bleeding problems
- ulcers
- stomach problems such as heartburn, upset stomach, or stomach pain that do not go away or recur
- a migraine so severe as to require bed rest
- problems or serious side effects from taking pain relievers or fever reducers

Ask a doctor or pharmacist before use if you are

taking a prescription drug for:
- anticoagulation (thinning of the blood)
- diabetes
- gout
- arthritis

Stop use and ask a doctor if

- an allergic reaction occurs. Seek medical help right away.
- your migraine is not relieved or worsens after first dose
- new or unexpected symptoms occur
- ringing in the ears or loss of hearing occurs

If pregnant or breast-feeding, ask a health professional before use. It is especially important not to use aspirin during the last 3 months of pregnancy unless definitely directed to do so by a doctor because it may cause problems in the unborn child or complications during delivery.

Keep out of reach of children.

Overdose warning: Taking more than the recommended dose can cause serious health problems. In case of overdose, get medical help or contact a Poison Control Center right away. Quick medical attention is critical for adults as well as for children even if you do not notice any signs or symptoms.

Directions:

- do not use more than directed (see overdose warning)
- adults: take 2 (tablets, caplets or geltabs) with a glass of water
- if symptoms persist or worsen, ask your doctor
- do not take more than 2 (tablets, caplets, or geltabs) in 24 hours, unless directed by a doctor
- under 18 years of age: ask a doctor

Overdose: **Acetylcysteine as an antidote for acetaminophen overdose.** See OVERDOSE PROFESSIONAL INFORMATION FOR COMTREX AND EXCEDRIN PRODUCTS section at the beginning of the Bristol-Myers Products listing.

How Supplied: EXCEDRIN® MIGRAINE is supplied as:

Coated white circular tablets or coated white caplets with letter "E" debossed on one side. Supplied in bottles of 24, 50, 100, and 250. Coated round geltabs–green on one side, white on the other, printed with black "E" on one side. Supplied in bottles of 24, 50, and 100 (2 bottles of 50 each).

Store at 20–25°C (68–77°F).

Shown in Product Identification Guide, page 506

EXCEDRIN PM®

[ĕx "cĕd 'rĭn]

Pain Reliever/Nighttime Sleep-Aid

Active Ingredients: Each tablet, caplet or geltab contains: Acetaminophen 500 mg and Diphenhydramine citrate 38 mg.

Inactive Ingredients: (Tablet and Caplet) benzoic acid, carnauba wax, croscarmellose sodium, D&C yellow #10 lake, FD&C blue #1 lake, hypromellose, magnesium stearate, methylparaben*, microcrystalline cellulose, mineral oil, polysorbate 20, povidone, pregelatinized starch, propylene glycol, propylparaben*, simethicone emulsion, sodium citrate, sorbitan monolaurate, stearic acid, titanium dioxide

---

*may contain these ingredients

(Geltab) benzoic acid, croscarmellose sodium, D&C red #33 lake, edetate disodium, FD&C blue #1, FD&C blue #1 lake, gelatin, glycerin, hypromellose, magnesium stearate, methylparaben*, microcrystalline cellulose, mineral oil, polysorbate 20, povidone, pregelatinized starch, propylene glycol, propylparaben*, simethicone emulsion, sorbitan monolaurate, stearic acid, titanium dioxide

---

*may contain these ingredients

Uses: For temporary relief of occasional headaches and minor aches and pains with accompanying sleeplessness.

Continued on next page

Excedrin P.M.—Cont.

Warnings:

Alcohol warning: If you consume 3 or more alcoholic drinks every day, ask your doctor whether you should take acetaminophen or other pain relievers/fever reducers. Acetaminophen may cause liver damage.

Do not use
• in children under 12 years of age
• with any other product containing diphenhydramine, even one used on skin
• with any other products containing acetaminophen. Taking more than directed may cause liver damage

Ask a doctor before use if you have
• glaucoma
• a breathing problem such as emphysema or chronic bronchitis
• trouble urinating due to an enlarged prostate gland

Ask a doctor or pharmacist before use if you are taking sedatives or tranquilizers

When using this product
• avoid alcoholic drinks
• drowsiness may occur
• be careful when driving a motor vehicle or operating machinery

Stop use and ask a doctor if
• new symptoms occur
• sleeplessness lasts continuously for more than 2 weeks. Insomnia may be a symptom of serious underlying medical illness.
• pain gets worse or lasts for more than 10 days
• painful area is red or swollen
• fever gets worse or lasts for more than 3 days

If pregnant or breast-feeding, ask a health professional before use.

Keep out of reach of children.

Overdose warning: Taking more than the recommended dose can cause serious health problems. In case of overdose, get medical help or contact a Poison Control Center right away. Quick medical attention is critical for adults as well as for children even if you do not notice any signs or symptoms.

Directions:
• do not use more than directed (see overdose warning)
• children under 12 years of age: consult a doctor
• adults and children 12 years and over: take 2 tablets, caplets or geltabs at bedtime, if needed, or as directed by a doctor.

Overdose: Acetylcysteine as an antidote for acetaminophen overdose. See OVERDOSE PROFESSIONAL INFORMATION FOR COMTREX AND EXCEDRIN PRODUCTS section at the beginning of the Bristol-Myers Products listing.

How Supplied: Excedrin PM is available in tablets, caplets and geltab in bottles of 24, 50 and 100. Tablets and caplets are coated light blue and debossed with PM on one side. Geltabs are gel coated light blue and white and imprinted with PM on one side.
Store at room temperature.

Shown in Product Identification Guide, page 506

Cadbury Adams USA LLC

**182 TABOR ROAD
MORRIS PLAINS, NJ 07950**

Direct Inquiries to:
1-(800) 524-2854

For Consumer Product Information Call:
1-(800) 524-2854 .

HALLS FRUIT BREEZERS™
Pectin Throat Drops

Active Ingredient (in each drop):
Pectin 7 mg

Purpose:
Oral Demulcent

Uses: temporarily relieves the following symptoms associated with sore mouth and sore throat:
• minor discomfort
• irritated areas

Warnings:

Sore throat warning: if sore throat is severe, persists for more than 2 days, is accompanied or followed by fever, headache, rash, swelling, nausea, or vomiting, consult a doctor promptly. These may be serious.

Stop use and ask a doctor if
• sore mouth does not improve in 7 days
• irritation, pain, or redness persists or worsens

Keep out of reach of children.

Directions:
• adults and children 5 years and over: dissolve 1 or 2 drops (one at a time) slowly in the mouth. Repeat as needed.
• children under 5 years: ask a doctor

Cool Berry
Inactive Ingredients: FD&C blue no. 2, FD&C red no. 40, flavors, glucose syrup, partially hydrogenated cottonseed oil, sucrose, titanium dioxide, water
Tropical Chill
Inactive Ingredients: beta carotene, FD&C red no. 40, FD&C yellow no. 5 (tartrazine), FD&C yellow no. 6, flavors, glucose syrup, partially hydrogenated cottonseed oil, soy lecithin, sucrose, titanium dioxide, water
Cool Citrus Blend
Inactive Ingredients: beta carotene, flavors, glucose syrup, partially hydrogenated cottonseed oil, soy lecithin, sucrose, titanium dioxide, water
Cool Creamy Orange
Inactive Ingredients: beta carotene, carboxymethylcellulose sodium, FD&C red no. 40, FD&C yellow no. 5 (tartrazine), FD&C yellow no. 6, flavors, glucose syrup, sodium chloride, soy lecithin, sucrose, titanium dioxide, water
Cool Creamy Strawberry
Inactive Ingredients: beta carotene, carboxymethylcellulose sodium, FD&C blue no. 2, FD&C red no. 40, flavors, glucose syrup, sodium chloride, soy lecithin, sucrose, titanium dioxide, water

How Supplied: Halls Fruit Breezers are available in five flavors: Cool Berry, Cool Citrus Blend, Tropical Chill, Cool Creamy Orange and Cool Creamy Strawberry in bags of 25 drops and blisters of 8 (Cool Berry and Tropical Chill).
Shown in Product Identification Guide, page 506

HALLS® MENTHO–LYPTUS®
Cough Suppressant/Oral Anesthetic Drops
[*Hols*]

Active Ingredient: *MENTHO-LYPTUS®:* Menthol 6.5 mg per drop. *CHERRY:* Menthol 7 mg per drop. *HONEY-LEMON:* Menthol 8 mg per drop. *ICE BLUE™ PEPPERMINT:* Menthol 10 mg per drop. *SPEARMINT:* Menthol 5.6 mg per drop. *STRAWBERRY:* Menthol 3.1 mg per drop. *TROPICAL FRUIT:* Menthol 3.1 mg per drop.

Purposes: Cough suppressant, Oral anesthetic

Uses: temporarily relieves: • cough due to a cold • occasional minor irritation or sore throat

Warnings:

Sore throat warning: if sore throat is severe, persists for more than 2 days, is accompanied or followed by fever, headache, rash, swelling, nausea, or vomiting, consult a doctor promptly. These may be serious.

Ask a doctor if you have • persistent or chronic cough such as occurs with smoking, asthma, or emphysema • cough accompanied by excessive phlegm (mucus)

Stop use and ask a doctor if • cough persists for more than 1 week, tends to recur, or is accompanied by fever, rash, or persistent headache. These could be signs of a serious condition. • sore mouth does not improve in 7 days • irritation, pain, or redness persists or worsens

Keep out of reach of children.

Directions: *MENTHO-LYPTUS®, CHERRY, HONEY-LEMON, ICE BLUE™ PEPPERMINT and SPEARMINT:* • adults and children 5 years and over: dissolve 1 drop slowly in the mouth. Repeat every 2 hours as needed. • children under 5 years: ask a doctor.

STRAWBERRY and TROPICAL FRUIT: • adults and children 5 years and over: dissolve 2 drops (one at a time) slowly in the mouth. Repeat every 2 hours as needed. • children under 5 years: ask a doctor

Inactive Ingredients: *MENTHO-LYPTUS®:* flavors, glucose syrup, sucrose, water. *CHERRY:* FD&C blue no. 2, FD&C red no. 40, flavors, glucose syrup, sucrose, water. *HONEY-LEMON:* beta carotene, flavors, glucose syrup, honey, soy lecithin, sucrose, water. *ICE BLUE™ PEPPERMINT:* FD&C blue no. 1, flavors, glucose syrup, sucrose, water. *SPEARMINT:* beta carotene, FD&C blue no. 1, flavors, glucose syrup, soy lecithin, sucrose, water. *STRAWBERRY*: FD&C red no. 40, flavors, glucose syrup, sucrose, water. *TROPICAL FRUIT*: FD&C red no. 40, flavors, glucose syrup, sucrose, water.

How Supplied: Halls® *Mentho-Lyptus®* Cough Suppressant Drops are available in single sticks of 9 drops each and in bags of 30. They are available in seven flavors: *Regular Mentho-Lyptus®, Cherry, Honey-Lemon, Ice Blue™ Peppermint, Spearmint, Strawberry* and *Tropical Fruit.* Regular Mentho-Lyptus®, Cherry, Honey-Lemon, Strawberry flavors are also available in bags of 80 drops. *Mentho-Lyptus®, Cherry,* and *Strawberry* are also available in bags of 200 drops.

Shown in Product Identification Guide, page 506

HALLS® PLUS
Cough Suppressant/Oral Anesthetic Drops
[*Hols*]

Active Ingredients: Each drop contains Menthol 10 mg.
Purposes: Cough suppressant, Oral anesthetic

Uses: temporarily relieves: • cough due to a cold • occasional minor irritation or sore throat

Warnings: Sore throat warning: if sore throat is severe, persists for more than 2 days, is accompanied or followed by fever, headache, rash, swelling, nausea, or vomiting, consult a doctor promptly. These may be serious.
Ask a doctor before use if you have • persistent or chronic cough such as occurs with smoking, asthma, or emphysema • cough accompanied by excessive phlegm (mucus)
Stop use and ask a doctor if • cough persists for more than 1 week, tends to recur, or is accompanied by fever, rash, or persistent headache. These could be signs of a serious condition. • sore mouth does not improve in 7 days • irritation, pain, or redness persists or worsens
Keep out of reach of children.

Directions: • adults and children 5 years and over: dissolve 1 drop slowly in the mouth. Repeat every 2 hours as needed. • children under 5 years: ask a doctor

Inactive Ingredients: MENTHO-LYPTUS®: carrageenan, flavors, glucose syrup, glycerin, partially hydrogenated cottonseed oil, pectin, soy lecithin, sucrose, water. CHERRY: carrageenan, FD&C blue no. 2, FD&C red no. 40, flavors, glucose syrup, glycerin, partially hydrogenated cottonseed oil, pectin, soy lecithin, sucrose, water. HONEY-LEMON: beta carotene, carrageenan, flavors, glucose syrup, glycerin, honey, partially hydrogenated cottonseed oil, pectin, sucrose, water.

How Supplied: Halls® Plus Cough Suppressant / Throat Drops are available in single sticks of 10 drops each and in bags of 25 drops. They are available in three flavors: Regular Mentho-Lyptus®, Cherry and Honey-Lemon.

Shown in Product Identification Guide, page 506

HALLS® SUGAR FREE
HALLS® SUGAR FREE SQUARES
MENTHO-LYPTUS®
Cough Suppressant/Oral Anesthetic Drops
[*Hols*]

Active Ingredient: Halls® Sugar Free: BLACK CHERRY and CITRUS BLEND™: Menthol 5 mg per drop. MOUNTAIN MENTHOL™: Menthol 5.8 mg per drop. HONEY-LEMON: 9.5 mg per drop.
Halls® Sugar Free Squares: BLACK CHERRY: Menthol 5.8 mg per drop. MOUNTAIN MENTHOL™: Menthol 6.8 mg per drop.
Purposes: Cough suppressant, Oral anesthetic

Uses: temporarily relieves: • cough due to a cold • occasional minor irritation or sore throat

Warnings:
Sore throat warning: if sore throat is severe, persists for more than 2 days, is accompanied or followed by fever, headache, rash, swelling, nausea, or vomiting, consult a doctor promptly. These may be serious.
Ask a doctor before use if you have • persistent or chronic cough such as occurs with smoking, asthma, or emphysema • cough accompanied by excessive phlegm (mucus)
Stop use and ask a doctor if • cough persists for more than 1 week, tends to recur, or is accompanied by fever, rash or persistent headache. These could be signs of a serious condition. • sore mouth does not improve in 7 days • irritation, pain, or redness persists or worsens
Keep out of reach of children.

Directions: • adults and children 5 years and over: dissolve 1 drop slowly in mouth. Repeat every 2 hours as needed. • children under 5 years: ask a doctor

Additional Information:
Halls® Sugar Free:
Exchange Information*:
1 Drop = Free Exchange
10 Drops = 1 Fruit
*The dietary exchanges are based on the *Exchange Lists for Meal Planning,* Copyright ©1989 by the American Diabetes Association, Inc. and the American Dietetic Association.
Excess consumption may have a laxative effect.

Inactive Ingredients: Halls Sugar Free BLACK CHERRY: acesulfame potassium, aspartame, carboxymethylcellulose sodium, FD&C blue no. 1, FD&C

red no. 40, flavors, isomalt, water **Phenylketonurics: Contains Phenylalanine 2 mg Per Drop.** CITRUS BLEND™: acesulfame potassium, aspartame, carboxymethylcellulose sodium, flavors, isomalt, yellow 5 (tartrazine), water **Phenylketonurics: Contains Phenylalanine 2 mg Per Drop.** MOUNTAIN MENTHOL™: acesulfame potassium, aspartame, carboxymethylcellulose sodium, flavors, isomalt, water **Phenylketonurics: Contains Phenylalanine 2 mg Per Drop.** HONEY-LEMON: acesulfame potassium, aspartame, beta carotene, carboxymethylcellulose sodium, flavors, isomalt, water **Phenylketonurics: Contains Phenylalanine 2 mg Per Drop.**

How Supplied: Halls® Sugar Free: Halls® Sugar Free Mentho-Lyptus® Cough Suppressant Drops are available in bags of 25 drops. They are available in four flavors: Black Cherry, Citrus Blend™ and Mountain Menthol™ and Honey-Lemon. Halls® Sugar Free Squares: Halls® Sugar Free Squares Mentho-Lyptus® Cough Suppressant Drops are available in single sticks of 9 drops each. They are available in two flavors: Black Cherry and Mountain Menthol™.

Shown in Product Identification Guide, page 506

HALLS DEFENSE® MULTI-BLEND SUPPLEMENT DROPS

Supplement Facts/Ingredients:
Supplement Facts
Serving Size 1 Drop

	Amount Per Drop	% Daily Value*
Calories	15	
Sodium	10 mg	<1%*
Total Carbohydrate	4 g	1%*
Sugars	3 g	†
Vitamin C	60 mg	100%
Zinc	1.5 mg	10%
Standard Echinacea Root Extract	15 mg	†

(Echinacea angustifolia and Echinacea purpurea)

* Percent Daily Values (DV) are based on a 2,000 calorie diet.
† Daily Value (DV) not established.

Other Ingredients: Sugar; Glucose Syrup; Sodium Ascorbate; Citric Acid; Partially Hydrogenated Cottonseed Oil; Natural Flavoring; Ascorbic Acid; Zinc Sulfate; Red 40; Oils of Angelica Root, Anise Star, Ginger, Lemon Grass, Sage and White Thyme; Blue 1.

Continued on next page

Halls Defense Drops—Cont.

Description: Halls Defense® Multi-Blend Supplement Drops help you keep going. Each drop provides 100% of the Daily Value of Vitamin C, Zinc to help support your natural resistance system**, plus Echinacea.

> **** This statement has not been evaluated by the Food & Drug Administration. This product is not intended to diagnose, treat, cure, or prevent any disease.**

Indications: Dietary Supplementation

Warnings: Do not use if you have a severe systemic illness such as tuberculosis, leukosis, collagen disease, multiple sclerosis or similar condition. Do not use if you have allergies to the daisy family (Asteraceae). Do not use if you are pregnant or breast-feeding. Keep out of the reach of children.

Suggested Use: As a dietary supplement, take one drop 4 times per day. Not recommended for use for more than 8 weeks consecutively.

How Supplied: Halls Defense® Multi-Blend Supplement Drops are available in Harvest Cherry in bags of 25 drops.
Shown in Product Identification Guide, page 506

HALLS DEFENSE® Vitamin C Supplement Drops
[Hols]

Ingredients: *ASSORTED CITRUS:* Sugar, Glucose Syrup, Sodium Ascorbate, Citric Acid, Natural Flavoring, Ascorbic Acid, Color Added (with Soy Lecithin) and Red 40. *STRAWBERRY:* Sugar, Glucose Syrup, Sodium Ascorbate, Citric Acid, Ascorbic Acid, Natural and Artificial Flavoring, Blue 2, Red 40. *WATERMELON:* Sugar, Glucose Syrup, Sodium Ascorbate, Citric Acid, Malic Acid, Ascorbic Acid, Potassium Citrate, Artificial Flavor, Red 40.

Description: Halls Defense® Vitamin C Supplement Drops are a delicious way to get 100% of the Daily Value of Vitamin C. Each drop provides 60 mg of Vitamin C (100% of the Daily Value).

Indications: Dietary Supplementation.

How Supplied: Halls Defense® Vitamin C Supplement Drops are available in Assorted Citrus (lemon, sweet grapefruit, orange) with all natural flavors, Strawberry and Watermelon in 9 drop sticks and bags of 30. Halls Defense® Assorted Citrus and Strawberry are available in bags of 80.
Shown in Product Identification Guide, page 506

TRIDENT® FOR KIDS
Sugarless Gum with Recaldent
[Tri-dent for kids]

Ingredients: *BERRY BUBBLE GUM:* Sorbitol, Gum Base, Mannitol, Glycerin, Artificial and Natural Flavoring, Xylitol, Calcium Casein Peptone-Calcium Phosphate (Lactose-Free Milk Derivative)**, Soy Lecithin, Acetylated Monoglycerides, Sucralose, Red 40 Lake and Blue 2 Lake. **Contains a Milk-Based Ingredient.**
RECALDENT™**: A patented ingredient derived from casein, a bovine phosphoprotein found in milk. RECALDENT is a trademark of Bonlac Bioscience PTY Ltd.

Description: Trident® For Kids is a dental care gum that remineralizes tooth enamel by safely delivering calcium and phosphate directly to teeth. In addition to strengthening teeth, chewing Trident for Kids™ may reduce the risk of tooth decay.

Directions: Trident® For Kids chewed after meals provides an ideal way to deliver the benefits of Recaldent™, to help remove food particles that may adhere to teeth, and to help minimize plaque acids.

How Supplied: Trident® For Kids with Recaldent is available in Berry Bubble Gum Flavor in an 8-stick pack.
Shown in Product Identification Guide, page 506

TRIDENT WHITE®
[Tri-dent White]
Sugarless Gum with Recaldent

Ingredients: *PEPPERMINT*: Sorbitol, Gum Base, Maltitol, Mannitol, Artificial and Natural Flavoring; Less Than 2% of: Acacia, Acesulfame Potassium, Aspartame, BHT (To Maintain Freshness), Calcium Casein Peptone-Calcium Phosphate (Lactose-Free Milk Derivative)**, Candelilla Wax, Sodium Stearate and Titanium Dioxide (Color). **Contains a Milk Derived Ingredient. Phenylketonurics: Contains Phenylalanine.**

Ingredients: *WINTERGREEN:* Sorbitol, Gum Base, Maltitol, Mannitol, Artificial and Natural Flavoring; Less Than 2% of: Acacia, Acesulfame Potassium, Aspartame, BHT (To Maintain Freshness), Calcium Casein Peptone-Calcium Phosphate (Lactose-Free Milk Derivative)**, Candelilla Wax, Glycerin, Sodium Stearate, Soy Lecithin and Titanium Dioxide (Color). **Contains a Milk Derived Ingredient. Phenylketonurics: Contains Phenylalanine.**

Ingredients: *SPEARMINT:* Sorbitol, Gum Base, Maltitol, Mannitol, Artificial and Natural Flavoring; Less Than 2% of: Acacia, Acesulfame Potassium, Aspartame, BHT (To Maintain Freshness), Calcium Casein Peptone-Calcium Phos-

---

phate (Lactose-Free Milk Derivative)**, Candelilla Wax, Sodium Stearate, Soy Lecithin and Titanium Dioxide (Color). **Contains a Milk Derived Ingredient. Phenylketonurics: Contains Phenylalanine.**

Ingredients: *COOL RUSH:* Gum Base, Sorbitol, Maltitol, Mannitol, Natural and Artificial Flavoring; Less Than 2% of: Acacia, Acesulfame Potassium, Aspartame, BHT (To Maintain Freshness), Calcium Casein Peptane-Calcium Phosphate (Lactose-Free Milk Derivative)**, Candelilla Wax, Sodium Stearate and Titanium Dioxide (Color). **Contains a Milk Derived Ingredient. Phenylketonurics: Contains Phenylalanine.**
RECALDENT**: A patented ingredient derived from casein, a bovine phosphoprotein found in milk. RECALDENT is a trademark of Bonlac Bioscience International PTY LTD.

Description: Trident White® is a whitening gum that uses proprietary surfactant technology to help break up and gently remove stains from teeth. In addition to whitening teeth, chewing Trident White® remineralizes tooth enamel by delivering calcium and phosphate beneath the tooth's surface.

Directions: When used as a part of a daily oral care regimen, Trident White helps gently remove stains caused by common beverages and food items consumed every day.

How Supplied: Trident White® is available in Peppermint, Wintergreen Spearmint flavors and Cool Rush in a 12-pellet blister foil.
Shown in Product Identification Guide, page 507

Celltech
Pharmaceuticals, Inc.
**PO BOX 31766
ROCHESTER, NY 14603**

Direct Inquiries to:
Customer Service Department
P.O. Box 31766
Rochester, NY 14603
(585) 274-5300
(888) 963-3382

**DELSYM®
(dextromethorphan polistirex)
Extended-Release Suspension
12-Hour Cough Suppressant
DELSYM®
(dextromethorphan polistirex)
Extended-Release Suspension
12 Cough Cough Suppressant for Children**

Active Ingredient (in each 5 mL teaspoonful): dextromethorphan polistirex equivalent to 30 mg dextromethorphan hydrobromide.

Purpose: Cough suppressant

Use: Temporarily relieves cough due to minor throat and bronchial irritation as may occur with the common cold or inhaled irritants.

Warnings: Do not use if you are now taking a prescription monoamine oxidase inhibitor (MAOI) (certain drugs for depression, psychiatric or emotional conditions, or Parkinson's disease), or for 2 weeks after stopping the MAOI drug. If you do not know if your prescription drug contains an MAOI, ask a doctor or pharmacist before taking this product.
Ask a doctor before use if you have
• chronic cough that lasts as occurs with smoking, asthma or emphysema
• cough that occurs with too much phlegm (mucus)
Stop use and ask a doctor if cough lasts more than 7 days, cough comes back, or occurs with fever, rash or headache that lasts. These could be signs of a serious condition.
If pregnant or breast-feeding, ask a health professional before use.
Keep out of reach of children. In case of overdose, get medical help or contact a Poison Control Center right away.

Directions:
• shake bottle well before use
• dose as follows or as directed by a doctor

adults and children 12 years of age and over	2 teaspoonfuls every 12 hours, not to exceed 4 teaspoonfuls in 24 hours
children 6 to under 12 years of age	1 teaspoonful every 12 hours, not to exceed 2 teaspoonfuls in 24 hours
children 2 to under 6 years of age	½ teaspoonful every 12 hours, not to exceed 1 teaspoonful in 24 hours
children under 2 years of age	consult a doctor

Other Information:
• **each 5 mL teaspoonful contains:** sodium 5 mg
• store at 20°–25°C (68°–77°F)

Inactive Ingredients: alcohol 0.26%, citric acid, ethylcellulose, FD&C Yellow No. 6, flavor, high fructose corn syrup, methylparaben, polyethylene glycol 3350, polysorbate 80, propylene glycol, propylparaben, purified water, sucrose, tragacanth, vegetable oil, xanthan gum.

How Supplied:
89 mL (3 fl oz.) bottles
NDC 53014-842-61
148 ml (5 fl oz.) bottles
NDC 53014-842-56
Celltech Pharmaceuticals, Inc.
Rochester, NY 14623 USA
®Celltech Manufacturing, Inc.

Effcon™ Laboratories, Inc.

P.O. BOX 7499
MARIETTA, GA 30065-1499

Address Inquiries to:
Brad Rivet
(800-722-2428)
Fax: (770-428-6811)

PIN-X®
Pinworm Treatment

Description: Each 1 mL of liquid for oral administration contains:
Pyrantel pamoate .... 144.10 mg
(equivalent to 50 mg pyrantel base)
Also contains citric acid, flavor, glycerin, lecithin, magnesium aluminum silicate, methylparaben, polysorbate 80, povidone, propylene glycol, propylparaben, purified water, saccharin sodium, simethicone emulsion, sodium benzoate, sorbitol solution and xanthan gum.

Indications and Usage: For the treatment of pinworms.

Contraindications: Hypersensitivity to any of the ingredients.

Warnings: KEEP THIS AND ALL DRUGS OUT OF THE REACH OF CHILDREN. In case of accidental overdose, seek professional assistance or contact a Poison Control Center immediately.
Abdominal cramps, nausea, vomiting, diarrhea, headache, or dizziness sometimes occur after taking this drug. If any of these conditions persist, consult a doctor. If you are pregnant or have liver disease, do not take this product unless directed by a doctor.

Directions for Use: Read package insert carefully before taking this medication. Take only according to directions and do not exceed the recommended dosage unless directed by a doctor. Medication should only be taken one time as a single dose; do not repeat treatment unless directed by a doctor. When one individual in a household has pinworms, the entire household should be treated unless otherwise advised. See **Warnings**. If any worms other than pinworms are present before or after treatment, consult a doctor. If any symptoms or pinworms are still present after treatment, consult a doctor. This product can be taken any time of day, with or without meals. It may be taken alone or with milk or fruit juice. Use of a laxative is not necessary prior to, during, or after medication.
Adults and children 2 years to under 12 years of age: oral dosage is a single dose of 5 milligrams of pyrantel base per pound, or 11 milligrams per kilogram, of body weight not to exceed 1 gram. Dosage information is summarized on the following schedule:

Weight	Dosage (taken as a single dose)
Less than 25 pounds (11 kg) or under 2 years old	Do not use unless directed by a doctor
25 to 37 pounds (11 to 16 kg)	½ teaspoonful
38 to 62 pounds (17 to 28 kg)	1 teaspoonful
63 to 87 pounds (29 to 39 kg)	1 ½ teaspoonfuls
88 to 112 pounds (40 to 50 kg)	2 teaspoonfuls
113 to 137 pounds (51 to 62 kg)	2 ½ teaspoonfuls
138 to 186 pounds (63 to 73 kg)	3 teaspoonfuls (1 tablespoonful)
163 to 187 pounds (74 to 84 kg)	3 ½ teaspoonfuls
188 pounds and over (85 kg and over)	4 teaspoonfuls

SHAKE WELL BEFORE USING

How Supplied: Pin-X is supplied as an opaque yellow, caramel-flavored suspension, which contains pyrantel pamoate 144.10 mg (equivalent to 50 mg pyrantel base) per mL, in bottles of 30 mL (1 fl oz), NDC 55806-024-10 and in bottles of 60 mL (2 fl oz), NDC 55806-024-11. Store at 15°-30°C (59°-86°F).
Marketed by:
Effcon™ Laboratories, Inc.
Marietta, GA 30065-1499

8181003
Rev 6/03
R0

Shown in Product Identification Guide, page 507

EDUCATIONAL MATERIAL

Patient Education Brochures—Pin-X® Pinworm Treatment

Effcon Laboratories provides complimentary Patient Education Brochures for patient counseling regarding the treatment and prevention of pinworm infestation. Brochures are available for all healthcare professionals and may be requested by phone (800-722-2428); fax (770-428-6811); or through Effcon's web page (www.effcon.com).

**IF YOU SUSPECT
AN INTERACTION. . .**
The 1,800-page
PDR Companion Guide™ can help.
Use the order form
in the front of this book.

Fleming & Company
1733 GILSINN LANE
FENTON, MO 63026

Direct Inquiries to:
Tom Johnson
636 343-5306
800-633-1886
FAX (636) 343-5322
www.flemingcompany.com

OCEAN® Nasal Spray
(buffered isotonic saline)

Description: A 0.65% special saline made isotonic by the addition of a dual preservative system and buffering excipients prevent nasal irritation.
Ingredients: 0.65% Sodium Chloride and Phenylcarbinol and Benzalkonium Chloride as preservatives.

Action and Uses: For dry nasal membranes including rhinitis medicamentosa, rhinitis sicca and atrophic rhinitis. OCEAN® may also be used as a mist or drop. Upright delivers a spray; horizontally a stream; upside down a drop.

Administration and Dosage: For dry nasal membranes, two squeezes in each nostril P.R.N.

Supplied: White plastic 45cc spray bottles with orange cap (0256-0152-01). Also in pints (0256-0152-02).

PURGE
(Flavored Castor Oil Stimulant Laxative)

Composition: Contains 95% castor oil (USP) in a sweetened lemon flavored base that completely masks the odor and taste of the oil.

Indications: Preparation of the bowel for x-ray, surgery and proctological procedures, IVPs, and constipation.

Dosage: Adults and children 12 years of age and over: 15–60 mL (1–4 tbsp) in a single dose. Children 2 to under 12 years of age: 5–15 mL (1–3 tsp) in a single dose. Children under 2 years: consult a physician.

Precaution: Not indicated when nausea, vomiting, abdominal pain or symptoms of appendicitis occur. Pregnancy, use only on advice of physician.

Supplied: Plastic 1 oz. & 2 oz. bottles.

**IF YOU SUSPECT
AN INTERACTION. . .**
The 1,800-page
PDR Companion Guide™ can help.
Use the order form
in the front of this book.

GlaxoSmithKline Consumer Healthcare, L.P.
P.O. BOX 1467
PITTSBURGH, PA 15230

Direct Inquiries to:
Consumer Affairs
1-800-245-1040
For Medical Emergencies Contact:
Consumer Affairs
1-800-245-1040

ABREVA®
Cold Sore/Fever Blister Treatment Cream
Docosanol 10% Cream

Uses:
- Treats cold sore/fever blisters on the face or lips
- Shortens healing time and duration of symptoms: tingling, pain, burning, and/or itching

Active Ingredient: **Purpose:**
Docosanol 10% ... Cold sore/fever blister treatment

Inactive Ingredients: Benzyl alcohol, light mineral oil, propylene glycol, purified water, sucrose distearate, sucrose stearate.

Directions:
- **adults and children 12 years or over:**
  - wash hands before and after applying cream
  - apply to affected area on face or lips at the first sign of cold sore/fever blister (tingle). **Early treatment ensures the best results.**
  - rub in gently but completely
  - use 5 times a day until healed
- **children under 12 years:** ask a doctor

Warnings:
For external use only.
Do not use
- if you are allergic to any ingredient in this product
When using this product
- apply only to affected areas
- do not use in or near the eyes
- avoid applying directly inside your mouth
- do not share this product with anyone. This may spread infection.
Stop use and ask a doctor if
- your cold sore gets worse or the cold sore is not healed within 10 days
- **Keep out of reach of children.** If swallowed, get medical help or contact a poison control center right away.
Other Information:
- store at 20°–25°C (68°–77°F)
- do not freeze

How Supplied: Abreva Cream is supplied in 2.0 g [.07 oz] tubes.
Question? Call 1-877-709-3539 weekdays

*Shown in Product Identification
Guide, page 507*

BC® POWDER
ARTHRITIS STRENGTH BC® POWDER
BC® COLD POWDER LINE

Description: BC® POWDER: **Active Ingredients:** Each powder contains Aspirin 650 mg, Salicylamide 195 mg and Caffeine 33.3 mg. **Inactive Ingredients:** Docusate Sodium, Fumaric Acid, Lactose Monohydrate and Potassium Chloride. ARTHRITIS STRENGTH BC® POWDER: **Active Ingredients:** Each powder contains Aspirin 742 mg, Salicylamide 222 mg and Caffeine 38 mg. **Inactive Ingredients:** Docusate Sodium, Fumaric Acid, Lactose Monohydrate and Potassium Chloride.
BC® ALLERGY SINUS COLD POWDER

Active Ingredients: Aspirin 650 mg, Pseudoephedrine Hydrochloride 60 mg and Chlorpheniramine Maleate 4 mg per powder. **Inactive Ingredients:** Fumaric Acid, Glycine, Lactose, Potassium Chloride, Silica, Sodium Lauryl Sulfate. BC® SINUS COLD POWDER. **Active Ingredients:** Aspirin 650 mg and Pseudoephedrine Hydrochloride 60 mg. per powder. **Inactive Ingredients:** Colloidal Silicon Dioxide, Microcrystalline Cellulose, Povidone, Pregelatinized Starch, Stearic Acid.

Indications: BC Powder is for relief of simple headache; for temporary relief of minor arthritic pain, for relief of muscular aches, discomfort and fever of colds; and for relief of normal menstrual pain and pain of tooth extraction.
Arthritis Strength BC Powder is specially formulated to fight occasional minor pain and inflammation of arthritis. Like Original Formula BC, Arthritis Strength BC provides fast temporary relief of minor arthritis pain and inflammation, relief of muscular aches, discomfort and fever of colds; and pain of tooth extraction.
BC Allergy Sinus Cold Powder is for relief of multiple symptoms such as body aches, fever, nasal congestion, sneezing, running nose, and watery itchy eyes associated with allergy and sinus attacks and the onset of colds. BC Sinus Cold Powder is for relief of such symptoms as body aches, fever, and nasal congestion.

BC Powder®, Arthritis Strength BC® Powder and BC Cold Powder Line:

Warnings: **Children and teenagers should not use this medicine for chicken pox or flu symptoms before a doctor is consulted about Reye's Syndrome, a rare but serious illness reported to be associated with aspirin. Keep this and all medicines out of children's reach. In case of accidental overdose, contact a physician or poison control center immediately.**
As with any drug, if you are pregnant or nursing a baby seek the advice of a health professional before using this product.

IT IS ESPECIALLY IMPORTANT NOT TO USE ASPIRIN DURING THE LAST 3 MONTHS OF PREGNANCY UNLESS SPECIFICALLY DIRECTED TO DO SO BY A DOCTOR BECAUSE IT MAY CAUSE PROBLEMS IN THE UNBORN CHILD OR COMPLICATIONS DURING DELIVERY.

Alcohol Warning: If you consume 3 or more alcoholic drinks every day, ask your doctor whether you should take aspirin or other pain relievers/fever reducers. Aspirin may cause stomach bleeding.

Allergy Alert: Aspirin may cause a severe allergic reaction which may include hives, facial swelling, shock or asthma (wheezing). **Ask a doctor before use if you have** asthma, ulcers, a bleeding problem, stomach problems that last or come back such as heartburn, upset stomach or pain. **Ask a doctor or pharmacist before use** if you are taking a prescription drug for gout, diabetes, arthritis or anticoagulation (blood thinning). **Stop use and ask a doctor if** an allergic reaction occurs, ringing in ears or loss of hearing occurs, pain gets worse or persists for more than 10 days, fever lasts more than 3 days, redness or swelling is present, or new symptoms occur.

For BC Powder and Arthritis Strength BC Powder:

When using these products limit the use of caffeine containing drugs, foods, or drinks, because too much caffeine may cause nervousness, irritability, sleeplessness, and occasionally, rapid heartbeat.

For BC Cold Powder Line:

Do not exceed recommended dosage. If nervousness, dizziness, or sleeplessness occur, discontinue use and consult a doctor. If symptoms do not improve within 7 days, or are accompanied by fever that lasts more than 3 days, or if new symptoms occur, consult a physician before continuing use. Do not take BC if you are sensitive to aspirin, or have heart disease, high blood pressure, thyroid disease, diabetes, asthma, glaucoma, emphysema, chronic pulmonary disease, shortness of breath, difficulty in breathing or difficulty in urination due to enlargement of the prostate gland, or if you are presently taking a prescription antihypertensive or antidepressant drug unless directed by a doctor. *"Drug interaction precaution.* Do not use this product if you are now taking a prescription monoamine oxidase inhibitor (MAOI) (certain drugs for depression, psychiatric or emotional conditions, or Parkinson's disease), or for 2 weeks after stopping the MAOI drug. If you are uncertain whether your prescription drug contains an MAOI, consult a health professional before taking this product." BC Allergy Sinus Cold Powder with antihistamine may cause drowsiness. Avoid alcoholic beverages when taking this product because it may increase drowsiness. Use caution when driving a motor vehicle or operating machinery. May cause excitability, especially in children.

Overdosage: In case of accidental overdosage, contact a physician or poison control center immediately.

Dosage and Administration: BC® Powder, Arthritis Strength BC® Powder, BC® Cold Powder Line:
Place one powder on tongue and follow with liquid. If you prefer, stir powder into glass of water or other liquid.
For BC Powder and Arthritis Strength BC Powder:
Adults and children 12 years and over: Take one powder every 3–4 hours not to exceed 4 powders in 24 hours.
For BC Cold Powder Line:
Adults and children 12 years and over: Take one powder every 6 hours not to exceed 4 powders in 24 hours. For children under 12, consult a physician.

How Supplied: BC Powder: Available in tamper evident overwrapped envelopes of 2 or 6 powders, as well as tamper evident boxes of 24 and 50 powders.
Arthritis Strength BC Powder: Available in tamper evident over wrapped envelopes of 6 powders, and tamper evident overwrapped boxes of 24 and 50 powders.
BC Cold Powder Line:
Available in tamper-evident overwrapped envelopes of 6 powders, as well as tamper-evident boxes of 12 powders (For BC Allergy Sinus Cold Powder only).

Orange Flavor
CITRUCEL®
[sĭt 'rə-sĕl]
(Methylcellulose)
Bulk-forming Fiber Laxative

Description: Each 19 g adult dose (approximately one heaping measuring tablespoonful) contains Methylcellulose 2 g. Each 9.5 g child's dose (one-half the adult dose) contains Methylcellulose 1 g. Methylcellulose is a nonallergenic fiber. Also contains: Citric Acid, FD&C Yellow No. 6 Lake, Orange Flavors (natural and artificial), Potassium Citrate, Riboflavin, Sucrose, and other ingredients. Each adult dose contains approximately 3 mg of sodium and contributes 60 calories from Sucrose.

Actions: Promotes elimination by providing additional fiber (bulk) to the diet. This product generally produces bowel movement in 12 to 72 hours.

Indications: For relief of constipation (irregularity). May also be used for relief of constipation associated with other bowel disorders such as irritable bowel syndrome, diverticular disease, and hemorrhoids as well as for bowel management during postpartum, postsurgical, and convalescent periods when recommended by a physician.

Contraindications: Intestinal obstruction, fecal impaction, known hypersensitivity to formula ingredients.

Warnings: Patients should be instructed to consult their physician before using any laxative if they have noticed a sudden change in bowel habits which persists for two weeks. Unless directed by a physician, patients should be advised not to use laxative products when abdominal pain, nausea, or vomiting is present. Patients should also be advised to discontinue use and consult a physician if rectal bleeding or failure to have a bowel movement occurs after use of any laxative product. Unless recommended by a physician, patients should not exceed the recommended maximum daily dose. Patients should not use laxative products for a period longer than one week unless as directed by a physician. **TAKING THIS PRODUCT WITHOUT ADEQUATE FLUID MAY CAUSE IT TO SWELL AND BLOCK YOUR THROAT OR ESOPHAGUS AND MAY CAUSE CHOKING. DO NOT TAKE THIS PRODUCT IF YOU HAVE DIFFICULTY IN SWALLOWING. IF YOU EXPERIENCE CHEST PAIN, VOMITING, OR DIFFICULTY IN SWALLOWING OR BREATHING AFTER TAKING THIS PRODUCT, SEEK IMMEDIATE MEDICAL ATTENTION. KEEP THIS AND ALL DRUGS OUT OF THE REACH OF CHILDREN.**

Dosage and Administration: Adult Dose: dissolve one leveled scoop (one heaping tablespoon – 19g) in 8 ounces of cold water up to three times daily at the first sign of constipation. Children age 6 to 12 years of age: *one-half the adult dose* stirred briskly in 8 ounces of cold water, once daily at the first sign of constipation. The mixture should be administered promptly and drinking another glass of water is highly recommended (see warnings). Children under 6 years of age: *Use only as directed by a physician.* Continued use for 12 to 72 hours may be necessary for full benefit.
TAKE THIS PRODUCT (CHILD OR ADULT DOSE) WITH AT LEAST 8 OZ. (A FULL GLASS) OF WATER OR OTHER FLUID. TAKING THIS PRODUCT WITHOUT ENOUGH LIQUID MAY CAUSE CHOKING. SEE WARNINGS.

How Supplied: 16 oz., 30 oz., and 50 oz. containers.
Boxes of 20-single-dose packets.
Store below 86°F (30°C). Protect contents from humidity; keep tightly closed.
Shown in Product Identification Guide, page 507

Sugar Free Orange Flavor
CITRUCEL®
[sĭt 'rə-sĕl]
(Methylcellulose)
Bulk-forming Fiber Laxative

Description: Each 10.2 g adult dose (approximately one rounded measuring tablespoonful) contains Methylcellulose

Continued on next page

Citrucel Sugar Free—Cont.

2 g. Each 5.1 g child's dose (one-half the adult dose) contains Methylcellulose 1 g. Methylcellulose is a nonallergenic fiber. Also contains: Aspartame, Dibasic Calcium Phosphate, FD&C Yellow No. 6 Lake, Malic Acid, Maltodextrin, Orange Flavors (natural and artificial), Potassium Citrate, and Riboflavin. Each 10.2 g dose contains approximately 3 mg of sodium and contributes 24 calories from Maltodextrin.

Actions: Promotes elimination by providing additional fiber (bulk) to the diet. This product generally produces bowel movement in 12 to 72 hours.

Indications: For relief of constipation (irregularity). May also be used for relief of constipation associated with other bowel disorders such as irritable bowel syndrome, diverticular disease, and hemorrhoids as well as for bowel management during postpartum, postsurgical, and convalescent periods when recommended by a physician.

Contraindications and Warnings: See entry for "Orange Flavor Citrucel".

Phenylketonurics: CONTAINS PHENYLALANINE 52 mg per adult dose. Individuals with phenylketonuria and other individuals who must restrict their intake of phenylalanine should be warned that each 10.2 g adult dose contains aspartame which provides 52 mg of phenylalanine.

Dosage and Administration: Adult Dose: dissolve one leveled scoop (one rounded measuring tablespoon – 10.2 g) in 8 ounces of cold water up to three times daily at the first sign of constipation. Children age 6 to 12 years of age: *one-half the adult dose* stirred briskly into at least 8 ounces of cold water, once daily at the first sign of constipation. The mixture should be administered promptly and drinking another glass of water is highly recommended (see warnings). Children under 6 years of age: *Use only as directed by a physician.* Continued use for 12 to 72 hours may be necessary for full benefit. **TAKE THIS PRODUCT (CHILD OR ADULT DOSE) WITH AT LEAST 8 OZ. (A FULL GLASS) OF WATER OR OTHER FLUID. TAKING THIS PRODUCT WITHOUT ENOUGH LIQUID MAY CAUSE CHOKING. SEE WARNINGS.**

How Supplied:
8.6 oz, 16.9 oz, and 32 oz containers. Boxes of 20 single-dose packets. Store below 86°F (30°C). Protect contents from humidity; keep tightly closed.
Shown in Product Identification Guide, page 507

CITRUCEL®
(methylcellulose)
Soluble Fiber Caplet
Bulk-Forming Fiber Laxative

Uses: Helps restore and maintain regularity. Helps relieve constipation. Also useful in treatment of constipation (irregularity) associated with other bowel disorders when recommended by a physician. This product generally produces a bowel movement in 12 to 72 hours.

Active Ingredient: Each caplet contains 500mg Methylcellulose.

Inactive Ingredients: Crospovidone, Dibasic Calcium Phosphate, FD&C Yellow No. 6 Aluminum Lake, Magnesium Stearate, Maltodextrin, Povidone, Sodium Lauryl Sulfate.

Directions: Adult dose: Take two caplets as needed with 8 ounces of liquid, up to six times daily. Children (6–12 years): Take one caplet with 8 ounces of liquid, up to six times per day. The dosage requirement may vary according to the severity of constipation. Children under 6 years: consult a physician. **TAKE THIS PRODUCT (CHILD OR ADULT DOSE) WITH AT LEAST 8 OUNCES (A FULL GLASS) OF WATER OR OTHER FLUID. TAKING THIS PRODUCT WITHOUT ENOUGH LIQUID MAY CAUSE CHOKING. SEE WARNINGS.**

Directions for Use: Take each dose with 8oz. of liquid.

Age	Dose	Daily Maximum
Adults & Children over 12 years	2 Caplets	Up to 6 times daily*
Children (6 to 12 years)	1 Caplet	Up to 6 times daily*
Children under 6 years	Consult a physician	

*Refer to directions below.

Warnings: Consult a physician before using any laxative product if you have noticed a sudden change in bowel habits which persists for two weeks. Unless directed by a physician, do not use laxative products when abdominal pain, nausea, or vomiting are present. Discontinue use and consult a physician if rectal bleeding or failure to produce a bowel movement occurs after use of any laxative product. Unless recommended by a physician, do not exceed recommended maximum daily dose. Laxative products should not be used for a period longer than a weak unless directed by a physician. If sensitive to any of the ingredients, do not use. **TAKING THIS PRODUCT WITHOUT ADEQUATE FLUID MAY CAUSE IT TO SWELL AND BLOCK YOUR THROAT OR ESOPHAGUS AND MAY CAUSE CHOKING. DO NOT TAKE THIS PRODUCT IF YOU HAVE DIFFICULTY IN SWALLOWING. IF YOU EXPERIENCE CHEST PAIN, VOMITING, OR DIFFICULTY IN SWALLOWING OR BREATHING AFTER TAKING**

THIS PRODUCT, SEEK IMMEDIATE MEDICAL ATTENTION. KEEP THIS AND ALL DRUGS OUT OF THE REACH OF CHILDREN.
Store at room temperature 15–30°C (59–86°F). Protect contents from moisture.
Tamper evident feature: Bottle sealed with printed foil under cap. Do not use if foil is torn or broken.

How Supplied: Bottles of 100 and 164 caplets
Questions or comments?
Call toll-free 1-800-897-6081 weekdays.
Patents Pending
The various Citrucel Logos and design elements of the packaging are Registered Trademarks of GlaxoSmithKline.
©2001 GlaxoSmithKline
Distributed by:
GlaxoSmithKline Consumer Healthcare
GlaxoSmithKline Consumer Healthcare, L.P.
Moon Township, PA 15108, Made in Canada.

CONTAC® Non-Drowsy
Decongestant
12 Hour Cold Caplets

Product Information: Each Maximum Strength Contac 12 Hour Cold Caplet provides up to 12 hours of relief. Part of the caplet goes to work right away for fast relief; the rest is released gradually to provide up to 12 hours of prolonged relief. With just one caplet in the morning and one at bedtime, you feel better all day, sleep better at night, breathing freely without congestion or sinus pressure.

Indications: Temporarily relieves nasal congestion due to the common cold, hay fever or other upper respiratory allergies and associated with sinusitis. Helps decongest sinus openings and passages; temporarily relieves sinus congestion and pressure.

Directions: Adults and children over 12 years of age: One caplet every 12 hours, not to exceed 2 caplets in 24 hours, or as directed by a doctor. Children under 12 years of age: consult a doctor.
TAMPER-EVIDENT PACKAGING FEATURES FOR YOUR PROTECTION:
Each caplet is encased in a plastic cell with a foil back; do not use if cell or foil is broken.

Warnings: Do not exceed the recommended dosage. If nervousness, dizziness, or sleeplessness occur, discontinue use and consult a doctor. If symptoms do not improve within 7 days or are accompanied by high fever, consult a doctor. Do not take this product, unless directed by a doctor, if you have heart disease, high blood pressure, thyroid disease, diabetes, glaucoma or difficulty in urination due to enlargement of the prostate gland. KEEP THIS AND ALL DRUGS OUT OF REACH OF CHILDREN. IN CASE OF ACCIDENTAL OVERDOSE, SEEK PROFESSIONAL ASSISTANCE OR CONTACT A POISON CONTROL CENTER IMMEDIATELY. As with any drug, if you are pregnant or nursing a baby, seek the advice of a health professional before using this product.

Drug Interaction Precaution: Do not use this product if you are now taking a prescription monoamine oxidase inhibitor (MAOI) (certain drugs for depression, psychiatric or emotional conditions, or Parkinson's disease), or for 2 weeks after stopping the MAOI drug. If you are uncertain whether your prescription drug contains an MAOI, consult a health professional before taking this product.

Active Ingredient: Pseudoephedrine Hydrochloride 120 mg.

Store at 15° to 25°C (59° to 77°F) in a dry place and protest from light.

Each Caplet Also Contains: Carnauba Wax, Colloidal Silicon Dioxide, Dibasic Calcium Phosphate, Hypromellose, Magnesium Stearate, Microcrystalline Cellulose, Polyethylene Glycol, Polysorbate 80, Titanium Dioxide.

How Supplied: Consumer packages of 10 and 20 caplets.
Note: There are other CONTAC products. Make sure this is the one you are interested in. See the table below for all of the products in the CONTAC line.
Shown in Product Identification Guide, page 507

**CONTAC® Non-Drowsy
Timed Release-Maximum Strength
12 Hour Cold Caplets**

Indications: For the temporary relief of nasal congestion due to the common cold, hay fever or other upper respiratory allergies, and nasal congestion associated with sinusitis. Promotes nasal and/or sinus drainage; temporarily relieves sinus congestion and pressure. Temporarily restores freer breathing through the nose.
Each Maximum Strength Contac 12-Hour Cold caplet provides up to 12 hours of relief. Part of the caplet goes to work right away for fast relief; the rest is released gradually to provide up to 12 hours of prolonged relief. With just one caplet in the morning and one at bedtime, you feel better all day, sleep better at night, breathing freely without congestion or sinus pressure.

Active Ingredient: Each coated extended-release caplet contains Pseudoephedrine Hydrochloride 120 mg.

Inactive Ingredients: carnauba wax, collodial silicon dioxide, dibasic calcium

phosphate, hypromellose, magnesium stearate, microcrystalline cellulose, polyethylene glycol, polysorbate 80, titanium dioxide.

Directions: Adults and children 12 years of age and over – One caplet every 12 hours, not to exceed two caplets in 24 hours. This product is not recommended for children under 12 years of age.

Warnings: Do not exceed recommended dosage. If nervousness, dizziness, or sleeplessness occur, discontinue use and consult a doctor. If symptoms do not improve within 7 days or are accompanied by fever, consult a doctor. Do not take this product if you have heart disease, high blood pressure, thyroid disease, diabetes, or difficulty in urination due to enlargement of the prostate gland unless directed by a doctor. As with any drug, if you are pregnant or nursing a baby, seek the advice of a health professional before using this product.

Drug Interaction Precaution: Do not use this product if you are now taking a prescription monoamine oxidase inhibitor (MAOI) (certain drugs for depression, psychiatric or emotional conditions, or Parkinson's disease), or for 2 weeks after stopping the MAOI drug. If you are uncertain whether your prescription contains an MAOI, consult a health professional before taking this product.
KEEP THIS AND ALL DRUGS OUT OF THE REACH OF CHILDREN. In case of accidental overdose, seek professional assistance or contact a Poison Control Center immediately.
Store at 15° to 25°C (59° to 77°F) in a dry place and protect from light.

How Supplied: Packets of 10 and 20 Caplets
U.S. Patent No. 5,895,663
Comments or questions?
Call toll-free 1-800-245-1040 weekdays.

**CONTAC®
Severe Cold and Flu
Caplets Maximum Strength
Analgesic• Decongestant
Antihistamine• Cough Suppressant
CONTAC®
Severe Cold and Flu
Caplets Non-Drowsy
Nasal Decongestant • Analgesic•
Cough Suppressant**

Active Ingredients: Each *Non-Drowsy Caplet* contains Acetaminophen 325 mg, Psudoephedrine HCl 30 mg and Dextromethorphan Hydrobromide 15 mg.
Each *Maximum Strength Caplet* contains Acetaminophen 500 mg, Dextromethorphan Hydrobromide 15 mg, Pseudoephedrine HCl 30 mg and chlorpheniromine Maleate 2 mg.

Product Information: Two caplets every 6 hours to help relieve the dis-

comforts of severe colds with flu-like symptoms.

Indications: *Non-Drowsy & Maximum Strength Caplets:* Temporarily relieves nasal congestion & coughing due to the common cold. Provides temporary relief of fever, sore throat, headache & minor aches associated with the common cold or the flu.
Maximum Strength Caplets: Temporarily relieves runny nose, sneezing, itchy and watery eyes due to the common cold.

Directions: Adults (12 years and older): Two caplets every 6 hours, not to exceed 8 caplets in any 24-hour period, or as directed by a doctor. Children under 12 years of age: consult a doctor.
TAMPER-EVIDENT PACKAGING FEATURES FOR YOUR PROTECTION:
Caplets are encased in a plastic cell with a foil back. Do not use if cell or foil is broken. The letters ND SCF for non-drowsy and SCF for maximum strength appear on each caplet; do not use this product if these letters are missing.

Warnings: For *Non-Drowsy and Maximum Strength Caplets:* Do not exceed recommended dosage. If nervousness, dizziness, or sleeplessness occur, discontinue use and consult a doctor. If symptoms do not improve or are accompanied by fever that lasts for more than 3 days, or if new symptoms occur, consult a doctor. If sore throat is severe, persists for more than 2 days, is accompanied or followed by fever, headache, rash, nausea, or vomiting, consult a doctor promptly. A persistent cough may be a sign of a serious condition. If cough persists for more than 7 days, tends to recur, or is accompanied by rash, persistent headache, fever that lasts for more than 3 days, or if new symptoms occur, consult a doctor. Do not take this product for persistent or chronic cough such as occurs with smoking, asthma, emphysema, or if cough is accompanied by excessive phlegm (mucus) unless directed by a doctor. Do not take this product if you have heart disease, high blood pressure, thyroid disease, diabetes, glaucoma or difficulty in urination due to enlargement of the prostate gland unless directed by a doctor. **Alcohol Warning:** If you consume 3 or more alcoholic drinks every day, ask your doctor whether you should take acetaminophen or other pain relievers/fever reducers. Acetaminophen may cause liver damage. **KEEP THIS AND ALL DRUGS OUT OF THE REACH OF CHILDREN.** Prompt medical attention is critical for adults as well as for children even if you do not notice any signs or symptoms. In case of accidental overdose, seek professional assistance or contact a Poison Control Center immediately. As with any drug, if you are pregnant or nursing a baby, seek the advice of a health professional before using this product.

Continued on next page

PDR For Nonprescription Drugs

	CONTAC Non-Drowsy 12 Hour Cold Caplets	CONTAC 12 Hour Cold Capsules	CONTAC Severe Cold and Flu Caplets Maximum Strength (each 2 caplet dose)	CONTAC Severe Cold and Flu Non-Drowsy Caplets (each 2 caplet dose)	CONTAC Day & Night Cold & Flu Day Caplets	CONTAC Day & Night Cold & Flu Night Caplets
Phenylpropanolamine HCl	—	75.0 mg	—	—	—	—
Chlorpheniramine Maleate	—	8.0 mg	4.0 mg	—	—	—
Pseudoephedrine HCl	120 mg	—	60 mg	60.0 mg	60.0 mg	60.0 mg
Acetaminophen	—	—	1000.0 mg	650.0 mg	650.0 mg	650.0 mg
Dextromethorphan Hydrobromide	—	—	30.0 mg	30.0 mg	30.0 mg	—
Diphenhydramine HCl	—	—	—	—	—	50.0 mg

Contac Sev. Cold/Flu—Cont.

Additional Warnings for *Maximum Strength Caplets:* May cause excitability especially in children. Do not take this product, unless directed by a doctor, if you have a breathing problem such as emphysema or chronic bronchitis. May cause marked drowsiness: alcohol, sedatives, and tranquilizers may increase the drowsiness effect. Avoid taking alcoholic beverages while taking this product. Do not take this product if you are taking sedatives or tranquilizers, without first consulting your doctor. Use caution when driving a motor vehicle or operating machinery.

Drug Interaction Precaution: Do not use this product if you are now taking a prescription monoamine oxidase inhibitor (MAOI) (certain drugs for depression, psychiatric or emotional conditions, or Parkinson's disease), or for 2 weeks after stopping the MAOI drug. If you are uncertain whether your prescription drug contains an MAOI, consult a health professional before taking this product.

Inactive Ingredients: Each *Non-Drowsy and Maximum Strength Caplet* contains: Carnauba Wax, Colloidal Silicon Dioxide, Hypromellose, Magnesium stearate, Microcrystalline Cellulose, Polyethylene Glycol, Polysorbate 80, Starch, Stearic Acid, Titanium Dioxide. Each *Maximum Strength Caplet* also contains: FD&C Blue #1 Al Lake.

Avoid storing at high temperature (greater than 100°F).

How Supplied: *Non-Drowsy:* Consumer packages of 16.
Maximum Strength: Consumer packages of 16 & 30.

Product Change: Maximum Strength Caplets now with new decongestant (pseudoephedrine HCl).

Note: There are other CONTAC products. Make sure this is the one you are interested in. See the table below for all of the products in the CONTAC line.

[See table above]
Shown in Product Identification Guide, page 507

DEBROX® Drops
Ear Wax Removal Aid

Active Ingredient: **Purpose:**
Carbamide peroxide
6.5% non USP* .. Earwax removal aid

Actions: DEBROX®, used as directed, cleanses the ear with sustained microfoam. DEBROX Drops foam on contact with earwax due to the release of oxygen (there may be an associated crackling sound). DEBROX Drops provide a safe, nonirritating method of softening and removing ear wax.

Uses: For occasional use as an aid to soften, loosen, and remove excessive earwax.

Directions: Adults and children over 12 years of age: tilt head sideways and place 5 to 10 drops into ear. Tip of applicator should not enter ear canal. Keep drops in ear for several minutes by keeping head tilted or placing cotton in the ear. Use twice daily for up to four days if needed, or as directed by a doctor. Any wax remaining after treatment may be removed by gently flushing the ear with warm water, using a soft rubber bulb ear syringe. Children under 12 years of age: consult a doctor.

Warnings: FOR USE IN THE EAR ONLY. Do not use if you have ear drainage or discharge, ear pain, irritation or rash in the ear, or are dizzy; consult a doctor. Do not use if you have an injury or perforation (hole) of the eardrum or after ear surgery unless directed by a doctor. Do not use for more than four days. If excessive earwax remains after use of this product, consult a doctor. Avoid contact with the eyes. In case of accidental ingestion, seek professional assistance or contact a poison control center immediately.

Other Information: Avoid exposing bottle to excessive heat and direct sunlight. Keep tip on bottle when not in use.

Product foams on contact with earwax due to release of oxygen. There may be an associated "crackling" sound. Keep this and all drugs out of the reach of children.

Inactive Ingredients: citric acid, flavor, glycerin, propylene glycol, sodium lauroyl sarcosinate, sodium stannate, water

How Supplied: DEBROX Drops are available in ½-fl-oz or 1-fl-oz (15 or 30 ml) plastic squeeze bottles with applicator spouts.
Questions or comments? 1-800-245-1040 weekdays.
Shown in Product Identification Guide, page 507

ECOTRIN
Enteric-Coated Aspirin
Antiarthritic, Antiplatelet
COMPREHENSIVE PRESCRIBING INFORMATION

Description: Ecotrin enteric coated aspirin (acetylsalicylic acid) tablets available in 81mg, 325mg and 500 mg tablets for oral administration. The 325 mg and 500 mg tablets contain the following inactive ingredients: Carnuba Wax, Colloidal Silicon Dioxide, FD&C Yellow No. 6, Hypromellose, Methacrylic Acid Copolymer, Microcrystalline Cellulose, Pregelatinized Starch, Propylene Glycol, Simethicone, Sodium Starch Glycolate, Stearic Acid, Talc, Titanium Dioxide, and Triethyl Citrate. The 81 mg tablets contain Carnuba Wax, Corn Starch, D&C Yellow No. 10, FD&C Yellow No. 6, Hypromellose, Methacrylic Acid Copolymer, Microcrystalline Cellulose, Propylene Glycol, Simethicone, Stearic Acid, Talc and Triethyl Citrate.
Aspirin is an odorless white, needle-like crystalline or powdery substance. When exposed to moisture, aspirin hydrolyzes into salicylic and acetic acids, and gives off a vinegary-odor. It is highly lipid soluble and slightly soluble in water.

Clinical Pharmacology: Mechanism of Action: Aspirin is a more potent inhibitor of both prostaglandin synthesis and platelet aggregation than other salicylic acid derivatives. The differences in activity between aspirin and salicylic acid are thought to be due to the acetyl group on the aspirin molecule. This acetyl group is responsible for the inactivation of cyclooxygenase via acetylation.

PHARMACOKINETICS

Absorption: In general, immediate release aspirin is well and completely absorbed from the gastrointestinal (GI) tract. Following absorption, aspirin is hydrolyzed to salicylic acid with peak plasma levels of salicylic acid occurring within 1–2 hours of dosing (see Pharmacokinetics—Metabolism). The rate of absorption from the GI tract is dependent upon the dosage form, the presence or absence of food, gastric pH (the presence or absence of GI antacids or buffering agents), and other physiologic factors. Enteric coated aspirin products are erratically absorbed from the GI tract.

Distribution: Salicylic acid is widely distributed to all tissues and fluids in the body including the central nervous system (CNS), breast milk, and fetal tissues. The highest concentrations are found in the plasma, liver, renal cortex, heart, and lungs. The protein binding of salicylate is concentration-dependent, i.e., non-linear. At low concentrations (< 100 mcg/mL) approximately 90 percent of plasma salicylate is bound to albumin while at higher concentrations (> 400 mcg/mL), only about 75 percent is bound. The early signs of salicylic overdose (salicylism), including tinnitus (ringing in the ears), occur at plasma concentrations approximating 200 mcg/mL. Severe toxic effects are associated with levels > 400 mcg/mL (See Adverse Reactions and Overdosage.)

Metabolism: Aspirin is rapidly hydrolyzed in the plasma to salicylic acid such that plasma levels of aspirin are essentially undetectable 1–2 hours after dosing. Salicylic acid is primarily conjugated in the liver to form salicyluric acid, a phenolic glucuronide, an acyl glucuronide, and a number of minor metabolites. Salicylic acid has a plasma half-life of approximately 6 hours. Salicylate metabolism is saturable and total body clearance decreases at higher serum concentrations due to the limited ability of the liver to form both salicyluric acid and phenolic glucuronide. Following toxic doses (10–20 grams (g)), the plasma half-life may be increased to over 20 hours.

Elimination: The elimination of salicylic acid follows zero order pharmacokinetics; (i.e., the rate of drug elimination is constant in relation to plasma concentration). Renal excretion of unchanged drug depends upon urine pH. As urinary pH rises above 6.5, the renal clearance of free salicylate increases from < 5 percent to > 80 percent. Alkalinization of the urine is a key concept in the management of salicylate overdose. (See Overdosage.) Following therapeutic doses, approximately 10 percent is found excreted in the urine as salicylic acid, 75 percent as salicyluric acid, and 10 percent phenolic and 5 percent acyl glucuronides of salicylic acid.

Pharmacodynamics: Aspirin affects platelet aggregation by irreversibly inhibiting prostaglandin cyclo-oxygenase. This effect lasts for the life of the platelet and prevents the formation of the platelet aggregating factor thromboxane A2. Non-acetylated salicylates do not inhibit this enzyme and have no effect on platelet aggregation. At somewhat higher doses, aspirin reversibly inhibits the formation of prostaglandin 1_2 (prostacyclin), which is an arterial vasodilator and inhibits platelet aggregation.

At higher doses aspirin is an effective anti-inflammatory agent, partially due to inhibition of inflammatory mediators via cyclooxygenase inhibition in peripheral tissues. In vitro studies suggest that other mediators of inflammation may also be suppressed by aspirin administration, although the precise mechanism of action has not been elucidated. It is this non-specific suppression of cyclooxygenase activity in peripheral tissues following large doses that leads to its primary side effect of gastric irritation. (See Adverse Reactions.)

Clinical Studies: Ischemic Stroke and Transient Ischemic Attack (TIA): In clinical trials of subjects with TIA's due to fibrin platelet emboli or ischemic stroke, aspirin has been shown to significantly reduce the risk of the combined endpoint of stroke or death and the combined endpoint of TIA, stroke, or death by about 13–18 percent.

Suspect Acute Myocardial Infarction (MI): In a large, multi-center study of aspirin, streptokinase, and the combination of aspirin and streptokinase in 17,187 patients with suspected acute MI, aspirin treatment produced a 23-percent reduction in the risk of vascular mortality. Aspirin was also shown to have an additional benefit in patients given a thrombolytic agent.

Prevention of Recurrent MI and Unstable Angina Pectoris: These indications are supported by the results of six large, randomized, multi-center, placebo-controlled trials of predominantly male post-MI subjects and one randomized placebo-controlled study of men with unstable angina pectoris. Aspirin therapy in MI subjects was associated with a significant reduction (about 20 percent) in the risk of the combination endpoint of subsequent death and/or nonfatal reinfarction in these patients. In aspirin-treated unstable angina patients the event rate was reduced to 5 percent from the 10 percent rate in the placebo group.

Chronic Stable Angina Pectoris: In a randomized, multi-center, double-blind trial designed to assess the role of aspirin for prevention of MI in patients with chronic stable angina pectoris, aspirin significantly reduced the primary combined endpoint of nonfatal MI, fatal MI, and sudden death by 34 percent. The secondary endpoint for vascular events (first occurrence of MI, stroke, or vascular death) was also significantly reduced (32 percent).

Revascularization Procedures: Most patients who undergo coronary artery revascularization procedures have already had symptomatic coronary artery disease for which aspirin is indicated. Similarly, patients with lesions of the carotid bifurcation sufficient to require carotid endarterectomy are likely to have had a precedent event. Aspirin is recommended for patients who undergo revascularization procedures if there is a pre-existing condition for which aspirin is already indicated.

Rheumatologic Diseases: In clinical studies in patients with rheumatoid arthritis, juvenile rheumatoid arthritis, ankylosing spondylitis and osteoarthritis, aspirin has been shown to be effective in controlling various indices of clinical disease activity.

Animal Toxicology: The acute oral 50 percent lethal dose in rats is about 1.5 g/kg and in mice 1.1 g/kg. Renal papillary necrosis and decreased urinary concentrating ability occur in rodents chronically administered high doses. Dose-dependent gastric mucosal injury occurs in rats and humans. Mammals may develop aspirin toxicosis associated with GI symptoms, circulatory effects, and central nervous system depression. (See Overdosage.)

Indications and Usage: Vascular Indications (Ischemic Stroke, TIA, Acute MI, Prevention of Recurrent MI, Unstable Angina Pectoris, and Chronic Stable Angina Pectoris): Aspirin is indicated to: (1) Reduce the combined risk of death and nonfatal stroke in patients who have had ischemic stroke or transient ischemia of the brain due to fibrin platelet emboli, (2) reduce the risk of vascular mortality in patients with a suspected acute MI, (3) reduce the combined risk of death and nonfatal MI in patients with a previous MI or unstable angina pectoris, and (4) reduce the combined risk of MI and sudden death in patients with chronic stable angina pectoris.

Revascularization Procedures (Coronary Artery Bypass Graft (CABG), Percutaneous Transluminal Coronary Angioplasty (PTCA), and Carotid Endarterectomy): Aspirin is indicated in patients who have undergone revascularization procedures (i.e., CABG, PTCA, or carotid endarterectomy) when there is a pre-existing condition for which aspirin is already indicated.

Rheumatologic Disease Indications (Rheumatoid Arthritis, Juvenile Rheumatoid Arthritis, Spondyloarthropathies, Osteoarthritis, and the Arthritis and Pleurisy of Systemic Lupus Erythematosus (SLE)): Aspirin is indicated for the relief of the signs and symptoms of rheumatoid arthritis, juvenile rheu-

Continued on next page

Ecotrin—Cont.

matoid arthritis, osteoarthritis, spondyloarthropathies, and arthritis and pleurisy associated with SLE.

Contraindications: Allergy: Aspirin is contraindicated in patients with known allergy to nonsteroidal anti-inflammatory drug products and in patients with the syndrome of asthma, rhinitis, and nasal polyps. Aspirin may cause severe urticaria, angioedema, or bronchospasm (asthma).

Reye's Syndrome: Aspirin should not be used in children or teenagers for viral infections, with or without fever, because of the risk of Reye's syndrome with concomitant use of aspirin in certain viral illnesses.

Warnings: Alcohol Warning: Patients who consume three or more alcoholic drinks every day should be counseled about the bleeding risks involved with chronic, heavy alcohol use while taking aspirin.

Coagulation Abnormalities: Even low doses of aspirin can inhibit platelet function leading to an increase in bleeding time. This can adversely affect patients with inherited (hemophilia) or acquired (liver disease or vitamin K deficiency) bleeding disorders.

GI Side Effects: GI side effects include stomach pain, heartburn, nausea, vomiting, and gross GI bleeding. Although minor upper GI symptoms, such as dyspepsia, are common and can occur anytime during therapy, physicians should remain alert for signs of ulceration and bleeding, even in the absence of previous GI symptoms. Physicians should inform patients about the signs and symptoms of GI side effects and what steps to take if they occur.

Peptic Ulcer Disease: Patients with a history of active peptic ulcer disease should avoid using aspirin, which can cause gastric mucosal irritation and bleeding.

Precautions
General

Renal Failure: Avoid aspirin in patients with severe renal failure (glomerular filtration rate less than 10 mL/minute).

Hepatic Insufficiency: Avoid aspirin in patients with severe hepatic insufficiency.

Sodium Restricted Diets: Patients with sodium-retaining states, such as congestive heart failure or renal failure, should avoid sodium-containing buffered aspirin preparations because of their high sodium content.

Laboratory Tests: Aspirin has been associated with elevated hepatic enzymes, blood urea nitrogen and serum creatinine, hyperkalemia, proteinuria, and prolonged bleeding time.

Drug Interactions

Angiotensin Converting Enzyme (ACE) Inhibitors: The hyponatremic and hypotensive effects of ACE inhibitors may be diminished by the concomitant administration of aspirin due to its direct effect on the renin-angiotensin conversion pathway.

Acetazolamide: Concurrent use of aspirin and acetazolamide can lead to high serum concentrations of acetazolamide (and toxicity) due to competition at the renal tubule for secretion.

Anticoagulant Therapy (Heparin and Warfarin): Patients on anticoagulation therapy are at increased risk for bleeding because of drug-drug interactions and the effect on platelets. Aspirin can displace warfarin from protein binding sites, leading to prolongation of both the prothrombin time and the bleeding time. Aspirin can increase the anticoagulant activity of heparin, increasing bleeding risk.

Anticonvulsants: Salicylate can displace protein-bound phenytoin and valproic acid, leading to a decrease in the total concentration of phenytoin and an increase in serum valproic acid levels.

Beta Blockers: The hypotensive effects of beta blockers may be diminished by the concomitant administration of aspirin due to inhibition of renal prostaglandins, leading to decreased renal blood flow, and salt and fluid retention.

Diuretics: The effectiveness of diuretics in patients with underlying renal or cardiovascular disease may be diminished by the concomitant administration of aspirin due to inhibition of renal prostaglandins, leading to decreased renal blood flow and salt and fluid retention.

Methotrexate: Salicylate can inhibit renal clearance of methotrexate, leading to bone marrow toxicity, especially in the elderly or renal impaired.

Nonsteroidal Anti-inflammatory Drugs (NSAID's): The concurrent use of aspirin with other NSAID's should be avoided because this may increase bleeding or lead to decreased renal function.

Oral Hypoglycemics: Moderate doses of aspirin may increase the effectiveness of oral hypoglycemic drugs, leading to hypoglycemia.

Uricosuric Agents (Probenecid and Sulfinpyrazone): Salicylates antagonize the uricosuric action of uricosuric agents.

Carcinogenesis, Mutagenesis, Impairment of Fertility: Administration of aspirin for 68 weeks at 0.5 percent in the feed of rats was not carcinogenic. In the Ames Salmonella assay, aspirin was not mutagenic; however, aspirin did induce chromosome aberrations in cultured human fibroblasts. Aspirin inhibits ovulation in rats. (See Pregnancy.)

Pregnancy: Pregnant women should only take aspirin if clearly needed. Because of the known effects of NSAID's on the fetal cardiovascular system (closure of the ductus arteriosus), use during the third trimester of pregnancy should be avoided. Salicylate products have also been associated with alterations in maternal and neonatal hemostasis mechanisms, decreased birth weight, and with perinatal mortality.

Labor and Delivery: Aspirin should be avoided 1 week prior to and during labor and delivery because it can result in excessive blood loss at delivery. Prolonged gestation and prolonged labor due to prostaglandin inhibition have been reported.

Nursing Mothers: Nursing mothers should avoid using aspirin because salicylate is excreted in breast milk. Use of high doses may lead to rashes, platelet abnormalities, and bleeding in nursing infants.

Pediatric Use: Pediatric dosing recommendations for juvenile rheumatoid arthritis are based on well-controlled clinical studies. An initial dose of 90–130 mg/kg/day in divided doses, with an increase as needed for anti-inflammatory efficacy (target plasma salicylate levels of 150–300 mcg/mL) are effective. At high doses (i.e., plasma levels of greater than 200 mg/mL), the incidence of toxicity increases.

Adverse Reactions: Many adverse reactions due to aspirin ingestion are dose-related. The following is a list of adverse reactions that have been reported in the literature. (See Warnings.)

Body as a Whole: Fever, hypothermia, thirst.

Cardiovascular: Dysrhythmias, hypotension, tachycardia.

Central Nervous System: Agitation, cerebral edema, coma, confusion, dizziness, headache, subdural or intracranial hemorrhage, lethargy, seizures.

Fluid and Electrolyte: Dehydration, hyperkalemia, metabolic acidosis, respiratory alkalosis.

Gastrointestinal: Dyspepsia, GI bleeding, ulceration and perforation, nausea, vomiting, transient elevations of hepatic enzymes, hepatitis, Reye's Syndrome, pancreatitis.

Hematologic: Prolongation of the prothrombin time, disseminated intravascular coagulation, coagulopathy, thrombocytopenia.

Hypersensitivity: Acute anaphylaxis, angioedema, asthma, bronchospasm, laryngeal edema, urticaria.

Musculoskeletal: Rhabdomyolysis.

Metabolism: Hypoglycemia (in children), hyperglycemia.

Reproductive: Prolonged pregnancy and labor, stillbirths, lower birth weight infants, antepartum and postpartum bleeding.

Respiratory: Hyperpnea, pulmonary edema, tachypnea.

Special Senses: Hearing loss, tinnitus. Patients with high frequency hearing loss may have difficulty perceiving tinnitus. In these patients, tinnitus cannot be used as a clinical indicator of salicylism.

Urogenital: Interstitial nephritis, papillary necrosis, proteinuria, renal insufficiency and failure.

Drug Abuse and Dependence: Aspirin is non-narcotic. There is no known potential for addiction associated with the use of aspirin.

Overdosage: Salicylate toxicity may result from acute ingestion (overdose) or chronic intoxication. The early signs of salicylic overdose (salicylism), including tinnitus (ringing in the ears), occur at plasma concentrations approaching 200 mcg/mL. Plasma concentrations of aspirin above 300 mcg/mL are clearly toxic. Severe toxic effects are associated with levels above 400 mcg/mL. (See Clinical Pharmacology.) A single lethal dose of aspirin in adults is not known with certainty but death may be expected at 30 g. For real or suspected overdose, a Poison Control Center should be contacted immediately. Careful medical management is essential.

Signs and Symptoms: In acute overdose, severe acid-base and electrolyte disturbances may occur and are complicated by hyperthermia and dehydration. Respiratory alkalosis occurs early while hyperventilation is present, but is quickly followed by metabolic acidosis.

Treatment: Treatment consists primarily of supporting vital functions, increasing salicylate elimination, and correcting the acid-base disturbance. Gastric emptying and/or lavage is recommended as soon as possible after ingestion, even if the patient has vomited spontaneously. After lavage and/or emesis, administration of activated charcoal, as a slurry, is beneficial, if less than 3 hours have passed since ingestion. Charcoal adsorption should not be employed prior to emesis and lavage.

Severity of aspirin intoxication is determined by measuring the blood salicylate level. Acid-base status should be closely followed with serial blood gas and serum pH measurements. Fluid and electrolyte balance should be maintained.

In severe cases, hyperthermia and hypovolemia are the major immediate threats to life. Children should be sponged with tepid water. Replacement fluid should be administered intravenously and augmented with correction of acidosis. Plasma electrolytes and pH should be monitored to promote alkaline diuresis of salicylate if renal function is normal. Infusion of glucose may be required to control hypoglycemia.

Hemodialysis and peritoneal dialysis can be performed to reduce the body drug content. In patients with renal insufficiency or in cases of life-threatening intoxication, dialysis is usually required. Exchange transfusion may be indicated in infants and young children.

Dosage and Administration: Each dose of aspirin should be taken with a full glass of water unless patient is fluid restricted. Anti-inflammatory and analgesic dosages should be individualized. When aspirin is used in high doses, the development of tinnitus may be used as a clinical sign of elevated plasma salicylate levels except in patients with high frequency hearing loss.

Ischemic Stroke and TIA: 50–325 mg once a day. Continue therapy indefinitely.

Suspected Acute MI: The initial dose of 160–162.5 mg is administered as soon as an MI is suspected. The maintenance dose of 160–162.5 mg a day is continued for 30 days post infarction. After 30 days, consider further therapy based on dosage and administration for prevention of recurrent MI.

Prevention of Recurrent MI: 75–325 mg once a day. Continue therapy indefinitely.

Unstable Angina Pectoris: 75–325 mg once a day. Continue therapy indefinitely.

Chronic Stable Angina Pectoris: 75–325 mg once a day. Continue therapy indefinitely.

CABG: 325 mg daily starting 6 hours post-procedure. Continue therapy for 1 year post-procedure.

PTCA: The initial dose of 325 mg should be given 2 hours pre-surgery. Maintenance dose is 160–325 mg daily. Continue therapy indefinitely.

Carotid Endarterectomy: Doses of 80 mg once daily to 650 mg twice daily, started presurgery, are recommended. Continue therapy indefinitely.

Rheumatoid Arthritis: The initial dose is 3 g a day in divided doses. Increase as needed for anti-inflammatory efficacy with target plasma salicylate levels of 150–300 mcg/mL. At high doses (i.e., plasma levels of greater than 200 mg/mL), the incidence of toxicity increases.

Juvenile Rheumatoid Arthritis: Initial dose is 90–130 mg/kg/day in divided doses. Increase as needed for anti-inflammatory efficacy with target plasma salicylate levels of 150–300 mcg/mL. At high doses (i.e., plasma levels of greater than 200 mg/mL), the incidence of toxicity increases.

Spondyloarthropathies: Up to 4 g per day in divided doses.

Osteoarthritis: Up to 3 g per day in divided doses.

Arthritis and Pleurisy of SLE: The initial dose is 3 g a day in divided doses. Increase as needed for anti-inflammatory efficacy with target plasma salicylate levels of 150–300 mcg/mL. At high doses (i.e., plasma levels of greater than 200 mg/mL), the incidence of toxicity increases.

How Supplied: 81 mg convex orange film coated tablet with ECOTRIN LOW printed in black ink on one side of the tablet. Available as follows

NDC 0108-0117-82 Bottle of 36 tablets
NDC 0108-0117-83 Bottle of 120 tablets
325 mg convex orange film coated tablet with ECOTRIN REG printed in black ink on one side of the tablet. Available as follows:

NDC 0108-0014-26 Bottle of 100 tablets
NDC 0108-0014-29 Bottle of 250 tablets
500 mg convex orange film coated tablet with ECOTRIN MAX printed in black ink on one side of the tablet. Available as follows:

NDC 0108-0016-23 Bottle of 60 tablets
NDC 0108-0016-27 Bottle of 150 tablets

Store in a tight container at 25°C (77° F); excursions permitted to 15–30° C (59–86° F).

Shown in Product Identification Guide, page 507

GAVISCON® Regular Strength Antacid Tablets
[găv 'ĭs-kŏn]

Composition: Each chewable tablet contains the following active ingredients: Aluminum hydroxide dried gel... 80 mg Magnesium trisilicate .... 20 mg and the following inactive ingredients: alginic acid, calcium stearate, flavor, sodium bicarbonate, starch (may contain corn starch), and sucrose.

Actions: Unique formulation produces soothing foam which floats on stomach contents. Foam containing antacid precedes stomach contents into the esophagus when reflux occurs to help protect the sensitive mucosa from further irritation. GAVISCON® acts locally without neutralizing entire stomach contents to help maintain integrity of the digestive process. Endoscopic studies indicate that GAVISCON Antacid Tablets are equally as effective in the erect or supine patient.

Indications: GAVISCON is specifically formulated for the temporary relief of heartburn (acid indigestion) due to acid reflux. GAVISCON is not indicated for the treatment of peptic ulcers.

Directions: Chew 2 to 4 tablets four times a day or as directed by a physician. Tablets should be taken after meals and at bedtime or as needed. For best results follow by a half glass of water or other liquid. DO NOT SWALLOW WHOLE.

Warnings: Do not take more than 16 tablets in a 24-hour period or 16 tablets daily for more than 2 weeks, except under the advice and supervision of a physician. Do not use this product except under the advice and supervision of a physician if you are on a sodium-restricted diet. Each GAVISCON Tablet contains approximately 19 mg of sodium.

Drug Interaction Precaution: Antacids may interact with certain prescription drugs. If you are presently taking a prescription drug, do not take this product without checking with your physician or other health professional.

Store at a controlled room temperature in a dry place.

Keep this and all drugs out of the reach of children. In case of accidental overdose, seek professional assistance or contact a poison control center immediately.

How Supplied: Bottles of 100 tablets and in foil-wrapped 2s in boxes of 30 tablets.

Shown in Product Identification Guide, page 508

Continued on next page

GAVISCON® EXTRA STRENGTH
Antacid Tablets

[găv 'ĭs-kŏn]

Composition: Each chewable tablet contains the following active ingredients:
Aluminum hydroxide .... 160 mg
Magnesium carbonate .... 105 mg
and the following inactive ingredients: alginic acid, calcium stearate, flavor, sodium bicarbonate, and sucrose. May contain stearic acid. Contains sorbitol or mannitol. May contain starch.

Actions: Gavison's unique antacid foam barrier neutralizes stomach acid.

Indications: For the relief of heartburn, sour stomach, acid indigestion and upset stomach associated with these conditions.

Directions: Chew 2 to 4 tablets four times a day or as directed by a physician. Tablets should be taken after meals and at bedtime or as needed. For best results follow by a half glass of water or other liquid. DO NOT SWALLOW WHOLE.

Warnings: Do not take more than 16 tablets in a 24-hour period or 16 tablets daily for more than 2 weeks, except under the advice and supervision of a physician. Do not use this product except under the advice and supervision of a physician if you are on a sodium-restricted diet. Each Extra Strength Gaviscon tablet contains approximately 19 mg of sodium.

Drug Interaction Precaution: Antacids may interact with certain prescription drugs. If you are presently taking a prescription drug, do not take this product without checking with your physician or other health professional.

Store at a controlled room temperature in a dry place.

Keep this and all drugs out of the reach of children. In case of accidental overdose, seek professional assistance or contact a poison control center immediately.

How Supplied: Bottles of 100 tablets and in foil-wrapped 2s in boxes of 6 and 30 tablets.

Shown in Product Identification Guide, page 508

GAVISCON® Regular Strength
Liquid Antacid

[găv 'ĭs-kŏn]

Composition: Each tablespoonful (15 ml) contains the following active ingredients:
Aluminum hydroxide .... 95 mg
Magnesium carbonate .... 358 mg
and the following inactive ingredients: Benzyl alcohol, D&C Yellow #10, edetate disodium, FD&C Blue #1, flavor, glycerin, saccharin sodium, sodium alginate, sorbitol solution, water, and xanthan gum.

Actions: Gaviscon's unique antacid foam barrier neutralizes stomach acid.

Indications: For the relief of heartburn, sour stomach, acid indigestion and upset stomach associated with these conditions.

Directions: SHAKE WELL BEFORE USING. Take 1 or 2 tablespoonfuls four times a day or as directed by a physician. GAVISCON Regular Strength Liquid should be taken after meals and at bedtime. Dispense product only by spoon or other measuring device.

Warnings: Except under the advice and supervision of a physician, do not take more than 8 tablespoonfuls in a 24-hour period or 8 tablespoonfuls daily for more than 2 weeks. May have laxative effect. Do not use this product if you have a kidney disease. Do not use this product if you are on a sodium-restricted diet except under the advice and supervision of a physician. Each tablespoonful of GAVISCON Regular Strength Liquid contains approximately 1.7 mEq sodium.

Keep this and all drugs out of the reach of children. In case of accidental overdose, seek professional assistance or contact a poison control center immediately.

Drug Interaction Precaution: Antacids may interact with certain prescription drugs. If you are presently taking a prescription drug, do not take this product without checking with your physician or other health professional.

Keep tightly closed. Avoid freezing. Store at a controlled room temperature.

How Supplied: 12 fluid oz (355 ml) bottles.

Shown in Product Identification Guide, page 507

GAVISCON® EXTRA STRENGTH
Liquid Antacid

[găv 'ĭs-kŏn]

Composition: Each 2 teaspoonfuls (10 mL) contains the following active ingredients:
Aluminum hydroxide .... 508 mg
Magnesium carbonate .... 475 mg
and the following inactive ingredients: Benzyl alcohol, edetate disodium, flavor, glycerin, saccharin sodium, simethicone emulsion, sodium alginate, sorbitol solution, water, and xanthan gum.

Actions: Gaviscon's unique antacid foam barrier neutralizes stomach acid.

Indications: For the relief of heartburn, sour stomach, acid indigestion and upset stomach associated with these conditions.

Directions: SHAKE WELL BEFORE USING. Take 2 to 4 teaspoonfuls four times a day or as directed by a physician. GAVISCON Extra Strength Liquid should be taken after meals and at bedtime. Dispense product only by spoon or other measuring device.

Warnings: Except under the advice and supervision of a physician, do not take more than 16 teaspoonfuls in a 24-hour period or 16 teaspoonfuls daily for more than 2 weeks. May have laxative effect. Do not use this product if you have a kidney disease. Do not use this product if you are on a sodium-restricted diet except under the advice and supervision of a physician. Each teaspoonful contains approximately 0.9 mEq sodium.

Keep this and all drugs out of the reach of children. In case of accidental overdose, seek professional assistance or contact a poison control center immediately.

Drug Interaction Precaution: Antacids may interact with certain prescription drugs. If you are presently taking a prescription drug, do not take this product without checking with your physician or other health professional.

Keep tightly closed. Avoid freezing. Store at a controlled room temperature.

How Supplied: 12 fl oz (355 mL) bottles.

Shown in Product Identification Guide, page 508

GLY–OXIDE® Liquid

Description/Active Ingredient: GLY-OXIDE® Liquid contains carbamide peroxide 10%.

Actions: Gly-Oxide is specially formulated to release peroxide and oxygen bubbles in your mouth. The peroxide and oxygen-rich microfoam help:
- gently remove unhealthy tissue, then cleanse and soothe canker sores and minor wounds and inflammations so natural healing can better occur.
- kill odor-forming germs.
- foam and flush out food particles ordinary brushing can miss.
- clean stains from orthodontics/dentures/bridgework/etc. better than brushing alone.

Indications For Temporary Use: Gly-Oxide liquid is for temporary use in cleansing canker sores and minor wound or gum inflammation resulting from minor dental procedures, dentures, orthodontic appliances, accidental injury, or other irritations of the mouth and gums. Gly-Oxide can also be used to guard against the risk of infections in the mouth and gums.

Everyday Uses: Gly-Oxide may be used routinely to improve oral hygiene as an aid to regular brushing or when regular brushing is inadequate or impossible such as total care geriatrics, etc. Gly-Oxide kills germs to reduce mouth odors and/or odors on dental appliances. Gly-Oxide penetrates between teeth and other areas of the mouth to flush out food particles ordinary brushing can miss. This can be especially useful when brushing is made more difficult by the presence of orthodontics or other dental appliances. Plus, Gly-Oxide helps remove stains on dental appliances to improve appearance.

Directions For Temporary Use: Do not dilute. Replace tip on bottle when not in use. **Adults and children 2 years of age and older:** Apply several drops directly from bottle onto affected area; spit out after 2 to 3 minutes. Use up to four times daily after meals and at bedtime or as directed by dentist or doctor. OR place 10 drops on tongue, mix with saliva, swish for several minutes, and then spit out. Use by children under 12 years of age should be supervised. **Children under 2 years of age:** Consult a dentist or doctor.

Directions For Everyday Use: The product may be used following the temporary use directions above. OR apply Gly-Oxide to the toothbrush (it will sink into the brush), cover with toothpaste, brush normally, and spit out.

Warnings: Severe or persistent oral inflammation, denture irritation, or gingivitis may be serious. If sore mouth symptoms do not improve in 7 days, or if irritation, pain, or redness persists or worsens, or if swelling, rash, or fever develops, discontinue use of product and see your dentist or doctor promptly. Avoid contact with eyes. **KEEP THIS AND ALL DRUGS OUT OF THE REACH OF CHILDREN.** In case of accidental overdose, seek professional assistance or contact a poison control center immediately.

Inactive Ingredients: Citric Acid, Flavor, Glycerin, Propylene Glycol, Sodium Stannate, Water, and Other Ingredients.
Protect from excessive heat and direct sunlight.

How Supplied: GLY-OXIDE® Liquid is available in ½-fl-oz and 2-fl-oz plastic squeeze bottles with applicator spouts. Comments or Questions? Call Toll-free 1-800-245-1040 Weekdays
SmithKline Beecham Consumer Healthcare, L.P.
Moon Township, PA 15108

Made in U.S.A.

Shown in Product Identification Guide, page 508

GOODY'S
Body Pain Formula Powder

Indications: For temporary relief of minor body aches & pains due to muscular aches, arthritis & headaches.

Directions: Adults: Place one powder on tongue and follow with liquid, or stir powder into a glass of water or other liquid. May be repeated in 4 to 6 hours. Do not take more than 4 powders in any 24-hour period. Children under 12 years of age: Consult a doctor.

Warnings: Children and teenagers should not use this medicine for chicken pox or flu symptoms before a doctor is consulted about Reye's Syndrome, a rare but serious illness reported to be associated with aspirin. Do not use with any other product containing acetaminophen. Ask a doctor before use if you have asthma, ulcers, a bleeding problem, stomach problems that last or come back such as heartburn, upset stomach or pain. Ask a doctor or pharmacist before use if you are taking a prescription drug for gout, diabetes, arthritis or anticoagulation (blood thinning). Stop use and ask a doctor if an allergic reaction occurs, ringing in ears or loss of hearing occurs, pain gets worse or persists for more than 10 days, fever lasts more than 3 days, redness or swelling occur. As with any drug, if you are pregnant, or nursing a baby, seek the advice of a health professional before using this product.
IT IS ESPECIALLY IMPORTANT NOT TO USE ASPIRIN DURING THE LAST 3 MONTHS OF PREGNANCY UNLESS SPECIFICALLY DIRECTED TO DO SO BY A DOCTOR BECAUSE IT MAY CAUSE PROBLEMS IN THE UNBORN CHILD OR COMPLICATIONS DURING DELIVERY.
Alcohol Warning: If you consume 3 or more alcoholic drinks every day, ask your doctor whether you should take acetaminophen and aspirin or other pain relievers/fever reducers. Acetaminophen and aspirin may cause liver damage and stomach bleeding.
Keep this and all medicines out of the reach of children. Overdose warning: Taking more than the recommended dose can cause serious health problems. In case of overdose, contact a doctor or poison control center immediately.

Active Ingredients: Each powder contains: 500 mg. aspirin and 325 mg. acetaminophen.

Inactive Ingredients: Each powder contains: Lactose Monohydrate and Potassium Chloride.

GOODY'S®
Extra Strength Headache Powder

Indications: For Temporary Relief of Minor Aches & Pains Due to Headaches, Arthritis, Colds & Fever

Directions: Adults: Place one powder on tongue and follow with liquid or stir powder into a glass of water or other liquid. May be repeated in 4 to 6 hours. Do not take more than 4 powders in any 24-hour period. Children under 12 years of age: Consult a doctor.

Warnings: Children and teenagers should not use this medicine for chicken pox or flu symptoms before a doctor is consulted about Reye's Syndrome, a rare but serious illness reported to be associated with aspirin. Do not use with any other product containing acetaminophen. **Ask a doctor before use if you have** asthma, ulcers, a bleeding problem, stomach prob-

lems that last or come back such as heartburn, upset stomach or pain. **Ask a doctor or pharmacist before use** if you are taking a prescription drug for gout, diabetes, arthritis or anticoagulation (blood thinning). **When using this product** limit the use of caffeine containing drugs, foods, or drinks, because too much caffeine may cause nervousness, irritability, sleeplessness, and occasionally, rapid heartbeat. **Stop use and ask a doctor if** an allergic reaction occurs, ringing in ears or loss of hearing occurs, pain gets worse or persists for more than 10 days, fever lasts for more than 3 days, redness or swelling is present, or new symptoms occur. As with any drug, if you are pregnant, or nursing a baby, seek the advice of a health professional before using this product.
IT IS ESPECIALLY IMPORTANT NOT TO USE ASPIRIN DURING THE LAST 3 MONTHS OF PREGNANCY UNLESS SPECIFICALLY DIRECTED TO DO SO BY A DOCTOR BECAUSE IT MAY CAUSE PROBLEMS IN THE UNBORN CHILD OR COMPLICATIONS DURING DELIVERY.
Alcohol Warning: If you consume 3 or more alcoholic drinks every day, ask your doctor whether you should take acetaminophen and aspirin or other pain relievers/fever reducers. Acetaminophen and aspirin may cause liver damage and stomach bleeding. **Keep this and all medicines out of the reach of children. Overdose warning:** Taking more than the recommended dose can cause serious health problems. In case of overdose, contact a doctor or poison control center immediately.

Active Ingredients: Each Powder contains 520 mg. aspirin in combination with 260 mg. acetaminophen and 32.5 mg. caffeine.

Inactive Ingredients: Lactose Monohydrate and Potassium Chloride.

GOODY'S®
Extra Strength Pain Relief Tablets

Indications: Goody's EXTRA STRENGTH tablets are a specially developed pain reliever that provide fast & effective temporary relief from minor aches & pain due to headaches, arthritis, colds or "flu," muscle strain, backache & menstrual discomfort. It is recommended for temporary relief of toothaches and to reduce fever.

Dosage: Adults: Two tablets with water or other liquid. May be repeated in 4 to 6 hours. Do not take more than 8 tablets in any 24-hour period. Children under 12 years of age: Consult a doctor.

Warnings: Children and teenagers should not use this medicine for chicken pox or flu symptoms before a doctor is consulted about Reye's Syndrome, a rare but serious illness

Continued on next page

Goody's Pain Relief—Cont.

reported to be associated with aspirin. **Do not use** with any other product containing acetaminophen. **Ask a doctor before use if you have** asthma, ulcers, a bleeding problem, stomach problems that last or come back such as heartburn, upset stomach or pain. **Ask a doctor or pharmacist before use** if you are taking a prescription drug for gout, diabetes, arthritis or anticoagulation (blood thinning) **When using this product** limit the use of caffeine containing drugs, foods, or drinks, because too much caffeine may cause nervousness, irritability, sleeplessness, and occasionally, rapid heartbeat. **Stop use and ask a doctor if** an allergic reaction occurs, ringing in ears or loss of hearing occurs, pain gets worse or persists for more than 10 days, fever lasts more than 3 days, redness or swelling is present, or new symptoms occur.

As with any drug, if you are pregnant, or nursing a baby, seek the advice of a health professional before using this product. IT IS ESPECIALLY IMPORTANT NOT TO USE ASPIRIN DURING THE LAST 3 MONTHS OF PREGNANCY UNLESS SPECIFICALLY DIRECTED TO DO SO BY A DOCTOR BECAUSE IT MAY CAUSE PROBLEMS IN THE UNBORN CHILD OR COMPLICATIONS DURING DELIVERY. **Alcohol Warning:** If you consume 3 or more alcoholic drinks every day, ask your doctor whether you should take acetaminophen and aspirin or other pain relievers/fever reducers. Acetaminophen and aspirin may cause liver damage and stomach bleeding. **Keep this and all medicines out of the reach of children. Overdose warning:** Taking more than the recommended dose can cause serious health problems. In case of overdose, contact a doctor or poison control center immediately. **Active Ingredients:** Each tablet contains 260 mg. aspirin in combination with 130 mg. acetaminophen and 16.25 mg. caffeine. **Inactive Ingredients:** Corn Starch, Crospovidone, Povidone, Pregelatinized Starch and Stearic Acid.

GOODY'S PM® POWDER
For Pain with Sleeplessness

Indications: For temporary relief of occasional headaches and minor aches and pains with accompanying sleeplessness.

Directions: Adults and children 12 years of age and older: One dose (2 powders). Take both powders at bedtime, if needed, or as directed by a doctor. Place powders on tongue and follow with liquid. If you prefer, stir powders into glass of water or other liquid.

Warnings: Keep this and all medicines out of the reach of children. Overdose Warning: Taking more than the recommended dose can cause serious health problems. In case of accidental overdose, contact a doctor or poison control center immediately. Prompt medical attention is critical for adults as well as for children even if you do not notice any signs or symptoms.

As with any drug, if you are pregnant or nursing a baby, seek the advice of a health professional before using this product. Do not give this product to children under 12 years of age. Do not use for more than 10 days or for fever for more than 3 days unless directed by a doctor. Consult your doctor if redness or swelling is present, symptoms persist or get worse or new ones occur. If sleeplessness persists continuously for more than 2 weeks consult your doctor. Insomnia may be a symptom of serious underlying medical illness. Do not take this product, unless directed by a doctor, if you have a breathing problem such as emphysema or chronic bronchitis or if you have glaucoma or difficulty in urination due to enlargement of the prostate gland. **Do Not Use** with any other product containing diphenhydramine, including one applied topically, or with any other product containing acetaminophen. Avoid alcoholic beverages while taking this product. Do not use this product if you are taking sedatives or tranquilizers without first consulting your doctor. **Alcohol Warning:** If you consume 3 or more alcoholic drinks every day, ask your doctor whether you should take acetaminophen or other pain relievers/fever reducers. Acetaminophen may cause liver damage.

Caution: This product will cause drowsiness. Do not drive a motor vehicle or operate machinery after use.

Active Ingredients: Each powder contains 500 mg. Acetaminophen and 38 mg. Diphenhydramine Citrate.

Inactive Ingredients: Citric Acid, Docusate Sodium, Fumaric Acid, Glycine, Lactose Monohydrate, Magnesium Stearate, Potassium Chloride, Silica Gel, Sodium Citrate Dihydrate.

MASSENGILL®
[mas 'sen-gil]
Baby Powder Scent Soft Cloth Towelette

Ingredients: Purified Water, Octoxynol-9, Lactic Acid, Disodium Edta, Fragrance, Potassium Sorbate, Cetylpyridinium Chloride, and Sodium Bicarbonate.

Indications: For cleansing and refreshing the external vaginal area.

Actions: Massengill Baby Powder Scent Soft Cloth Towelette safely cleanse the external vaginal area. The towelette delivery system makes the application soft and gentle.

Directions: Remove towelette from foil packet, unfold, and gently wipe from front to back. After towelette has been used once, return towelette to foil packet and throw it away. Safe to use daily as often as needed. For external use only.

How Supplied: 50 individually sealed soft cloth towelettes per carton. Comments, questions or for information about STD's and vaginal health, call toll free 1-800-245-1040 weekdays.

MASSENGILL Feminine Cleansing Wash, Floral
[mas 'sen-gil]

Ingredients: Purified Water, sodium laureth sulfate, magnesium laureth sulfate, sodium laureth-8 sulfate, magnesium laureth-8 sulfate, sodium oleth sulfate, magnesium oleth sulfate, lauramidopropyl betaine, myristamine oxide, lactic acid, PEG-120 methyl glucose dioleate, fragrance, sodium methylparaben, sodium ethylparaben, sodium propylparaben, methylchloroisothiazolinone, methylisothiazolinone, D&C Red #33.

Indications: For cleansing and refreshing of external vaginal area.

Actions: Massengill feminine cleansing wash safely and gently cleanses the external vaginal area.

Directions: Pour small amount into palm of hand or wash cloth and lather into wet skin. Rinse clean. Safe to use daily. For external use only.

How Supplied: 8 fl. oz plastic flip-top bottle.
Shown in Product Identification Guide, page 508

EDUCATIONAL MATERIAL

"The facts about Vaginal Infections and STDs"
A guide for women on vaginal infections and sexually transmitted diseases (STDs).
Free to physicians, pharmacists and patients in limited quantities by writing GlaxoSmithKline Consumer Healthcare, L.P. PO Box 1469, Pittsburgh, PA 15230 or calling 1-800-366-8900.
GlaxoSmithKline Consumer Healthcare, L.P.
1000 GSK Drive
Moon Township, PA 15108

NICODERM® CQ®
Nicotine Transdermal System/Stop Smoking Aid

Formerly available only by prescription Available as:

Step 1 - 21 mg/24 hours
Step 2 - 14 mg/24 hours
Step 3 - 7 mg/24 hours

If you smoke:
More than 10 Cigarettes per Day:
Start with Step 1
10 Cigarettes a Day or Less:
Start with Step 2
WHAT IS THE NICODERM CQ PATCH AND HOW IS IT USED?
NicoDerm CQ is a small, nicotine containing patch. When you put on a NicoDerm CQ patch, nicotine passes through the skin and into your body. NicoDerm CQ is very thin and uses special material to control how fast nicotine passes through the skin. Unlike the sudden jolts of nicotine delivered by cigarettes, the amount of nicotine you receive remains relatively smooth throughout the 24 or 16 hours period you wear the NicoDerm CQ patch. This helps to reduce cravings you may have for nicotine.

Active Ingredient: Nicotine

Purpose: Stop Smoking Aid

Use: reduces withdrawal symptoms, including nicotine craving, associated with quitting smoking

Directions:
• **if you are under 18 years of age, ask a doctor before use**
• before using this product, read the enclosed user's guide for complete directions and other information
• stop smoking completely when you begin using the patch
• **if you smoke more than 10 cigarettes per day**, use according to the following 10 week schedule:

STEP 1	STEP 2	STEP 3
Use one 21 mg patch/day	Use one 14 mg patch/day	Use one 7 mg patch/day
Weeks 1–6	Weeks 7–8	Weeks 9–10

• if you smoke **10 or less cigarettes per day**, do not use **STEP 1 (21 mg)**. Start with **STEP 2 (14 mg)** for 6 weeks, then **STEP 3 (7 mg)** for two weeks and then stop.
• steps 2 and 3 allow you to gradually reduce your level of nicotine. Completing the full program will increase your chances of quitting successfully.
• apply one new patch every 24 hours on skin that is dry, clean and hairless
• remove backing from patch and immediately press onto skin. Hold for 10 seconds.
• wash hands after applying or removing patch. Throw away the patch in the enclosed disposal tray. See enclosed user's guide for safety and handling.
• you may wear the patch for 16 or 24 hours
• if you crave cigarettes when you wake up, wear the patch for 24 hours
• if you have vivid dreams or other sleep disturbances, you may remove the patch at bedtime and apply a new one in the morning
• the used patch should be removed and a new one applied to a different skin site at the same time each day
• do not wear more than one patch at a time
• do not cut patch in half or into smaller pieces

• do not leave patch on for more than 24 hours because it may irritate your skin and loses strength after 24 hours
• stop using the patch at the end of 10 weeks. If you started with **STEP 2**, stop using the patch at the end of 8 weeks. If you still feel the need to use the patch talk to your doctor.

Warnings:
If you are pregnant or breast-feeding, only use this medicine on the advice of your health care provider. Smoking can seriously harm your child. Try to stop smoking without using any nicotine replacement medicine. This medicine is believed to be safer than smoking. However, the risks to your child from this medicine are not fully known.

Do Not Use
• if you continue to smoke, chew tobacco, use snuff, or use a nicotine gum or other nicotine containing products

Ask a doctor before use if you have
• heart disease, recent heart attack, or irregular heartbeat. Nicotine can increase your heart rate.
• high blood pressure not controlled with medication. Nicotine can increase your blood pressure.
• an allergy to adhesive tape or skin problems because you are more likely to get rashes

Ask a doctor or pharmacist before use if you are
• using a non-nicotine stop smoking drug
• taking a prescription medication for depression or asthma. Your prescription dose may need to be adjusted.

When using this product
• do not smoke even when not wearing the patch. The nicotine in your skin will still be entering your blood stream for several hours after you take off the patch.
• if you have vivid dreams or other sleep disturbances remove this patch at bedtime

Stop use and ask a doctor if
• skin redness caused by the patch does not go away after four days, or if skin swells, or you get a rash
• irregular heartbeat or palpitations occur
• you get symptoms of nicotine overdose such as nausea, vomiting, dizziness, weakness and rapid heartbeat

Keep out of reach of children and pets. Used patches have enough nicotine to poison children and pets. If swallowed, get medical help or contact a Poison Control Center right away. Dispose of the used patches by folding sticky ends together and inserting in disposal tray in this box.

READ THE LABEL
Read the carton and the User's Guide before using this product. Keep the carton and User's Guide. They contain important information.

Inactive Ingredients: Ethylene vinyl acetate-copolymer, polyisobutylene and high density polyethylene between pigmented and clear polyester backings.
Store at 20–25°C (68–77°F)

TO INCREASE YOUR SUCCESS IN QUITTING:
1. You must be motivated to quit.

2. Complete the full treatment program, applying a new patch every day.
3. Use with a support program as described in the Users Guide.

NicoDerm CQ User's Guide
KEYS TO SUCCESS
1) You must really want to quit smoking for **NicoDerm® CQ®** to help you.
2) Complete the full program, applying a new patch every day.
3) **NicoDerm CQ** works best when used together with a support program: See page 3 for details.
4) If you have trouble using **NicoDerm CQ**, ask your doctor or pharmacist or call GlaxoSmithKline 1-800-834-5895 weekdays (10:00 am 4:30 pm EST).

SO, YOU'VE DECIDED TO QUIT.
Congratulations. Your decision to stop smoking is one of the most important things you can do to improve your health. Quitting smoking is a two-part process that involves:
1) overcoming your physical need for nicotine, and
2) breaking your smoking habit.
NicoDerm CQ helps smokers quit by reducing nicotine withdrawal symptoms.
Many NicoDerm CQ users will be able to stop smoking for a few days but often will start smoking again. Most smokers have to try to quit several times before they completely stop.
Your own chances of quitting smoking depend on how strongly you are addicted to nicotine, how much you want to quit, and how closely you follow a quitting plan like the one that comes with NicoDerm CQ.

QUITTING SMOKING IS HARD!
If you find you cannot stop or if you start smoking again after using NicoDerm CQ please talk to a health care professional who can help you find a program that may work better for you. Breaking this addiction doesn't happen overnight.
Because NicoDerm CQ provides some nicotine, the NicoDerm CQ patch will help you stop smoking by reducing nicotine withdrawal symptoms such as nicotine craving, nervousness and irritability.
This User's Guide will give you support as you become a non-smoker. It will answer common questions about NicoDerm CQ and give tips to help you stop smoking, and should be referred to often.

WHERE TO GET HELP.
You are more likely to stop smoking by using NicoDerm CQ with a support program that helps you break your smoking habit. There may be support groups in your area for people trying to quit. Call your local chapter of the American Lung Association, American Cancer Society or American Heart Association for further information. Toll free phone numbers are printed on the wallet card on the back cover of this User's Guide.
If you find you cannot stop smoking or if you start smoking again after using NicoDerm CQ, remember breaking this addiction doesn't happen overnight. You may want to talk to a health care profes-

Continued on next page

Nicoderm CQ—Cont.

sional who can help you improve your chances of quitting the next time you try NicoDerm CQ or another method.

LET'S GET ORGANIZED.

Your reason for quitting may be a combination of concerns about health, the effect of smoking on your appearance, and pressure from your family and friends to stop smoking. Or maybe you're concerned about the dangerous effect of second-hand smoke on the people you care about.

All of these are good reasons. You probably have others. Decide your most important reasons, and write them down on the wallet card inside the back cover of this User's Guide. Carry this card with you. In difficult moments, when you want to smoke, the card will remind you why you are quitting.

WHAT YOU'RE UP AGAINST.

Smoking is addictive in two ways. Your need for nicotine has become both physical and mental. You must overcome both addictions to stop smoking. So while NicoDerm CQ will lessen your body's craving for nicotine, you've got to want to quit smoking to overcome the mental dependence on cigarettes. Once you've decided that you're going to quit, it's time to get started. But first, there are some important cautions you should consider.

SOME IMPORTANT WARNINGS.

This product is only for those who want to stop smoking.

If you are pregnant or breast-feeding, only use this medicine on the advice of your health care provider. Smoking can seriously harm your child. Try to stop smoking without using any nicotine replacement medicine. This medicine is believed to be safer than smoking. However, the risks to your child from this medicine are not fully known.

Do not use
- if you continue to smoke, chew tobacco, use snuff or use a nicotine gum or other nicotine products.

Ask a doctor before use if you have:
- heart disease, recent heart attack, or irregular heartbeat. Nicotine can increase your heart rate.
- high blood pressure not controlled with medication. Nicotine can increase your blood pressure.
- an allergy to adhesive tape or have skin problems because you are more likely to get rashes.

Ask a doctor or pharmacist before use if you are
- using a non-nicotine stop smoking drug
- taking a prescription medication for asthma or depression. Your prescription dose may need to be adjusted.

When using this product:
- do not smoke even when not wearing the patch. The nicotine in your skin will still be entering your bloodstream for several hours after you take off the patch.
- you have vivid dreams or other sleep disturbances remove this patch at bedtime.

Stop use and ask a doctor if:
- skin redness caused by the patch does not go away after four days, or if your skin swells or you get a rash.
- irregular heartbeat or palpitations occur
- you get symptoms of nicotine overdose, such as nausea, vomiting, dizziness, weakness and rapid heartbeat.

Keep out of reach of children and pets. Used patches have enough nicotine to poison children and pets. If swallowed, get medical help or contact a Poison Control Center right away. Dispose of the used patches by folding sticky ends together and inserting in the disposal tray in this box.

LET'S GET STARTED.

If you are under 18 years of age, ask a doctor before use.

Becoming a non-smoker starts today. Your first step is to read through this entire User's Guide carefully.

First, check that you bought the right starting dose.

If you smoke more than 10 cigarettes a day, begin with Step 1 (21 mg). As the carton indicates, people who smoke 10 or less cigarettes per day should not use Step 1 (21 mg). They should start with Step 2 (14 mg). Throughout this User's Guide we will give specific instructions for people who smoke 10 or less cigarettes per day.

Next, set your personalized quitting schedule.

Take out a calendar that you can use to track your progress. Pick a quit date, and mark this on your calendar using the stickers in the middle of this User's Guide, as described below.

DIRECTIONS: FOR PEOPLE WHO SMOKE MORE THAN 10 CIGARETTES PER DAY

STEP 1. (Weeks 1–6). Your quit date (and the day you'll start using Nico-Derm CQ patch).

Choose your quit date (it should be soon).

This is the day you will quit smoking cigarettes entirely and begin using NicoDerm CQ to reduce your cravings for nicotine. Place the Step 1 sticker on this date. For the first six weeks, you'll use the highest-strength (21 mg) NicoDerm CQ patches. Be sure to follow the directions on page 10.

Completing the full program will increase your chances of quitting successfully. This is done by changing over to the Step 2 (14mg) patch for 2 weeks followed by a final 2 weeks with the Step 3 (7mg) patch. The Step 2 and Step 3 treatment periods allow you to gradually reduce the amount of nicotine you get, rather than stopping suddenly, and will increase your chances of quitting.

STEP 2. (Weeks 7–8). The day you'll start reducing your use of NicoDerm CQ patch.

Switching to Step 2 (14mg) patches after 6 weeks begins to gradually reduce your nicotine usage. Place the Step 2 sticker on this date (the first day of week seven). Use the 14mg patches for two weeks.

STEP 3. (Weeks 9–10). The day you'll further start reducing your use of Nico-Derm CQ patch.

After eight weeks, nicotine intake is further reduced by moving down to Step 3 (7mg) patches. Place the Step 3 sticker on this date (the first day of week nine). Use the 7 mg patches for two weeks.

THE NICODERM CQ PROGRAM

STEP 1	STEP 2	STEP 3
Use one 21 mg patch/day	Use one 14 mg patch/day	Use one 7 mg patch/day
Weeks 1–6	Weeks 7–8	Weeks 9–10

STOP USING NICODERM CQ AT THE END OF WEEK 10. If you still feel the need to use the patch after Week 10, talk with your doctor or health professional.

DIRECTIONS: FOR PEOPLE WHO SMOKE 10 OR LESS CIGARETTES PER DAY

Do not use Step 1 (21 mg).

Begin with STEP 2 – Initial Treatment Period (Weeks 1–6): 14mg patches.

Choose our quit date (it should be soon). This is the Day you will quit smoking cigarettes entirely and begin using NicoDerm CQ to reduce your cravings for nicotine. Place the Step 2 sticker on this date. For the first six weeks, you'll use the Step 2 (14mg) NicoDerm CQ patches. Be sure to follow the directions on page 10.

Continue with STEP 3 – Step Down Treatment Period (Weeks 7–8): 7mg patches.

Completing the full program will increase your chances of quitting successfully. This is done by changing over to the Step 3 (7mg) patches for 2 weeks. The two week step down treatment period allows you to gradually reduce the amount of nicotine you get, rather than stopping suddenly, and will increase your chances of quitting. Place the Step 3 sticker on the first day of week seven. Use the 7mg patches for two weeks. People who smoke 10 or less cigarettes per day should not use NicoDerm CQ for longer than 8 weeks. If you still feel the need to use NicoDerm CQ after 8 weeks, talk with your doctor.

PLAN AHEAD.

Because smoking is an addiction, it is not easy to stop. After you've given up nicotine, you may still have a strong urge to smoke. Plan ahead NOW for these times, so you're not tempted to start smoking again in a moment of weakness. The following tips may help:
- Keep the phone numbers of supportive friends and family members handy.
- Keep a record of your quitting process. In the event that you slip, immediately stop smoking and resume your quit attempt with the NicoDerm CQ patch. If you smoke at all, write down what you think caused the slip.
- Put together an Emergency Kit that includes items that will help take your mind off occasional urges to smoke. You might include cinnamon gum or lemon drops to suck on, a relaxing cassette tape, and something for your hands to play with, like a smooth rock, rubber band or small metal balls.

- Set aside some small rewards, like a new magazine or a gift certificate from your favorite store, which you'll "give" yourself after passing difficult hurdles.
- Think now about the times when you most often want a cigarette, and then plan what else you might do instead of smoking. For instance, you might plan to take your coffee break in a new location, or take a walk right after dinner, so you won't be tempted to smoke.

HOW NICODERM CQ WORKS.

NicoDerm CQ patches provide nicotine to your system. They work as a temporary aid to help you quit smoking by reducing nicotine withdrawal symptoms, including nicotine craving. NicoDerm CQ provides a lower level of nicotine to your blood than cigarettes, and allows you to gradually do away with your body's need for nicotine.

Because NicoDerm CQ does not contain the tar or carbon monoxide of cigarette smoke, it does not have the same health dangers as tobacco. However, it still delivers nicotine, the addictive part of cigarette smoke. Nicotine can cause side effects such as headache, nausea, upset stomach, and dizziness.

HOW TO USE NICODERM CQ PATCHES.

Read all the following instructions, and the instructions on the outer carton, before using NicoDerm CQ. Refer to them often to make sure you're using NicoDerm CQ correctly. Please refer to the CD for additional help.

1) Stop smoking completely before you start using NicoDerm CQ.
2) To reduce nicotine craving and other withdrawal symptoms, use NicoDerm CQ according to the directions on pages 6–8.
3) Insert used NicoDerm CQ patches in the child resistant disposal tray provided in the box – safely away from children and pets.

When to apply and remove NicoDerm CQ patches.

Each day apply a new patch to a different place on skin that is dry, clean and hairless. **You can wear a NicoDerm CQ patch for either 16 or 24 hours.** If you crave cigarettes when you wake up, wear the patch for 24 hours. If you begin to have vivid dreams or other disruptions of your sleep while wearing the patch 24 hours, try taking the patch off at bedtime (after about 16 hours) and putting on a new one when you get up the next day.

PLACE THESE STICKERS ON YOUR CALENDAR

STEP 1
A new 21 mg patch every day AT THE BEGINNING OF WEEK #1 (QUIT DAY)

STEP 2
A new 14 mg patch every day AT THE BEGINNING OF WEEK #7

For people who smoke 10 or less cigarettes per day: Do not use STEP 1 (21 mg). Use STEP 2 (14 mg) at the beginning of week #1 and STEP 3 (7 mg) at the beginning of week #7.

PLACE THESE STICKERS ON YOUR CALENDAR

STEP 3
A new 7 mg patch every day AT THE BEGINNING OF WEEK #9

EX-SMOKER
WHEN YOU HAVE COMPLETED YOUR QUITTING PROGRAM

Do not smoke even when you are not wearing the patch.

Remove the used patch and put on a new patch at the same time every day. Applying the patch at about the same time each day (first thing in the morning, for instance) will help you remember when to put on a new patch. Do not leave the same NicoDerm CQ patch on for more than 24 hours because it may irritate your skin and because it loses strength after 24 hours.

Do not use NicoDerm CQ continuously for more than 10 weeks (8 weeks for people who smoke 10 or less cigarettes per day).

How to apply a NicoDerm CQ patch.

1. Do not remove the NicoDerm CQ patch from its sealed protective pouch until you are ready to use it. NicoDerm CQ patches will lose nicotine to the air if you store them out of the pouch.
2. Choose a non-hairy, clean, dry area of skin. Do not put a NicoDerm CQ patch on skin that is burned, broken out, cut, or irritated in any way. Make sure your skin is free of lotion and soap before applying a patch.
3. A clear, protective liner covers the sticky back side of the NicoDerm CQ patch—the side that will be put on your skin. The liner has a slit down the middle to help you remove it from the patch. With the sticky back side facing you, pull half the liner away from the NicoDerm CQ patch starting at the middle slit, as shown in the illustration above. Hold the NicoDerm CQ patch at one of the outside edges (touch the sticky side as little as possible), and pull off the other half of the protective liner.
Place this liner in the slot in the disposable tray provided in the NicoDerm CQ package where it will be out of reach of children and pets.
4. Immediately apply the sticky side of the NicoDerm CQ patch to your skin. **Press the patch firmly on your skin with the heel of your hand for at least 10 seconds.** Make sure it sticks well to your skin, especially around the edges.
5. Wash your hands when you have finished applying the NicoDerm CQ patch. Nicotine on your hands could get into your eyes and nose, and cause stinging, redness, or more serious problems.
6. After 24 or 16 hours, remove the patch you have been wearing. Fold the used NicoDerm CQ patch in half with the sticky side together. Carefully dispose of the used patch in the slot of the disposal tray provided in the NicoDerm CQ package where it will be out of the reach of children and pets. Even used patches have enough nicotine to poison children and pets. Wash your hands.
7. Chose a different place on your skin to apply the next NicoDerm CQ patch and repeat Steps 1 to 6. Do not apply a new patch to a previously used skin site for at least one week.

If your NicoDerm CQ patch gets wet during wearing.
Water will not harm the NicoDerm CQ patch you are wearing if applied properly. You can bathe, swim, or shower for short periods while you are wearing the NicoDerm CQ patch.

If your NicoDerm CQ patch comes off while wearing.
NicoDerm CQ patches generally stick well to most people's skin. However, a patch may occasionally come off. If your NicoDerm CQ patch falls off during the day, put on a new patch, making sure you select a non-hairy, non-irritated area of the skin that is clean and dry.
If the soap you use has lanolin or moisturizers, the patch may not stick well. Using a different soap may help. Body creams, lotions and sunscreens can also cause problems with keeping your patch on. Do not apply creams or lotions to the place on your skin where you will put the patch.
If you have followed the directions and the patch still does not stick to you, try using medical adhesive tape over the patch.

Disposing of NicoDerm CQ patches.
Fold the used patch in half with the sticky side together.
Carefully dispose of the patch in the disposal slot of the tray provided in the NicoDerm CQ package where it will be out of the reach of children and pets. Small amounts of nicotine, even from a used patch, can poison children and pets. **Keep all nicotine patches away from children and pets.** Wash your hands after disposing of the patch.

If your skin reacts to the NicoDerm CQ patch.
When you first put on a NicoDerm CQ patch, mild itching, burning, or tingling is normal and should go away within an hour. After you remove a NicoDerm CQ patch, the skin under the patch might be somewhat red. Your skin should not stay red for more than a day after removing the patch. **Stop use and ask a doctor if skin redness caused by the patch does not go away after four days, or if your skin swells, or you get a rash. Do not put on a new patch.**

Storage Instructions
Keep each NicoDerm CQ patch in its protective pouch, unopened, until you are ready to use it, because the patch will lose nicotine to the air if it's outside the pouch.
Store NicoDerm CQ patches at 20–25 C (68–77 F) because they are sensitive to heat. Remember, the inside of your car can reach temperatures much higher than this. A slight yellowing of the sticky side of the patch is normal. Do not use NicoDerm CQ patches stored in pouches that are open or torn.

TIPS TO MAKE QUITTING EASIER.
Within the first few weeks of giving up smoking, you may be tempted to smoke for pleasure, particularly after completing a difficult task, or at a party or bar.

Continued on next page

Nicoderm CQ—Cont.

Hear are some tips to help get you through the important first stages of becoming a nonsmoker:

On Your Quit Date:

- Ask your family, friends and co-workers to support you in your efforts to stop smoking.
- Throw away all your cigarettes, matches, lighters, ashtrays, etc.
- Keep busy on your quit day. Exercise. Go to a movie. Take a walk. Get together with friends.
- Figure out how much money you'll save by not smoking. Most ex-smokers can save more than $1,000 a year on the price of cigarettes alone.
- Write down what you will do with the money you save.
- Know your high risk situations and plan ahead how you will deal with them.
- Visit your dentist and have your teeth cleaned to get rid of the tobacco stains.

Right after Quitting:

- During the first few days after you've stopped smoking, spend as much time as possible at places where smoking is not allowed.
- Drink large quantities of water and fruit juices.
- Try to avoid alcohol, coffee and other beverages you associate with smoking.
- Remember that temporary urges to smoke will pass, even if you don't smoke a cigarette.
- Keep your hands busy with something like a pencil or a paper clip.
- Find other activities that help you relax without cigarettes. Swim, jog, take a walk, play basketball.
- Don't worry too much about gaining weight. Watch what you eat, take time for daily exercise, and change your eating habits if you need to.
- Laughter helps. Watch or read something funny

WHAT TO EXPECT.

The First Few Days.

Your body is now coming back into balance. During the first few days after you stop smoking, you might feel edgy and nervous and have trouble concentrating. You might get headaches, feel dizzy and a little out of sorts, feel sweaty or have stomach upsets. You might even have trouble sleeping at first. These are typical nicotine withdrawal symptoms that will go away with time. Your smoker's cough will get worse before it gets better. But don't worry, that's a good sign. Coughing helps clear the tar deposits out of your lungs.

After A Week Or Two.

By now you should be feeling more confident that you can handle those smoking urges. Many of your nicotine withdrawal symptoms have left by now, and you should be noticing some positive signs: less coughing, better breathing and an improved sense of taste and smell, to name a few.

After A Month.

You probably have the urge to smoke much less often now. But urges may still occur, and when they do, they are likely to be powerful ones that come out of no-

where. Don't let them catch you off guard. Plan ahead for these difficult times.

Concentrate on the ways non-smokers are more attractive than smokers. Their skin is less likely to wrinkle. Their teeth are whiter, cleaner. Their breath is fresher.

Their hair and clothes smell better. That cough that seems to make even a laugh sound more like a rattle is a thing of the past. Their children and others around them are healthier, too.

What To Do About Relapse.

What should you do if you slip and start smoking again? The answer is simple. A lapse of one or two or even a few cigarettes should not spoil your efforts! Throw away your cigarettes, forgive yourself and continue with the program. Listen to the Compact Disc and re-read the User's Guide to ensure that you're using NicoDerm CQ correctly and following the other important tips for dealing with the mental and social dependence on nicotine. Your doctor, pharmacist or other health professional can also provide useful counseling on the importance of stopping smoking. You should consider them partners in your quit attempt.

What To Do About Relapse After a Successful Quit Attempt.

If you have taken up regular smoking again, don't be discouraged. Research shows that the best thing you can do is try again, since several quitting attempts may be needed before you're successful. And your chances of quitting successfully increase with each quit attempt.

The important thing is to learn from your last attempt.

- Admit that you've slipped, but don't treat yourself as a failure.
- Try to identify the "trigger" that caused you to slip, and prepare a better plan for dealing with this problem next time.
- Talk positively to yourself – tell yourself that you have learned something from this experience.
- Make sure you used NicoDerm CQ patches correctly
- Remember that it takes practice to do anything, and quitting smoking is no exception.

WHEN THE STRUGGLE IS OVER.

Once you've stopped smoking, take a second and pat yourself on your back. Now do it again. You deserve it. Remember now why you decided to stop smoking in the first place. Look at your list of reasons. Read them again. And smile.

Now think about all the money you are saving and what you'll do with it. All the non-smoking places you can go, and what you might do there. All those years you may have added to your life, and what you'll do with them. Remember that temptation may not be gone forever. However, the hard part is behind you so look forward with a positive attitude, and enjoy your new life as a non-smoker.

QUESTIONS & ANSWERS

1. How will I feel when I stop smoking and start using NicoDerm CQ?

You'll need to prepare yourself for some nicotine withdrawal symptoms. These begin almost immediately after you stop smoking, and are usually at their worst during the first three or four days. Understand that any of the following is possible:

- craving for nicotine
- anxiety, irritability, restlessness, mood changes, nervousness
- disruptions of your sleep
- drowsiness
- trouble concentrating
- increased appetite and weight gain
- headaches, muscular pain, constipation, fatigue.

NicoDerm CQ reduces nicotine withdrawal symptoms such as irritability and nervousness, as well as the craving for nicotine you used to satisfy by having a cigarette.

2. Is NicoDerm CQ just substituting one form of nicotine for another?

NicoDerm CQ does contain nicotine. The purpose of NicoDerm CQ is to provide you with enough nicotine to reduce the physical withdrawal symptoms so you can deal with the mental aspects of quitting.

3. Can I be hurt by using NicoDerm CQ?

For most adults, the amount of nicotine delivered from the patch is less than from smoking. If you believe you may be sensitive to even this amount of nicotine, you should not use this product without advice from your doctor. There are also some important warnings in this User's Guide (See page 4).

4. Will I gain weight?

Many people do tend to gain a few pounds the first 8–10 weeks after they stop smoking. This is a very small price to pay for the enormous gains that you will make in your overall health and attractiveness. If you continue to gain weight after the first two months, try to analyze what you're doing differently. Reduce your fat intake, choose healthy snacks, and increase your physical activity to burn off the extra calories. Drink lots of water. This is good for your body and skin, and also helps to reduce the amount you eat.

5. Is NicoDerm CQ more expensive than smoking?

The total cost of NicoDerm CQ program is similar to what a person who smokes one and a half packs of cigarettes a day would spend on cigarettes for the same period of time. Also, use of NicoDerm CQ is only a short-term cost, while the cost of smoking is a long-term cost, including the health problems smoking causes.

6. What if I slip up?

Discard your cigarettes, forgive yourself and then get back on track. Don't consider yourself a failure or punish yourself. In fact, people who have already tried to quit are more likely to be successful the next time.

GOOD LUCK!

WALLET CARD

My most important reasons to quit smoking are:

WALLET CARD
Where to call for Help:

American Lung Association	American Cancer Society	American Heart Association
800-586-4872	800-227-2345	800-242-8721

For people who smoke more than 10 cigarettes per day:

STEP 1	STEP 2	STEP 3
Use one 21 mg patch/day	Use one 14 mg patch/day	Use one 7 mg patch/day
Weeks 1–6	Weeks 7–8	Weeks 9–10

People who smoke 10 or less cigarettes per day. Do not use STEP 1 (21 mg). Use STEP 2 (14 mg) for six weeks and STEP 3 (7 mg) for two weeks and then stop.

Copyright © 2002 GlaxoSmithKline

For your family's protection, NicoDerm CQ patches are supplied in child resistant pouches. Do not use if individual pouch is open or torn.

Manufactured by ALZA Corporation, Mountain View, CA 94043 for GlaxoSmithKline Consumer Healthcare, L.P. Comments or Questions? Call 1–800–834–5895 Weekdays. (10 a.m.–4:30 p.m. EST).

- **Not for sale to those under 18 years of age.**
- **Proof of age required.**
- **Not for sale in vending machines or from any source where proof of age cannot be verified.**

Available as

NicoDerm CQ Step 1 (21 mg/24 hours)–7 Patches*

NicoDerm CQ Step 1 (21 mg/24 hours)–14 Patches*

NicoDerm CQ Step 2 (14 mg/24 hours)–14 Patches*

NicoDerm CQ Step 3 (7 mg/24 hours)–14 Patches**

NicoDerm CQ Clear Step 1 (21 mg/24 hours)–7 Patches*

NicoDerm CQ Clear Step 1 (21 mg/24 hours)–14 Patches*

NicoDerm CQ Clear Step 1 (21 mg/24 hours)–21 Patches*

NicoDerm CQ Clear Step 2 (14 mg/24 hours)–14 Patches*

NicoDerm CQ Clear Step 3 (7 mg/24 hours)–14 Patches**

* User's Guide, CD & Child Resistant Disposal Tray

** User's Guide, & Child Resistant Disposal Tray

Shown in Product Identification Guide, page 508

NICODERM® CQ® CLEAR
Nicotine Transdermal System/Stop Smoking Aid

Formerly available only by prescription
Available as:

       Step 1 - 21 mg/24 hours
       Step 2 - 14 mg/24 hours
       Step 3 - 7 mg/24 hours

If you smoke:
More than 10 Cigarettes per Day:
Start with Step 1
10 Cigarettes a Day or Less:
Start with Step 2

WHAT IS THE NICODERM CQ PATCH AND HOW IS IT USED?
NicoDerm CQ is a small, nicotine containing patch. When you put on a NicoDerm CQ patch, nicotine passes through the skin and into your body. NicoDerm CQ is very thin and uses special material to control how fast nicotine passes through the skin. Unlike the sudden jolts of nicotine delivered by cigarettes, the amount of nicotine you receive remains relatively smooth throughout the 24 or 16 hours period you wear the NicoDerm CQ patch. This helps to reduce cravings you may have for nicotine.

Active Ingredient: Nicotine

Purpose: Stop Smoking Aid

Use: reduces withdrawal symptoms, including nicotine craving, associated with quitting smoking

Directions:
- **if you are under 18 years of age, ask a doctor before use**
- before using this product, read the enclosed user's guide for complete directions and other information
- stop smoking completely when you begin using the patch
- **if you smoke more than 10 cigarettes per day**, use according to the following 10 week schedule:

STEP 1	STEP 2	STEP 3
Use one 21 mg patch/day	Use one 14 mg patch/day	Use one 7 mg patch/day
Weeks 1–6	Weeks 7–8	Weeks 9–10

- if you smoke **10 or less cigarettes per day**, do not use **STEP 1 (21 mg)**. Start with **STEP 2 (14 mg)** for 6 weeks, then **STEP 3 (7 mg)** for two weeks and then stop.
- steps 2 and 3 allow you to gradually reduce your level of nicotine. Completing the full program will increase your chances of quitting successfully.
- apply one new patch every 24 hours on skin that is dry, clean and hairless
- remove backing from patch and immediately press onto skin. Hold for 10 seconds.
- wash hands after applying or removing patch. Throw away the patch in the enclosed disposal tray. See enclosed user's guide for safety and handling.
- you may wear the patch for 16 or 24 hours
- if you crave cigarettes when you wake up, wear the patch for 24 hours
- if you have vivid dreams or other sleep disturbances, you may remove the patch at bedtime and apply a new one in the morning
- the used patch should be removed and a new one applied to a different skin site at the same time each day
- do not wear more than one patch at a time
- do not cut patch in half or into smaller pieces

- do not leave patch on for more than 24 hours because it may irritate your skin and loses strength after 24 hours
- stop using the patch at the end of 10 weeks. If you started with **STEP 2**, stop using the patch at the end of 8 weeks. If you still feel the need to use the patch talk to your doctor.

Warnings:
If you are pregnant or breast-feeding, only use this medicine on the advice of your health care provider. Smoking can seriously harm your child. Try to stop smoking without using any nicotine replacement medicine. This medicine is believed to be safer than smoking. However, the risks to your child from this medicine are not fully known.

Do Not Use
- if you continue to smoke, chew tobacco, use snuff, or use a nicotine gum or other nicotine containing products

Ask a doctor before use if you have
- heart disease, recent heart attack, or irregular heartbeat. Nicotine can increase your heart rate.
- high blood pressure not controlled with medication. Nicotine can increase your blood pressure.
- an allergy to adhesive tape or skin problems because you are more likely to get rashes

Ask a doctor or pharmacist before use if you are
- using a non-nicotine stop smoking drug
- taking a prescription medication for depression or asthma. Your prescription dose may need to be adjusted.

When using this product
- do not smoke even when not wearing the patch. The nicotine in your skin will still be entering your blood stream for several hours after you take off the patch.
- if you have vivid dreams or other sleep disturbances remove this patch at bedtime

Stop use and ask a doctor if
- skin redness caused by the patch does not go away after four days, or if skin swells, or you get a rash
- irregular heartbeat or palpitations occur
- you get symptoms of nicotine overdose such as nausea, vomiting, dizziness, weakness and rapid heartbeat

Keep out of reach of children and pets. Used patches have enough nicotine to poison children and pets. If swallowed, get medical help or contact a Poison Control Center right away. Dispose of the used patches by folding sticky ends together and inserting in disposal tray in this box.

READ THE LABEL
Read the carton and the User's Guide before using this product. Keep the carton and User's Guide. They contain important information.

Inactive Ingredients: Ethylene vinyl acetate-copolymer, polyisobutylene and high density polyethylene between clear polyester backings.

Store at 20–25°C (68–77°F)

Continued on next page

Nicoderm CQ Clear—Cont.

TO INCREASE YOUR SUCCESS IN QUITTING:
1. You must be motivated to quit.
2. Complete the full treatment program, applying a new patch every day.
3. Use with a support program as described in the Users Guide.

NicoDerm CQ User's Guide
KEYS TO SUCCESS
1) You must really want to quit smoking for **NicoDerm® CQ®** to help you.
2) Complete the full program, applying a new patch every day.
3) **NicoDerm CQ** works best when used together with a support program: See page 3 for details.
4) If you have trouble using **NicoDerm CQ**, ask your doctor or pharmacist or call GlaxoSmithKline 1-800-834-5895 weekdays (10:00 am 4:30 pm EST).

SO, YOU'VE DECIDED TO QUIT.
Congratulations. Your decision to stop smoking is one of the most important things you can do to improve your health. Quitting smoking is a two-part process that involves:
1) overcoming your physical need for nicotine, and
2) breaking your smoking habit.
NicoDerm CQ helps smokers quit by reducing nicotine withdrawal symptoms.
Many NicoDerm CQ users will be able to stop smoking for a few days but often will start smoking again. Most smokers have to try to quit several times before they completely stop.
Your own chances of quitting smoking depend on how strongly you are addicted to nicotine, how much you want to quit, and how closely you follow a quitting plan like the one that comes with NicoDerm CQ.

QUITTING SMOKING IS HARD!
If you find you cannot stop or if you start smoking again after using NicoDerm CQ please talk to a health care professional who can help you find a program that may work better for you. Breaking this addiction doesn't happen overnight.
Because NicoDerm CQ provides some nicotine, the NicoDerm CQ patch will help you stop smoking by reducing nicotine withdrawal symptoms such as nicotine craving, nervousness and irritability.
This User's Guide will give you support as you become a non-smoker. It will answer common questions about NicoDerm CQ and give tips to help you stop smoking, and should be referred to often.

WHERE TO GET HELP.
You are more likely to stop smoking by using NicoDerm CQ with a support program that helps you break your smoking habit. There may be support groups in your area for people trying to quit. Call your local chapter of the American Lung Association, American Cancer Society or American Heart Association for further information. Toll free phone numbers are printed on the wallet card on the back cover of this User's Guide.
If you find you cannot stop smoking or if you start smoking again after using NicoDerm CQ, remember breaking this addiction doesn't happen overnight. You may want to talk to a health care professional who can help you improve your chances of quitting the next time you try NicoDerm CQ or another method.

LET'S GET ORGANIZED.
Your reason for quitting may be a combination of concerns about health, the effect of smoking on your appearance, and pressure from your family and friends to stop smoking. Or maybe you're concerned about the dangerous effect of second-hand smoke on the people you care about.
All of these are good reasons. You probably have others. Decide your most important reasons, and write them down on the wallet card inside the back cover of this User's Guide. Carry this card with you. In difficult moments, when you want to smoke, the card will remind you why you are quitting.

WHAT YOU'RE UP AGAINST.
Smoking is addictive in two ways. Your need for nicotine has become both physical and mental. You must overcome both addictions to stop smoking. So while NicoDerm CQ will lessen your body's craving for nicotine, you've got to want to quit smoking to overcome the mental dependence on cigarettes. Once you've decided that you're going to quit, it's time to get started. But first, there are some important cautions you should consider.

SOME IMPORTANT WARNINGS.
This product is only for those who want to stop smoking.
If you are pregnant or breast-feeding, only use this medicine on the advice of your health care provider. Smoking can seriously harm your child. Try to stop smoking without using any nicotine replacement medicine. This medicine is believed to be safer than smoking. However, the risks to your child from this medicine are not fully known.

Do not use
• if you continue to smoke, chew tobacco, use snuff or use a nicotine gum or other nicotine products.

Ask a doctor before use if you have:
• heart disease, recent heart attack, or irregular heartbeat, Nicotine can increase your heart rate.
• high blood pressure not controlled with medication. Nicotine can increase your blood pressure.
• an allergy to adhesive tape or have skin problems because you are more likely to get rashes.

Ask a doctor or pharmacist before use if you are
• using a non-nicotine stop smoking drug
• taking a prescription medication for asthma or depression. Your prescription dose may need to be adjusted.

When using this product:
• do not smoke even when not wearing the patch. The nicotine in your skin will still be entering your bloodstream for several hours after you take off the patch.
• you have vivid dreams or other sleep disturbances remove this patch at bedtime.

Stop use and ask a doctor if:
• skin redness caused by the patch does not go away after four days, or if your skin swells or you get a rash.
• irregular heartbeat or palpitations occur
• you get symptoms of nicotine overdose, such as nausea, vomiting, dizziness, weakness and rapid heartbeat.

Keep out of reach of children and pets. Used patches have enough nicotine to poison children and pets. If swallowed, get medical help or contact a Poison Control Center right away. Dispose of the used patches by folding sticky ends together and inserting in the disposal tray in this box.

LET'S GET STARTED.
If you are under 18 years of age, ask a doctor before use.
Becoming a non-smoker starts today. Your first step is to read through this entire User's Guide carefully.
First, check that you bought the right starting dose.
If you smoke more than 10 cigarettes a day, begin with Step 1 (21 mg). As the carton indicates, people who smoke 10 or less cigarettes per day should not use Step 1 (21 mg). They should start with Step 2 (14 mg). Throughout this User's Guide we will give specific instructions for people who smoke 10 or less cigarettes per day.
Next, set your personalized quitting schedule.
Take out a calendar that you can use to track your progress. Pick a quit date, and mark this on your calendar using the stickers in the middle of this User's Guide, as described below.

DIRECTIONS: FOR PEOPLE WHO SMOKE MORE THAN 10 CIGARETTES PER DAY
STEP 1. (Weeks 1–6). Your quit date (and the day you'll start using NicoDerm CQ patch).
Choose your quit date (it should be soon).
This is the day you will quit smoking cigarettes entirely and begin using NicoDerm CQ to reduce your cravings for nicotine. Place the Step 1 sticker on this date. For the first six weeks, you'll use the highest-strength (21 mg) NicoDerm CQ patches. Be sure to follow the directions on page 10.
Completing the full program will increase your chances of quitting successfully. This is done by changing over to the Step 2 (14mg) patch for 2 weeks followed by a final 2 weeks with the Step 3 (7mg) patch. The Step 2 and Step 3 treatment periods allow you to gradually reduce the amount of nicotine you get, rather than stopping suddenly, and will increase your chances of quitting.
STEP 2. (Weeks 7–8). The day you'll start reducing your use of NicoDerm CQ patch.
Switching to Step 2 (14mg) patches after 6 weeks begins to gradually reduce your nicotine usage. Place the Step 2 sticker on this date (the first day of week seven). Use the 14mg patches for two weeks.

STEP 3. (Weeks 9–10). The day you'll further start reducing your use of Nico-Derm CQ patch.

After eight weeks, nicotine intake is further reduced by moving down to Step 3 (7mg) patches. Place the Step 3 sticker on this date (the first day of week nine). Use the 7 mg patches for two weeks.

THE NICODERM CQ PROGRAM

STEP 1	STEP 2	STEP 3
Use one	Use one	Use one
21 mg	14 mg	7 mg
patch/day	patch/day	patch/day
Weeks 1–6	Weeks 7–8	Weeks 9–10

STOP USING NICODERM CQ AT THE END OF WEEK 10. If you still feel the need to use the patch after Week 10, talk with your doctor or health professional.

DIRECTIONS: FOR PEOPLE WHO SMOKE 10 OR LESS CIGARETTES PER DAY

Do not use Step 1 (21 mg).

Begin with STEP 2 – Initial Treatment Period (Weeks 1–6): 14mg patches.

Choose our quit date (it should be soon). This is the Day you will quit smoking cigarettes entirely and begin using NicoDerm CQ to reduce your cravings for nicotine. Place the Step 2 sticker on this date. For the first six weeks, you'll use the Step 2 (14mg) NicoDerm CQ patches. Be sure to follow the directions on page 10.

Continue with STEP 3 – Step Down Treatment Period (Weeks 7–8): 7mg patches.

Completing the full program will increase your chances of quitting successfully. This is done by changing over to the Step 3 (7mg) patches for 2 weeks. The two week step down treatment period allows you to gradually reduce the amount of nicotine you get, rather than stopping suddenly, and will increase your chances of quitting. Place the Step 3 sticker on the first day of week seven. Use the 7mg patches for two weeks.

People who smoke 10 or less cigarettes per day should not use NicoDerm CQ for longer than 8 weeks. If you still feel the need to use NicoDerm CQ after 8 weeks, talk with your doctor.

PLAN AHEAD.

Because smoking is an addiction, it is not easy to stop. After you've given up nicotine, you may still have a strong urge to smoke. Plan ahead NOW for these times, so you're not tempted to start smoking again in a moment of weakness. The following tips may help:

- Keep the phone numbers of supportive friends and family members handy.
- Keep a record of your quitting process. In the event that you slip, immediately stop smoking and resume your quit attempt with the NicoDerm CQ patch. If you smoke at all, write down what you think caused the slip.
- Put together an Emergency Kit that includes items that will help take your mind off occasional urges to smoke. You might include cinnamon gum or lemon drops to suck on, a relaxing cassette tape, and something for your hands to play with, like a smooth rock, rubber band or small metal balls.
- Set aside some small rewards, like a new magazine or a gift certificate from your favorite store, which you'll "give" yourself after passing difficult hurdles.
- Think now about the times when you most often want a cigarette, and then plan what else you might do instead of smoking. For instance, you might plan to take your coffee break in a new location, or take a walk right after dinner, so you won't be tempted to smoke.

HOW NICODERM CQ WORKS.

NicoDerm CQ patches provide nicotine to your system. They work as a temporary aid to help you quit smoking by reducing nicotine withdrawal symptoms, including nicotine craving. NicoDerm CQ provides a lower level of nicotine to your blood than cigarettes, and allows you to gradually do away with your body's need for nicotine.

Because NicoDerm CQ does not contain the tar or carbon monoxide of cigarette smoke, it does not have the same health dangers as tobacco. However, it still delivers nicotine, the addictive part of cigarette smoke. Nicotine can cause side effects such as headache, nausea, upset stomach, and dizziness.

HOW TO USE NICODERM CQ PATCHES.

Read all the following instructions, and the instructions on the outer carton, before using NicoDerm CQ. Refer to them often to make sure you're using NicoDerm CQ correctly. Please refer to the CD for additional help.

1) Stop smoking completely before you start using NicoDerm CQ.
2) To reduce nicotine craving and other withdrawal symptoms, use NicoDerm CQ according to the directions on pages 6–8.
3) Insert used NicoDerm CQ patches in the child resistant disposal tray provided in the box – safely away from children and pets.

When to apply and remove NicoDerm CQ patches.

Each day apply a new patch to a different place on skin that is dry, clean and hairless. **You can wear a NicoDerm CQ patch for either 16 or 24 hours.** If you crave cigarettes when you wake up, wear the patch for 24 hours. If you begin to have vivid dreams or other disruptions of your sleep while wearing the patch 24 hours, try taking the patch off at bedtime (after about 16 hours) and putting on a new one when you get up the next day.

PLACE THESE STICKERS ON YOUR CALENDAR

STEP 1	STEP 2
A new 21 mg patch every day AT THE BEGINNING OF WEEK #1 (QUIT DAY)	A new 14 mg patch every day AT THE BEGINNING OF WEEK #7

For people who smoke 10 or less cigarettes per day: Do not use STEP 1 (21 mg). Use STEP 2 (14 mg) at the beginning of week #1 and STEP 3 (7 mg) at the beginning of week #7.

PLACE THESE STICKERS ON YOUR CALENDAR

STEP 3	EX-SMOKER
A new 7 mg patch every day AT THE BEGINNING OF WEEK #9	WHEN YOU HAVE COMPLETED YOUR QUITTING PROGRAM

Do not smoke even when you are not wearing the patch.

Remove the used patch and put on a new patch at the same time every day. Applying the patch at about the same time each day (first thing in the morning, for instance) will help you remember when to put on a new patch. Do not leave the same NicoDerm CQ patch on for more than 24 hours because it may irritate your skin and because it loses strength after 24 hours.

Do not use NicoDerm CQ continuously for more than 10 weeks (8 weeks for people who smoke 10 or less cigarettes per day).

How to apply a NicoDerm CQ patch.

1. Do not remove the NicoDerm CQ patch from its sealed protective pouch until you are ready to use it. NicoDerm CQ patches will lose nicotine to the air if you store them out of the pouch.
2. Choose a non-hairy, clean, dry area of skin. Do not put a NicoDerm CQ patch on skin that is burned, broken out, cut, or irritated in any way. Make sure your skin is free of lotion and soap before applying a patch.
3. A clear, protective liner covers the sticky back side of the NicoDerm CQ patch—the side that will be put on your skin. The liner has a slit down the middle to help you remove it from the patch. With the sticky back side facing you, pull half the liner away from the NicoDerm CQ patch starting at the middle slit, as shown in the illustration above. Hold the NicoDerm CQ patch at one of the outside edges (touch the sticky side as little as possible), and pull off the other half of the protective liner.
Place this liner in the slot in the disposable tray provided in the NicoDerm CQ package where it will be out of reach of children and pets.
4. Immediately apply the sticky side of the NicoDerm CQ patch to your skin. **Press the patch firmly on your skin with the heel of your hand for at least 10 seconds.** Make sure it sticks well to your skin, especially around the edges.
5. Wash your hands when you have finished applying the NicoDerm CQ patch. Nicotine on your hands could get into your eyes and nose, and cause stinging, redness, or more serious problems.
6. After 24 or 16 hours, remove the patch you have been wearing. Fold the used NicoDerm CQ patch in half with the sticky side together. Carefully dispose of the used patch in the slot of the disposal tray provided in the NicoDerm CQ package where it will be out of the reach of children and pets. Even used patches have enough nicotine to poison children and pets. Wash your hands.
7. Chose a different place on your skin to apply the next NicoDerm CQ patch and

Continued on next page

Nicoderm CQ Clear—Cont.

repeat Steps 1 to 6. Do not apply a new patch to a previously used skin site for at least one week.

If your NicoDerm CQ patch gets wet during wearing.

Water will not harm the NicoDerm CQ patch you are wearing if applied properly. You can bathe, swim, or shower for short periods while you are wearing the NicoDerm CQ patch.

If your NicoDerm CQ patch comes off while wearing.

NicoDerm CQ patches generally stick well to most people's skin. However, a patch may occasionally come off. If your NicoDerm CQ patch falls off during the day, put on a new patch, making sure you select a non-hairy, non-irritated area of the skin that is clean and dry.

If the soap you use has lanolin or moisturizers, the patch may not stick well. Using a different soap may help. Body creams, lotions and sunscreens can also cause problems with keeping your patch on. Do not apply creams or lotions to the place on your skin where you will put the patch.

If you have followed the directions and the patch still does not stick to you, try using medical adhesive tape over the patch.

Disposing of NicoDerm CQ patches.

Fold the used patch in half with the sticky side together.

Carefully dispose of the patch in the disposal slot of the tray provided in the NicoDerm CQ package where it will be out of the reach of children and pets. Small amounts of nicotine, even from a used patch, can poison children and pets. **Keep all nicotine patches away from children and pets.** Wash your hands after disposing of the patch.

If your skin reacts to the NicoDerm CQ patch.

When you first put on a NicoDerm CQ patch, mild itching, burning, or tingling is normal and should go away within an hour. After you remove a NicoDerm CQ patch, the skin under the patch might be somewhat red. Your skin should not stay red for more than a day after removing the patch. **Stop use and ask a doctor if skin redness caused by the patch does not go away after four days, or if your skin swells, or you get a rash. Do not put on a new patch.**

Storage Instructions

Keep each NicoDerm CQ patch in its protective pouch, unopened, until you are ready to use it, because the patch will lose nicotine to the air if it's outside the pouch.

Store NicoDerm CQ patches at 20–25 C (68–77 F) because they are sensitive to heat. Remember, the inside of your car can reach temperatures much higher than this. A slight yellowing of the sticky side of the patch is normal. Do not use NicoDerm CQ patches stored in pouches that are open or torn.

TIPS TO MAKE QUITTING EASIER.

Within the first few weeks of giving up smoking, you may be tempted to smoke for pleasure, particularly after completing a difficult task, or at a party or bar. Hear are some tips to help get you through the important first stages of becoming a nonsmoker:

On Your Quit Date:

- Ask your family, friends and co-workers to support you in your efforts to stop smoking.
- Throw away all your cigarettes, matches, lighters, ashtrays, etc.
- Keep busy on your quit day. Exercise. Go to a movie. Take a walk. Get together with friends.
- Figure out how much money you'll save by not smoking. Most ex-smokers can save more than $1,000 a year on the price of cigarettes alone.
- Write down what you will do with the money you save.
- Know your high risk situations and plan ahead how you will deal with them.
- Visit your dentist and have your teeth cleaned to get rid of the tobacco stains.

Right after Quitting:

- During the first few days after you've stopped smoking, spend as much time as possible at places where smoking is not allowed.
- Drink large quantities of water and fruit juices.
- Try to avoid alcohol, coffee and other beverages you associate with smoking.
- Remember that temporary urges to smoke will pass, even if you don't smoke a cigarette.
- Keep your hands busy with something like a pencil or a paper clip.
- Find other activities that help you relax without cigarettes. Swim, jog, take a walk, play basketball.
- Don't worry too much about gaining weight. Watch what you eat, take time for daily exercise, and change your eating habits if you need to.
- Laughter helps. Watch or read something funny

WHAT TO EXPECT.

The First Few Days.

Your body is now coming back into balance. During the first few days after you stop smoking, you might feel edgy and nervous and have trouble concentrating. You might get headaches, feel dizzy and a little out of sorts, feel sweaty or have stomach upsets. You might even have trouble sleeping at first. These are typical nicotine withdrawal symptoms that will go away with time. Your smoker's cough will get worse before it gets better. But don't worry, that's a good sign. Coughing helps clear the tar deposits out of your lungs.

After A Week Or Two.

By now you should be feeling more confident that you can handle those smoking urges. Many of your nicotine withdrawal symptoms have left by now, and you should be noticing some positive signs: less coughing, better breathing and an improved sense of taste and smell, to name a few.

After A Month.

You probably have the urge to smoke much less often now. But urges may still occur, and when they do, they are likely to be powerful ones that come out of nowhere. Don't let them catch you off guard. Plan ahead for these difficult times.

Concentrate on the ways non-smokers are more attractive than smokers. Their skin is less likely to wrinkle. Their teeth are whiter, cleaner. Their breath is fresher.

Their hair and clothes smell better. That cough that seems to make even a laugh sound more like a rattle is a thing of the past. Their children and others around them are healthier, too.

What To Do About Relapse.

What should you do if you slip and start smoking again? The answer is simple. A lapse of one or two or even a few cigarettes should not spoil your efforts! Throw away your cigarettes, forgive yourself and continue with the program. Listen to the Compact Disc again and re-read the User's Guide to ensure that you're using NicoDerm CQ correctly and following the other important tips for dealing with the mental and social dependence on nicotine. Your doctor, pharmacist or other health professional can also provide useful counseling on the importance of stopping smoking. You should consider them partners in your quit attempt.

What To Do About Relapse After a Successful Quit Attempt.

If you have taken up regular smoking again, don't be discouraged. Research shows that the best thing you can do is try again, since several quitting attempts may be needed before you're successful. And your chances of quitting successfully increase with each quit attempt.

The important thing is to learn from your last attempt.

- Admit that you've slipped, but don't treat yourself as a failure.
- Try to identify the "trigger" that caused you to slip, and prepare a better plan for dealing with this problem next time.
- Talk positively to yourself – tell yourself that you have learned something from this experience.
- Make sure you used NicoDerm CQ patches correctly
- Remember that it takes practice to do anything, and quitting smoking is no exception.

WHEN THE STRUGGLE IS OVER.

Once you've stopped smoking, take a second and pat yourself on your back. Now do it again. You deserve it. Remember now why you decided to stop smoking in the first place. Look at your list of reasons. Read them again. And smile.

Now think about all the money you are saving and what you'll do with it. All the non-smoking places you can go, and what you might do there. All those years you may have added to your life, and what you'll do with them. Remember that temptation may not be gone forever. However, the hard part is behind you so look forward with a positive attitude, and enjoy your new life as a non-smoker.

QUESTIONS & ANSWERS

1. How will I feel when I stop smoking and start using NicoDerm CQ?

You'll need to prepare yourself for some nicotine withdrawal symptoms. These begin almost immediately after you stop smoking, and are usually at their worst during the first three or four days. Understand that any of the following is possible:

- craving for nicotine
- anxiety, irritability, restlessness, mood changes, nervousness
- disruptions of your sleep
- drowsiness
- trouble concentrating
- increased appetite and weight gain
- headaches, muscular pain, constipation, fatigue.

NicoDerm CQ reduces nicotine withdrawal symptoms such as irritability and nervousness, as well as the craving for nicotine you used to satisfy by having a cigarette.

2. Is NicoDerm CQ just substituting one form of nicotine for another?

NicoDerm CQ does contain nicotine. The purpose of NicoDerm CQ is to provide you with enough nicotine to reduce the physical withdrawal symptoms so you can deal with the mental aspects of quitting.

3. Can I be hurt by using NicoDerm CQ?

For most adults, the amount of nicotine delivered from the patch is less than from smoking. If you believe you may be sensitive to even this amount of nicotine, you should not use this product without advice from your doctor. There are also some important warnings in this User's Guide (See page 4).

4. Will I gain weight?

Many people do tend to gain a few pounds the first 8–10 weeks after they stop smoking. This is a very small price to pay for the enormous gains that you will make in your overall health and attractiveness. If you continue to gain weight after the first two months, try to analyze what you're doing differently. Reduce your fat intake, choose healthy snacks, and increase your physical activity to burn off the extra calories. Drink lots of water. This is good for your body and skin, and also helps to reduce the amount you eat.

5. Is NicoDerm CQ more expensive than smoking?

The total cost of NicoDerm CQ program is similar to what a person who smokes one and a half packs of cigarettes a day would spend on cigarettes for the same period of time. Also, use of NicoDerm CQ is only a short-term cost, while the cost of smoking is a long-term cost, including the health problems smoking causes.

6. What if I slip up?

Discard your cigarettes, forgive yourself and then get back on track. Don't consider yourself a failure or punish yourself. In fact, people who have already tried to quit are more likely to be successful the next time.

GOOD LUCK!

WALLET CARD

My most important reasons to quit smoking are:

WALLET CARD

Where to call for Help:

American Lung Association 800-586-4872	American Cancer Society 800-227-2345	American Heart Association 800-242-8721

For people who smoke more than 10 cigarettes per day:

STEP 1 Use one 21 mg patch/day Weeks 1–6	STEP 2 Use one 14 mg patch/day Weeks 7–8	STEP 3 Use one 7 mg patch/day Weeks 9–10

People who smoke 10 or less cigarettes per day. Do not use STEP 1 (21 mg). Use STEP 2 (14 mg) for six weeks and STEP 3 (7 mg) for two weeks and then stop.

Copyright © 2002 GlaxoSmithKline

For your family's protection, NicoDerm CQ patches are supplied in child resistant pouches. Do not use if individual pouch is open or torn.

Manufactured by ALZA Corporation, Mountain View, CA 94043 for GlaxoSmithKline Consumer Healthcare, L.P. Comments or Questions? Call 1–800–834–5895 Weekdays. (10 a.m.–4:30 p.m. EST).

- **Not for sale to those under 18 years of age.**
- **Proof of age required.**
- **Not for sale in vending machines or from any source where proof of age cannot be verified.**

Available as

NicoDerm CQ Step 1 (21 mg/24 hours)–7 Patches*

NicoDerm CQ Step 1 (21 mg/24 hours)–14 Patches*

NicoDerm CQ Step 2 (14 mg/24 hours)–14 Patches*

NicoDerm CQ Step 3 (7 mg/24 hours)–14 Patches**

NicoDerm CQ Clear Step 1 (21 mg/24 hours)–7 patches*

NicoDerm CQ Clear Step 1 (21 mg/24 hours)–14 patches*

NicoDerm CQ Clear Step 1 (21 mg/24 hours)–21 patches*

NicoDerm CQ Clear Step 2 (14 mg/24 hours)–14 patches*

NicoDerm CQ Clear Step 3 (7 mg/24 hours)–14 patches**

* User's Guide, CD & Child Resistant Disposal Tray

** User's Guide, & Child Resistant Disposal Tray

NICORETTE®
Nicotine Polacrilex Gum/Stop Smoking Aid
Available in Original 2mg and 4mg Strengths,
Mint 2mg and 4mg Strengths and Orange 2mg and 4mg Strengths

IF YOU SMOKE LESS THAN 25 CIGARETTES A DAY: Use 2 mg
IF YOU SMOKE 25 OR MORE CIGARETTES A DAY: Use 4 mg

Action: Stop Smoking Aid

Drug Facts:

Active Ingredient: (In each chewing piece)	Purpose:
Nicotine polacrilex, 2 or 4 mg	Stop smoking aid

Use:
- reduces withdrawal symptoms, including nicotine craving, associated with quitting smoking

Warnings:

If you are pregnant or breast-feeding, only use this medicine on the advice of your health care provider. Smoking can seriously harm your child. Try to stop smoking without using any nicotine replacement medicine. This medicine is believed to be safer than smoking. However, the risks to your child from this medicine are not fully known.

Do not use:
- if you continue to smoke, chew tobacco, use snuff, or use a nicotine patch or other nicotine containing products

Ask a doctor before use if you have:
- heart disease, recent heart attack, or irregular heartbeat. Nicotine can increase your heart rate.
- high blood pressure not controlled with medication. Nicotine can increase blood pressure.
- stomach ulcer or diabetes

Ask a doctor or pharmacist before use if you are:
- using a non-nicotine stop smoking drug
- taking prescription medicine for depression or asthma. Your prescription dose may need to be adjusted.

Stop use and ask a doctor if:
- mouth, teeth or jaw problems occur
- irregular heartbeat or palpitations occur
- you get symptoms of nicotine overdose such as nausea, vomiting, dizziness, diarrhea, weakness and rapid heartbeat

Keep out of reach of children and pets. Pieces of nicotine gum may have enough nicotine to make children and pets sick. Wrap used pieces of gum in paper and throw away in the trash. In case of overdose, get medical help or contact a Poison Control Center right away.

Directions:
- if you are under 18 years of age, ask a doctor before use
- before using this product, read the enclosed User's Guide for complete directions and other important information
- stop smoking completely when you begin using the gum
- if you smoke 25 or more cigarettes a day; use 4 mg nicotine gum
- if you smoke less than 25 cigarettes a day; use 2 mg nicotine gum

Use according to the following 12 week schedule:

[See table at bottom of next page]

- nicotine gum is a medicine and must be used a certain way to get the best results

Continued on next page

Nicorette—Cont.

- chew the gum slowly until it tingles. Then park it between your cheek and gum. When the tingle is gone, begin chewing again, until the tingle returns.
- repeat this process until most of the tingle is gone (about 30 minutes)
- do not eat or drink for 15 minutes before chewing the nicotine gum, or while chewing a piece
- to improve your chances of quitting, use at least 9 pieces per day for the first 6 weeks
- if you experience strong or frequent cravings, you may use a second piece within the hour. However, do not continuously use one piece after another since this may cause you hiccups, heartburn, nausea or other side effects.
- do not use more than 24 pieces a day
- stop using the nicotine gum at the end of 12 weeks. If you still feel the need to use nicotine gum, talk to your doctor.

Other Information:
- store at 20–25°C (68–77°F)
- protect from light

Inactive Ingredients:

Original [2 mg] Inactive Ingredients: Flavors, glycerin, gum base, sodium carbonate, sorbitol, sodium bicarbonate.

Original [4 mg] Inactive Ingredients: Flavors, glycerin, gum base, sodium carbonate, sorbitol, D&C Yellow 10.

Mint [2 mg] Inactive Ingredients: Gum base, magnesium oxide, menthol, peppermint oil, sodium bicarbonate, sodium carbonate, xylitol.

Mint [4 mg] Inactive Ingredients: Gum base, magnesium oxide, menthol, peppermint oil, sodium carbonate, xylitol, D&C yellow #10 Al. lake.

Orange [2 mg] Inactive Ingredients: Flavor, gum base, magnesium oxide, sodium bicarbonate, sodium carbonate, xylitol

Orange [4 mg] Inactive Ingredients: Flavor, gum base, magnesium oxide, sodium carbonate, xylitol, D&C Yellow #10 Al. lake.

TO INCREASE YOUR SUCCESS IN QUITTING:
1. You must be motivated to quit.
2. Use Enough—Chew **at least 9 pieces** of Nicorette per day during the first six weeks.
3. Use Long Enough—Use Nicorette for the full 12 weeks.
4. Use with a support program as directed in the enclosed User's Guide.*

*The American Cancer Society supports the use of a stop smoking aid and counseling as effective tools when quitting smoking but does not endorse any specific product. GlaxoSmithKline pays a fee to the American Cancer Society for the use of its logo.

To remove the gum, tear off single unit.

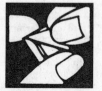

Peel off backing starting at corner with loose edge.

Push gum through foil.

Blister packaged for your protection. **Do not use if individual seals are open or torn.**

- **not for sale to those under 18 years of age**
- **proof of age required**
- **not for sale in vending machines or from any source where proof of age cannot be verified**

READ THE LABEL
Read the carton and the User's Guide before taking this product. Do not discard carton or User's Guide. They contain important information.

How Supplied: Nicorette Original and Mint are available in:
  2 mg or 4 mg Starter kit*—110 pieces
  2 mg or 4 mg Refill—48 pieces, 168 pieces or 192 pieces
Nicorette Orange is available in:
  2 mg or 4 mg Starter kit*—110 pieces
  2 mg or 4 mg Refill—48 pieces
*User's Guide and CD included in kit
Questions or comments? call **1-800-419-4766** weekdays (10:00 a.m.– 4:30 p.m. EST)

Manufactured by Pharmacia AB, Stockholm, Sweden for
GlaxoSmithKline Consumer Healthcare, L.P.
Moon Township, PA 15108

USER'S GUIDE:
HOW TO USE NICORETTE TO HELP YOU QUIT SMOKING
KEYS TO SUCCESS:
1) You must really want to quit smoking for **Nicorette®** to help you.
2) You can greatly increase your chances for success by using at least 9 to 12 pieces every day when you start using **Nicorette**.
3) You should continue to use **Nicorette** as explained in the User's Guide for 12 full weeks.
4) **Nicorette** works best when used together with a support program.
5) If you have trouble using **Nicorette**, ask your doctor or pharmacist or call GlaxoSmithKline at 1-800-419-4766 weekdays (10:00am–4:30pm EST).

SO YOU DECIDED TO QUIT
Congratulations. Your decision to stop smoking is an important one. That's why you've made the right choice in choosing **Nicorette** gum. Your own chances of quitting smoking depend on how much you want to quit, how strongly you are addicted to tobacco, and how closely you follow a quitting program like the one that comes with **Nicorette**.

QUITTING SMOKING IS HARD!
If you've tried to quit before and haven't succeeded, don't be discouraged! Quitting isn't easy. It takes time, and most people try a few times before they are successful. The important thing is to try again until you succeed. This User's Guide will give you support as you become a non-smoker. It will answer common questions about **Nicorette** and give tips to help you stop smoking, and should be referred to often.

WHERE TO GET HELP
You are more likely to stop smoking by using **Nicorette** with a support program that helps you break your smoking habit. There may be support groups in your area for people trying to quit. Call your local chapter of the American Lung Association (1-800-586-4872), American Cancer Society (1-800-227-2345) or American Heart Association (1-800-242-8721) for further information. If you find you cannot stop smoking or if you start smoking again after using **Nicorette**, remember breaking this addiction doesn't happen overnight. You may want to talk to a health care professional who can help you improve your chances of quitting the next time you try **Nicorette** or another method.

LET'S GET ORGANIZED
Your reason for quitting may be a combination of concerns about health, the effect of smoking on your appearance, and pressure from your family and friends to stop smoking. Or maybe you're concerned about the dangerous effect of second-hand smoke on the people you care about. All of these are good reasons. You

Weeks 1 to 6	Weeks 7 to 9	Weeks 10 to 12
1 piece every 1 to 2 hours	1 piece every 2 to 4 hours	1 piece every 4 to 8 hours

probably have others. Decide your most important reasons, and write them down on the wallet card inside the back cover of the User's Guide. Carry this card with you. In difficult moments, when you want to smoke, the card will remind you why you are quitting.

WHAT YOU'RE UP AGAINST

Smoking is addictive in two ways. Your need for nicotine has become both physical and mental. You must overcome both addictions to stop smoking. So while **Nicorette** will lessen your body's physical addition to nicotine, you've got to want to quit smoking to overcome the mental dependence on cigarettes. Once you've decided that you're going to quit, it's time to get started. But first, there are some important cautions you should consider.

SOME IMPORTANT WARNINGS. This product is only for those who want to stop smoking.

If you are pregnant or breast-feeding, only use this medicine on the advice of your health care provider. Smoking can seriously harm your child. Try to stop smoking without using any nicotine replacement medicine. This medicine is believed to be safer than smoking. However, the risks to your child from this medicine are not fully known.

Do not use
- if you continue to smoke, chew tobacco, use snuff, or use a nicotine patch or other nicotine containing products.

Ask a doctor before use if you have
- heart disease, recent heart attack, or irregular heartbeat. Nicotine can increase your heart rate.
- high blood pressure not controlled with medication. Nicotine can increase your blood pressure.
- stomach ulcer or diabetes

Ask a doctor or pharmacist before use if you are
- using a non-nicotine stop smoking drug
- taking a prescription medicine for depression or asthma. Your prescription dose may need to be adjusted.

Stop use and ask a doctor if
- mouth, teeth or jaw problems occur
- irregular heartbeat or palpitations occur
- you get symptoms of nicotine overdose such as nausea, vomiting, dizziness, diarrhea, weakness and rapid heartbeat

Keep out of reach of children and pets. Pieces of nicotine gum may have enough nicotine to make children and pets sick. Wrap used pieces of gum in paper and throw away in the trash. In case of overdose, get medical help or contact a Poison Control Center right away.

LET'S GET STARTED

Becoming a non-smoker starts today. First, check that you bought the right starting dose. **If you smoke 25 or more cigarettes a day**, use 4 mg nicotine gum. **If you smoke less than 25 cigarettes a day**, use 2 mg nicotine gum. Next read through the entire User's Guide carefully. Then, set your personalized quitting schedule. Take out a calendar that

you can use to track your progress, and identify four dates, using the stickers in the User's Guide.

STEP 1: (Weeks 1–6) Your quit date (and the day you'll start using Nicorette gum). Choose your quit date (it should be soon). This is the day you will quit smoking cigarettes entirely and begin using **Nicorette** to satisfy your cravings for nicotine. For the first six weeks, you'll use a piece of **Nicorette** every hour or two. Be sure to follow the directions starting on pages 9 and 11 of the User's Guide. Place the Step 1 sticker on this date.

STEP 2: (Weeks 7–9) The day you'll start reducing your use of Nicorette. After six weeks, you'll begin gradually reducing your **Nicorette** usage to one piece every two to four hours. Place the Step 2 sticker on this date (the first day of week seven).

STEP 3: (Weeks 10–12) The day you'll further reduce your use of Nicorette. Nine weeks after you begin using **Nicorette**, you will further reduce your nicotine intake by using one piece every four to eight hours. Place the Step 3 sticker on this date (the first day of week ten). For the next three weeks, you'll use a piece of **Nicorette** every four to eight hours. **End of treatment: The day you'll complete Nicorette therapy.**

Nicorette should not be used for longer than twelve weeks. Identify the date thirteen weeks after the date you chose in Step 1 and place the "EX-Smoker" sticker on your calendar.

PLAN AHEAD

Because smoking is an addiction, it is not easy to stop. After you've given up cigarettes, you will still have a strong urge to smoke. Plan ahead NOW for these times, so you're not defeated in a moment of weakness. The following tips may help:
- Keep the phone numbers of supportive friends and family members handy.
- Keep a record of your quitting process. Track the number of **Nicorette** pieces you use each day, and whether you feel a craving for cigarettes. In the event that you slip, immediately stop smoking and resume your quit attempt with **Nicorette**.
- Put together an Emergency Kit that includes items that will help take your mind off occasional urges to smoke. Include cinnamon gum or lemon drops to suck on, a relaxing cassette tape and something for your hands to play with, like a smooth rock, rubber band or small metal balls.
- Set aside some small rewards, like a new magazine or a gift certificate from your favorite store, which you'll 'give' yourself after passing difficult hurdles.
- Think now about the times when you most often want a cigarette, and then plan what else you might do instead of smoking. For instance, you might plan to take your coffee break in a new location, or take a walk right after dinner, so you won't be tempted to smoke.

HOW NICORETTE GUM WORKS

Nicorette's sugar-free chewing pieces provide nicotine to your system—they work as a temporary aid to help you quit

smoking by reducing nicotine withdrawal symptoms. **Nicorette** provides a lower level of nicotine to your blood than cigarettes, and allows you to gradually do away with your body's need for nicotine. Because **Nicorette** does not contain the tar or carbon monoxide of cigarette smoke, it does not have the same health dangers as tobacco. However, it still delivers nicotine, the addictive part of cigarette smoke. Nicotine can cause side effects such as headache, nausea, upset stomach and dizziness.

HOW TO USE NICORETTE GUM

If you are under 18 years of age, ask a doctor before use.

Before you can use **Nicorette** correctly, you have to practice! That sounds silly, but it isn't.

Nicorette isn't like ordinary chewing gum. It's a medicine, and must be chewed a certain way to work right. Chewed like ordinary gum, **Nicorette** won't work well and can cause side effects. An overdose can occur if you chew more than one piece of **Nicorette** at the same time, or if you chew many pieces one after another. Read all the following instructions before using **Nicorette**. Refer to them often to make sure you're using **Nicorette** gum correctly. If you chew too fast, or do not chew correctly, you may get hiccups, heartburn, or other stomach problems. Don't eat or drink for 15 minutes before using **Nicorette**, or while chewing a piece. The effectiveness of **Nicorette** may be reduced by some foods and drinks, such as coffee, juices, wine or soft drinks.

1. Stop smoking completely before you start using **Nicorette**.
2. To reduce craving and other withdrawal symptoms, use **Nicorette** according to the dosage schedule on page 11 of the User's Guide.
3. Chew each **Nicorette** piece <u>very slowly several times.</u>
4. Stop chewing when you notice a peppery taste, or a slight tingling in your mouth. (This usually happens after about 15 chews, but may vary from person to person.)
5. "PARK" the **Nicorette** piece between your cheek and gum and leave it there.
6. When the peppery taste or tingle is almost gone (in about a minute), start to chew a few times slowly again. When the taste or tingle returns, stop again.
7. Park the **Nicorette** piece again (in a different place in your mouth).
8. Repeat steps 3 to 7 (chew, chew, park) until most of the nicotine is gone from the **Nicorette** piece (usually happens in about half an hour; the peppery taste or tingle won't return).
9. Wrap the used **Nicorette** in paper and throw away in the trash.

See the chart in the **"DIRECTIONS"** section above for the recommended usage schedule for **Nicorette**.

[See table at top of next page]

To improve your chances of quitting, use at least 9 pieces of **Nicorette** a day. If you experience strong or frequent cravings you may use a second piece within the

Continued on next page

Nicorette—Cont.

hour. However, do not continuously use one piece after another, since this may cause you hiccups, heartburn, nausea or other side effects.

HOW TO REDUCE YOUR NICORETTE USAGE

The goal of using **Nicorette** is to slowly reduce your dependence on nicotine. The schedule for using **Nicorette** will help you reduce your nicotine craving gradually. Here are some tips to help you cut back during each step:

- After a while, start chewing each **Nicorette** piece for only 10 to 15 minutes, instead of half an hour. Then gradually begin to reduce the number of pieces used.
- Or, try chewing each piece for longer than half an hour, but reduce the number of pieces you use each day.
- Substitute ordinary chewing gum for some of the **Nicorette** pieces you would normally use. Increase the number of pieces of ordinary gum as you cut back on the **Nicorette** pieces.

STOP USING NICORETTE AT THE END OF WEEK 12. If you still feel the need to use **Nicorette** after Week 12, talk with your doctor.

TIPS TO MAKE QUITTING EASIER

Within the first few weeks of giving up smoking, you may be tempted to smoke for pleasure, particularly after completing a difficult task, or at a party or bar. Here are some tips to help get you through the important first stages of becoming a non-smoker:

On your Quit Date:

- Ask your family, friends, and co-workers to support you in your efforts to stop smoking.
- Throw away all your cigarettes, matches, lighters, ashtrays, etc.
- Keep busy on your quit day. Exercise. Go to a movie. Take a walk. Get together with friends.
- Figure out how much money you'll save by not smoking. Most ex-smokers can save more than $1,000 a year.
- Write down what you will do with the money you save.
- Know your high risk situations and plan ahead how you will deal with them.
- Keep **Nicorette** gum near your bed, so you'll be prepared for any nicotine cravings when you wake up in the morning.
- Visit your dentist and have your teeth cleaned to get rid of the tobacco stains.

Right after Quitting:

- During the first few days after you've stopped smoking, spend as much time as possible at places where smoking is not allowed.
- Drink large quantities of water and fruit juices.
- Try to avoid alcohol, coffee and other beverages you associate with smoking.
- Remember that temporary urges to smoke will pass, even if you don't smoke a cigarette.
- Keep your hands busy with something like a pencil or a paper clip.
- Find other activities which help you relax without cigarettes. Swim, jog, take a walk, play basketball.

The following chart lists the recommended usage schedule for **Nicorette**e:

Weeks 1 through 6	Weeks 7 through 9	Weeks 10 through 12
1 piece every 1 to 2 hours	1 piece every 2 to 4 hours	1 piece every 4 to 8 hours

DO NOT USE MORE THAN 24 PIECES PER DAY.

- Don't worry too much about gaining weight. Watch what you eat, take time for daily exercise, and change your eating habits if you need to.
- Laughter helps. Watch or read something funny.

WHAT TO EXPECT

Your body is now coming back into balance. During the first few days after you stop smoking, you might feel edgy and nervous and have trouble concentrating. You might get headaches, feel dizzy and a little out of sorts, feel sweaty or have stomach upsets. You might even have trouble sleeping at first. These are typical withdrawal symptoms that will go away with time. Your smoker's cough will get worse before it gets better. But don't worry, that's a good sign. Coughing helps clear the tar deposits out of your lungs.

After a Week or Two.

By now you should be feeling more confident that you can handle those smoking urges. Many of your withdrawal symptoms have left by now, and you should be noticing some positive signs: less coughing, better breathing and an improved sense of taste and smell, to name a few.

After a Month.

You probably have the urge to smoke much less often now. But urges may still occur, and when they do, they are likely to be powerful ones that come out of nowhere. Don't let them catch you off guard. Plan ahead for these difficult times. Concentrate on the ways non-smokers are more attractive than smokers. Their skin is less likely to wrinkle. Their teeth are whiter, cleaner. Their breath is fresher. Their hair and clothes smell better. That cough seems to make even a laugh sound more like a rattle is a thing of the past. Their children and others around them are healthier, too.

What To Do About Relapse.

What should you do if you slip and start smoking again? The answer is simple. A lapse of one or two or even a few cigarettes has not spoiled your efforts! Discard your cigarettes, forgive yourself and try again. If you start smoking again, keep your box of **Nicorette** for your next quit attempt. If you have taken up regular smoking again, don't be discouraged. Research shows that the best thing you can do is to try again. The important thing is to learn from your last attempt.

- Admit that you've slipped, but don't treat yourself as a failure.
- Try to identify the 'trigger' that caused you to slip, and prepare a better plan for dealing with this problem next time.

- Talk positively to yourself—tell yourself that you have learned something from this experience.
- Make sure you used **Nicorette** gum correctly over the full 12 weeks to reduce your craving for nicotine.
- Remember that it takes practice to do anything, and quitting smoking is no exception.

WHEN THE STRUGGLE IS OVER

Once you've stopped smoking, take a second and pat yourself on the back. Now do it again. You deserve it. Remember now why you decided to stop smoking in the first place. Look at your list of reasons. Read them again. And smile. Now think about all the money you are saving and what you'll do with it. All the non-smoking places you can go, and what you might do there. All those years you may have added to your life, and what you'll do with them. Remember that temptation may not be gone forever. However, the hard part is behind you, so look forward with a positive attitude and enjoy your new life as a non-smoker.

QUESTIONS & ANSWERS

1. How will I feel when I stop smoking and start using Nicorette? You'll need to prepare yourself for some nicotine withdrawal symptoms. These begin almost immediately after you stop smoking, and are usually at their worst during the first three to four days. Understand that any of the following is possible:

- craving for cigarettes
- anxiety, irritability, restlessness, mood changes, nervousness
- drowsiness
- trouble concentrating
- increased appetite and weight gain
- headaches, muscular pain, constipation, fatigue.

Nicorette can help provide relief from withdrawal symptoms such as irritability and nervousness, as well as the craving for nicotine you used to satisfy by having a cigarette.

2. Is Nicorette just substuting one form of nicotine for another? **Nicorette** does contain nicotine. The purpose of **Nicorette** is to provide you with enough nicotine to help control the physical withdrawal symptoms so you can deal with the mental aspects of quitting. During the 12 week program, you will gradually reduce your nicotine intake by switching to fewer pieces each day. Remember, don't use **Nicorette** together with nicotine patches or other nicotine containing products.

3. Can I be hurt by using Nicorette? For most adults, the amount of nicotine in the gum will be less than from smoking. Some people will be sensitive to even this amount of nicotine and should not use this product without advice from their doctor (see page 4 of User's Guide). Because **Nicorette** is a gum-based product, chewing it can cause dental fillings to loosen and aggravate other mouth, tooth and jaw problems. **Nicorette** can also cause hiccups, heartburn and other stomach problems especially if chewed too quickly or not chewed correctly.

4. Will I gain weight? Many people do tend to gain a few pounds in the first 8–10 weeks after they stop smoking. This is a very small price to pay for the enormous gains that you will make in your overall health and attractiveness. If you continue to gain weight after the first two months, try to analyze what you're doing differently. Reduce your fat intake, choose healthy snacks, and increase your physical activity to burn off the extra calories.

5. Is Nicorette more expensive than smoking? The total cost of **Nicorette** for the twelve week program is about equal to what a person who smokes one and a half packs of cigarettes a day would spend on cigarettes for the same period of time. Also use of **Nicorette** is only a short-term cost, while the cost of smoking is a long-term cost, because of the health problems smoking causes.

6. What if I slip up? Discard your cigarettes, forgive yourself and then get back on track. Don't consider yourself a failure or punish yourself. In fact, people who have already tried to quit are more likely to be successful the next time. **GOOD LUCK!**
[End User's Guide]
Copyright © 2001 GlaxoSmithKline Consumer Healthcare, L.P.
Shown in Product Identification Guide, page 508

Maximum Strength
NYTOL® QUICKGELS® SOFTGELS

Indication: For relief of occasional sleeplessness.

Directions: Adults and children 12 years of age and over: oral dosage is one softgel (50 mg) at bedtime if needed, or as directed by a doctor.

Warnings: Do not give to children under 12 years of age. If sleeplessness persists continuously for more than two weeks, consult your doctor. Insomnia may be a symptom of serious underlying medical illness. **Do not take this product, unless directed by a doctor, if you have a breathing problem such as emphysema or chronic bronchitis, or if you have glaucoma or difficulty in urination due to enlargement of the prostate gland. Do not use** with any other product containing diphenhydramine, including one applied topically. Avoid alcoholic beverages while taking this product. Do not take this product if you are taking sedatives or tranquilizers, without first consulting your doctor. In case of accidental overdose, seek professional assistance or contact a Poison Control Center immediately. As with any drug, if you are pregnant or nursing a baby, seek the advice of a health professional before using this product. Keep out of reach of children.

Drug Interactions: Alcohol and other drugs which cause CNS depression will heighten the depressant effect of this product. Monoamine oxidase (MAO) inhibitors will prolong and intensify the anticholinergic effects of antihistamines.

Symptoms and Treatment of Oral Overdosage: In adults overdose may cause CNS depression resulting in hypnosis and coma. In children CNS hyperexcitability may follow sedation; the stimulant phase may bring tremor, delirium and convulsions. Gastrointestinal reactions may include dry mouth, appetite loss, nausea and/or vomiting. Respiratory distress and cardiovascular complications (hypotension) may be evident. Treatment includes inducing emesis and controlling symptoms.

Active Ingredient: Diphenhydramine Hydrochloride 50 mg per softgel.

Inactive Ingredients: Edible Ink, Gelatin, Glycerin, Polyethylene Glycol, Purified Water, Sorbitol.

How Supplied: Available in packages of 8 and 16 softgels.
Shown in Product Identification Guide, page 508

NYTOL® QUICKCAPS® CAPLETS

Indication: For relief of occasional sleeplessness.

Directions: Adults and children 12 years of age and over: oral dosage is two caplets (50 mg) at bedtime if needed, or as directed by a doctor.

Warnings: Do not give to children under 12 years of age. If sleeplessness persists continuously for more than two weeks, consult your doctor. Insomnia may be a symptom of serious underlying medical illness. **Do not take this product, unless directed by a doctor, if you have a breathing problem such as emphysema or chronic bronchitis, or if you have glaucoma or difficulty in urination due to enlargement of the prostate gland. Do not use** with any other product containing diphenhydramine, including one applied topically. Avoid alcoholic beverages while taking this product. Do not take this product if you are taking sedatives or tranquilizers, without first consulting your doctor. In case of accidental overdose, seek professional assistance or contact a Poison Control Center immediately. As with any drug, if you are pregnant or nursing a baby, seek the advice of a health professional before using this product. Keep out of reach of children.

Drug Interactions: Alcohol and other drugs which cause CNS depression will heighten the depressant effect of this product. Monoamine oxidase (MAO) inhibitors will prolong and intensify the anticholinergic effects of antihistamines.

Symptoms and Treatment of Oral Overdosage: In adults, overdose may cause CNS depression resulting in hyp-
nosis and coma. In children, CNS hyperexcitability may follow sedation; the stimulant phase may bring tremor, delirium and convulsions. Gastrointestinal reactions may include dry mouth, appetite loss, nausea and/or vomiting. Respiratory distress and cardiovascular complications (hypotension) may be evident. Treatment includes inducing emesis and controlling symptoms.

Active Ingredient: Diphenhydramine Hydrochloride 25 mg per caplet.

Inactive Ingredients: Corn Starch, Lactose, Microcrystalline Cellulose, Silica, Stearic Acid.

How supplied: Available in tamper-evident packages of 16, 32 and 72 caplets.
Shown in Product Identification Guide, page 508

Quick Dissolve
PHAZYME®–125 MG Chewable Tablets
[fay-zime]

Description: A great tasting, smooth cool mint chewable tablet containing simethicone, an antiflatulent to alleviate or relieve the symptoms referred to as gas. Uniquely formulated to dissolve quickly and completely in your mouth. It has no known side effects or drug interactions.

Active Ingredient: Each tablet contains simethicone 125 mg.

Inactive Ingredients: Aspartame, citricacid, colloidal silicon dioxide, crospovidone, dextrates, maltodextrin, mannitol, peppermint flavor, pregelatinized starch, sodium bicarbonate, sorbitol, talc, tribasic calcium phosphate.

Actions: Simethicone minimizes gas formation and relieves gas entrapment in both the stomach and the lower G.I. tract. This action combats the distress due to gastrointestinal gas.
Other Information: Each tablet contains sodium 8 mg. Phenylketonurics: contains phenylalanine 0.4 mg per tablet.

Indication: Relieves pressure, bloating or fullness commonly referred to as gas.

Warnings: Keep this and all drugs out of the reach of children. If condition persists, consult your physician.
Store at room temperature 59°–86°F (15°–30°C).

Dosage: Directions: Chew one or two tablets thoroughly, as needed after a meal]. Do not exceed four tablets per day except under the advice and supervision of a physician.

How Supplied: White, bevel-edged tablets imprinted with "Phazyme 125" in 18 count and 48 count bottles.
Shown in Product Identification Guide, page 509

Continued on next page

Ultra Strength
PHAZYME®–180 MG Softgels
[fay-zime]

Description: An orange, easy to swallow softgel, containing simethicone, an antiflatulent to alleviate or relieve the symptoms referred to as gas. It has no known side effects or drug interactions.
Active Ingredient: Each softgel contains simethicone 180 mg.
Inactive Ingredients: FD&C Yellow No. 6, gelatin, glycerin, and white edible ink.

Actions: Simethicone minimizes gas formation and relieves gas entrapment in both the stomach and the lower G.I. tract. This action combats the distress due to gastrointestinal gas.

Indication: Relieves pressure, bloating or fullness commonly referred to as gas.

Warnings: Keep this and all drugs out of the reach of children. If condition persists, consult your physician.
Store at room temperature 59°–86°F (15°–30°C).

Dosage: Directions: Swallow one or two softgels as needed after a meal. Do not exceed two softgels per day except under the advice and supervision of a physician.

How Supplied: Orange softgel imprinted with "PZ 180" in 12 count and 36 count blister pack, 60 count and 100 count bottles.

Shown in Product Identification Guide, page 508

SENSODYNE® FRESH MINT
SENSODYNE® FRESH IMPACT
SENSODYNE® COOL GEL
SENSODYNE® WITH BAKING SODA
SENSODYNE® TARTAR CONTROL
SENSODYNE® TARTAR CONTROL PLUS WHITENING
SENSODYNE® ORIGINAL FLAVOR
SENSODYNE® EXTRA WHITENING
Anticavity toothpaste for sensitive teeth

Active Ingredients: "Fresh Impact" Potassium Nitrate 5% Sodium Fluoride 0.15% w/v fluoride ion 5% Potassium Nitrate and 0.15% w/v Sodium Monofluorophosphate (Extra Whitening) or Sodium Fluoride (Fresh Mint, 0.15% w/v; Baking Soda, 0.15% w/v; Cool Gel, 0.13% w/v; Tartar Control, 0.13% w/v; Tartar Control Plus Whitening 0.145% w/v; Original Flavor, 0.13% w/v), or Sodium Fluoride 0.15% w/v fluoride ion (Fresh Impact). Sensodyne Fresh Mint, Sensodyne Fresh Impact, Sensodyne Cool Gel, Sensodyne with Baking Soda, Sensodyne Tartar Control, Sensodyne Tartar Control Plus Whitening, Sensodyne Original Flavor and Sensodyne Extra Whitening contain fluoride for cavity prevention and Potassium Nitrate clinically proven to reduce

pain sensitivity for relief of dentinal hypersensitivity resulting from the exposure of tooth dentin due to periodontal surgery, cervical (gum line) erosion, abrasion or recession which causes pain on contact with hot, cold, or tactile stimuli.

Inactive Ingredients: *Baking Soda:* Flavor, Glycerin, Hydrated Silica, Hydroxyethylcellulose, Methylparaben, Propylparaben, Silica, Sodium Bicarbonate, Sodium Lauryl Sulfate, Sodium Saccharin, Titanium Dioxide, Water.
Extra Whitening: Calcium Peroxide, Flavor, Glycerin, Hydrated Silica, PEG-12, PEG-75, Silica, Sodium Carbonate, Sodium Lauryl Sulfate, Sodium Saccharin, Titanium Dioxide, Water.
Tartar Control: Cellulose Gum, Cocamidopropyl Betaine, Flavor, Glycerin, Hydrated Silica, Silica, Sodium Bicarbonate, Sodium Saccharin, Tetrapotassium Pyrophosphate, Titanium Dioxide, Water.
Tartar Control Plus Whitening: Cellulose Gum, Flavor, Glycerin, Polyethylene Glycol, Silica, Sodium Lauryl Sulfate, Sodium Saccharin, Tetrapotassium Pyrophosphate, Titanium Dioxide, Water.
Cool Gel: Cellulose Gum, FD&C Blue #1, Flavor, Glycerin, Hydrated Silica, Silica, Sodium Methyl Cocoyl Taurate, Sodium Saccharin, Sorbitol, Trisodium Phosphate, Water. *Fresh Impact:* D&C yellow #10 lake, FD&C blue #1 lake, flavor, glycerin, hydrated silica, sodium benzoate, sodium hydroxide, sodium lauryl sulfate, sodium saccharin, sorbitol, titanium dioxide, water, xanthan gum
Fresh Mint: Inactive Ingredients: Carbomer, cellulose gum, D&C yellow #10, FD&C blue #1, flavor, glycerin, hydrated silica, octadecene/MA copolymer, poloxamer 407, potassium hydroxide, sodium lauroyl sarcosinate, sodium saccharin, sorbitol, titanium dioxide, water, xanthan gum.
Original Flavor: Cellulose Gum, D&C Red No. 28, Glycerin, Hydrated Silica, Peppermint Oil, Silica, Sodium Methyl Cocoyl Taurate, Sodium Saccharin, Sorbitol, Titanium Dioxide, Trisodium Phosphate, Water.

Actions: All Sensodyne Formulas significantly reduce tooth hypersensitivity, with response to therapy evident after two weeks of use. Controlled double-blind clinical studies provide substantial evidence of the safety and effectiveness of Potassium Nitrate. The current theory on mechanism of action is that potassium nitrate has an effect on neural transmission, interrupting the signal which would result in the sensation of pain. Fluorides are anticariogenic, forming fluoroapatite in the outer surface of the dental enamel which is resistant to acids and caries.

Warnings: Sensitive teeth may indicate a serious problem that may need prompt care by a dentist. See your dentist if the problem persists or worsens. Do not use this product longer than 4 weeks unless recommended by a dentist or physician. Keep this and all drugs

out of the reach of children. If accidentally swallow more than used for brushing, seek professional assistance or contact a Poison Control Center immediately.

Dosage and Administration: Adults and children 12 years of age and older: Apply a 1-inch strip of the product onto a soft bristle toothbrush. Brush teeth thoroughly for at least 1 minute twice a day (morning and evening) or as recommended by a dentist or physician. Make sure to brush all sensitive areas of the teeth. Children under 12 years of age: consult a dentist or physician.

How Supplied: All Sensodyne formulas are supplied in 2.1 oz. (60g), 4.0 oz. (113g) and 6.0 oz. (170g) tubes. Sensodyne Cool Gel is supplied in 4.0 oz. and 6.0 oz. tubes. Sensodyne Baking Soda is supplied in 4.0 oz and 6.0 oz. only.

SINGLET® For Adults
Nasal Decongestant/Antihistamine/Analgesic (pain reliever)/Antipyretic (fever reducer)

Indications: For temporary relief of nasal congestion and sinus and headache pain associated with sinusitis or due to a cold, hay fever or other upper respiratory allergies. Also temporarily relieves nasal congestion, sinus headache, runny nose, sneezing, itching of the nose or throat, and itchy, watery eyes due to hay fever or other upper respiratory allergies. Also temporarily relieves fever due to the common cold.

Directions: Adults (12 years and older): 1 caplet every 4 to 6 hours, **not to exceed 4 caplets in any 24-hour period,** or as directed by a doctor. Children under 12 years of age: Consult a doctor.

Warnings: **Do not exceed recommended dosage.** If nervousness, dizziness, or sleeplessness occur, discontinue use and consult a doctor. Do not take this product for more than 10 days. If symptoms do not improve or are accompanied by fever that lasts for more than 3 days, or if new symptoms occur, consult a doctor. Do not take this product, unless directed by a doctor, if you have a breathing problem such as emphysema or chronic bronchitis, or if you have heart disease, high blood pressure, thyroid disease, diabetes, glaucoma or difficulty in urination due to enlargement of the prostate gland. May cause excitability especially in children. May cause drowsiness; alcohol, sedatives, and tranquilizers may increase the drowsiness effect. Avoid alcoholic beverages while taking this product. Do not take this product if you are taking sedatives or tranquilizers, without first consulting your doctor. Use caution when driving a motor vehicle or operating machinery. **KEEP THIS AND ALL DRUGS OUT OF THE REACH OF CHILDREN.** Prompt medical attention is critical for adults as well as for children even if you do not notice any signs or symptoms. In case of accidental overdose, seek professional assistance or contact a Poison Control Center immediately. As with any drug, if you are pregnant or nursing a baby, seek the advice of a health professional before using this product.

Alcohol Warning: If you consume 3 or more alcoholic drinks every day, ask your doctor whether you should take acetaminophen or other pain reliever/fever reducers. Acetaminophen may cause liver damage.

Drug Interaction Precaution: Do not use this product if you are now taking a prescription monoamine oxidase inhibitor (MAOI) (certain drugs for depression, psychiatric or emotional conditions, or Parkinson's disease), or for 2 weeks after stopping the MAOI drug. If you are uncertain whether your prescription drug contains an MAOI, consult a health professional before taking this product.

Active Ingredients: Each caplet contains: Pseudoephedrine Hydrochloride 60 mg, Chlorpheniramine Maleate 4 mg, Acetaminophen 650 mg.

Inactive Ingredients: D&C Red 27, D&C Yellow 10, FD&C Blue 1, Hydroxypropyl Cellulose, Hypromellose, Magnesium Stearate, Microcrystalline Cellulose, Polyethylene Glycol, Pregelatinized Corn Starch, Sodium Starch Glycolate, Sucrose and Titanium Dioxide.
Store at room temperature (59°–86°F). Avoid excessive heat and humidity.
Comments or Questions? Call toll-free 1-800-245-1040 weekdays
Distributed by: GlaxoSmithKline Consumer Healthcare, L.P.
Moon Township, PA 15108. Made in U.S.A.

SOMINEX Original Formula
Nighttime Sleep Aid
Doctor-preferred sleep ingredient

Indications: Helps to reduce difficulty falling asleep.

Directions: Adults and children 12 years and over: Take 2 tablets at bedtime if needed, or as directed by a doctor. For best results, take recommended dose. This will provide approximately six to eight hours of restful sleep.

Warnings: Do not give to children under 12 years of age. If sleeplessness persists continually for more than 2 weeks, consult your doctor. Insomnia may be a symptom of serious underlying medical illness. Do not take this product, unless directed by a doctor, if you have a breathing problem such as emphysema or chronic bronchitis, or if you have glaucoma or difficulty in urination due to enlargement of the prostate gland. Avoid alcoholic beverages while taking this product. Do not take this product if you are taking sedatives or tranquilizers,

without first consulting your doctor. As with any drug, if you are pregnant or nursing a baby, seek the advice of a health professional before using this product. **Keep this and all drugs out of the reach of children.** In case of accidental overdose, seek professional assistance or contact a poison control center immediately.

Active Ingredients: Each tablet contains 25 mg Diphenhydramine HCl.

Inactive Ingredients: Dibasic Calcium Phosphate, FD&C Blue #1, Magnesium Stearate, Microcrystalline Cellulose, Silicon Dioxide, Starch.
Tamper Evident Feature: Individually sealed in foil for your protection. Do not use if foil or plastic bubble is torn or punctured.
Store at room temperature, avoid excessive heat (greater than 100°F) or humidity.

How Supplied: Consumer Packages of 16, 32 and 72 tablets
Also Available in Maximum Strength Formula.
Comments or Questions? Call Toll-Free 1-800-245-1040 Weekdays.
GlaxoSmithKline Consumer Healthcare, L.P.
Moon Township, PA 15108. Made in U.S.A.

TAGAMET HB® 200
Cimetidine Tablets 200 mg/
Acid Reducer

Tagamet HB® 200 relieves and prevents heartburn, acid indigestion and sour stomach when used as directed. It contains the same ingredient found in prescription strength Tagamet. Tagamet HB 200 reduces the production of stomach acid.

Active Ingredient: Cimetidine, 200 mg.

Inactive Ingredients: Cellulose, cornstarch, hypromellose, magnesium stearate, polyethylene glycol, polysorbate 80, povidone, sodium lauryl sulfate, sodium starch glycolate, titanium dioxide.

Uses:
• For relief of heartburn associated with acid indigestion and sour stomach.
• For prevention of heartburn associated with acid indigestion and sour stomach brought on by eating or drinking certain food and beverages.

Directions:
• For **relief** of symptoms, swallow 1 tablet with a glass of water.
• For **prevention** of symptoms, swallow 1 tablet with a glass of water **right before or anytime up to 30 minutes before** eating food or drinking beverages that cause heartburn.
• Tagamet HB 200 can be used up to twice daily (up to 2 tablets in 24 hours).
• This product should not be given to children under 12 years old unless directed by a doctor.

Warnings:
Allergy Warning: Do not use if you are allergic to Tagamet HB 200 (cimetidine) or other acid reducers.

Ask a Doctor Before Use If You are Taking:
• theophylline (oral asthma medicine)
• warfarin (blood thinning medicine)
• phenytoin (seizure medicine)
If you are not sure whether your medication contains one of these drugs or have any other questions about medicines you are taking, call our consumer affairs specialist at 1-800-482-4394.
• Do not take the maximum daily dosage for more than 2 weeks continuously except under the advice and supervision of a doctor.
• If you have trouble swallowing, or persistent abdominal pain, see your doctor promptly. You may have a serious condition that may need a different treatment.
• As with any drug, if you are pregnant or nursing a baby, seek the advice of a health professional before using this product.
• Keep this and all medications out of the reach of children.
• In case of accidental overdose, seek professional assistance or contact a poison control center immediately.

READ THE LABEL
Read the directions and warnings before taking this medication.
Store at 15°–30°C (59°–86°F).

Comments or questions? Call Toll-Free 1-800-482-4394 weekdays.

PHARMACOKINETIC INTERACTIONS
Cimetidine at prescription doses is known to inhibit various P450 metabolizing isoenzymes, which could affect metabolism of other drugs and increase their blood concentration. Investigation of pharmacokinetic interactions at the recommended OTC doses of cimetidine have thus far shown only small effects.
A pharmacokinetic study conducted in 26 normal male subjects (mean age, 38 years) at steady state using the maximum recommended OTC dose level (200 mg twice a day), showed that Tagamet HB 200, on average, increased the 24 hour AUC of theophylline by 14% and increased peak theophylline levels by 15%. This interaction should be borne in mind in advising patients on the use of Tagamet HB 200. At the prescription doses of cimetidine, clinically significant pharmacokinetic interactions between cimetidine and warfarin, phenytoin, and theophylline have been reported. At prescription doses, pharmacokinetic interactions have been reported for a number of other drugs as well, such as with dihydropyridine calcium channel blockers or some short acting benzodiazepines. At the maximum recommended OTC dose level (200 mg twice a day), a pharmacokinetic study conducted in 21 normal male subjects (mean age, 38 years) showed that Tagamet HB 200, on average, increased the total AUC of triazolam by 26–28% and increased peak

Continued on next page

Tagamet HB 200—Cont.

triazolam levels by 11–23%. Tagamet HB 200 did not alter the apparent terminal elimination half-life of triazolam.

How Supplied: Tagamet HB 200 (Cimetidine Tablets 200 mg) is available in boxes of blister packs in 6, 30, 50, & 70 tablet sizes.

Shown in Product Identification Guide, page 509

TEGRIN® DANDRUFF SHAMPOO – EXTRA CONDITIONING

Description: Tegrin® Dandruff Shampoo contains 7% w/w Coal Tar Solution, USP, equivalent to 0.7% w/w coal tar, in a pleasantly scented, high-foaming, cleansing shampoo base with emollients, conditioners and other formula components.

Active Ingredients: **Purpose:**
7% w/w Coal tar .... Anti Dandruff
solution, USP   Anti Seborrheic
equivalent to 0.7%   Dermatitis
w/w Coal tar   Anti Psoriasis

Use: controls the flaking and itching of the scalp associated with dandruff, seborrheic dermatitis, and psoriasis.

Warnings: For external use only. Ask a doctor before use if you have psoriasis or seborrheic dermatitis that covers a large area of the body. **Ask a doctor or pharmacist if you are** using other forms of psoriasis therapy such as ultraviolet radiation or prescription drugs. **When using this product** • do not use for prolonged periods • avoid contact with eyes. If contact occurs, rinse eyes thoroughly with water. • use caution in exposing skin to sunlight after application. It may increase your tendency to sunburn for up to 24 hours after application. **Stop use and ask a doctor if** condition worsens or does not improve after regular use of this product as directed. **Keep out of reach of children.** If swallowed, get medical help or contact a Poison Control Center right away.

Directions: Shake well. Wet hair, lather, rinse, repeat. For best results use at least twice a week or as directed by a doctor.

Other Information:
Store at 20°–25°C (68°–77°F)

Inactive Ingredients:
Alcohol (7.0%), Ammonium Lauryl Sulfate, Citric Acid, FD&C Blue #1, Fragrance, Glycol Stearate (and) Sodium Laureth Sulfate (and) Hexylene Glycol, Guar Hydroxypropyltrimonium Chloride, Hydroxypropyl Methylcellulose, Lauramide DEA, Methylparaben, Propylparaben, Sodium Lauryl Sulfate, Water.

How Supplied: Tegrin® Dandruff Shampoo is available in Extra Conditioning and Fresh Herbal formulas and supplied in 7 fl. oz. (207 ml) plastic bottles.

Coal Tar is obtained in the destructive distillation of bituminous coal and is a highly effective agent for controlling the flaking and itching of the scalp associated with dandruff, seborrheic dermatitis, and psoriasis. The action of coal tar is believed to be keratolytic, antiseptic, antipruritic, and astringent. The coal tar solution used in Tegrin® Dandruff Shampoo is prepared in such a way as to reduce the itch and other irritant components found in crude coal tar without reduction in therapeutic potency.

Coal Tar Solution has been used clinically for many years as a remedy for dandruff and for scaling associated with scalp disorders such as seborrhea and psoriasis. Its mechanism of action has not been fully established, but it is believed to retard the rate of turnover of epidermal cells with regular use. A number of clinical studies have demonstrated the performance attributes of Tegrin® Dandruff Shampoo against dandruff and seborrheic dermatitis. In addition to relieving the above symptoms, Tegrin® Dandruff Shampoo, used regularly, maintains scalp and hair cleanliness and leaves the hair lustrous and manageable.

TEGRIN® DANDRUFF SHAMPOO-FRESH HERBAL

Description: Tegrin® Dandruff Shampoo contains 7% w/w Coal Tar Solution, USP, equivalent to 0.7% w/w coal tar, in a pleasantly scented, high-foaming, cleansing shampoo base with emollients, conditioners and other formula components.

Active Ingredients: **Purpose:**
7% w/w Coal tar
    solution, USP .... Anti Dandruff
equivalent to 0.7%
    w/w Coal tar   Anti Seborrheic
    Dermatitis Anti Psoriasis

Use: controls the flaking and itching of the scalp associated with dandruff, seborrheic dermatitis, and psoriasis.

Warnings:
For external use only
Ask a doctor before use if you have psoriasis or seborrheic dermatitis that covers a large area of the body
Ask a doctor or pharmacist if you are using other forms of psoriasis therapy such as ultraviolet radiation or prescription drugs
When using this product • do not use for prolonged periods
• avoid contact with eyes. If contact occurs, rinse eyes thoroughly with water.
• use caution in exposing skin to sunlight after application. It may increase your tendency to sunburn for up to 24 hours after application.
Stop use and ask a doctor if condition worsens or does not improve after regular use of this product as directed.
Keep out of reach of children. If swallowed, get medical help or contact a Poison Control center right away.

Directions: Shake well. Wet hair. Lather, rinse, repeat. For best results use at least twice a week or as directed by a doctor.

Other Information:
Store at 20°–25°C (68°–77°F)

Inactive Ingredients:
Alcohol (7.0%), Citric Acid, Cocamide DEA, FD&C Blue #1, Fragrance, Glycol Stearate (and) Sodium Laureth Sulfate (and) Hexylene Glycol, Hydroxypropyl Methylcellulose, Methylparaben, Propylparaben, Sodium Lauryl Sulfate, Water.

How Supplied: Tegrin® Dandruff Shampoo is available in Extra Conditioning and Fresh Herbal formulas and supplied in 7 fl. oz. (207 ml) plastic bottles.

Coal Tar is obtained in the destructive distillation of bituminous coal and is a highly effective agent for controlling the flaking and itching of the scalp associated with dandruff, seborrheic dermatitis and psoriasis. The action of coal tar is believed to be keratolytic, antiseptic, antipruritic, and astringent. The coal tar solution used in Tegrin® Dandruff Shampoo is prepared in such a way as to reduce the pitch and other irritant components found in crude coal tar without reduction in therapeutic potency.

Coal Tar Solution has been used clinically for many years as a remedy for dandruff and for scaling associated with scalp disorders such as seborrhea and psoriasis. Its mechanism of action has not been fully established, but it is believed to retard the rate of turnover of epidermal cells with regular use. A number of clinical studies have demonstrated the performance attributes of Tegrin® Dandruff Shampoo against dandruff and seborrheic dermatitis. In addition to relieving the above symptoms, Tegrin® Dandruff Shampoo, used regularly, maintains scalp and hair cleanliness and leaves the hair lustrous and manageable.

Shown in Product Identification Guide, page 509

TEGRIN® SKIN CREAM FOR PSORIASIS

Description: Tegrin® Skin Cream for Psoriasis contains 5% Coal Tar Solution, USP, equivalent to 0.8% Coal Tar and alcohol of 4.7%.

Active Ingredient: 5% Coal Tar Solution, USP, equivalent to 0.8% Coal Tar.

Use: relieves itching, flaking and irritation of the skin associated with psoriasis and seborrheic dermatitis.

Directions: Apply to affected areas one to four times daily or as directed by a doctor.

Warnings:
For external use only
Ask a doctor before use if you have psoriasis or seborrheic dermatitis that covers a large area of the body

Ask a doctor or pharmacist before use if you are using other forms of psoriasis therapy such as ultraviolet radiation or prescription drugs

When using this product
- avoid contact with eyes. If contact occurs, rinse eyes thoroughly with water.
- use caution in exposing skin to sunlight after application. It may increase tendency to sunburn for up to 24 hours after application.
- do not use for prolonged periods
- do not use in or around the rectum or in the genital area or groin

Stop use and ask a doctor if condition worsens or does not improve after regular use

Warning: This product contains a chemical known to the State of California to cause cancer.

Keep out of reach of children. If swallowed, get medical help or contact a Poison Control Center right away.

Inactive Ingredients: Acetylated Lanolin Alcohol, Alcohol (4.7%), Carbomer-934P, Ceteth-2, Ceteth-16, Cetyl Acetate, Cetyl Alcohol, D&C Red No. 28, Fragrance, Glyceryl Tribehenate, Laneth-16, Lanolin Alcohol, Laureth-23, Methyl Gluceth-20, Methylchloroisothiazolinone, Methylisothiazolinone, Mineral Oil, Octyldodecanol, Oleth-16, Petrolatum, Potassium Hydroxide, Purified Water, Steareth-16, Stearyl Alcohol, Titanium Dioxide.

How Supplied: Tegrin® Skin Cream for Psoriasis is available in a 2 oz (57g) tube.

Shown in Product Identification Guide, page 509

TUMS® Regular Antacid/Calcium Supplement Tablets
TUMS E–X® and TUMS E–X® Sugar Free Antacid/Calcium Supplement Tablets
TUMS ULTRA® Antacid/Calcium Supplement Tablets

Professional Labeling: Indicated for the symptomatic relief of hyperacidity associated with the diagnosis of peptic ulcer, gastritis, peptic esophagitis, gastric hyperacidity, and hiatal hernia.

Indications: For fast relief of acid indigestion, heartburn, sour stomach, and upset stomach associated with these symptoms.

Active Ingredient:
Tums, Calcium Carbonate 500 mg
Tums E-X, Calcium Carbonate 750 mg
Tums ULTRA, Calcium Carbonate 1000 mg

Actions: Tums provides rapid neutralization of stomach acid. Each Tums tablet has an acid-neutralizing capacity (ANC) of 10 mEq. Each Tums E-X tablet has an ANC of 15 mEq and each Tums ULTRA tablet, an ANC of 20 mEq. This high neutralization capacity makes Tums tablets an ideal antacid for management of conditions associated with hyperacidity. It effectively neutralizes free acid yet does not cause systemic alkalosis in the presence of normal renal function. A double-blind placebo-controlled clinical study demonstrated that calcium carbonate taken at a dosage of 16 Tums tablets daily for a two-week period was non-constipating/non-laxative.

Warnings: Tums: Do not take more than 15 tablets in a 24-hour period or use the maximum dosage of this product for more than 2 weeks, except under the advice and supervision of a physician. If symptoms persist for 2 weeks, stop using this product and see a physician. Keep this and all drugs out of the reach of children.

Tums E-X: Do not take more than 10 tablets in a 24-hour period or use the maximum dosage of this product for more than two weeks, except under the advice and supervision of a physician. If symptoms persist for two weeks, stop using this product and see a physician. Keep this and all drugs out of the reach of children.

Additionally, for Tums Ex Sugar Free: Phenylketonurics: Contains phenylalanine, less than 1 mg per tablet.

Tums ULTRA: Do not take more than 7 tablets in 24-hour period or use the maximum dosage of this product for more than two weeks, except under the advice and supervision of a physician. If symptoms persist for two weeks, stop using and see a physician. Keep this and all drugs out of the reach of children.

Drug Interaction Precaution: Antacids may interact with certain prescription drugs. If you are presently taking a prescription drug, do not take this product without checking with your physician or other health professional.

Dosage and Administration:
Tums: Chew 2-4 tablets as symptoms occur. Repeat hourly if symptoms return, or as directed by physician.
Tums E-X: Chew 2-4 tablets as symptoms occur. Repeat hourly if symptoms return, or as directed by a physician.
Tums ULTRA: Chew 2-3 tablets as symptoms occur. Repeat hourly if symptoms return, or as directed by a physician.

AS A DIETARY SUPPLEMENT:
Calcium Supplement Directions
Tums, Tums E-X, & Tums ULTRA:
USES: As a daily source of extra calcium.

Tums is recommended by the National Osteoporosis Foundation.

IMPORTANT INFORMATION ON OSTEOPOROSIS: Research shows that certain ethnic, age and other groups are at higher risk for developing osteoporosis, including Caucasian and Asian teen and young adult women, menopausal women, older persons and those persons with a family history of fragile bones.

A balanced diet with enough calcium and regular exercise throughout life will help you to build and maintain healthy bones and may reduce your risk of developing osteoporosis. Adequate calcium intake is important, but daily intakes above 2,000 mg are not likely to provide any additional benefit.

DIRECTIONS: Chew 2 tablets twice daily.

[See table above]

Ingredients (all variants except sugar free): Sucrose, Corn Starch, Talc, Mineral Oil, Flavors (natural and/or artificial), Sodium Polyphosphate. May also contain 1% or less of Adipic Acid, Blue 1 Lake, Yellow 6 Lake, Yellow 5 Lake, Red 40 Lake.

Ingredients (Sugar Free): Sorbitol, Acacia, Natural and Artificial Flavors, Calcium Stearate, Adipic Acid, Yellow 6 Lake, Aspartame.

How Supplied:

Tums: Peppermint flavor is available in 12-tablet rolls, 3-roll wraps, and bottles of 75, 150, and 180. **Assorted Flavors** (Cherry, Lemon, Orange, and Lime), are available in 12-tablet rolls, 3-roll wraps, and bottles of 75, 150, and 320.

Tums E-X: Wintergreen 3-roll wraps and bottles of 48, 96, and 116.

Tums E-X: Assorted Fruit, Assorted Tropical Fruit, and Assorted Berries, Fresh Blend 8 tablet rolls, 3-roll wraps, 6-roll wraps, and bottles of 48, 96, and 116. Assorted Tropical Fruit and Assorted Berries are also available in bottles of 200 tablets.

Tums EX Sugar Free: Orange Cream; bottles of 48 and 80 tablets.

Tums ULTRA: Assorted Berries, and **Spearmint** bottles of 160 tablets. **Assorted Fruit** and **Assorted Mint** bottles

Supplement Facts

	Tums 2 Tablets	Tums E-X 2 Tablets	Tums E-X Sugar Free 2 Tablets	Tums Ultra 2 Tablets
Serving Size	2 Tablets	2 Tablets	2 Tablets	2 Tablets
Amount Per Serving				
Calories	5	10	5	10
Sorbitol (g)	—	—	1	—
Sugars (g)	1	2	—	3
Calcium (mg)	400	600	600	800
% Daily Value	40	60	60	80
Sodium (mg)	—	5	—	10
% Daily Value	—	<1%	—	<1%

Continued on next page

Tums Antacid—Cont.

of 36, 72, and 86 tablets. Assorted Fruit also available in bottles of 160 tablets. **Tropical Fruit** bottles of 160 tablets.
Shown in Product Identification Guide, page 509

VIVARIN Tablets & Caplets
Alertness Aid with Caffeine
Maximum Strength

Each Tablet or Caplet Contains 200 mg. Caffeine, Equal to About Two Cups of Coffee
Take Vivarin for a safe, fast pick up anytime you feel drowsy and need to be alert. The caffeine in Vivarin is less irritating to your stomach than coffee, according to a government appointed panel of experts.

FDA APPROVED USES: Helps restore mental alertness or wakefulness when experiencing fatigue or drowsiness.

Active Ingredients: Caffeine 200 mg.

Inactive Ingredients: Tablet: Colloidal Silicon Dioxide, D&C Yellow #10 Al. Lake, Dextrose, FD&C Yellow #6 Al. Lake, Magnesium Stearate, Microcrystalline Cellulose, Starch.
Caplet: Carnauba Wax, Colloidal Silicon Dioxide, D&C Yellow #10 Al Lake, Dextrose, FD&C Yellow #6 Al Lake, Hypromellose, Magnesium Stearate, Microcrystalline Cellulose, Polyethylene Glycol, Polysorbate 80, Starch, Titanium Dioxide.

Directions: Adults and children 12 years and over: Take 1 tablet (200 mg) not more often than every 3 to 4 hours.

Warnings: The recommended dose of this product contains about as much caffeine as two cups of coffee. Limit the use of caffeine containing medications, foods, or beverages while taking this product because too much caffeine may cause nervousness, irritability, sleeplessness, and occasionally, rapid heartbeat. For occasional use only. Not intended for use as a substitute for sleep. If fatigue or drowsiness persists or continues to recur, consult a doctor. Do not give to children under 12 years of age. As with any drug, if you are pregnant or nursing a baby, seek the advice of a health professional before using this product. In case of accidental overdose, seek professional assistance or contact a poison control center immediately. Keep this and all drugs out of the reach of children.

Tamper Evident Feature: Individually sealed in foil for your protection. Do not use if foil or plastic bubble is torn or punctured.

Store at room temperature, avoid excessive heat (greater than 100°F) or humidity.

How Supplied:
Tablets: Consumer packages of 16, 40 and 80 tablets
Caplets: Consumer packages of 24 and 48 caplets

Comments or Questions? Call Toll-Free 1-800-245-1040 Weekdays.
GlaxoSmithKline Consumer Healthcare, L.P.
Moon Township, PA 15108. Made in U.S.A.
©1996 SmithKline Beecham
Shown in Product Identification Guide, page 509

Hyland's, Inc.

See Standard Homeopathic Company

Johnson & Johnson • MERCK
Consumer Pharmaceuticals Co.
7050 CAMP HILL ROAD
FORT WASHINGTON, PA 19034

Direct Inquiries to:
Consumer Relationship Center
Fort Washington, PA 19034
(800) 962-5357

PEPCID AC®
TABLETS, CHEWABLE TABLETS AND GELCAPS
(Maximum Strength PEPCID AC Tablets)

Description: Each Pepcid AC Tablet, Chewable tablet, and gelcap contain famotidine 10 mg as an active ingredient.

Inactive Ingredients: TABLETS: Hydroxypropyl cellulose, hypromellose, red iron oxide, magnesium stearate, microcrystalline cellulose, starch, talc, titanium dioxide.
CHEWABLE TABLETS: aspartame, cellulose acetate, flavors, hydroxypropyl cellulose, hypromellose, lactose, magnesium stearate, mannitol, microcrystalline cellulose, red ferric oxide.
GELCAPS: benzyl alcohol, black iron oxide, butylparaben, castor oil, edetate calcium disodium, FD&C red #40, gelatin, hypromellose, magnesium stearate, methylparaben, microcrystalline cellulose, pregelatinized corn starch, propylene glycol, propylparaben, sodium lauryl sulfate, sodium propionate, talc, titanium dioxide.
Each Maximum Strength Pepcid AC Tablet contains famotidine 20 mg as an active ingredient.

Inactive Ingredients: carnauba wax, hydroxypropyl cellulose, hypromellose, magnesium stearate, microcrystalline cellulose, pregelatinized starch, talc, titanium dioxide.

Product Benefits:
• **1 Tablet, Chewable Tablet or Gelcap** relieves heartburn associated with acid indigestion and sour stomach.
• prevents heartburn associated with acid indigestion and sour stomach brought on by eating or drinking certain food and beverages.
It contains famotidine, a prescription-proven medicine.
The ingredient in PEPCID AC and Maximum Strength Pepcid AC, famotidine, has been prescribed by doctors for years to treat millions of patients safely and effectively. The active ingredient in PEPCID AC and Maximum Strength Pepcid AC has been taken safely with many frequently prescribed medications.

Action: It is normal for the stomach to produce acid, especially after consuming food and beverages. However, acid in the wrong place (the esophagus), or too much acid, can cause burning pain and discomfort that interfere with everyday activities.
• **Heartburn—Caused by acid in the esophagus**

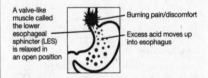

A valve-like muscle called the lower esophageal sphincter (LES) is relaxed in an open position
Burning pain/discomfort
Excess acid moves up into esophagus

In clinical studies, PEPCID AC and Maximum Strength Pepcid AC film-coated tablets were significantly better than placebo tablet (tablets without the medicine) in relieving and preventing heartburn. Pepcid AC and Maximum Strength Pepcid AC chewables contain the same active ingredient.

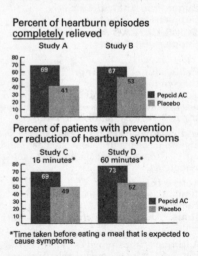

Percent of heartburn episodes completely relieved
Study A: Pepcid AC 69, Placebo 41
Study B: Pepcid AC 67, Placebo 53

Percent of patients with prevention or reduction of heartburn symptoms
Study C 15 minutes*: Pepcid AC 69, Placebo 49
Study D 60 minutes*: Pepcid AC 73, Placebo 52

*Time taken before eating a meal that is expected to cause symptoms.

Uses:
• **For Relief** of heartburn, associated with acid indigestion, and sour stomach;
• **For Prevention** of heartburn associated with acid indigestion and sour

stomach brought on by eating or drinking certain food and beverages.

Tips for Managing Heartburn:
- Do not lie flat or bend over soon after eating.
- Do not eat late at night, or just before bedtime.
- Certain foods or drinks are more likely to cause heartburn, such as rich, spicy, fatty, and fried foods, chocolate, caffeine, alcohol, and even some fruits and vegetables.
- Eat slowly and do not eat big meals.
- If you are overweight, lose weight.
- If you smoke, quit smoking.
- Raise the head of your bed.
- Wear loose fitting clothing around your stomach.

Warnings:

Allergy alert Do not use if you are allergic to famotidine or other acid reducers

Do not use:
- if you have trouble swallowing
- with other acid reducers
- if you have kidney disease, except under the advice and supervision of a doctor (for Maximum Strength Pepcid AC)

Stop use and ask a doctor if:
- stomach pain continues
- you need to take this product for more than 14 days

If pregnant or breast-feeding, ask a health professional before use.

Keep out of reach of children. In case of overdose, get medical help or contact a Poison Control Center right away.

Directions:
- Adults and children 12 years and over:
- Tablet: To relieve symptoms, swallow 1 tablet with a glass of water.
  Chewable Tablet: Do not swallow tablet whole: chew completely. To relieve symptoms, chew one tablet before swallowing.
  Gelcap: To relieve symptoms, swallow one gelcap with a glass of water.
- Tablet & Gelcap: To prevent symptoms, swallow one tablet or gelcap with a glass of water any time from 15 to 60 minutes before eating food or drinking beverages that cause heartburn.
- Chewable Tablet: To prevent symptoms, chew one chewable tablet with a glass of water at any time from 15 to 60 minutes before eating food or drinking beverages that cause heartburn.
- Do not use more than 2 tablets, chewable tablets or gelcaps in 24 hours.
- Children under 12 years: ask a doctor.

Other Information:
- read the directions and warnings before use
- store at 25°–30°C (77°–86°F)
- keep the carton and package insert, they contain important information
- protect from moisture

in addition to the above the following also applies to the chewable tablet
- do not use if individual pouch is open or torn
- phenylketonurics: contains phenylalanine 1.4 mg per chewable tablet

How Supplied:

Pepcid AC Tablet is available as a rose-colored tablet identified as 'PEPCID AC'. NDC 16837-872

Pepcid AC Gelcap is available as a rose and white gelatin coated, capsule shaped tablet identified as 'PEPCID AC'. NDC 16837-856

Pepcid AC Chewable Tablet is available as a rose-colored chewable tablet identified as 'PEPCID AC'. NDC 16837-873 Maximum Strength Pepcid AC Tablet is a white, "D" shaped, film coated tablet identified as "PAC 20." NDC 16837 855

Shown in Product Identification Guide, page 509

PEPCID® COMPLETE
Acid Reducer + Antacid
with DUAL ACTION
Reduces and Neutralizes Acid

Description:

Active Ingredients: (in each chewablet tablet)	**Purpose:**
Famotidine 10mg	Acid Reducer
Calcium Carbonate 800 mg	Antacid
Magnesium Hydroxide 165 mg	Antacid

Inactive Ingredients: Mint flavor: Cellulose acetate, corn starch, dextrates, flavors, hydroxypropyl cellulose, hypromellose, lactose, magnesium stearate, pregelatinized starch, red iron oxide, sodium lauryl sulfate, sugar Berry flavor: Cellulose acetate, corn starch, D&C red #7, dextrates, FD&C blue #1, FD&C red #40, flavors, hydroxypropyl cellulose, hypromellose, lactose, magnesium stearate, pregelatinized starch, sodium lauryl sulfate, sugar

Sodium Content:
Each chewable tablet contains 0.5 mg of sodium.

Acid Neutralizing Capacity:
Each chewable tablet contains 21.7 mEq of acid neutralizing capacity.

Product Benefits: Pepcid Complete combines an acid reducer (famotidine) with antacids (calcium carbonate and magnesium hydroxide) to relieve heartburn in two different ways: Acid reducers decrease the production of new stomach acid; antacids neutralize acid that is already in the stomach. The active ingredients in PEPCID COMPLETE have been used for years to treat acid-related problems in millions of people safely and effectively.

Uses: To relieve heartburn associated with acid indigestion and sour stomach.

Action: It is normal for the stomach to produce acid, especially after consuming food and beverages. However, acid in the stomach may move up into the wrong place (the esophagus), causing burning pain and discomfort that interfere with everyday activities.

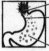

Heartburn—Caused by acid in the esophagus
- Burning pain/discomfort in esophagus
- A valve-like muscle called the lower esophageal sphincter (LES) is relaxed in an open position
- Acid moves up from stomach

Tips For Managing Heartburn
- Do not lie flat or bend over soon after eating.
- Do not eat late at night, or just before bedtime.
- Certain foods or drinks are more likely to cause heartburn, such as rich, spicy, fatty, and fried foods, chocolate, caffeine, alcohol, and even some fruits and vegetables.
- Eat slowly and do not eat big meals.
- If you are overweight, lose weight.
- If you smoke, quit smoking.
- Raise the head of your bed.
- Wear loose fitting clothing around your stomach.

PROVEN EFFECTIVE IN CLINICAL STUDIES
[See figure below]

Warnings:
- **Allergy alert:** Do not use if you are allergic to famotidine or other acid reducers.
- **Do not use:** if you have trouble swallowing.
- With other famotidine products or acid reducers.
- **Ask a doctor or pharmacist before use if you are** taking a prescription drug. Antacids may interact with certain prescription drugs.
- **Stop use and ask a doctor if** stomach pain continues
- You need to take this product for more than 14 days.
- **If pregnant or breast-feeding,** ask a health professional before use.
- **Keep out of reach of children.** In case of overdose, get medical help or contact a poison control center right away.

Continued on next page

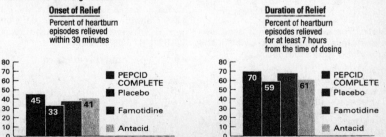

In clinical studies, PEPCID COMPLETE was significantly better than placebo pills tablets (without medicine) in relieving heartburn.

Onset of Relief
Percent of heartburn episodes relieved within 30 minutes

45 33 41

- PEPCID COMPLETE
- Placebo
- Famotidine
- Antacid

Duration of Relief
Percent of heartburn episodes relieved for at least 7 hours from the time of dosing

70 59 61

- PEPCID COMPLETE
- Placebo
- Famotidine
- Antacid

Pepcid Complete—Cont.

Directions:
- Adults and children 12 years and over:
  - **do not swallow tablet whole; chew completely.**
  - to relieve symptoms, **chew** 1 tablet before swallowing.
  - do not use more than 2 chewable tablets in 24 hours.
- Children under 12 years: ask a doctor.

Other Information:
- read the directions and warnings before use.
- keep the carton and package insert. They contain important information.
- store at 25°–30°C (77–86 F).
- protect from moisture.

How Supplied: Pepcid Complete is available as a rose-colored chewable tablet identified by 'P'. NDC 16837-888 – Mint flavor
Pepcid Complete Berry flavor
NDC 16837-291

Shown in Product Identification Guide, page 509

Lederle Consumer Healthcare

See Wyeth Consumer Healthcare

Lil' Drug Store Products
1201 CONTINENTAL PLACE NE CEDAR RAPIDS, IA 52402–2025

Direct Inquiries to:
Steve Bosking
phone: (319) 294-3766
www.ldsconsumerproducts.com

PRODIUM®
[prō-dē-um]
Phenazopyridine Hydrochloride 95mg
Urinary Pain Reliever

Description:
- Each Prodium® tablet contains phenazopyridine HCl 95mg.

Benefits:
- Fast relief of pain, urgency, frequency, and burning of urination.
- Prodium® contains phenazopyridine HCl, an ingredient doctors recommend most to help relieve the pain associated with Urinary Tract Discomfort.
- Easy-to-swallow tablet.
  Note: Phenazopyridine HCl produces a harmless orange to red color in the urine and may stain fabric.

Dosage:
- Adult Dosage is two tablets after meals, three times a day.
- Dosage administration should not exceed 12 tablets or 2 days of medication. Treatment of a urinary tract infection with phenazopyridine HCl should not exceed 2 days because there is a lack of evidence that the combined administration of phenazopyridine HCl and an antibacterial provides greater benefit than administration of the antibacterial alone after 2 days.
Note: Prodium® should be used for temporary relief, consult your doctor for underlying condition and for treatment.

Warnings:
- Phenazopyridine HCl should not be used in patients who have previously exhibited hypersensitivity to it or have Kidney trouble.
- The decline in renal function associated with advanced age should be kept in mind. A yellowish tinge of the skin or sclera may indicate accumulation due to impaired renal excretion and the need to discontinue therapy.
- Phenazopyridine HCl use is also contraindicated in patients with hepatitis or renal insufficiency.
- Individuals with any hepatic or renal trouble should not use this product unless directed by your doctor.
- As with any drug, if you are pregnant or nursing a baby, seek the advice of a health professional before using this product.
- Do not administer to children under 12 years of age unless directed by your doctor.
- If symptoms are severe or persist for more than two days, call your doctor.
- Staining of soft contact lenses has been reported.
- Phenazopyridine HCl is known to cause gastrointestinal upset in some individuals, discontinue use if symptoms occur. Taking with or following meals will reduce gastric upset.
- Keep this and all medicines out of the reach of children.
- In case of accidental overdose, get medical help right away.
- Carcinogenesis: Long-term administration of phenazopyridine HCl has induced neoplasia in rats (large intestine) and mice (liver). Although no association between phenazopyridine HCl and human neoplasia has been reported, adequate epidemiological studies along these lines have not been conducted.

Storage Instructions:
- Store at controlled room temperature 15°–30° C(59°–86° F)

Inactive Ingredients: lactose, magnesium silicate, magnesium stearate, microcrystalline cellulose, pharmaceutical glaze, sodium starch glycolate

Questions: **1-877-507-6516** or
www.ldsconsumerproducts.com

Manufactured for and Distributed by: LDS Consumer Products, 1201 Continental Place NE, Cedar Rapids, IA 52402 1-877-507-6516

www.ldsconsumerproducts.com

How Supplied:
- Prodium® is supplied in cartons of 30 tablets (NDC 10961-240-30) and 12 tablets (NDC 10961-240-12)

Shown in Product Identification Guide, page 510

REPLENS
[rē-plĕns]
Long Lasting Vaginal Moisturizer

Benefits:
- Replenish moisture for days with one application
- Soothing, immediate relief
- Estrogen Free

Uses: Replens provides safe, immediate, and long-lasting relief of vaginal itching, burning, and soreness associated with vaginal dryness.
One application provides moisture for up to three days.

Important: If the aluminum seal on the tube is damaged or opened, DO NOT USE and return entire contents to place of purchase. Store at room temperature (59°–86°F). Avoid exposure to extreme heat or cold.

Warnings: • Replens is not a contraceptive. • Keep out of reach of children. • If vaginal irritation occurs, discontinue use. If symptoms persist, contact your physician.

Ingredients: Purified water, glycerin, mineral oil, polycarbophil, carbomer 934P, hydrogenated palm oil glyceride, sorbic acid, methyparaben, sodium hydroxide

How Supplied: 8 Pre-Filled Applicators and 14 Applications with One Reusable Applicator.
Manufactured in the U.S.
For and Distributed By:
LDS Consumer Products
1201 Continental Place NE
Cedar Rapids, IA 52402
Questions?
Call 1-877-507-6516
or visit our website
www.replens.com

Shown in Product Identification Guide, page 510

WARTNER®
Wart Removal System

Removes warts with a single treatment. Wartner® is a fast and effective treatment for the removal of common warts and plantar warts. Wartner® freezes the wart on the spot, causing the wart to fall off within 10 to 14 days, usually after one application.
Wartner® is suitable for the removal of common warts and the removal of plantar warts on the bottom of the foot (**Read the Side Panel and Information Leaflet carefully for warnings and cautions**) in adults and children over the age of 4. This package can be used for up to 10 treatments.
Read the Label and Entire Information Leaflet Carefully Before Use. Keep for Reference.

Use: For the removal of common warts as well as the removal of plantar warts on the bottom of the foot. Common warts are skin-colored, usually appear on the hands and feet and are easily recognized by the rough "cauliflower-like" appearance of the surface. The plantar wart is recognized by its location only on the bottom of the foot, its tenderness, and the interruption of the footprint pattern.

Danger – Extremely Flammable. Contents Under Pressure. Keep away from fire, flame, and heat. Do not smoke while using this product. Protect from sunlight and do not expose to temperatures above 120°F. Store at room temperature away from heat.

Warnings: Keep Out of Reach of Children. Avoid Contact with Eyes. Do not inhale vapor/spray and use only in well-ventilated areas. Do Not Swallow. For External use Only. Use Wartner® only if you are sure the skin condition is a wart. If you are not sure, consult your Doctor. Do not use if you cannot see clearly to read the information on the container or the information leaflet. Do not use if you cannot see clearly the wart you are treating. Use only as directed. If Wartner® is not used exactly as instructed or if you mistakenly apply it directly to the skin or use it on conditions that are not warts, it may cause serious burns and permanent scarring of the skin.

Caution: Wartner® should only be used in combination with the applicators provided. Use one foam applicator for each wart. Do not reuse applicator. Do not treat each wart with Wartner® more than three times in total.

Instructions for Use: See Information Leaflet. If information leaflet is missing, contact your pharmacist or distributor for another copy before using this product. See toll-free number.

Contents: dimethyl ether and propane.

Manufacturer:
Wartner USA b.v.
World Trade Center
Beursplein 37 (Room 405)
3011 AA Rotterdam
The Netherlands
www.wartner-us.com
Distributor:
LDS Consumer Products
1201 Continental Place NE
Cedar Rapids, IA 52402
1-877-507-6516
www.ldsconsumerproducts.com
Shown in Product Identification Guide, page 510

**IF YOU SUSPECT
AN INTERACTION. . .**
The 1,800-page
PDR Companion Guide™ can help.
Use the order form
in the front of this book.

Matrixx Initiatives, Inc.
4742 NORTH 24TH STREET
SUITE 455
PHOENIX, AZ 85016

Direct Inquiries:
Phone: 602-385-8888
Fax: 602-385-8850
Web Site: www.matrixxinc.com

ZICAM® Allergy Relief
[zī′kăm]

Drug Facts:

Active Ingredients:	Purpose:
Luffa operculata 4x, 12x, 30x	
Galphimia glauca 12x, 30x	
Histanium hydrochloricum 12x, 30x, 200x	
Sulphur 12x, 30x, 200x	Upper respiratory allergy symptom relief

Uses:
• Relieves symptoms of hay fever and other upper respiratory allergies such as: *sinus pressure *runny nose *sneezing *itchy eyes *watery eyes *nasal congestion

Warnings: For nasal use only. Ask a doctor before use if you have ear, nose or throat sensitivity or if you are susceptible to nose bleeds. **When using this product** avoid contact with eyes. In case of accidental contact with eyes, flush with water and immediately seek professional help. The use of this container by more than one person may spread infection. **Stop use and ask a doctor** if symptoms persist. **If pregnant or breast-feeding,** ask a health professional before use. **Keep out of reach of children.** If swallowed, get medical help or contact a Poison Control Center right away.

Directions:
• Adults and children 6 years of age and older (with adult supervision):
  • Remove cap and safety clip.
  • Hold with thumb at bottom of bottle and nozzle between your fingers.
  • Before using the first time, prime pump by depressing several times.
  • Place tip of nozzle just past nasal opening (approximately 1/8").
  • While inside nasal opening, slightly angle nozzle outward.
  • Pump once into each nostril.
  • After application, press lightly on outside of each nostril for about 5 seconds.
  • Wait at least 30 seconds before blowing nose.
  • Use once every 4 hours.
  • Optimal results may not be seen for 1-2 weeks. After 1-2 weeks, may need to use only 1-2 times daily. For best results, use up to one week before contact with known causes of your allergies.
• Children under 6 years of age: Consult a doctor before use.

Inactive Ingredients: benzalkonium chloride, benzyl alcohol, edetate diso-

---

dium, glycerine, hydroxyethylcellulose, potassium chloride, potassium phosphate, purified water, sodium chloride, sodium phosphate

How Supplied: *ZICAM® Allergy Relief nasal pump:* 0.5 FL OZ (15 mL) pump bottle
Shown in Product Identification Guide, page 510

ZICAM® Cold Remedy
ZICAM® Cold Remedy Swabs
ZICAM® Cold Remedy Swabs Kids Size
ZICAM® Cold Remedy Oral Mist
ZICAM® Cold Remedy RapidMelts
ZICAM® Cold Remedy Chewables
[zī ′kăm]

Drug Facts:
ZICAM® Cold Remedy original pump, ZICAM® Cold Remedy Swabs, ZICAM® Cold Remedy Swabs Kids Size only:

Active Ingredient:	Purpose:
Zincum Gluconicum 2X	Reduces duration and severity of the common cold

ZICAM® Cold Remedy Oral Mist, ZICAM® Cold Remedy RapidMelts, ZICAM® Cold Remedy Chewables only:

Active Ingredient:	Purpose:
Zincum Gluconicum 1X	Reduces duration and severity of the common cold
Zincum Aceticum 2X	

Uses:
• Reduces duration of the common cold
• Reduces severity of cold symptoms:
* sore throat *stuffy nose *sneezing
* coughing *congestion

Warnings: *ZICAM® Cold Remedy original pump, ZICAM® Cold Remedy Swabs, ZICAM® Cold Remedy Swabs Kids Size only:*

For nasal use only. Ask a doctor before use if you have ear, nose or throat sensitivity or if you are susceptible to nose bleeds. **When using this product** avoid contact with eyes. In case of accidental contact with eyes, flush with water and immediately seek professional help. Temporary discomfort such as burning, stinging, sneezing, or increased nasal discharge may result from use of this product. To help avoid irritation, do not sniff up gel. The use of this container by more than one person may spread infection. **Stop use of this product and ask a doctor** if symptoms persist. ZICAM® Cold Remedy was formulated to shorten the duration of the common cold and may not be effective for flu or allergies. **If pregnant or breast-feeding,** ask a health professional before use. **Keep out of reach of children.** If swallowed, get medical help or contact a Poison Control Center right away.

Continued on next page

Zicam Cold—Cont.

ZICAM® Cold Remedy Oral Mist, ZICAM® Cold Remedy RapidMelts, ZICAM® Cold Remedy Chewables only:
For oral use only. Stop use and ask a doctor if symptoms persist. ZICAM® Cold Remedy was formulated to shorten the duration of the common cold and may not be effective for flu or allergies. **If pregnant or breast-feeding,** ask a health professional before use. **Keep out of reach of children.**

ZICAM® Cold Remedy Oral Mist only:
When using this product avoid contact with eyes. In case of accidental contact with eyes, flush with water and immediately seek professional help.

Directions: *ZICAM® Cold Remedy nasal pump:*
- Adults and children 3 years of age and older (with adult supervision):
  - Remove cap and safety cap.
  - Hold with thumb at bottom of bottle and nozzle between your fingers.
  - Before using the first time, prime pump by depressing several times.
  - Place tip of nozzle just past nasal opening (approximately 1/8").
  - While inside nasal opening, slightly angle nozzle outward.
  - Pump once into each nostril. To avoid possible irritation, do not sniff up gel.
  - After application, press lightly on outside of each nostril for about 5 seconds.
  - Wait at least 30 seconds before blowing nose.
  - Use once every 4 hours.
  - For best results, use at the first sign of a cold and continue to use for an additional 48 hours after symptoms subside.
- Children under 3 years of age: Consult a doctor before use.

ZICAM® Cold Remedy Swabs only:
- Adults and children 3 years of age and older (with adult supervision):
  - Separate one swab from the other.
  - Before opening:
    - Turn swab upside down to medication saturates swab head.
    - Return right side up and squeeze at blue dot to move medication away from dotted tear line.
  - To open:
    - Fold so arrow heads meet; then tear scross dotted line.
    - Slide plastic sleeve halfway down swab handle to expose swab tip.
  - Apply medication just inside of each nostril. During application, press lightly on outside of nostril for about 5 seconds. Do not insert swab more than ¼" past nasal opening.
  - Discard swab after use.
  - Wait at least 30 seconds before blowing nose.
  - Use one swab every 4 hours.
  - For best results, use at the first sign of a cold and continue to use for an additional 48 hours after symptoms subside.
- Children under 3 years of age: Consult a doctor before use.

ZICAM® Cold Remedy Swabs Kids Size only:
- Adults and children 3 years of age and older (with adult supervision):
  - Separate one swab from the other.
  - Before opening:
    - Turn swab upside down so medication saturates swab head.
    - Return right side up and squeeze at yellow dot to move medication away from dotted tear line.
  - To open:
    - Fold so arrow heads meet; then tear across dotted line.
    - Slide plastic sleeve halfway down swab handle to expose swab tip.
  - Apply medication just inside of first nostril. During application, press lightly on outside of nostril for about 5 seconds. Do not insert swab more than ¼" past nasal opening.
  - Re-moisten swab by pulling plastic sleeve back around swab tip. Then pull sleeve down and apply to second nostril.
  - Discard swab after use.
  - Wait at least 30 seconds before blowing nose.
  - Use one tube every 4 hours.
  - For best results, use at the first sign of a cold and continue to use for an additional 48 hours after symptoms subside.
- Children under 3 years of age: Consult a doctor before use.

ZICAM® Cold Remedy Oral Mist only:
- Adults and children 3 years of age and older:
  - Spray four times in mouth at the onset of symptoms. Spray on inside of cheeks, roof of mouth and gums. Retain 15 seconds. Swallow.
  - Repeat every three hours until symptoms are gone.
  - For best results, use for an additional 48 hours after symptoms subside.
  - To avoid minor stomach upset, do not take on an empty stomach.
  - Do not eat or drink for 15 minutes after use. Do not eat or drink citrus fruits or juices for 30 minutes before or after. Otherwise, drink plenty of fluids.
- Children under 3 years of age: Consult a doctor before use.

ZICAM® Cold Remedy RapidMelts only:
- Adults and children 3 years of age and older:
  - Dissolve entire tablet in mouth. Do not chew. Do not swallow whole.
  - Take one tablet at the onset of symptoms.
  - Repeat every three hours until symptoms are gone.
  - For best results, use for an additional 48 hours after symptoms subside.
  - To avoid minor stomach upset, do not take on an empty stomach.
  - Do not eat or drink for 15 minutes after use. Do not eat or drink citrus fruits or juices for 30 minutes before or after. Otherwise, drink plenty of fluids.
- Children under 3 years of age: Consult a doctor before use.

ZICAM® Cold Remedy Chewables only:
- Adults and children 6 years of age and older:
  - Take one square at the onset of symptoms. Chew thoroughly before swallowing.
  - Repeat every three hours until symptoms are gone.
  - For best results, use for an additional 48 hours after symptoms subside.
  - To avoid minor stomach upset, do not take on an empty stomach.
  - Do not eat or drink for 15 minutes after use. Do not eat or drink citrus fruits or juices for 30 minutes before or after. Otherwise, drink plenty of fluids.
  - This product is not recommended for children under 6 years of age due to the hazard of choking.

Inactive Ingredients:
ZICAM® Cold Remedy original pump, ZICAM® Cold Remedy Swabs, ZICAM® Cold Remedy Swabs Kids Size®: benzalkonium chloride, glycerin, hydroxyethylcellulose, purified water, sodium chloride, sodium hydroxide
ZICAM® Cold RemedyOral Mist only: benzalkonium chloride, fructose, glycerine, peppermint flavor, purified water
ZICAM® Cold RemedyRapidMelts only: crosspovidone, magnesium stearate, mannitol, microcrystalline cellulose, natural & artificial cherry flavor, polysorbate 80, polyvinyl pyrolidone, purified talc, silicon dioxide, sodium lauryl sulphate, sodium starch glycolate, sorbitan monosterate, sucralose
ZICAM® Cold Remedy Chewables only: FD&C red 40, glycerine, HPMC, lecithin, maltitol syrup, maltodextrin, mono and di-glycerides, natural & artificial strawberry flavor, partially hydrogenated cotton seed and soy oil, sugar

How Supplied: *ZICAM® Cold Remedy nasal pump:* 0.5 FL OZ (15 mL) pump bottle; *ZICAM® Cold Remedy Swabs and ZICAM® Cold Remedy Swabs Kids Size:* 20 medicated swabs; *ZICAM® Cold Remedy Oral Mist:* 1.0 FL OZ (30 mL) pump bottle; *ZICAM® Cold Remedy RapidMelts:* 25 quick dissolve tablets; *ZICAM® Cold Remedy Chewables:* 25 chewable squares

Shown in Product Identification Guide, page 510

ZICAM® Extreme Congestion Relief
ZICAM® Sinus Relief
[zī 'kăm]

Drug Facts:

Active Ingredient: **Purpose:**
Oxymetazoline HCl 0.05% .... Nasal decongestant

Uses:
- Temporarily relieves nasal congestion due to:
  *common cold *sinusitis *hay fever *upper respiratory allergies
- Helps clear nasal passages
- Shrink swollen membranes
- Temporarily relieves sinus congestion and pressure

Warnings: **For nasal use only. Ask a doctor before use if you have** heart disease, high blood pressure, thyroid disease, diabetes, trouble urinating due to enlarged prostrate gland. **When using this product do not use more than directed.** Do not use for more than 3 days. Use only as directed. Frequent or prolonged use may cause nasal congestion to recur or worsen. Temporary discomfort such as burning, stinging, sneezing, or an increase in nasal discharge may result. Use of this container by more than one person may spread infection. **Stop use and ask a doctor** if symptoms persist. **If pregnant or breast-feeding,** ask a health professional before use. **Keep out of reach of children. If swallowed,** get medical help or contact a Poison Control Center right away.

Directions: Adults and children 6 to under 12 years of age (with adult supervision): Pump 2 or 3 times in each nostril without tilting your head, not more often than once every 10 to 12 hours. Sniff deeply. Do not exceed 2 doses in any 24-hour period. Wipe nozzle clean after use. Children under 6 years of age: Consult a doctor.

To use pump:
Remove cap and safety clip.
Hold with thumb at bottom of bottle and nozzle between fingers.
Before using the first time, prime pump by depressing several times.

ZICAM® Extreme Congestion Relief only

Inactive Ingredients: alkoxylated diester, aloe barbadensis gel, benzalkonium chloride, benzyl alcohol, disodium EDTA, disodium phosphate, glycerine, hydroxyethylcellulose, hydroxylated lecithin, monosodium phosphate, purified water

ZICAM® Sinus Relief only

Inactive Ingredients: alkoxylated diester, aloe barbadensis gel, benzalkonium chloride, benzyl alcohol, disodium EDTA, disodium phosphate, di-alpha tocopherol, eucalyptol, glycerine, hydroxyethylcellulose, hydroxylated lecithin, menthol, monosodium phosphate, polysorbate 80, purified water

How Supplied: *ZICAM® Extreme Congestion Relief and ZICAM ® Sinus Relief nasal pump:* 0.5 FL OZ (15 mL) pump bottle
Shown in Product Identification Guide, page 510

UNKNOWN DRUG?
Consult the
Product Identification Guide
(Gray Pages)
for full-color photos of
leading over-the-counter
medications

McNeil Consumer and Specialty Pharmaceuticals
Division of McNeil-PPC, Inc.
FORT WASHINGTON, PA 19034

Direct Inquiries to:
Consumer Relationship Center
Fort Washington, PA 19034
(800) 962-5357

MAXIMUM STRENGTH GAS AID SOFTGELS

Description: Each softgel of Maximum Strength GasAid contains simethicone 125 mg.

Actions: Simethicone acts in the stomach and intestines by altering the surface tension of gas bubbles enabling them to coalesce, thereby freeing and eliminating the gas more easily by belching or passing flatus.

Uses: Relieves bloating, pressure, fullness or stuffed feeling commonly referred to as gas.

Directions: Adults and children 12 years and over: take 1–2 softgels as needed after meals and at bedtime. Do not take more than 4 softgels in 24 hours unless directed by a doctor.

Warnings:
Keep out of reach of children.

Other Information:
• **do not use if carton or any blister unit is open or broken**
• store at room temperature. Avoid high humidity and excessive heat (40°C). Protect from light

Inactive Ingredients: D&C yellow #10, FD&C blue #1, FD&C red #40, gelatin, glycerin, peppermint oil, titanium dioxide.

How Supplied: Softgels in 12s, 24s blister packaging. Each Maximum Strength GasAid softgel is oval, green in color, and imprinted with "I-G" on one side.
Shown in Product Identification Guide, page 510

IMODIUM® A–D LIQUID AND CAPLETS
(loperamide hydrochloride)

Description: Each 5 mL (teaspoon) of *IMODIUM® A-D* liquid contains loperamide hydrochloride 1 mg. *IMODIUM® A-D* liquid is stable, cherry-mint flavored, and clear in color.
Each caplet of *IMODIUM® A-D* contains 2 mg of loperamide hydrochloride and is scored and colored green.

Actions: *IMODIUM® A-D* contains a clinically proven antidiarrheal medication. Loperamide HCl acts by slowing in-

testinal motility and by affecting water and electrolyte movement through the bowel.

Uses: controls symptoms of diarrhea, including Travelers' Diarrhea.

Directions:
• **drink plenty of clear fluids to help prevent dehydration caused by diarrhea**
• find right dose on chart. If possible, use weight to dose; otherwise use age

adults and children 12 years and over	4 teaspoonfuls (1 dosage cup) or 2 caplets after the first loose stool; 2 teaspoonfuls or 1 caplet after each subsequent loose stool; but no more than 8 teaspoonfuls or 4 caplets in 24 hours
children 9–11 years (60–95 lbs)	2 teaspoonfuls (½ dosage cup) or 1 caplet after the first loose stool and 1 teaspoonful or ½ caplet after each subsequent loose stool but no more than 6 teaspoonfuls or 3 caplets in 24 hours
children 6–8 years (48–59 lbs)	2 teaspoonfuls (½ dosage cup) or 1 caplet after the first loose stool and 1 teaspoonful or ½ caplet after each subsequent loose stool but no more than 4 teaspoonfuls or 2 caplets in 24 hours
children under 6 years (up to 47 lbs)	ask a doctor

Imodium A-D Liquid Professional Dosage Schedule for children 2–5 years old (24–47 lbs): 1 teaspoonful after first loose bowel movement, followed by 1 after each subsequent loose bowel movement. Do not exceed 3 teaspoonfuls a day.

Warnings:
Allergy alert: Do not use if you have ever had a rash or other allergic reaction to loperamide HCl
Do not use if you have bloody or black stool
Ask a doctor before use if you have
• fever • mucus in the stool • a history of liver disease
Stop use and ask a doctor if
• symptoms get worse • diarrhea lasts for more than 2 days
If pregnant or breast feeding, ask a health professional before use. **Keep out of reach of children.** In case of overdose, get medical help or contact a Poison Control Center right away.

Continued on next page

Imodium A-D—Cont.

Other Information:

Liquid:
- **do not use if carton is opened or if printed plastic neck wrap is broken or missing**
- **store between 20–25°C (68–77°F)**

Caplets:
- **store between 20–25°C (68–77°F)**
- **do not use if carton or blister unit is open or torn**

Professional Information:

Overdosage Information

Overdosage of loperamide HCl in man may result in constipation, CNS depression and nausea. A slurry of activated charcoal administered promptly after ingestion of loperamide hydrochloride can reduce the amount of drug which is absorbed. If vomiting occurs spontaneously upon ingestion, a slurry of 100 grams of activated charcoal should be administered orally as soon as fluids can be retained. If vomiting has not occurred, and CNS depression is evident, gastric lavage should be performed followed by administration of 100 gms of the activated charcoal slurry through the gastric tube. In the event of overdosage, patients should be monitored for signs of CNS depression for at least 24 hours. Children may be more sensitive to central nervous system effects than adults. If CNS depression is observed, naloxone may be administered. If responsive to naloxone, vital signs must be monitored carefully for recurrence of symptoms of drug overdose for at least 24 hours after the last dose of naloxone.

Inactive Ingredients:

Liquid: benzoic acid, citric acid, flavors, glycerin, propylene glycol, purified water, sodium benzoate, sorbitol, sucrose, contains 0.5% alcohol.
Caplets: colloidal silicon dioxide, D&C yellow no. 10, dibasic calcium phosphate, FD&C blue no. 1, magnesium stearate, microcrystalline cellulose.

How Supplied:

Liquid: Cherry-mint flavored liquid (clear) 2 fl. oz. and 4 fl. oz. tamper evident bottles with child resistant safety caps and special dosage cups.
Caplets: Green scored caplets in 6s, 12s, 18s, 24s, 48s and 72s blister packaging which is tamper evident and child resistant.

Shown in Product Identification Guide, page 510

IMODIUM® ADVANCED
(loperamide HCl/simethicone)
Caplets & Chewable Tablets

Description: Each easy to swallow caplet and mint-flavored chewable tablet of *Imodium® Advanced* contains loperamide HCl 2 mg/simethicone 125 mg.

Actions: *Imodium® Advanced* combines original prescription strength Imodium® to control the symptoms of diarrhea plus simethicone to relieve bloating, pressure and cramps commonly referred to as gas. Loperamide HCl acts by slowing intestinal motility and by affecting water and electrolyte movement through the bowel. Simethicone acts in the stomach and intestines by altering the surface tension of gas bubbles enabling them to coalesce, thereby freeing and eliminating the gas more easily by belching or passing flatus.

Use: Controls symptoms of diarrhea plus bloating, pressure, and cramps commonly referred to as gas.

Directions:
- **drink plenty of clear fluids to help prevent dehydration caused by diarrhea**
- **find right dose on chart.** If possible, use weight to dose; otherwise use age

adults and children 12 years and over	swallow 2 caplets or chew 2 tablets after the first loose stool; 1 caplet/tablet after each subsequent loose stool; but no more than 4 caplets/tablets in 24 hours
children 9–11 years (60–95 lbs)	swallow 1 caplet or chew 1 tablet after the first loose stool; ½ caplet/tablet after each subsequent loose stool; but no more than 3 caplets/tablets in 24 hours
children 6–8 years (48–59 lbs)	swallow 1 caplet or chew 1 tablet after the first loose stool; ½ caplet/tablet after each subsequent loose stool; but no more than 2 caplets/tablets in 24 hours
children under 6 years (up to 47 lbs)	ask a doctor

Warnings:
Allergy alert: Do no use if you have ever had a rash or other allergic reaction to loperamide HCl
Do not use if you have bloody or black stool
Ask a doctor before use if you have • fever • mucus in the stool • a history of liver disease
Ask a doctor or pharmacist before use if you are taking antibiotics
Stop use and ask a doctor if • symptoms get worse • diarrhea lasts for more than 2 days
If pregnant or breast-feeding, ask a health professional before use.
Keep out of reach of children. In case of overdose, get medical help or contact a Poison Control Center right away.

Other Information:

Caplets:
- store between 20–25°C (68–77°F)
- protect from light

Blister statement:
- do not use if carton is open or if blister unit is open or torn

Bottle statement:
- do not use if carton if open or if printed foil seal under bottle cap is open or torn

Chewable Tablets:
- do not use if carton is opened or if blister unit is broken
- store between 20–25°C (68–77°F)

Professional Information:
Overdosage Information:

Overdosage of loperamide HCl in man may result in constipation, CNS depression and nausea. A slurry of activated charcoal administered promptly after ingestion of loperamide hydrochloride can reduce the amount of drug which is absorbed. If vomiting occurs spontaneously upon ingestion, a slurry of 100 grams of activated charcoal should be administered orally as soon as fluids can be retained. If vomiting has not occurred, and CNS depression is evident, gastric lavage should be performed followed by administration of 100 gms of the activated charcoal slurry through the gastric tube. In the event of overdosage, patients should be monitored for signs of CNS depression for at least 24 hours. Children may be more sensitive to central nervous system effects than adults. If CNS depression is observed, naloxone may be administered. If responsive to naloxone, vital signs must be monitored carefully for recurrence of symptoms of drug overdose for at least 24 hours after the last dose of naloxone. No treatment is necessary for the simethicone ingestion in this circumstance.

Inactive Ingredients:

Caplets: acesulfame K, cellulose, dibasic calcium phosphate, flavor, sodium starch glycolate, stearic acid **Chewable Tablets:** Cellulose acetate, corn starch, D&C Yellow No. 10, dextrates, FD&C Blue No. 1, flavors, microcrystalline cellulose, polymethacrylates, saccharin sodium, sorbitol, stearic acid, sucrose, tribasic calcium phosphate.

How Supplied: Mint Chewable Tablets in 6's, 12's, 18's, 30's, and blister packaging which is tamper evident and child resistant. Each Imodium® Advanced tablet is round, light green in color and has "IMODIUM" embossed on one side and "2/125" on the other side. Imodium Advanced Caplets are available in blister packs of 12's and 18's and bottles of 30's and 42's. Each Imodium® Advanced Caplet is oval, white color and has "IMO" embossed on one side and "2/125" on the other side.

Shown in Product Identification Guide, page 510

MOTRIN® IB ibuprofen Pain Reliever/ Fever Reducer Tablets, Caplets and Gelcaps

Description: Each *MOTRIN® IB Tablet, Caplet and Gelcap* contains ibuprofen 200 mg.

Uses: Temporarily relieves minor aches and pains due to:
• headache • muscular aches • minor pain of arthritis • toothache • backache • the common cold • menstrual cramps
Temporarily reduces fever

Directions:
• do not take more than directed

adults and children 12 years and older	• take 1 tablet, caplet, or gelcap every 4 to 6 hours while symptoms persist • if pain or fever does not respond to 1 tablet, caplet or gelcap, 2 tablets, caplets or gelcaps may be used, but do not exceed 6 tablets, caplets or gelcaps in 24 hours unless directed by a doctor • the smallest effective dose should be used
children under 12 years	• ask a doctor

Warnings:
Allergy alert: Ibuprofen may cause a severe allergic reaction which may include:
• hives • facial swelling
• asthma (wheezing) • shock
Alcohol Warning: If you consume 3 or more alcoholic drinks every day, ask your doctor whether you should take ibuprofen or other pain relievers/fever reducers. Ibuprofen may cause stomach bleeding.
Do not use if you have ever had an allergic reaction to any other pain reliever/ fever reducer.
Ask a doctor before use if you have
• stomach pain • problems or serious side effects from taking pain relievers or fever reducers.
Ask a doctor or pharmacist before use if you are
• under a doctor's care for any serious condition
• taking any other drug
• taking any other product that contains ibuprofen, or any other pain reliever/ fever reducer
When using this product give with food or milk if stomach upset occurs.
Stop use and ask a doctor if
• an allergic reaction occurs. Seek medical help right away.
• pain gets worse or lasts more than 10 days
• fever gets worse or lasts more than 3 days
• stomach pain or upset gets worse or lasts
• redness or swelling is present in the painful area
• any new symptoms appear.

If pregnant or breast-feeding, ask a health professional before use. It is especially important not to use ibuprofen during the last 3 months of pregnancy unless definitely directed to do so by a doctor because it may cause problems in the unborn child or complications during delivery.
Keep out of reach of children. In case of overdose, get medical help or contact a Poison Control Center right away.
Other Information
• **Do not use if neck wrap or foil inner seal imprinted "Safety Seal®" is broken or missing.**
• Store between 20°–25°C (68°–77°F)

Professional Information:
Overdosage Information for Adult Motrin®
IBUPROFEN
The *toxicity of ibuprofen* overdose is dependent upon the amount of drug ingested and the time elapsed since ingestion, though individual response may vary, which makes it necessary to evaluate each case individually. Although uncommon, serious toxicity and death have been reported in the medical literature with ibuprofen overdosage. The most frequently reported symptoms of ibuprofen overdose include abdominal pain, nausea, vomiting, lethargy and drowsiness. Other central nervous system symptoms include headache, tinnitus, CNS depression and seizures. Metabolic acidosis, coma, acute renal failure and apnea (primarily in very young children) may rarely occur. Cardiovascular toxicity, including hypotension, bradycardia, tachycardia and atrial fibrillation, also have been reported. The *treatment of acute ibuprofen overdose* is primarily supportive. Management of hypotension, acidosis and gastrointestinal bleeding may be necessary. In cases of acute overdose, the stomach should be emptied through ipecac-induced emesis or lavage. Emesis is most effective if initiated within 30 minutes of ingestion. Orally administered activated charcoal may help in reducing the absorption and reabsorption of ibuprofen. In children, the estimated amount of ibuprofen ingested per body weight may be helpful to predict the potential for development of toxicity although each case must be evaluated. Ingestion of less than 100 mg/kg is unlikely to produce toxicity. Children ingesting 100 to 200 mg/kg may be managed with induced emesis and a minimal observation time of four hours. Children ingesting 200 to 400 mg/kg of ibuprofen should have immediate gastric emptying and at least four hours observation in a health care facility. Children ingesting greater than 400 mg/kg require immediate medical referral, careful observation and appropriate supportive therapy. Ipecac-induced emesis is not recommended in overdoses greater than 400 mg/kg because of the risk of convulsions and the potential for aspiration of gastric contents. In adult patients the history of the dose reportedly ingested does not appear to be predictive of toxicity. The need for

referral and follow-up must be judged by the circumstances at the time of the overdose ingestion. Symptomatic adults should be admitted to a health care facility for observation.
Our Adult MOTRIN® combination products contain pseudoephedrine in addition to ibuprofen. For basic overdose information regarding pseudoephedrine, please see below. For additional emergency information, please contact your local poison control center.
PSEUDOEPHEDRINE
Symptoms from pseudoephedrine overdose consist most often of mild anxiety, tachycardia and/or mild hypertension. Symptoms usually appear within 4 to 8 hours and are transient, usually requiring no treatment.

Inactive Ingredients:
Tablets and Caplets: carnauba wax, corn starch, FD&C Yellow #6, hypromellose, iron oxide, polydextrose, polyethylene glycol, silicon dioxide, stearic acid, titanium dioxide.
Gelcaps: benzyl alcohol, butylparaben, castor oil, cellulose, corn starch, edetate calcium disodium, FD&C Yellow No. 6, gelatin, hypromellose, iron oxide, methylparaben, povidone, propylparaben, silicon dioxide, sodium lauryl sulfate, sodium propionate, sodium starch glycolate, titanium dioxide.

How Supplied:
Tablets: (orange, printed "MOTRIN IB" in black) in tamper evident packaging of 24, 50, 100, and 165.
Caplets: (orange, printed "MOTRIN IB" in black) in tamper evident packaging of 24, 50, 100, 165, 250, 300 and
Gelcaps: (colored orange and white, printed "MOTRIN IB" in black) in tamper evident packaging of 24, 50 and 100.

Shown in Product Identification Guide, page 512

MOTRIN® COLD & SINUS CAPLETS

Description: Each MOTRIN® Cold & Sinus Caplet contains ibuprofen 200 mg and pseudoephedrine HCl 30 mg.

Uses: temporarily relieves these symptoms associated with the common cold, sinusitis, and flu:
• headache • nasal congestion
• fever • minor body aches and pains

Directions:

Adults and children 12 years and older	• take 1 caplet every 4 to 6 hours while symptoms persist • If symptoms do not respond to 1 caplet, 2 caplets may be used.

Continued on next page

Motrin Cold & Sinus—Cont.

	• do not use more than 6 caplets in any 24-hour period unless directed by a doctor • the smallest effective dose should be used
Children under 12 years of age	Consult a doctor

Warnings:
Allergy alert: Ibuprofen may cause a severe allergic reaction which may include:
• hives • facial swelling
• asthma (wheezing) • shock

Alcohol warning: If you consume 3 or more alcoholic drinks every day, ask your doctor whether you should take ibuprofen or other pain relievers/fever reducers. Ibuprofen may cause stomach bleeding.

Do not use if you
• have ever had an allergic reaction to any other pain reliever/fever reducer
• are now taking a prescription monoamine oxidase inhibitor (MAOI) (certain drugs for depression, psychiatric or emotional conditions, or Parkinson's disease), or for 2 weeks after stopping the MAOI drug. If you do not know if your prescription drug contains an MAOI, ask a doctor or pharmacist before taking this product.

Ask a doctor before use if you have
• heart disease • high blood pressure
• thyroid disease • diabetes
• trouble urinating due to an enlarged prostate gland
• had serious side effects from taking any pain reliever/fever reducers.

Ask a doctor or pharmacist before use if you are
• taking any other product that contains ibuprofen or pseudoephedrine.
• taking any other pain reliever/fever reducer or nasal decongestant
• under a doctor's care for any continuing medical condition
• taking other drugs on a regular basis

When using this product
• do not use more than directed
• give with food or milk if stomach upset occurs

Stop use and ask a doctor if
• an allergic reaction occurs. Seek medical help right away
• you get nervous, dizzy, or sleepless
• nasal congestion lasts for more than 7 days
• fever lasts for more than 3 days
• symptoms continue or get worse
• new or unexpected symptoms occur
• stomach pain occurs with use of this product or even if mild symptoms persist

If pregnant or breast-feeding, ask a health professional before use. It is especially important not to use this product during the last 3 months of pregnancy unless definitely directed to do so by a doctor because it may cause problems in the unborn child or complications during delivery.

Keep out of reach of children. In case of overdose, get medical help or contact a Poison Control Center right away.

Other Information:
• **do not use if blister unit is broken or open**
• Store at 20–25°C (68–77°F).
• avoid excessive heat above 40°C (104°F)
• read all warnings and directions before use. Keep carton.

Professional Information:
Overdosage Information:
For overdosage information, please refer to pg. 669

Inactive Ingredients: Caplets: carnauba wax, cellulose, corn starch, FD&C Red #40, hypromellose, silicon dioxide, sodium lauryl sulfate, sodium starch glycolate, stearic acid, titanium dioxide, triacetin.

How Supplied: Caplets: (white, printed "Cold & Sinus" in red) in blister packs of 20 and 40.

Shown in Product Identification Guide, page 512

Infants' MOTRIN® ibuprofen Concentrated Drops
Children's MOTRIN® ibuprofen Oral Suspension and Chewable Tablets
Junior Strength MOTRIN® ibuprofen Caplets and Chewable Tablets

Product information for all dosages of Children's MOTRIN have been combined under this heading

Description: *Infants' MOTRIN® Concentrated Drops* are available in an alcohol-free, berry-flavored suspension and a non-staining, dye-free, berry-flavored suspension. Each 1.25 mL contains ibuprofen 50 mg. *Children's MOTRIN® Oral Suspension* is available as an alcohol-free, berry, dye-free berry, bubblegum or grape-flavored suspension. Each 5 mL (teaspoon) of *Children's MOTRIN® Oral Suspension* contains ibuprofen 100 mg. Each *Children's MOTRIN® Chewable Tablet* contains 50 mg of ibuprofen and is available as orange or grape-flavored chewable tablets. *Junior Strength MOTRIN® Chewable Tablets* and *Junior Strength MOTRIN® Caplets* contain ibuprofen 100 mg. *Junior Strength MOTRIN® Chewable Tablets* are available in orange or grape flavors. *Junior Strength MOTRIN® Caplets* are available as easy-to-swallow caplets (capsule-shaped tablet).

Uses:
temporarily:
• reduces fever
• relieves minor aches and pains due to the common cold, flu, sore throat, headaches and toothaches

Directions:
See Table 2: Children's Motrin Dosing Chart on pg. 673

Warnings:
Allergy alert: Ibuprofen may cause a severe allergic reaction which may include:
• hives • facial swelling
• asthma (wheezing) • shock

Sore throat warning: Severe or persistent sore throat or sore throat accompanied by high fever, headache, nausea, and vomiting may be serious. Consult doctor promptly. Do not use more than 2 days or administer to children under 3 years of age unless directed by doctor.

Do not use if the child has ever had an allergic reaction to any other fever reducer/pain reliever

Ask a doctor before use if the child has
• not been drinking fluids
• lost a lot of fluid due to continued vomiting or diarrhea
• stomach pain
• problems or serious side effects from taking fever reducers or pain relievers

Ask a doctor or pharmacist before use if the child
• under a doctor's care for any serious condition
• taking any other drug
• taking any other product that contains ibuprofen, or any other fever reducer/pain reliever

When using this product
• mouth or throat burning may occur; give with food or water (*Children's MOTRIN® Chewable Tablets and Junior Strength MOTRIN® Chewable Tablets* only)
• give with food or milk if stomach upset occurs

Stop use and ask a doctor if
• an allergic reaction occurs. Seek medical help right away.
• fever or pain gets worse or lasts more than 3 days
• the child does not get any relief within first day (24 hours) of treatment
• stomach pain or upset gets worse or lasts
• redness or swelling is present in the painful area
• any new symptoms appear

Keep out of reach of children. In case of overdose, get medical help or contact a Poison Control Center right away.

Other Information: *Infants', Children's and Junior Strength MOTRIN® products:*
• Store at 20–25°C (68–77°F)
Infants' MOTRIN® Concentrated Drops:
• **do not use if plastic carton wrap or bottle wrap imprinted "Safety Seal®" and "Use with Enclosed Dosage Device" is broken or missing.**
Children's MOTRIN® Suspension Liquid:
• **do not use if plastic carton wrap or bottle wrap imprinted "Safety Seal®" is broken or missing**
Children's MOTRIN® Chewable Tablets:
• Phenylketonurics: Contains phenylalanine 1.4 mg per tablet
• **do not use if neck wrap or foil inner seal imprinted "Safety Seal®" is broken or missing**
Junior Strength MOTRIN® Caplets and Chewable Tablets:
• **do not use if neck wrap or foil inner seal imprinted "Safety Seal®" is broken or missing**

Junior Strength MOTRIN® Chewable Tablets:
• phenylketonurics: contains phenylalanine 2.8 mg per tablet (tablet only)

Professional Information:
Overdosage Information for all Infants', Children's & Junior Strength Motrin® Products

IBUPROFEN: The *toxicity of ibuprofen* overdose is dependent upon the amount of drug ingested and the time elapsed since ingestion, though individual response may vary, which makes it necessary to evaluate each case individually. Although uncommon, serious toxicity and death have been reported in the medical literature with ibuprofen overdosage. The most frequently reported symptoms of ibuprofen overdose include abdominal pain, nausea, vomiting, lethargy and drowsiness. Other central nervous system symptoms include headache, tinnitus, CNS depression and seizures. Metabolic acidosis, coma, acute renal failure and apnea (primarily in very young children) may rarely occur. Cardiovascular toxicity, including hypotension, bradycardia, tachycardia and atrial fibrillation, also have been reported.

The *treatment of acute ibuprofen overdose* is primarily supportive. Management of hypotension, acidosis and gastrointestinal bleeding may be necessary. In cases of acute overdose, the stomach should be emptied through ipecac-induced emesis or lavage. Emesis is most effective if initiated within 30 minutes of ingestion. Orally administered activated charcoal may help in reducing the absorption and reabsorption of ibuprofen. In children, the estimated amount of ibuprofen ingested per body weight may be helpful to predict the potential for development of toxicity although each case must be evaluated. Ingestion of less than 100 mg/kg is unlikely to produce toxicity. Children ingesting 100 to 200 mg/kg may be managed with induced emesis and a minimal observation time of four hours. Children ingesting 200 to 400 mg/kg of ibuprofen should have immediate gastric emptying and at least four hours observation in a health care facility. Children ingesting greater than 400 mg/kg require immediate medical referral, careful observation and appropriate supportive therapy. Ipecac-induced emesis is not recommended in overdoses greater than 400 mg/kg because of the risk of convulsions and the potential for aspiration of gastric contents.

In adult patients the history of the dose reportedly ingested does not appear to be predictive of toxicity. The need for referral and follow-up must be judged by the circumstances at the time of the overdose ingestion. Symptomatic adults should be admitted to a health care facility for observation.

Our Children's MOTRIN® Cold products contain pseudoephedrine in addition to ibuprofen. The following is basic overdose information regarding pseudoephedrine.

PSEUDOEPHEDRINE: Symptoms from pseudoephedrine overdose consist most often of mild anxiety, tachycardia and/or mild hypertension. Symptoms usually appear within 4 to 8 hours of ingestion and are transient, usually requiring no treatment.

For additional emergency information, please contact your local poison control center.

Inactive Ingredients:
Infants' MOTRIN® Concentrated Drops:
Berry-Flavored: citric acid, corn starch, FD&C Red #40, flavors, glycerin, polysorbate 80, purified water, sodium benzoate, sorbitol, sucrose, xanthan gum. **Dye-Free Berry-Flavored:** artificial flavors, citric acid, corn starch, glycerin, polysorbate 80, purified water, sodium benzoate, sorbitol, sucrose, xanthan gum.
Children's MOTRIN® Oral Suspension:
Berry-Flavored: acesulfame potassium, citric acid, corn starch, D&C Yellow #10, FD&C Red #40, glycerin, natural and artificial flavors, polysorbate 80, purified water, sodium benzoate, sucrose, xanthan gum. **Dye-Free Berry-Flavored:** acesulfame potassium, citric acid, corn starch, glycerin, natural and artificial flavors, polysorbate 80, purified water, sodium benzoate, sucrose, xanthan gum. **Bubble Gum-Flavored:** acesulfame potassium, citric acid, corn starch, FD&C Red #40, glycerin, natural and artificial flavors, polysorbate 80, purified water, sodium benzoate, sucrose, xanthan gum. **Grape-Flavored:** acesulfame potassium, citric acid, corn starch, D&C Red #33, FD&C Blue #1, FD&C Red #40, glycerin, natural and artificial flavors, polysorbate 80, purified water, sodium benzoate, sucrose, xanthan gum.
Children's MOTRIN® Chewable Tablets:
Orange-Flavored: acesulfame K, aspartame, cellulose, citric acid, FD&C Yellow #6, flavor, fumaric acid, hydroxyethyl cellulose, hydroxypropyl methylcellulose, magnesium stearate, mannitol, povidone, sodium lauryl sulfate, sodium starch glycolate. **Grape-Flavored:** acesulfame K, aspartame, cellulose, citric acid, D&C Red #7, D&C Red #30, FD&C Blue #1, flavor, fumaric acid, hydroxyethyl cellulose, hydroxypropyl methylcellulose, magnesium stearate, mannitol, povidone, sodium lauryl sulfate, sodium starch glycolate.
Junior Strength MOTRIN® Chewable Tablets: **Orange-Flavored:** acesulfame K, aspartame, cellulose, citric acid, FD&C yellow #6, flavor, fumaric acid, hydroxyethyl cellulose, hydroxypropyl methylcellulose, magnesium stearate, mannitol, povidone, sodium lauryl sulfate, sodium starch glycolate. **Grape-Flavored:** acesulfame K, aspartame, cellulose, citric acid, D&C Red #7, D&C Red #30, FD&C Blue #1, flavor, fumaric acid, hydroxyethyl cellulose, hydroxypropyl methylcellulose, magnesium stearate, mannitol, povidone, sodium lauryl sulfate, sodium starch glycolate. **Easy-To-Swallow Caplets:** carnauba wax, cellulose, corn starch, D&C Yellow #10, FD&C Yellow #6, hydroxypropyl methylcellulose, polydextrose, polyethylene glycol, propylene glycol, silicon dioxide, sodium starch glycolate, titanium dioxide, triacetin.

How Supplied:
Infants' MOTRIN® Concentrated Drops: Berry-flavored, pink-colored liquid and Berry-Flavored, Dye-Free, white-colored liquid in ½ fl. oz. bottles w/calibrated plastic syringe.
Children's MOTRIN® Oral Suspension: Berry-flavored, pink-colored; (2 and 4 fl. oz) Berry-Flavored, Dye-Free white-colored, Bubble Gum-flavored, pink-colored and Grape-flavored, purple-colored liquid in tamper evident bottles (4 fl. oz.)
Children's MOTRIN® Chewable Tablets: Orange-flavored, orange-colored and Grape-flavored, purple-colored chewable tablets in 24 count bottles.
Junior Strength MOTRIN® Chewable Tablets: Orange-flavored, orange-colored chewable tablets or Grape-flavored, purple-colored chewable tablets in 24 count bottles.
Junior Strength MOTRIN® Caplets: Easy-to-swallow caplets (capsule shaped tablets) in 24 count bottles.
Shown in Product Identification Guide, page 511

**Children's MOTRIN® Cold
ibuprofen/pseudoephedrine HCl
Oral Suspension**

Description: *Children's MOTRIN® Cold Oral Suspension* is an alcohol-free berry, dye-free berry, or grape-flavored suspension. Each 5 mL (teaspoonful) contains the pain reliever/fever reducer ibuprofen 100 mg and the nasal decongestant pseudoephedrine HCl 15 mg.

Uses: temporarily relieves these cold, sinus and flu symptoms:
•nasal and sinus congestion
•stuffy nose •headache •sore throat
•minor body aches and pains •fever

Directions:
See Table 2: Children's Motrin Dosing Chart on pg. 673.

Warnings:
Allergy alert: Ibuprofen may cause a severe allergic reaction which may include:
•hives •facial swelling
•asthma (wheezing) •shock
Sore throat warning: Severe or persistent sore throat or sore throat accompanied by high fever, headache, nausea, and vomiting may be serious. Consult a doctor promptly. Do not use more than 2 days or administer to children under 3 years of age unless directed by doctor.

Continued on next page

Motrin Children's—Cont.

Do not use
- if the child has ever had an allergic reaction to any other pain reliever/fever reducer and/or nasal decongestant
- in a child who is taking a prescription monoamine oxidase inhibitor [MAOI] (certain drugs for depression, psychiatric or emotional conditions, or Parkinson's disease), or for 2 weeks after stopping the MAOI drug. If you do not know if your child's prescription drug contains an MAOI, ask a doctor or pharmacist before giving this product.

Ask a doctor before use if the child has
- not been drinking fluids
- lost a lot of fluid due to continued vomiting or diarrhea
- problems or serious side effects from taking pain relievers, fever reducers or nasal decongestants
- stomach pain
- heart disease
- high blood pressure
- thyroid disease
- diabetes

Ask a doctor or pharmacist before use if the child is
- under a doctor's care for any continuing medical condition
- taking any other drug
- taking any other product that contains ibuprofen or pseudoephedrine
- taking any other pain reliever/fever reducer and/or nasal decongestant

When using this product
- **do not exceed recommended dosage**
- give with food or milk if stomach upset occurs

Stop use and ask a doctor if
- an allergic reaction occurs. Seek medical help right away.
- the child does not get any relief within first day (24 hours) of treatment
- fever, pain or nasal congestion gets worse, or lasts for more than 3 days
- stomach pain or upset gets worse or lasts
- symptoms continue or get worse
- redness or swelling is present in the painful area
- the child gets nervous, dizzy, sleepless or sleepy
- any new symptoms appear

Keep out of reach of children. In case of overdose, get medical help or contact a Poison Control Center right away.

Other Information:
- **do not use if plastic carton wrap or bottle wrap imprinted "Safety Seal®" is broken or missing.**
- Store at 20–25°C (68–77°F)

Professional Information:
Overdosage Information
For overdosage information, please refer to pg. 671

Inactive Ingredients: Berry Flavor: acesulfame potassium, citric acid, corn starch, D&C yellow #10, FD&C red #40, flavors, glycerin, polysorbate 80, purified water, sodium benzoate, sucrose, xanthan gum. **Dye-Free Berry Flavor:** acesulfame potassium, citric acid, corn starch, flavors, glycerin, polysorbate 80, purified water, sodium benzoate, sucrose, xanthan gum. **Grape Flavor:** acesulfame potassium, citric acid, corn starch, D&C red #33, FD&C blue #1, FD&C red #40, flavors, glycerin, polysorbate 80, purified water, sodium benzoate, sucrose, xanthan gum.

How Supplied: Berry-flavored, pink-colored; Grape-flavored, purple-colored, and Dye-Free Berry-flavored, white-colored liquid in child resistant tamper-evident bottles of 4 fl. oz.

Shown in Product Identification Guide, page 511

Children's Motrin® Dosing Chart
[See table 2 on next page]

NIZORAL® A-D
KETOCONAZOLE SHAMPOO 1%

Description: *Nizoral® A-D (Ketoconazole Shampoo 1%) Anti-Dandruff Shampoo* is a light-blue liquid for topical application, containing the broad spectrum synthetic antifungal agent Ketoconazole in a concentration of 1%.

Use: Controls flaking, scaling, and itching associated with dandruff.

Directions:

Adults and children 12 years and over:	• wet hair thoroughly • apply shampoo, generously lather, rinse thoroughly. Repeat. • use every 3–4 days for up to 8 weeks or as directed by a doctor. Then use only as needed to control dandruff.
children under 12 years	• ask a doctor

Warnings:
• **For external use only**
Do Not Use
- on scalp that is broken or inflamed
- if you are allergic to ingredients in this product

When Using This Product
- avoid contact with eyes
- if product gets into eyes, rinse thoroughly with water

Stop use and ask a doctor if
- rash appears
- condition worsens or does not improve in 2–4 weeks

If pregnant or breast-feeding, ask a doctor before use.

Keep out of the reach of children.
If swallowed get medical help or contact a Poison Control Center right away.

Other Information:
- store between 35° and 86°F (2° and 30°C)
- protect from light • protect from freezing

Professional Information:
Overdosage Information *Nizoral® A-D (Ketoconazole) 1% Shampoo* is intended for external use only. In the event of accidental ingestion, supportive measures should be employed. Induced emesis and gastric lavage should usually be avoided.

Inactive Ingredients: acrylic acid polymer (carbomer 1342), butylated hydroxytoluene, cocamide MEA, FD&C Blue #1, fragrance, glycol distearate, polyquaternium-7, quaternium-15, sodium chloride, sodium cocoyl sarcosinate, sodium hydroxide and/or hydrochloric acid, sodium laureth sulfate, tetrasodium EDTA, water.

How Supplied: Available in 4 and 7 fl oz bottles
Shown in Product Identification Guide, page 512

ST. JOSEPH 81 mg Aspirin
ST. JOSEPH 81 mg Adult Low Strength Aspirin Chewable & Enteric Coated Tablets

Description: Each St. Joseph Adult Low Strength Aspirin tablet contains 81 mg of aspirin.

Uses:
- temporarily relieves minor aches and pains or as recommended by your doctor
- ask your doctor about other uses for St. Joseph Adult 81 mg Aspirin

Directions:
- drink a full glass of water with each dose
- **adults and children 12 years and over:**
  - take 4 to 8 tablets every 4 hours while symptoms persist
  - do not exceed 48 tablets in 24 hours or as directed by a doctor
- **children under 12:**
  - do not use unless directed by a doctor

Warnings:
Reye's syndrome: Children and teenagers should not use this drug for chicken pox or flu symptoms before a doctor is consulted about Reye's syndrome, a rare but serious illness reported to be associated with aspirin.

Allergy alert: Aspirin may cause a severe allergic reaction which may include:
- hives
- facial swelling
- asthma (wheezing)
- shock

Alcohol warning: If you consume 3 or more alcoholic drinks every day, ask your doctor whether you should take aspirin or other pain relievers/fever reducers. Aspirin may cause stomach bleeding.

Do not use
- If you have ever had an allergic reaction to any other pain reliever/fever reducer
- for at least 7 days after tonsillectomy or oral surgery unless directed by a doctor (*chewable tablet formulation only*)

Table 2. Children's Motrin Dosing Chart

AGE GROUP*		0-5 mos*	6-11 mos	12-23 mos	2-3 yrs	4-5 yrs	6-8 yrs	9-10 yrs	11 yrs	Maximum doses/ 24 hrs
WEIGHT	(if possible use weight to dose; otherwise use age)	6-11 lbs	12-17 lbs	18-23 lbs	24-35 lbs	36-47 lbs	48-59 lbs	60-71 lbs	72-95 lbs	
PRODUCT FORM	INGREDIENTS	Dose to be administered based on weight or age†								
Infants' Drops	Per 1.25 mL									
Infants' Motrin Concentrated Drops	Ibuprofen 50 mg	—	1.25 mL	1.875 mL	—	—	—	—	—	4 times in 24 hrs
Children's Liquid	Per 5 mL teaspoonful (TSP)									
Children's Motrin Suspension	Ibuprofen 100 mg	—	—	—	1 TSP	1 ½ TSP	2 TSP	2 ½ TSP	3 TSP	4 times in 24 hrs
Children's Motrin Cold Suspension Liquid†	Ibuprofen 100 mg Pseudoephedrine HCl 15 mg	—	—	—	1 TSP	1 TSP	2 TSP	2 TSP	2 TSP	4 times in 24 hrs
Children's Tablets & Caplets	Per tablet/ caplet									
Children's Motrin Chewable Tablets	Ibuprofen 50 mg	—	—	—	2 tablets	3 tablets	4 tablets	5 tablets	6 tablets	4 times in 24 hrs
Junior Strength Motrin Chewable Tablets	Ibuprofen 100 mg	—	—	—	—	—	2 tablets	2 ½ tablets	3 tablets	4 times in 24 hrs
Junior Strength Motrin Caplets	Ibuprofen 100 mg	—	—	—	—	—	2 caplets	2 ½ caplets	3 caplets	4 times in 24 hrs

† Do not give, take or chew more than directed. If needed, repeat dose every 6-8 hours; except for Children's Motrin Cold which is every 6 hours.

* Under 6 mos, call a doctor.

- Infants' Motrin Drops are more concentrated than Children's Motrin Liquids. The Infants' Concentrated Drops have been specifically designed for use only with enclosed dosing device. Do not use any other dosing device with this product.
- Children's Motrin Liquids are less concentrated than Infants' Motrin Drops. The Children's Motrin Liquids have been specifically designed for use with the enclosed measuring cup. Use only enclosed measuring cup to dose this product.
- Children's Motrin Chewable Tablets are not the same concentration as Junior Strength Motrin Chewable Tablets.
- Junior Strength Motrin Chewable Tablets contain twice as much medicine as Children's Motrin Chewable Tablets.

St. Joseph Aspirin—Cont.

Ask a doctor before use if you have
- asthma
- ulcers
- bleeding problems
- stomach problems that last or come back such as heartburn, upset stomach or pain

Ask a doctor or pharmacist before use if you are
- Taking a prescription drug for:
  - anticoagulation (blood thinning)
  - gout
  - diabetes
  - arthritis

Stop use and ask a doctor if
- allergic reaction occurs. Seek medical help right away.
- ringing in the ears or loss of hearing occurs
- pain gets worse or lasts more than 10 days
- new symptoms occur
- redness or swelling is present

If pregnant or breast-feeding, ask a health professional before use. It is especially important not to use aspirin during the last three months of pregnancy unless definitely directed to do so by a doctor because it may cause problems in the unborn child or complications during delivery.

Keep out of reach of children. In case of overdose, get medical help or contact a Poison Control Center right away.

Other Information:
- **do not use if carton is opened or neck wrap or foil inner seal imprinted with "Safety Seal®" is broken**
- store at room temperature. Avoid high humidity and excessive heat (40° C).

Inactive Ingredients: *St. Joseph 81 mg Adult Low Strength Aspirin Chewable Tablets:* corn starch, FD&C yellow #6 aluminum lake, flavor, mannitol, saccharin, silicon dioxide, stearic acid. *Enteric Coated Tablets:* cellulose, corn starch, FD&C Red #40, FD&C Yellow #6, glyceryl monostearate, iron oxide, methacrylic acid, silicon dioxide, simethicone, stearic acid, triethyl citrate.

How Supplied: *St. Joseph 81 mg Adult Low Strength Chewable Aspirin Tablets:* tamper evident bottles of 36 and 108 (Tri-Pack). *Enteric Coated Tablets:* tamper evident bottles of 36 100, and 180.

Comprehensive Prescribing Information
Description: St. Joseph Adult Low Strength Aspirin Chewable & Enteric Coated Tablets (acetylsalicylic acid) are available in 81 mg for oral administration. *St. Joseph 81 mg Adult Low Strength Aspirin Chewable Tablets* contain the following inactive ingredients: corn starch, FD&C yellow #6 aluminum lake, flavor, mannitol, saccharin, silicon dioxide, stearic acid. *St. Joseph 81 mg Adult Low Strength Aspirin Enteric Coated Tablets* contain the following inactive ingredients: cellulose, corn starch, FD&C Red #40, FD&C Yellow #6, glyceryl monostearate, iron oxide, methacrylic acid, silicon dioxide, simethicone,

stearic acid, triethyl citrate. Aspirin is an odorless white, needle-like crystalline or powdery substance. When exposed to moisture, aspirin hydrolyzes into salicylic and acetic acids, and gives off a vinegary-odor. It is highly lipid soluble and slightly soluble in water.

Clinical Pharmacology:
Mechanism of Action: Aspirin is a more potent inhibitor of both prostaglandin synthesis and platelet aggregation than other salicylic acid derivatives. The differences in activity between aspirin and salicylic acid are thought to be due to the acetyl group on the aspirin molecule. This acetyl group is responsible for the inactivation of cyclo-oxygenase via acetylation.

Pharmacokinetics: Absorption: In general, immediate release aspirin is well and completely absorbed from the gastrointestinal (GI) tract. Following absorption, aspirin is hydrolyzed to salicylic acid with peak plasma levels of salicylic acid occurring within 1–2 hours of dosing (see Pharmacokinetics—Metabolism). The rate of absorption from the GI tract is dependent upon the dosage form, the presence or absence of food, gastric pH (the presence or absence of GI antacids or buffering agents), and other physiologic factors. Enteric coated aspirin products are erratically absorbed from the GI tract.

Distribution: Salicylic acid is widely distributed to all tissues and fluids in the body including the central nervous system (CNS), breast milk, and fetal tissues. The highest concentrations are found in the plasma, liver, renal cortex, heart, and lungs. The protein binding of salicylate is concentration-dependent, i.e., nonlinear. At low concentrations (100 μg/mL), approximately 90 percent of plasma salicylate is bound to albumin while at higher concentrations (>400 μg/mL), only about 75 percent is bound. The early signs of salicylic overdose (salicylism), including tinnitus (ringing in the ears), occur at plasma concentrations approximating 200 μg/mL. Severe toxic effects are associated with levels >400 μg/mL. (See Adverse Reactions and Overdosage.)

Metabolism: Aspirin is rapidly hydrolyzed in the plasma to salicylic acid such that plasma levels of aspirin are essentially undetectable 1–2 hours after dosing. Salicylic acid is primarily conjugated in the liver to form salicyluric acid, a phenolic glucuronide, an acyl glucuronide, and a number of minor metabolites. Salicylic acid has a plasma half-life of approximately 6 hours. Salicylate metabolism is saturable and total body clearance decreases at higher serum concentrations due to the limited ability of the liver to form both salicyluric acid and phenolic glucuronide. Following toxic doses (10–20 grams (g)), the plasma half-life may be increased to over 20 hours.

Elimination: The elimination of salicylic acid follows zero order pharmacokinetics; (i.e., the rate of drug elimination

is constant in relation to plasma concentration). Renal excretion of unchanged drug depends upon urine pH. As urinary pH rises above 6.5, the renal clearance of free salicylate increases from 5 percent to >80 percent. Alkalinization of the urine is a key concept in the management of salicylate overdose. (See Overdosage.) Following therapeutic doses, approximately 10 percent is found excreted in the urine as salicylic acid, 75 percent as salicyluric acid, and 10 percent phenolic and 5 percent acyl glucuronides of salicylic acid.

Pharmacodynamics: Aspirin affects platelet aggregation by irreversibly inhibiting prostaglandin cyclo-oxygenase. The effect lasts for the life of the platelet and prevents the formation of the platelet aggregating factor thromboxane A2. Nonacetylated salicylates do not inhibit this enzyme and have no effect on platelet aggregation. At somewhat higher doses, aspirin reversibly inhibits the formation of prostaglandin I2 (prostacyclin), which is an arterial vasodilator and inhibits platelet aggregation. At higher doses, aspirin is an effective anti-inflammatory agent, partially due to inhibition of inflammatory mediators via cyclo-oxygenase inhibition in peripheral tissues. In vitro studies suggest that other mediators of inflammation may also be suppressed by aspirin administration, although the precise mechanism of action has not been elucidated. It is this nonspecific suppression of cyclo-oxygenase activity in peripheral tissues following large doses that leads to its primary side effect of gastric irritation. (See Adverse Reactions.)

Clinical Studies: Ischemic Stroke and Transient Ischemic Attack (TIA): In clinical trials of subjects with TIA's due to fibrin platelet emboli or ischemic stroke, aspirin has been shown to significantly reduce the risk of the combined endpoint of stroke or death and the combined endpoint of TIA, stroke, or death by about 13–18 percent.

Suspected Acute Myocardial Infarction (MI): In a large, multi-center study of aspirin, streptokinase, and the combination of aspirin and streptokinase in 17,187 patients with suspected acute MI, aspirin treatment produced a 23-percent reduction in the risk of vascular mortality. Aspirin was also shown to have an additional benefit in patients given a thrombolytic agent.

Prevention of Recurrent MI and Unstable Angina Pectoris: These indications are supported by the results of six large, randomized, multi-center, placebo-controlled trials of predominantly male post-MI subjects and one randomized placebo-controlled study of men with unstable angina pectoris. Aspirin therapy in MI subjects was associated with a significant reduction (about 20 percent) in the risk of the combined endpoint of subsequent death and/or nonfatal reinfarction in these patients. In aspirin-treated unstable angina patients, the event rate was reduced to 5 percent from the 10 percent rate in the placebo group.

Chronic Stable Angina Pectoris: In a randomized, multi-center, double-blind trial designed to assess the role of aspirin for prevention of MI in patients with chronic stable angina pectoris, aspirin significantly reduced the primary combined endpoint of nonfatal MI, fatal MI, and sudden death by 34 percent. The secondary endpoint for vascular events (first occurrence of MI, stroke, or vascular death) was also significantly reduced (32 percent).

Revascularization Procedures: Most patients who undergo coronary artery revascularization procedures have already had symptomatic coronary artery disease for which aspirin is indicated. Similarly, patients with lesions of the carotid bifurcation sufficient to require carotid endarterectomy are likely to have had a precedent event. Aspirin is recommended for patients who undergo revascularization procedures if there is a preexisting condition for which aspirin is already indicated.

Rheumatologic Diseases: In clinical studies in patients with rheumatoid arthritis, juvenile rheumatoid arthritis, ankylosing spondylitis and osteoarthritis, aspirin has been shown to be effective in controlling various indices of clinical disease activity.

Animal Toxicology: Ischemic Stroke and Transient Ischemic Attack (TIA): In clinical trials of subjects with TIA's due to fibrin platelet emboli or ischemic stroke, aspirin has been shown to significantly reduce the risk of the combined endpoint of stroke or death and the combined endpoint of TIA, stroke, or death by about 13–18 percent. The acute oral 50 percent lethal dose in rats is about 1.5 g/kilogram (kg) and in mice 1.1 g/kg. Renal papillary necrosis and decreased urinary concentrating ability occur in rodents chronically administered high doses. Dose-dependent gastric mucosal injury occurs in rats and humans. Mammals may develop aspirin toxicosis associated with GI symptoms, circulatory effects, and central nervous system depression. (See Overdosage.)

Indications and Usage: Vascular Indications (Ischemic Stroke, TIA, Acute MI, Prevention of Recurrent MI, Unstable Angina Pectoris, and Chronic Stable Angina Pectoris): Aspirin is indicated to: (1) Reduce the combined risk of death and nonfatal stroke in patients who have had ischemic stroke or transient ischemia of the brain due to fibrin platelet emboli, (2) reduce the risk of vascular mortality in patients with a suspected acute MI, (3) reduce the combined risk of death and nonfatal MI in patients with a previous MI or unstable angina pectoris, and (4) reduce the combined risk of MI and sudden death in patients with chronic stable angina pectoris.

Rheumatologic Disease Indications (Rheumatoid Arthritis, Juvenile Rheumatoid Arthritis, Spondyloarthropathies, Osteoarthritis, and the Arthritis and Pleurisy of Systemic Lupus Erythematosus (SLE)): Aspirin is indicated for the relief of the signs and symptoms of rheumatoid arthritis, juvenile rheumatoid arthritis, osteoarthritis, spondyloarthropathies, and arthritis and pleurisy associated with SLE.

Contraindications: Allergy: Aspirin is contraindicated in patients with known allergy to nonsteroidal anti-inflammatory drug products in patients with the syndrome of asthma, rhinitis, and nasal polyps. Aspirin may cause severe urticaria, angioedema, or bronchospasm (asthma).

Reye's Syndrome: Aspirin should not be used in children or teenagers for viral infections, with or without fever, because of the risk of Reye's syndrome with concomitant use of aspirin in certain viral illnesses.

Warnings: Alcohol Warning: Patients who consume three or more alcoholic drinks every day should be counseled about the bleeding risks involved with chronic, heavy alcohol use while taking aspirin.

Coagulation Abnormalities: Even low doses of aspirin can inhibit platelet function leading to an increase in bleeding time. This can adversely affect patients with inherited (hemophilia) or acquired (liver disease or vitamin K deficiency) bleeding disorders.

GI Side Effects: GI side effects include stomach pain, heartburn, nausea, vomiting, and gross GI bleeding. Although minor upper GI symptoms, such as dyspepsia, are common and can occur anytime during therapy, physicians should remain alert for signs of ulceration and bleeding, even in the absence of previous GI symptoms. Physicians should inform patients about the signs and symptoms of GI side effects and what steps to take if they occur.

Peptic Ulcer Disease: Patients with a history of active peptic ulcer disease should avoid using aspirin, which can cause gastric mucosal irritation and bleeding.

Precautions:

General: Renal Failure: Avoid aspirin in patients with severe renal failure (glomerular filtration rate less than 10 mL/minute)

Hepatic Insufficiency: Avoid aspirin in patients with severe hepatic insufficiency.

Sodium Restricted Diets: Patients with sodium-retaining states, such as congestive heart failure or renal failure, should avoid sodium-containing buffered aspirin preparations because of their high sodium content.

Laboratory Tests: Aspirin has been associated with elevated hepatic enzymes, blood urea nitrogen and serum creatinine, hyperkalemia, proteinuria, and prolonged bleeding time.

Drug Interactions: Angiotensin Converting Enzyme (ACE) Inhibitors: The hyponatremic and hypotensive effects of ACE inhibitors may be diminished by the concomitant administration of aspirin due to its indirect effect on the renin-angiotensin conversion pathway.

Acetazolamide: Concurrent use of aspirin and acetazolamide can lead to high serum concentrations of acetazolamide (and toxicity) due to competition at the renal tubule for secretion.

Anticoagulant Therapy (Heparin and Warfarin): Patients on anticoagulation therapy are at increased risk for bleeding because of drug-drug interactions and the effect on platelets. Aspirin can displace warfarin from protein binding sites, leading to prolongation of both the prothrombin time and the bleeding time. Aspirin can increase the anticoagulant activity of heparin, increasing bleeding risk.

Anticonvulsants: Salicylate can displace protein-bound phenytoin and valproic acid, leading to a decrease in the total concentration of phenytoin and an increase in serum valproic acid levels.

Beta Blockers: The hypotensive effects of beta blockers may be diminished by the concomitant administration of aspirin due to inhibition of renal prostaglandins, leading to decreased renal blood flow, and salt and fluid retention.

Diuretics: The effectiveness of diuretics in patients with underlying renal or cardiovascular disease may be diminished by the concomitant administration of aspirin due to inhibition of renal prostaglandins, leading to decreased renal blood flow and salt and fluit retention.

Methotrexate: Salicylate can inhibit renal clearance of methotrexate, leading to bone marrow toxicity, especially in the elderly or renal impaired.

Nonsteroidal Anti-Inflammatory Drugs (NSAID's): The concurrent use of aspirin with other NSAID's should be avoided because this may increase bleeding or lead to decreased renal function.

Oral Hypoglycemics: Moderate doses of aspirin may increase the effectiveness of oral hypoglycemic drugs, leading to hypoglycemia.

Uricosuric Agents (Probenecid and Sulfinpyrazone): Salicylates antagonize the uricosuric action of uricosuric agents.

Carcinogenesis, Mutagenesis, Impairment of Fertility: Administration of aspirin for 68 weeks at 0.5 percent in the feed of rats was not carcinogenic. In the Ames Salmonella assay, aspirin was not mutagenic; however, aspirin did induce chromosome aberrations in cultured human fibroblasts. Aspirin inhibits ovulation in rats. (See Pregnancy.)

Pregnancy: Pregnant women should only take aspirin if clearly needed. Because of the known effects of NSAID's on the fetal cardiovascular system (closure of the ductus arteriosus), use during the third trimester of pregnancy should be avoided. Salicylate products have also been associated with alterations in maternal and neonatal hemostasis mecha-

Continued on next page

St. Joseph Aspirin—Cont.

nisms, decreased birth weight, and with perinatal mortality.

Labor and Delivery: Aspirin should be avoided 1 week prior to and during labor and delivery because it can result in excessive blood loss at delivery. Prolonged gestation and prolonged labor due to prostaglandin inhibition have been reported.

Nursing Mothers: Nursing mothers should avoid using aspirin because salicylate is excreted in breast milk. Use of high doses may lead to rashes, platelet abnormalities, and bleeding in nursing infants.

Pediatric Use: Pediatric dosing recommendations for juvenile rheumatoid arthritis are based on well-controlled clinical studies. An initial dose of 90–130 mg/kg/day in divided doses, with an increase as needed for anti-inflammatory efficacy (target plasma salicylate levels of 150–300 µg/mL) are effective. At high doses (i.e., plasma levels of greater than 200 µg/mL), the incidence of toxicity increases.

Adverse Reactions: Many adverse reactions due to aspirin ingestion are dose-related. The following is a list of adverse reactions that have been reported in the literature. (See Warnings.)

Body as a Whole: Fever, hypothermia, thirst.

Cardiovascular: Dysrhythmias, hypotension, tachycardia.

Central Nervous System: Agitation, cerebral edema, coma, confusion, dizziness, headache, subdural or intracranial hemorrhage, lethargy, seizures.

Fluid and Electrolyte: Dehydration, hyperkalemia, metabolic acidosis, respiratory alkalosis.

Gastrointestinal: Dyspepsia, GI bleeding, ulceration and perforation, nausea, vomiting, transient elevations of hepatic enzymes, hepatitis, Reye's Syndrome, pancreatitis.

Hematologic: Prolongation of the prothrombin time, disseminated intravascular coagulation, coagulopathy, thrombocytopenia.

Hypersensitivity: Acute anaphylaxis, angioedema, asthma, bronchospasm, laryngeal edema, urticaria.

Musculoskeletal: Rhabdomyolysis.

Metabolism: Hypoglycemia (in children), hyperglycemia.

Reproductive: Prolonged pregnancy and labor, stillbirths, lower birth weight infants, antepartum and postpartum bleeding.

Special Senses: Hearing loss, tinnitus. Patients with high frequency hearing loss may have difficulty perceiving tinnitus. In these patients, tinnitus cannot be used as a clinical indicator of salicylism.

Urogenital: Interstitial nephritis, papillary necrosis, proteinuria, renal insufficiency and failure.

Drug Abuse and Dependence: Aspirin is nonnarcotic. There is no known po-

tential for addiction associated with the use of aspirin.

Overdosage: Salicylate toxicity may result from acute ingestion (overdose) or chronic intoxication. The early signs of salicylic overdose (salicylism), including tinnitus (ringing in the ears), occur at plasma concentrations approaching 200 µg/mL. Plasma concentrations of aspirin above 300 µg/mL are clearly toxic. Severe toxic effects are associated with levels above 400 µg/mL (See Clinical Pharmacology.) A single lethal dose of aspirin in adults is not known with certainty but death may be expected at 30 g. For real or suspected overdose, a Poison Control Center should be contacted immediately. Careful medical management is essential.

Signs and Symptoms: In acute overdose, severe acid-base and electrolyte disturbances may occur and are complicated by hyperthermia and dehydration. Respiratory alkalosis occurs early while hyperventilation is present, but is quickly followed by metabolic acidosis.

Treatment: Treatment consists primarily of supporting vital functions, increasing salicylate elimination, and correcting the acid-base disturbance. Gastric emptying and/or lavage is recommended as soon as possible after ingestion, even if the patient has vomited spontaneously. After lavage and/or emesis, administration of activated charcoal, as a slurry, is beneficial, if less than 3 hours have passed since ingestion. Charcoal adsorption should not be employed prior to emesis and lavage. Severity of aspirin intoxication is determined by measuring the blood salicylate level. Acid-base status should be closely followed with serial blood gas and serum pH measurements. Fluid and electrolyte balance should also be maintained. In severe cases, hyperthermia and hypovolemia are the major immediate threats to life. Children should be sponged with tepid water. Replacement fluids should be administered intravenously and augmented with correction of acidosis. Plasma electrolytes and pH should be monitored to promote alkaline diuresis of salicylate if renal function is normal. Infusion of glucose may be required to control hypoglycemia. Hemodialysis and peritoneal dialysis can be performed to reduce the body drug content. In patients with renal insufficiency or in cases of life-threatening intoxication, dialysis is usually required. Exchange transfusion may be indicated in infants and young children.

Dosage and Administration: Each dose of aspirin should be taken with a full glass of water unless the patient is fluid restricted. Anti-inflammatory and analgesic dosages should be individualized. When aspirin is used in high doses, the development of tinnitus may be used as a clinical sign of elevated plasma salicylate levels except in patients with high frequency hearing loss.

Ischemic Stroke and TIA: 50–325 mg once a day. Continue therapy indefinitely

Suspected Acute MI: The initial dose of 160–162.5 mg is administered as soon as an MI is suspected. The maintenance dose of 160–162.5 mg a day is continued for 30 days post-infarction. After 30 days, consider further therapy based on dosage and administration for prevention of recurrent MI.

Prevention of Recurrent MI: 75–325 mg once a day. Continue therapy indefinitely.

Unstable Angina Pectoris: 75–325 mg once a day. Continue therapy indefinitely.

Chronic Stable Angina Pectoris: 75–325 mg once a day. Continue therapy indefinitely.

CABG: 325 mg daily starting 6 hours post-procedure. Continue therapy for 1 year post-procedure.

PTCA: The initial dose of 325 mg daily should be given 2 hours pre-surgery. Maintenance dose is 160–325 mg daily. Continue therapy indefinitely.

Carotid Endarterectomy: Doses of 80 mg once daily to 650 mg twice daily, started presurgery, are recommended. Continue therapy indefinitely.

Rheumatoid Arthritis: The initial dose is 3 g a day in divided doses. Increase as needed for anti-inflammatory efficacy with target plasma salicylate levels of 150–300 µg/mL. At high doses (i.e., plasma levels of greater than 200 µg/mL), the incidence of toxicity increases.

Juvenile Rheumatoid Arthritis: Initial dose is 90–130 mg/kg/day in divided doses. Increase as needed for anti-inflammatory efficacy with target plasma salicylate levels of 150–300 µg/mL. At high doses (i.e., plasma levels of greater than 200 µg/mL), the incidence of toxicity increases.

Spondyloarthropathies: Up to 4 g per day in divided doses.

Osteoarthritis: Up to 3 g per day in divided doses.

Arthritis and Pleurisy of SLE: The initial dose is 3 g a day in divided doses. Increase as needed for anti-inflammatory efficacy with target plasma salicylate levels of 150–300 µg/mL. At high doses (i.e., plasma levels of greater than 200 µg/mL), the incidence of toxicity increases.

How Supplied: *St. Joseph Adult Low Strength Aspirin Chewable Tablets* are round, concave, orange-flavored, orange-colored tablets that are debossed with the "SJ" logo. Available as follows:

NDC 50580-173-36 Bottle of 36 tablets
NDC Coated Tablets 50580-173-08 Tri-Pack

St Joseph Adult Low Strength Enteric Coated Tablets are round, concave, pink-coated tablets that are printed with the "St J" logo. Available as follows:

NDC 50580-126-36 Bottle of 36 tablets
NDC 50580-126-10 Bottle of 100 tablets
NDC 50580-126-18 Bottle of 180 tablets

Store in tight container at 25 deg.C (77 deg.F); excursions permitted to 15–30 deg.C (59–86 deg.F).

Shown in Product Identification Guide, page 512

SIMPLY COUGH™ LIQUID

Description: *Simply Cough™ Liquid* is Cherry Berry-flavored and contains no alcohol or aspirin. Each teaspoonful (5 mL) contains dextromethorphan HBr 5 mg.

Actions: *Simply Cough™ Liquid* is a single ingredient product that contains the cough suppressant dextromethorphan hydrobromide to provide fast, effective, temporary relief of your child's cough.

Uses: temporarily relieves cough occurring with a cold

Directions:
• find right dose on chart below. If possible, use weight to dose; otherwise use age.
• only use with enclosed measuring cup
• if needed, repeat dose every 4 hours
• do not use more than 4 times in 24 hours

AccuDose™ Chart

Weight (lb)	Age (yr)	Dose (tsp)
under 24	under 2	call a doctor
24–47	2–5	1 tsp
48–95	6–11	2 tsp

Professional Dosage Schedule: 4–11 mos (12–17 lbs): ½ teaspoonful; 12–23 mos (18–23 lbs): ¾ teaspoonful; 2–3 years (24–35 lbs) 1 teaspoonful; 4–5 yrs (36–47 lbs): 1½ teaspoonsful; 6–8 yrs (48–59 lbs): 2 teaspoonsful; 9–10 yrs (60–71 lbs): 2½ teaspoonsful; 11 yrs (72–95 lbs): 3 teaspoonsful.
If needed, repeat dose every 4 to 6 hours. Do not use more than 4 times in 24 hours.

Precautions: If a rare sensitivity reaction occurs, the drug should be discontinued.

Warnings: Do not use in a child who is taking a prescription monoamine oxidase inhibitor (MAOI) (certain drugs for depression, psychiatric or emotional conditions, or Parkinson's disease), or for 2 weeks after stopping the MAOI drug. If you do not know if your child's prescription drug contains an MAOI, ask a doctor or pharmacist before giving this product.
Ask a doctor before use if this child has
• cough that occurs with too much phlegm (mucus)
• chronic cough that lasts or occurs with asthma
Stop use and ask a doctor if
• cough gets worse or lasts for more than 5 days, comes back or occurs with fever, rash or headache that lasts. These could be signs of a serious condition.
Keep out of reach of children.
In case of overdose, get medical help or contact a Poison Control Center right away.
Other Information:
• **do not use if carton is opened, or if neck wrap or foil inner seal imprinted with "Safety Seal®" is broken or missing**
• store at room temperature

Professional Information:
Overdosage Information:
Acute dextromethorphan overdose usually does not result in serious signs and symptoms unless massive amounts have been ingested. Signs and symptoms of a substantial overdose may include nausea and vomiting, visual disturbances, CNS disturbances and urinary retention.

Inactive Ingredients: citric acid, corn syrup, FD&C Red #40, flavor, glycerin, purified water, sodium benzoate, sucralose

How Supplied: Cherry Berry flavored liquid in child resistant tamper-evident bottles of 4 fl. oz.
Shown in Product Identification Guide, page 512

SIMPLY SLEEP™
Nighttime Sleep Aid

Description: *SIMPLY SLEEP™* is a non habit-forming nighttime sleep aid. Each *SIMPLY SLEEP™* Caplet contains diphenhydramine HCl 25 mg.

Actions: *SIMPLY SLEEP™* contains an antihistamine (diphenhydramine HCl) which has sedative properties.

Use: relief of occasional sleeplessness

Directions:

adults and children 12 years and over	take 2 caplets at bedtime if needed or as directed by a doctor
children under 12 years	do not use

Warnings:
Do not use
• with any other product containing diphenhydramine, even one used on skin
• in children under 12 years of age
Ask a doctor before use if you have
• a breathing problem such as emphysema or chronic bronchitis
• trouble urinating due to an enlarged prostate gland
• glaucoma
Ask a doctor or pharmacist before use if you are taking sedatives or tranquilizers
When using this product
• drowsiness may occur
• avoid alcoholic drinks
• do not drive a motor vehicle or operate machinery
Stop use and ask a doctor if
• sleeplessness persists continuously for more than 2 weeks. Insomnia may be a symptom of serious underlying medical illness.
If pregnant or breast-feeding, ask a health professional before use.
Keep out of reach of children. In case of overdose, get medical help or contact a Poison Control Center right away.
Other Information:
• **Do not use if blister carton is opened or if blister unit is broken.**

• Store at room temperature
• see side panel for lot number and expiration date

Inactive Ingredients: carnauba wax, cellulose, croscarmellose sodium, dibasic calcium phosphate, FD&C blue #1, hypromellose, magnesium stearate, polyethylene glycol, polysorbate 80, titanium dioxide.

How Supplied: Light blue mini-caplets embossed with "SL" on one side in blister packs of 24 and 48.
Shown in Product Identification Guide, page 512

SIMPLY STUFFY™ LIQUID

Description: *Simply Stuffy™ Liquid* is Cherry Berry-flavored and contains no alcohol or aspirin. Each teaspoonful (5 mL) contains pseudoephedrine HCL 15 mg.

Actions: *Simply Stuffy™ Liquid* is a single ingredient product that contains the decongestant pseudoephedrine hydrochloride to provide fast, effective, temporary relief of your child's nasal congestion.

Uses: temporarily relieves nasal congestion due to:
• the common cold • hay fever • upper respiratory allergies • sinusitis

Directions:
• find right dose on chart below. If possible, use weight to dose; otherwise use age.
• only use with enclosed measuring cup
• if needed, repeat dose every 4 to 6 hours
• do not use more than 4 times in 24 hours

AccuDose™ Chart

Weight (lb)	Age (yr)	Dose (tsp)
under 24	under 2	call a doctor
24–47	2–5	1 tsp
48–95	6–11	2 tsp

Professional Dosage Schedule: 4–11 mos (12–17 lbs): ½ teaspoonful; 12–23 mos (18–23 lbs): ¾ teaspoonful; 2–3 yrs (24–35 lbs) 1 teaspoonful; 4–5 yrs (36–47 lbs): 1½ teaspoonsful; 6–8 yrs (48–59 lbs): 2 teaspoonsful; 9–10 yrs (60–71 lbs): 2½ teaspoonsful; 11 yrs (72–95 lbs): 3 teaspoonsful
If needed, repeat dose every 4 to 6 hours. Do not use more than 4 times in 24 hours.

Precautions: If a rare sensitivity reaction occurs, the drug should be discontinued.

Warnings: Do not use in a child who is taking a prescription monoamine oxidase inhibitor (MAOI) (certain drugs for depression, psychiatric or emotional conditions, or Parkinson's disease), or for 2 weeks after stopping the MAOI drug. If

Continued on next page

Simply Stuffy—Cont.

you do not know if your child's prescription drug contains an MAOI, ask a doctor or pharmacist before giving this product.
Ask a doctor before use if this child has
- heart disease • high blood pressure • thyroid disease • diabetes

When using this product
- **do not exceed recommended dosage**

Stop use and ask a doctor if
- nervousness, dizziness, or sleeplessness occur
- symptoms do not get better within 7 days or occur with a fever

Keep out of reach of children.
In case of overdose, get medical help or contact a Poison Control Center right away.
Other Information:
- **do not use if carton is opened, of if neck wrap or foil inner seal imprinted with "Safety Seal®" is broken or missing**
- store at room temperature

Professional Information:
Overdosage Information:
Symptoms from pseudoephedrine overdose consist most often of mild anxiety, tachycardia and/or mild hypertension. Symptoms usually appear within 4 to 8 hours of ingestion and are transient, usually requiring no treatment.

Inactive Ingredients: citric acid, corn syrup, FD&C Red #40, flavor, glycerin, purified water, sodium benzoate, sucralose

How Supplied: Cherry Berry flavored liquid in child resistant tamper-evident bottles of 4 fl. oz.

Shown in Product Identification Guide, page 512

Regular Strength TYLENOL® acetaminophen Tablets

Extra Strength TYLENOL® acetaminophen Gelcaps, Geltabs, Caplets, Tablets

Extra Strength TYLENOL® acetaminophen Adult Liquid Pain Reliever

TYLENOL® acetaminophen Arthritis Pain Extended Relief Caplets

TYLENOL® 8 Hour Acetaminophen Extended Release Geltabs/Caplets

Product information for all dosage forms of Adult TYLENOL actaminophen have been combined under this heading.

Description: *Each Regular Strength TYLENOL® Tablet contains acetaminophen 325 mg. Each Extra Strength TYLENOL® Gelcap, Geltab, Caplet, or Tablet contains acetaminophen 500 mg. Extra Strength TYLENOL® Adult Liquid is alcohol-free and each 15 mL (1/2 fl oz or one tablespoonful) contains 500 mg acetaminophen. Each TYLENOL®*
Arthritis Pain Extended Relief Caplet and each TYLENOL® 8 Hour Extended Release Geltab/caplet contains acetaminophen 650 mg.

Actions: Acetaminophen is a clinically proven analgesic/antipyretic. Acetaminophen produces analgesia by elevation of the pain threshold and antipyresis through action on the hypothalamic heat-regulating center. Acetaminophen is equal to aspirin in analgesic and antipyretic effectiveness and it is unlikely to produce many of the side effects associated with aspirin and aspirin-containing products. *Tylenol Arthritis Pain Extended Relief* and *TYLENOL 8 Hour Extended Release* use a unique, patented, bilayer caplet. The first layer dissolves quickly to provide prompt relief while the second layer is time released to provide up to 8 hours of relief.

Uses: *Regular Strength TYLENOL® Tablets, Extra Strength TYLENOL® Gelcaps, Geltabs, Caplets, or Tablets:* temporarily relieves minor aches and pains due to:
- headache • muscular aches • backache • arthritis
- the common cold • toothache • menstrual cramps
- reduces fever

Extra Strength TYLENOL® Adult Liquid: temporarily relieves minor aches and pains due to:
- headache • muscular aches • backache • arthritis
- the common cold • toothache • menstrual cramps
- reduces fever

TYLENOL® Arthritis Pain Extended Relief Caplets: temporarily relieves minor aches and pains due to:
- arthritis • the common cold • headache • toothache
- muscular aches • backache • menstrual cramps

TYLENOL® 8 Hour Extended Release Geltabs/Caplets: temporarily relieves minor aches and pains due to:
- muscular aches • backache • headache • toothache • the common cold
- menstrual cramps • minor pain of arthritis
- temporarily reduces fever

Directions:

Regular Strength TYLENOL® Tablets:
- **do not take more than directed (see overdose warning)**

adults and children 12 years and over	• take 2 tablets every 4 to 6 hours as needed • do not take more than 12 tablets in 24 hours
children 6–11 years	• take 1 tablet every 4 to 6 hours as needed • do not take more than 5 in 24 hours

children under 6 years	do not use this Regular Strength product in children under 6 years of age; this will provide more than the recommended dose (overdose) of TYLENOL® may cause liver damage

Extra Strength TYLENOL® Gelcaps, Geltabs, Caplets, or Tablets:
- **do not take more than directed (see overdose warning)**

adults and children 12 years and over	• take 2 every 4 to 6 hours as needed • do not take more than 8 in 24 hours
children under 12 years	do not use this Extra Strength product in children under 12 years of age; this will provide more than the recommended dose (overdose) of TYLENOL® and may cause liver damage

Extra Strength TYLENOL® Adult Liquid:
- **do not take more than directed (see overdose warning)**

adults and children 12 years and over	• take 2 tablespoons (tbsp.) in dose cup provided every 4 to 6 hours as needed • do not take more than 8 tablespoons in 24 hours
children under 12 years	do not use this adult Extra Strength product in children under 12 years of age; this will provide more than the recommended dose (overdose) of TYLENOL® and may cause liver damage

TYLENOL® 8 Hour Extended Release Geltabs/Caplets
- **do not take more than directed (see overdose warning)**

adults and children 12 years and over	• take 2 geltabs/caplets every 8 hours with water • swallow whole – do not crush, chew or dissolve • do not take more than 6 geltabs/caplets in 24 hours • do not use for more than 10 days unless directed by a doctor
children under 12 years	• ask a doctor

TYLENOL® Arthritis Pain Extended Relief Caplets
- **do not take more than directed (see overdose warning)**

adults	• take 2 every 8 hours with water • swallow whole – do not crush, chew or dissolve • do not take more than 6 in 24 hours • do not use for more than 10 days unless directed by a doctor
under 18 years of age	• ask a doctor

Precautions: If a rare sensitivity reaction occurs, the drug should be discontinued.

Warnings: *Regular Strength TYLENOL® Tablets, Extra Strength TYLENOL® Gelcaps, Geltabs, Caplets, or Tablets, Extra Strength TYLENOL® Liquid*
Alcohol warning: If you consume 3 or more alcoholic drinks every day, ask your doctor whether you should take acetaminophen or other pain relievers/fever reducers. Acetaminophen may cause liver damage.
Do not use:
- with any other product containing acetaminophen.

Stop using and ask a doctor if:
- new symptoms occur
- redness or swelling is present
- pain gets worse or lasts for more than 10 days
- fever gets worse or lasts for more than 3 days

If pregnant or breast-feeding, ask a health professional before use.
Keep out of reach of children.
Overdose warning: Taking more than the recommended dose (overdose) may cause liver damage. In case of overdose, get medical help or contact a Poison Control Center right away. Quick medical attention is critical for adults as well as for children even if you do not notice any signs of symptoms.
TYLENOL® Arthritis Pain Extended Relief Caplets:
Alcohol warning: If you consume 3 or more alcoholic drinks every day, ask your doctor whether you should take acetaminophen or other pain relievers/fever reducers. Acetaminophen may cause liver damage.
Do not use
- with any other product containing acetaminophen.

Stop use and ask a doctor if
- New symptoms occur
- Redness or swelling is present
- Pain gets worse or lasts for more than 10 days

If pregnant or breast-feeding, ask a health professional before use.
Keep out of reach of children.
Overdose warning: Taking more than the recommended dose (overdose) may

cause liver damage. In case of overdose, get medical help or contact a Poison Control Center right away. Quick medical attention is critical for adults as well as for children even if you do not notice any signs or symptoms.
TYLENOL® 8 Hour Extended Release Geltab/Caplets: **Alcohol warning:** If you consume 3 or more alcoholic drinks every day, ask your doctor whether you should take acetaminophen or other pain relievers/fever reducers. Acetaminophen may cause liver damage.
Do not use
- with any other product containing acetaminophen.

Stop use and ask a doctor if
- New symptoms occur
- Redness or swelling is present
- Pain gets worse or lasts for more than 10 days
- Fever gets worse or lasts for more than 3 days

If pregnant or breast-feeding, ask a health professional before use.
Keep out of reach of children.
Overdose warning: Taking more than the recommended dose (overdose) may cause liver damage. In case of overdose, get medical help or contact a Poison Control Center right away. Quick medical attention is critical for adults as well as for children even if you do not notice any signs or symptoms.
Other Information:
Regular Strength TYLENOL® Tablets
- **do not use if carton is opened or red neck wrap or foil inner seal imprinted with "Safety Seal®" is broken**
- store at room temperature

Extra Strength TYLENOL® Gelcaps, Geltabs, Caplets or Tablets
- **do not use if carton is opened or red neck wrap or foil inner seal imprinted with "Safety Seal®" is broken**
- store at room temperature (*tablet and caplet*)
- store at room temperature; avoid high humidity and excessive heat 40°C (104°F). (*Gelcap and Geltab*)

Extra Strength TYLENOL® Adult Liquid
- **do not use if carton is opened, or if bottle wrap or foil inner seal imprinted "Safety Seal®" is broken or missing.**
- Store at room temperature

TYLENOL® Arthritis Pain Extended Relief Caplets and *TYLENOL® 8 Hour Extended Release Geltabs/Caplets*
- **do not use if carton is opened or red neck wrap or foil inner seal with "Safety Seal®" is broken**
- store at 20–25°C (68–77°F)
- avoid excessive heat at 40°C (104°F)

Professional Information:
Overdosage Information for all Adult Tylenol products
ACETAMINOPHEN: Acetaminophen in massive overdosage may cause hepatic toxicity in some patients. In adults and adolescents ($\geq$ 12 years of age), hepatic toxicity may occur following ingestion of greater than 7.5 to 10 grams over a period of 8 hours or less. Fatalities are infrequent (less than 3–4% of untreated cases) and have rarely been reported with overdoses of less than 15 grams. In

children (<12 years of age), an acute overdosage of less than 150 mg/kg has not been associated with hepatic toxicity. Early symptoms following a potentially hepatotoxic overdose may include: nausea, vomiting, diaphoresis and general malaise. Clinical and laboratory evidence of hepatic toxicity may not be apparent until 48 to 72 hours postingestion. In adults and adolescents, any individual presenting with an unknown amount of acetaminophen ingested or with a questionable or unreliable history about the time of ingestion should have a plasma acetaminophen level drawn and be treated with *N*-acetylcysteine. For full prescribing information, refer to the *N*-acetylcysteine package insert. Do not await results of assays for plasma acetaminophen levels before initiating treatment with *N*-acetylcysteine. The following additional procedures are recommended: Promptly initiate gastric decontamination of the stomach. A plasma acetaminophen assay should be obtained as early as possible, but no sooner than four hours following ingestion. If an acetaminophen *extended release* product is involved, it may be appropriate to obtain an additional plasma acetaminophen level 4–6 hours following the initial acetaminophen level. If either acetaminophen level plots above the treatment line on the acetaminophen overdose nomogram, *N*-acetylcysteine treatment should be continued for a full course of therapy. Liver function studies should be obtained initially and repeated at 24-hour intervals. Serious toxicity or fatalities have been extremely infrequent following an acute acetaminophen overdose in young children, possibly because of differences in the way they metabolize acetaminophen. In children, the maximum potential amount ingested can be more easily estimated. If more than 150 mg/kg or an unknown amount was ingested, obtain a plasma acetaminophen level as soon as possible, but no sooner than 4 hours following ingestion. If an acetaminophen *extended release* product is involved, it may be appropriate to obtain an additional plasma acetaminophen level 4–6 hours following the initial acetaminophen level. If either acetaminophen level plots above the treatment line on the acetaminophen overdose nomogram, *N*-acetylcysteine treatment should be initiated and continued for a full course of therapy. If an assay cannot be obtained and the estimated acetaminophen ingestion exceeds 150 mg/kg, dosing with *N*-acetylcysteine should be initiated and continued for a full course of therapy. For additional emergency information, call your regional poison center or call the Rocky Mountain Poison Center toll-free, (1-800-525-6115).
Our adult Tylenol® combination products contain active ingredients in addition to acetaminophen. The following is basic overdose information regarding those ingredients.

Continued on next page

Tylenol Reg. Strength—Cont.

CHLORPHENIRAMINE: Chlorpheniramine toxicity should be treated as you would an anthihistamine/anticholinergic overdose and is likely to be present within a few hours after acute ingestion.

DEXTROMETHORHPHAN: Acute dextromethorphan overdose usually does not result in serious signs and symptoms unless massive amounts have been ingested. Signs and symptoms of a substantial overdose may include nausea and vomiting, visual disturbances, CNS disturbances and urinary retention.

DIPHENHYDRAMINE: Diphenhydramine toxicity should be treated as you would an antihistamine/anticholinergic overdose and is likely to be present within a few hours after acute ingestion.

DOXYLAMINE: Doxylamine toxicity should be treated as you would an antihistamine/anticholinergic overdose and is likely to be present within a few hours after acute ingestion.

GUAIFENESIN: Guaifenesin should be treated as a nontoxic ingestion.

PAMABROM: Acute overexposure of diuretics is primarily associated with fluid and electrolyte loss. Fluid loss should be treated with the appropriate intravenous and/or oral fluids.

PSEUDOEPHEDRINE: Symptoms from pseudoephedrine overdose consist most often of mild anxiety, tachycardia and/or mild hypertension. Symptoms usually appear within 4 to 8 hours of ingestion and are transient, usually requiring no treatment.

For additional emergency information, please contact your local poison control center.

Alcohol Information: Chronic heavy alcohol abusers may be at increased risk of liver toxicity from excessive acetaminophen use, although reports of this event are rare. Reports usually involve cases of severe chronic alcoholics and the dosages of acetaminophen most often exceed recommended doses and often involve substantial overdose. Healthcare professionals should alert their patients who regularly consume large amounts of alcohol not to exceed recommended doses of acetaminophen.

Inactive Ingredients:
Regular Strength TYLENOL® Tablets: cellulose, corn starch, magnesium stearate, sodium starch glycolate.
Extra Strength TYLENOL® **Tablets**: cellulose, corn starch, magnesium stearate, sodium starch glycolate. **Caplets:** cellulose, corn starch, FD&C Red #40, hypromellose, magnesium stearate, polyethylene glycol, sodium starch glycolate. **Gelcaps:** benzyl alcohol, butylparaben, castor oil, cellulose, corn starch, D&C Yellow #10, edetate calcium disodium, FD&C Blue #1, FD&C Blue #2, FD&C Red #40, gelatin, hypromellose, magnesium stearate, methylparaben, propylparaben, sodium lauryl sulfate, sodium propionate, sodium starch glycolate, titanium dioxide. **Geltabs:** benzyl

alcohol, butylparaben, castor oil, cellulose, corn starch, D&C Yellow #10, edetate calcium disodium, FD&C Blue #1, FD&C Blue #2, FD&C Red #40, gelatin, hypromellose, magnesium stearate, methylparaben, propylparaben, sodium lauryl sulfate, sodium propionate, sodium starch glycolate, titanium dioxide. *Extra Strength TYLENOL® Adult Liquid:* citric acid, D&C Red #33, FD&C Red #40, flavor, high fructose corn syrup, polyethylene glycol, propylene glycol, purified water, saccharin sodium, sodium benzoate, sorbitol

TYLENOL® Arthritis Pain Extended Relief Caplets: corn starch, hydroxyethyl cellulose, hypromellose, magnesium stearate, microcrystalline cellulose, povidone, powdered cellulose, pregelatinized starch, sodium starch glycolate, titanium dioxide, triacetin *TYLENOL® 8 Hour Extended Release Geltabs:* FD&C Blue #1, FD&C Blue #2, FD&C Red #40, gelatin, hydroxyethyl cellulose, hypromellose, magnesium stearate, methylparaben, povidone, propylparaben, sodium lauryl sulfate, sodium propionate, sodium starch glycolate, titanium dioxide

Tylenol 8 Hour Inactives (caplet): corn starch, hydroxyethyl cellulose, magnesium stearate, microcrystalline cellulose, povidone, powdered cellulose, pregelatinized starch, sodium starch glycolate, titanium dioxide, polyethylene glycol, polyvinyl alcohol, sucralose, talc, D&C Yellow #10, FD&C Red #40, FD&C Yellow #6.

Tylenol 8 Hour Geltab inactives: benzyl alcohol, butylparaben, castor oil, cellulose, corn starch, edetate calcium disodium, FD & C Blue #1, FD & C Blue #2, FD & C Red #40, gelatin, hydroxyethyl cellulose, hypromellose, magnesium stearate, methylparaben, povidone, propylparaben, sodium lauryl sulfate, sodium propionate, sodium starch glycolate, titanium dioxide

How Supplied:
Regular Strength TYLENOL® Tablets: (colored white, scored, imprinted "TYLENOL" and "325")—tamper-evident bottles of 100.
Extra Strength TYLENOL® Tablets: (colored white, imprinted "TYLENOL" and "500")—tamper-evident bottles of 30, 60, 100, and 200. *Caplets* (colored white, imprinted "TYLENOL 500 mg")— vials of 10, and tamper-evident bottles of 8, 16, 40, 325, 24, 50, 100, 150, and 250. *Gelcaps* (colored yellow and red, imprinted "Tylenol 500") tamper-evident bottles of 16, 40, 24, 50, 100, 150 and 225. *Geltabs* (colored yellow and red, imprinted "Tylenol 500") tamper-evident bottles of 24, 50, 16, 40, 100, and 150.
Extra Strength TYLENOL® Adult Liquid: Cherry-flavored liquid (colored red) 8 fl. oz. tamper-evident bottle with child resistant safety cap and special dosage cup.
TYLENOL® Arthritis Pain Extended Relief Caplets: (colored white, engraved "TYLENOL ER") tamper-evident bottles

of 24, 50, and 100, 150, 250 and 290 *TYLENOL® 8 Hour Extended Release Geltabs/caplet:* (colored white and red, imprinted "8 HOUR") tamper-evident bottles of 20, 40 and 80. colored red caplets available in 24's, 200's.

Shown in Product Identification Guide, page 513 & 514

TYLENOL® Severe Allergy Caplets

Maximum Strength

TYLENOL® Allergy Sinus Night Time Caplets

Maximum Strength

TYLENOL® Allergy Sinus Day Time Caplets, Gelcaps and Geltabs

Product information for all dosage forms of TYLENOL Allergy have been combined under this heading.

Description: Each *TYLENOL® Severe Allergy Relief Caplet* contains acetaminophen 500 mg and diphenhydramine HCl 12.5 mg. Each *Maximum Strength TYLENOL® Allergy Sinus Night Time Caplet* contains acetaminophen 500 mg, diphenhydramine HCl 25 mg, and pseudoephedrine HCl 30 mg. Each *Maximum Strength TYLENOL® Allergy Sinus Day Time Caplet Gelcap and Geltab* contains acetaminophen 500 mg, chlorpheniramine maleate 2 mg, and pseudoephedrine HCl 30 mg.

Actions:
TYLENOL® Severe Allergy Caplets contain a clinically proven analgesic-antipyretic and antihistamine. Acetaminophen produces analgesia by elevation of the pain threshold and antipyresis through action on the hypothalamic heat regulating center. Acetaminophen is equal to aspirin in analgesic and antipyretic effectiveness, and it is unlikely to produce many of the side effects associated with aspirin and aspirin-containing products. Diphenhydramine HCl is an antihistamine which helps provide temporary relief of itchy, watery eyes, runny nose, sneezing, itching of the nose or throat due to hay fever or other respiratory allergies.

Maximum Strength TYLENOL® Allergy Sinus Night Time Caplets contain, in addition to the above ingredients, a decongestant, pseudoephedrine HCl. Pseudoephedrine is a sympathomimetic amine which provides temporary relief of nasal and sinus congestion.

Maximum Strength TYLENOL® Allergy Sinus Day Time Caplets, Gelcaps and Geltabs contain acetaminophen, pseudoephedrine HCl and the antihistamine, chlorpheniramine maleate. Chlorpheniramine is an antihistamine which helps provide temporary relief of runny nose, sneezing and watery and itchy eyes.

Uses:

TYLENOL® Severe Allergy: temporarily relieves these symptoms due to hay fever or other respiratory allergies:

- itchy, watery eyes • runny nose
- sneezing • sore throat
- itching of nose or throat

Maximum Strength TYLENOL® Allergy Sinus Night Time and TYLENOL® Allergy Sinus Day Time: temporarily relieves these symptoms due to hay fever or other upper respiratory allergies:

- nasal congestion • sinus pressure
- sinus pain • headache
- runny nose • sneezing
- itchy, watery eyes • itchy throat

Precautions: If a rare sensitivity reaction occurs, the drug should be discontinued.

Directions:

TYLENOL® Severe Allergy:
- **do not take more than directed (see overdose warning)**

adults and children 12 years and over	• take 2 caplets every 4 to 6 hours as needed • do not take more than 8 caplets in 24 hours
children under 12 years	• do not use this adult product in children under 12 years of age; this will provide more than the recommended dose (overdose) and may cause liver damage.

Maximum Strength TYLENOL® Allergy Sinus Night Time:
- **do not take more than directed (see overdose warning)**

adults and children 12 years and over	• take 2 caplets every 4 to 6 hours as needed • do not take more than 8 caplets in 24 hours
children under 12 years	• do not use this adult product in children under 12 years of age; this will provide more than the recommended dose (overdose) and may cause liver damage.

Maximum Strength TYLENOL® Allergy Sinus Day Time:
- **do not take more than directed (see overdose warning)**

adults and children 12 years and over	• take two every 4 to 6 hours as needed • do not take more than 8 caplets in 24 hours
children under 12 years	• do not use this adult product in children under 12 years of age; this will provide more than the recommended dose (overdose) and may cause liver damage.

Warnings:

Alcohol warning: If you consume 3 or more alcoholic drinks every day, ask your doctor whether your should use acetaminophen or other pain relievers/fever reducers. Acetaminophen may cause liver damage.

Sore throat warning: If sore throat is severe, persists for more than 2 days, is accompanied or followed by fever, headache, rash, nausea or vomiting, consult a doctor promptly. *(applies to TYLENOL® Severe Allergy only)*

Do not use

- if you are now taking a prescription monoamine oxidase inhibitor (MAOI) (certain drugs for depression, psychiatric or emotional conditions, or Parkinson's disease) or for 2 weeks after stopping the MAOI drug. If you do not know if your prescription drug contains an MAOI, ask a doctor or pharmacist before taking this product (does not apply to *TYLENOL® Severe Allergy*)
- with any other product containing acetaminophen
- with any other product containing diphenhydramine, even one used on skin. (does not apply to TYLENOL® Allergy Sinus Day Time)

Ask a doctor or pharmacist before use if you are taking sedatives or tranquilizers

Stop use and ask a doctor if
- new symptoms occur
- redness or swelling is present
- pain gets worse or lasts for more than 7 days
- fever gets worse or lasts for more than 3 days
- you get nervous, dizzy or sleepless (does not apply to TYLENOL® Severe Allergy)

If pregnant or breast feeding, ask a health professional before use.

Keep out of reach of children.

Overdose warning: Taking more than the recommended dose (overdose) may cause liver damage. In case of overdose, get medical help or contact a Poison Control Center right away. Quick medical attention is critical for adults as well as for children even if you do not notice any signs or symptoms.

When using this product
- **do not exceed recommended dosage**
- marked drowsiness may occur (does not apply to TYLENOL® Allergy Sinus Day Time)
- drowsiness may occur (applies to TYLENOL® Allergy Sinus Day Time only)
- avoid alcoholic drinks
- alcohol, sedatives and tranquilizers may increase drowsiness
- be careful when driving a motor vehicle or operating machinery
- excitability may occur, especially in children

TYLENOL® Severe Allergy
Ask a doctor before use if you have
- glaucoma
- trouble urinating due to an enlarged prostate gland
- a breathing problem such as emphysema or chronic bronchitis

Maximum Strength TYLENOL® Allergy Sinus Night Time and Maximum Strength TYLENOL® Allergy Sinus Day Time
Ask a doctor before use if you have
- heart disease • glaucoma • diabetes
- thyroid disease • high blood pressure
- trouble urinating due to an enlarged prostate gland
- a breathing problem such as emphysema or chronic bronchitis

Other Information:
- **do not use if carton is opened or if blister unit is broken**

Tylenol Severe Allergy Caplets:
- store between 20–25°C (68–77°F)

TYLENOL® Allergy Sinus Day Time Caplet and TYLENOL® Allergy Sinus Night Time Caplet:
- store at room temperature

TYLENOL® Allergy Sinus Day Time Gelcap & Geltabs:
- store at room temperature; avoid high humidity and excessive heat 40°C (104°F)

Professional Information:
Overdosage Information:
For overdosage information, please refer to pgs. 679–680

Inactive Ingredients:
TYLENOL® Severe Allergy: **Caplets:** carnauba wax, cellulose, corn starch, D&C Yellow #10, FD&C Yellow #6, hydroxypropyl cellulose, hypromellose, iron oxide, magnesium stearate, polyethylene glycol, sodium citrate, sodium starch glycolate, titanium dioxide.

Maximum Strength TYLENOL® Allergy Sinus Night Time: **Caplets:** carnauba wax, cellulose, corn starch, D&C Yellow #10, FD&C Blue #1, hypromellose, iron oxide, magnesium stearate, polyethylene glycol, polysorbate 80, sodium citrate, sodium starch glycolate, titanium dioxide.

Maximum Strength TYLENOL® Allergy Sinus Day Time: **Caplets:** carnauba wax, cellulose, corn starch, D&C Yellow #10, FD&C Blue #1, FD&C Yellow #6, hydroxypropyl cellulose, hypromellose, iron oxide, magnesium stearate, polyethylene glycol, sodium starch glycolate, titanium dioxide. **Gelcaps and Geltabs:** benzyl alcohol, butylparaben, castor oil, cellulose, corn starch, D&C Yellow #10, edetate calcium disodium, FD&C Blue #1, FD&C Blue #2, gelatin, hypromellose, magnesium stearate, methylpara-

Continued on next page

Tylenol Severe Allergy—Cont.

ben, propylparaben, sodium lauryl sulfate, sodium propionate, sodium starch glycolate, titanium dioxide.

How Supplied:

TYLENOL® Severe Allergy: **Caplets:** Yellow film-coated, imprinted with "TYLENOL Severe Allergy" on one side—blister packs of 24.

Maximum Strength TYLENOL® Allergy Sinus Night Time: **Caplets:** Light blue film-coated, imprinted with "TYLENOL A/S Night Time" on one side—blister packs of 24.

Maximum Strength TYLENOL® Allergy Sinus Day Time: **Caplets:** Yellow film-coated, imprinted with "TYLENOL Allergy Sinus" on one side—blister packs of 24.

Gelcaps and Geltabs: Green and yellow-colored, imprinted with "TYLENOL A/S"—blister packs of 24 and 48.

These products are also available in a convenience pack containing Maximum Strength Tylenol Allergy Sinus Day (pack of 12) and Maximum Strength Tylenol Allergy Sinus Night (pack of 12).

Shown in Product Identification Guide, page 514

**Multi-Symptom
TYLENOL® Cold Day Non-Drowsy
Caplets and Gelcaps**

**Multi-Symptom
TYLENOL® Cold Night Time
Complete
Formula Caplets**

Product information for all dosage forms of TYLENOL Cold have been combined under this heading.

Description: Each *Multi-Symptom TYLENOL® Cold Day Non-Drowsy Caplet and Gelcap* contains acetaminophen 325 mg, dextromethorphan HBr 15 mg, and pseudoephedrine HCl 30 mg.

Each *Multi-Symptom TYLENOL® Cold Night Time Complete Formula Caplet* contains acetaminophen 325 mg, chlorpheniramine maleate 2 mg, dextromethorphan HBr 15 mg, and pseudoephedrine HCl 30 mg.

Actions: *Multi-Symptom TYLENOL® Cold Day Non-Drowsy* contains a clinically proven analgesic-antipyretic, a decongestant and a cough suppressant. Acetaminophen produces analgesia by elevation of the pain threshold and antipyresis through action on the hypothalamic heat regulating center. Acetaminophen is equal to aspirin in analgesic and antipyretic effectiveness and it is unlikely to produce many of the side effects associated with aspirin and aspirin-containing products. Pseudoephedrine is a sympathomimetic amine which provides temporary relief of nasal congestion. Dextromethorphan is a cough suppressant

which provides temporary relief of coughs due to minor throat irritations that may occur with the common cold.

Multi-Symptom TYLENOL® Cold Night Time Complete Formula Caplets contain, in addition to the above ingredients, an antihistamine. Chlorpheniramine is an antihistamine which helps provide temporary relief of runny nose, sneezing and watery and itchy eyes.

Uses: *Multi-Symptom TYLENOL® Cold Day Non-Drowsy:* temporarily relieves these cold symptoms:
• cough • sore throat • minor aches and pains • headaches • nasal congestion
• temporarily reduces fever

Multi-Symptom TYLENOL® Cold Night Time Complete Formula: temporarily relieves these cold symptoms:
• cough • sore throat • minor aches and pains • headache• nasal congestion
• runny nose • sneezing • watery and itchy eyes
• temporarily reduces fever

Directions: *Multi-Symptom TYLENOL® Cold Day Non-Drowsy and Multi-Symptom TYLENOL® Cold Night Time Complete Formula:*
• **do not take more than directed (see overdose warning)**

adults and children 12 years and over	• take 2 every 6 hours as needed • do not take more than 8 in 24 hours.
children under 12 years	• not intended for use in children under 12. Ask your doctor.

Precautions: If a rare sensitivity reaction occurs, the drug should be discontinued.

Warnings:

Alcohol Warning: If you consume 3 or more alcoholic drinks every day, ask your doctor whether you should take acetaminophen or other pain relievers/fever reducers. Acetaminophen may cause liver damage.

Sore throat warning: If sore throat is severe, persists for more than 2 days, is accompanied or followed by fever, headache, rash, nausea or vomiting, consult a doctor promptly.

Do not use
• if you are now taking a prescription monoamine oxidase inhibitor (MAOI) (certain drugs for depression, psychiatric or emotional conditions or Parkinson's disease), or for 2 weeks after stopping the MAOI drug. If you do not know if your prescription drug contains an MAOI, ask a doctor or pharmacist before taking this product.
• with any other product containing acetaminophen

Stop use and ask a doctor if
• new symptoms occur
• redness or swelling is present
• pain gets worse or lasts for more than 7 days

• fever gets worse or lasts for more than 3 days
• you get nervous, dizzy or sleepless
• cough lasts more than 7 days, comes back or occurs with fever, rash or headache that lasts. These could be signs of a serious condition.

If pregnant or breast-feeding, ask a health professional before use.

Keep out of reach of children.

Overdose warning: Taking more than the recommended dose (overdose) may cause liver damage. In case of overdose, get medical help or contact a Poison Control Center right away. Quick medical attention is critical for adults as well as for children even if you don't notice any signs or symptoms.

Multi-Symptom TYLENOL® Cold Day Non-Drowsy

Ask a doctor before use if you have
• heart disease • diabetes • thyroid disease • cough that occurs with too much phlegm (mucus) • high blood pressure • trouble urinating due to an enlarged prostate gland • chronic cough that lasts as occurs with smoking, asthma, chronic bronchitis or emphysema

When using this product
• do not exceed recommended dosage

Multi-Symptom TYLENOL® Cold Night Time Complete Formula:

Ask a doctor before use if you have
• heart disease • glaucoma • diabetes • thyroid disease • cough that occurs with too much phlegm (mucus) • high blood pressure • a breathing problem or chronic cough that lasts as occurs with smoking, asthma, chronic bronchitis or emphysema • trouble urinating due to an enlarged prostate gland

Ask a doctor or pharmacist before use if you are taking sedatives or tranquilizers

When using this product
• do not exceed recommended dosage
• drowsiness may occur • avoid alcoholic drinks • alcohol, sedatives and tranquilizers may increase drowsiness • be careful when driving a motor vehicle or operating machinery • excitability may occur, especially in children

Other Information:
• **do not use if carton is opened or if blister unit is broken**
• store at room temperature (avoid high humidity and excessive heat 40°C (104°F)—applies to TYLENOL® Cold Non-Drowsy Gelcap only)

Professional Information:

Overdosage Information

For overdosage information, please refer to pgs. 679–680

Inactive Ingredients: *Multi-Symptom TYLENOL® Cold Day Non Drowsy Formula:* **Caplets:** carnauba wax, cellulose, corn starch, D&C Yellow #10, FD&C Blue #1, hypromellose, iron oxide, magnesium stearate, sodium starch glycolate, titanium dioxide, triacetin.

Gelcaps: benzyl alcohol, butylparaben, castor oil, cellulose, corn starch, D&C Yellow #10, edetate calcium disodium, FD&C Red #40, gelatin, hypromellose, iron oxide, magnesium stearate, methyl-

paraben, propylparaben, sodium lauryl sulfate, sodium propionate, sodium starch glycolate, titanium dioxide.
Multi-Symptom TYLENOL® Cold Night Time Complete Formula: **Caplets:** carnauba wax, cellulose, corn starch, D&C Yellow #10, FD&C Blue #1, FD&C Yellow #6, hypromellose, iron oxide, magnesium stearate, sodium starch glycolate, titanium dioxide, triacetin.

How Supplied: *Multi-Symptom TYLENOL® Cold Day Non Drowsy* Caplets: White-colored, imprinted with "TYLENOL Cold"—blister packs of 12 & 24. Gelcaps: Red- and tan-colored, imprinted with "TYLENOL COLD"—blister packs of 24.
Multi-Symptom TYLENOL® Cold Night Time Complete Formula Caplets: Yellow-colored, imprinted with "TYLENOL Cold"—blister packs of 12 & 24.
These products are also available in a convenience pack containing Multi-Symptom TYLENOL® Cold Day Non-Drowsy (pack of 12) and Multi-Symptom TYLENOL® Cold Night Time Complete Formula (pack of 12).

Shown in Product Identification Guide, page 514

Multi-Symptom TYLENOL® COLD Severe Congestion Non-Drowsy

Description: Each *Multi-Symptom TYLENOL® Cold Severe Congestion Non-Drowsy Caplet* contains acetaminophen 325 mg, dextromethorphan HBr 15 mg, guaifenesin 200 mg and pseudoephedrine HCl 30 mg.

Actions: *Multi-Symptom TYLENOL® Cold Severe Congestion Non-Drowsy Caplets* contain a clinically proven analgesic-antipyretic, decongestant, expectorant and cough suppressant. Acetaminophen produces analgesia by elevation of the pain threshold and antipyresis through action on the hypothalamic heat regulating center. Acetaminophen is equal to aspirin in analgesic and antipyretic effectiveness and is unlikely to produce many of the side effects associated with aspirin and aspirin-containing products. Pseudoephedrine is a sympathomimetic amine which provides temporary relief of nasal congestion. Guaifenesin is an expectorant which helps loosen phlegm (mucus) and thin bronchial secretions to make coughs more productive. Dextromethorphan is a cough suppressant which provides temporary relief of coughs due to minor throat irritations that may occur with the common cold.

Uses: temporarily relieves these cold symptoms:
- cough • sore throat • minor aches and pains • headaches • nasal congestion
- helps loosen phlegm (mucus) and thin bronchial secretions to make coughs more productive
- temporarily reduces fever

Directions:

adults and children 12 years and over	• take 2 caplets every 6–8 hours as needed • do not take more than 8 caplets in 24 hours
children under 12 years	• not intended for use in children under 12. Ask your doctor.

Precautions: If a rare sensitivity reaction occurs, the drug should be discontinued.

Warnings:
Alcohol warning: If you consume 3 or more alcoholic drinks every day, ask your doctor whether you should take acetaminophen or other pain relievers/fever reducers. Acetaminophen may cause liver damage.
Sore throat warning: If sore throat is severe, persists for more than 2 days, is accompanied or followed by fever, headache, rash, nausea or vomiting, consult a doctor promptly.
Do not use
- if you are now taking a prescription monoamine oxidase inhibitor (MAOI) (certain drugs for depression, psychiatric or emotional conditions, or Parkinson's disease), or for 2 weeks after stopping the MAOI drug. If you do not know if your prescription drug contains an MAOI, ask a doctor or pharmacist before taking this product.
- with any other product containing acetaminophen

Ask a doctor before use if you have
- heart disease • diabetes • thyroid disease • cough that occurs with too much phlegm (mucus) • high blood pressure • trouble urinating due to an enlarged prostate gland • chronic cough that lasts as occurs with smoking, asthma, chronic bronchitis or emphysema

When using this product
- **do not exceed recommended dosage**
Stop use and ask a doctor if
- new symptoms occur
- redness or swelling is present
- pain gets worse or lasts for more than 7 days
- fever gets worse or lasts for more than 3 days
- you get nervous, dizzy or sleepless
- cough lasts more than 7 days, comes back or occurs with fever, rash or headache that lasts. These could be signs of a serious condition.
If pregnant or breast-feeding, ask a health professional before use.
Keep out of reach of children.
Overdose Warning:
Taking more than the recommended dose (overdose) may liver damage. In case of overdose, get medical help or contact a Poison Control Center right away. Quick medical attention is critical for adults as well as for children even if you do not notice any signs or symptoms.

Other Information:
- **do not use if carton is opened or if blister unit is broken**
- Store at room temperature.

Professional Information:
Overdosage Information: For overdosage information, please refer to pgs. 679–680.

Inactive Ingredients: carnauba wax, cellulose, corn starch, D&C Yellow #10, FD&C Blue #1, FD&C Yellow #6, hypromellose, iron oxide, povidone, silicon dioxide, sodium starch glycolate, stearic acid, titanium dioxide, triacetin

How Supplied: Caplets: Buttery-tan-colored, imprinted with "TYLENOL COLD SC" in green ink—blister packs of 24 & 48 ct.

Shown in Product Identification Guide, page 514

Maximum Strength TYLENOL® Flu Day Non-Drowsy Gelcaps
Maximum Strength TYLENOL® Flu NightTime Gelcaps
TYLENOL® NightTime Severe Cold & Flu Liquid

Product information for all dosage forms of TYLENOL Flu have been combined under this heading.

Description: Each *Maximum Strength TYLENOL® Flu Day Non-Drowsy Gelcap* contains acetaminophen 500 mg, dextromethorphan HBr 15 mg and pseudoephedrine HCl 30 mg. Each *Maximum Strength TYLENOL® Flu NightTime Gelcap* contains acetaminophen 500 mg, diphenhydramine HCl 25 mg and pseudoephedrine HCl 30 mg. *Maximum Strength TYLENOL® NightTime Severe Cold & Flu Liquid:* Each 30 mL (2 tablespoonsful) contains acetaminophen 1000 mg, dextromethorphan HBr 30 mg, doxylamine succinate 12.5 mg, and pseudoephedrine HCl 60 mg.

Actions: *Maximum Strength TYLENOL® Flu Day Non-Drowsy Gelcaps* contain a clinically proven analgesic-antipyretic, a decongestant and a cough suppressant. Acetaminophen produces analgesia by elevation of the pain threshold and antipyresis through action on the hypothalamic heat regulating center. Acetaminophen is equal to aspirin in analgesic and antipyretic effectiveness and it is unlikely to produce many of the side effects associated with aspirin and aspirin-containing products. Pseudoephedrine hydrochloride is a sympathomimetic amine which provides temporary relief of nasal congestion. Dextromethorphan is a cough suppressant which provides temporary relief of coughs due to minor throat irritations that may occur with the common cold.

Continued on next page

Tylenol Flu—Cont.

Maximum Strength TYLENOL® Flu NightTime Gelcaps contains the same clinically proven analgesic-antipyretic and decongestant as *Maximum Strength TYLENOL Flu Day Non-Drowsy Gelcaps* along with an antihistamine. Diphenhydramine is an antihistamine which helps provide temporary relief of runny nose and sneezing. *Maximum Strength TYLENOL® NightTime Severe Cold & Flu Liquid* contains the same clinically proven analgesic-antipyretic, decongestant and cough suppressant as *Maximum Strength TYLENOL Flu Day Non-Drowsy Gelcaps* along with an antihistamine. Doxylamine succinate is an antihistamine which helps provide temporary relief of runny nose and sneezing.

Uses:

Maximum Strength TYLENOL® Flu Day Non-Drowsy Gelcaps:

temporarily relieves these cold and flu symptoms:
- minor aches and pains • headaches
- sore throat • nasal congestion
- coughs
- temporarily reduces fever

Maximum Strength TYLENOL® Flu NightTime Gelcaps:

temporarily relieves these cold and flu symptoms:
- minor aches and pains • headaches
- sore throat • nasal congestion • runny nose • sneezing
- temporarily reduces fever

Maximum Strength TYLENOL® NightTime Severe Cold & Flu Liquid:

temporarily relieves these cold and flu symptoms:
- body aches and headaches • coughs
- nasal congestion • sore throat • runny nose • sneezing
- temporarily reduces fever

Directions:
- **do not take more than directed (see overdose warning)**

Maximum Strength TYLENOL® Flu Day Non-Drowsy Gelcaps:

adults and children 12 years and over	• take 2 gelcaps every 6 hours as needed • do not take more than 8 gelcaps in 24 hours
children under 12 years	• do not use this adult product in children under 12 years of age; this will provide more than the recommended dose (overdose) and may cause liver damage.

Maximum Strength TYLENOL® Flu NightTime Gelcaps:

adults and children 12 years and over	• take 2 gelcaps at bedtime • may repeat every 6 hours • do not take more than 8 gelcaps in 24 hours
children under 12 years	• do not use this adult product in children under 12 years of age; this will provide more than the recommended dose (overdose) and may cause liver damage.

Maximum Strength TYLENOL® NightTime Severe Cold & Flu Liquid:

adults and children 12 years and over	• take 2 tablespoons (tbsp) in dose cup provided every 6 hours as needed • do not take more than 8 tablespoons in 24 hours
children under 12 years	• do not use this adult product in children under 12 years of age; this will provide more than the recommended dose (overdose) and may cause serious liver damage.

Precautions: If a rare sensitivity reaction occurs, the drug should be discontinued.

Warnings:
Alcohol Warning: If you consume 3 or more alcoholic drinks every day, ask your doctor whether you should take acetaminophen or other pain relievers/fever reducers. Acetaminophen may cause liver damage.

Sore throat warning: If sore throat is severe, persists for more than 2 days, is accompanied or followed by fever, headache, rash, nausea or vomiting, consult a doctor promptly.

Do not use
- if you are now taking a prescription monoamine-oxidase inhibitor (MAOI) (certain drugs for depression, psychiatric or emotional conditions, or Parkinson's disease), or for 2 weeks after stopping the MAOI drug. If you do not know if your prescription drug contains an MAOI, ask a doctor or pharmacist before taking this product.
- with any other product containing acetaminophen

- with any other product containing diphenhydramine even one used on skin

If pregnant or breast-feeding, ask a health professional before use.

Keep out of reach of children.

Overdose warning: Taking more than the recommended dose (overdose) may cause liver damage. In case of overdose, get medical help or contact a Poison Control Center right away. Quick medical attention is critical for adults as well as for children even if you do not notice any signs or symptoms.

Maximum Strength TYLENOL® Flu Day Non-Drowsy Gelcaps

Ask a doctor before use if you have
- heart disease • diabetes • thyroid disease • cough that occurs with too much phlegm (mucus) • high blood pressure • trouble urinating due to an enlarged prostate gland • chronic cough that lasts as occurs with smoking, asthma, chronic bronchitis or emphysema

When using this product
- **do not exceed recommended dosage**

Stop use and ask a doctor if
- new symptoms occur
- redness or swelling is present
- pain gets worse or lasts for more than 7 days
- fever gets worse or lasts for more than 3 days
- you get nervous, dizzy or sleepless
- cough lasts more than 7 days, comes back or occurs with fever, rash or headache that lasts. These could be signs of a serious condition.

Maximum Strength TYLENOL® Flu NightTime Gelcaps

Ask a doctor before use if you have
- heart disease • glaucoma • diabetes
- thyroid disease • high blood pressure
- trouble urinating due to an enlarged prostate gland • a breathing problem such as emphysema or chronic bronchitis

Ask a doctor or pharmacist before use if you are taking sedatives or tranquilizers

When using this product
- **do not exceed recommended dosage**
- marked drowsiness may occur
- avoid alcoholic drinks
- alcohol, sedatives and tranquilizers may increase drowsiness
- be careful when driving a motor vehicle or operating machinery
- excitability may occur, especially in children

Stop use and ask a doctor if
- new symptoms occur
- redness or swelling is present
- pain gets worse or lasts for more than 7 days
- fever gets worse or lasts for more than 3 days
- you get nervous, dizzy or sleepless

Maximum Strength TYLENOL® NightTime Severe Cold & Flu Liquid

Ask a doctor before use if you have
- heart disease • glaucoma • diabetes
- thyroid disease • cough that occurs with too much phlegm (mucus)
- high blood pressure • a breathing problem such as emphysema or chronic bronchitis • trouble urinating due to an enlarged prostate gland

Ask a doctor or pharmacist before use if you are taking sedatives or tranquilizers

When using this product
- **do not exceed recommended dosage**
- marked drowsiness may occur
- avoid alcoholic drinks
- alcohol, sedatives and tranquilizers may increase drowsiness
- be careful when driving a motor vehicle or operating machinery
- excitability may occur, especially in children

Stop use and ask a doctor if
- new symptoms occur
- redness or swelling is present
- pain gets worse or lasts for more than 7 days
- fever gets worse or lasts for more than 3 days
- you get nervous, dizzy or sleepless
- cough lasts for more than 7 days, comes back or occurs with fever, rash or headache that lasts. These could be signs of a serious condition.

Other Information:
Maximum Strength TYLENOL® Flu Day Non-Drowsy Gelcaps and Maximum Strength TYLENOL® Flu NightTime Gelcaps:
- **do not use if carton is opened or if blister unit is broken**
- Store at room temperature; avoid high humidity and excessive heat 40°C (104°F)

Maximum Strength TYLENOL® Night-Time Severe Cold & Flu Liquid
- **do not use if carton is opened or if bottle wrap or foil inner seal imprinted "Safety Seal®" is broken or missing**
- Store at room temperature

Professional Information:
Overdosage Information
For overdosage information, please refer to pgs. 679–680

Inactive Ingredients: *Maximum Strength TYLENOL® Flu Day Non-Drowsy Gelcaps:* benzyl alcohol, butylparaben, castor oil, cellulose, corn starch, edetate calcium disodium, FD&C Blue #1, FD&C Red #40, gelatin, hypromellose, iron oxide, magnesium stearate, methylparaben, propylparaben, sodium lauryl sulfate, sodium propionate, sodium starch glycolate, titanium dioxide. *Maximum Strength TYLENOL® Flu NightTime Gelcaps:* benzyl alcohol, butylparaben, castor oil, cellulose, corn starch, D&C Red #28, edetate calcium disodium, FD&C Blue #1, gelatin, hypromellose, iron oxide, magnesium stearate, methylparaben, propylparaben, sodium citrate, sodium lauryl sulfate, sodium propionate, sodium starch glycolate, titanium dioxide. *Maximum Strength TYLENOL® Night-Time Severe Cold & Flu Liquid:* citric acid, corn syrup, D&C Red #33, FD&C Red #40, flavors, polyethylene glycol, propylene glycol, purified water, saccharin sodium, sodium benzoate, sorbitol.

How Supplied: *Maximum Strength TYLENOL® Flu Day Non-Drowsy* Gelcaps: Burgundy- and white-colored gelcap, imprinted with "TYLENOL FLU" in gray ink—blister packs of 12 & 24. *Maximum Strength TYLENOL® Flu NightTime:* **Gelcaps:** Blue and white-colored gelcap, imprinted with "TYLENOL FLU NT" gray ink—blister packs of 12 and 24. **Liquid:** Red-colored—bottles of 8 fl. oz with child resistant safety cap and tamper evident packaging.

These products are also available in a convenience pack containing *Maximum Strength TYLENOL Flu Day* (pack of 12) and *Maximum Strength TYLENOL Flu Night* (pack of 12).

Shown in Product Identification Guide, page 514 & 515

Extra Strength TYLENOL® PM Pain Reliever/Sleep Aid Caplets, Geltabs and Gelcaps

Description: Each *Extra Strength TYLENOL® PM Caplet, Geltab* or *Gelcap* contains acetaminophen 500 mg and diphenhydramine HCl 25 mg.

Actions: *Extra Strength TYLENOL® PM Caplets, Geltabs* and *Gelcaps* contain a clinically proven analgesic-antipyretic and an antihistamine. Maximum allowable non-prescription levels of acetaminophen and diphenhydramine provide temporary relief of occasional headaches and minor aches and pains accompanying sleeplessness. Acetaminophen is equal to aspirin in analgesic and antipyretic effectiveness and it is unlikely to produce many of the side effects associated with aspirin-containing products. Acetaminophen produces analgesia by elevation of the pain threshold. Diphenhydramine HCl is an antihistamine with sedative properties.

Uses:
temporary relief of occasional headaches and minor aches and pains with accompanying sleeplessness.

Directions:
- do not take more than directed adults and children 12 years and over: Take 2 caplets, geltabs or gelcaps at bedtime or as directed by a doctor. children under 12 years: Do not use this adult product in children under 12 years of age; this will provide more than the recommended dose (overdose) and may cause liver damage.

Precautions: If a rare sensitivity reaction occurs, the drug should be discontinued.

Warnings:
Alcohol Warning: If you consume 3 or more alcoholic drinks every day, ask your doctor whether you should take acetaminophen or other pain relievers/fever reducers. Acetaminophen may cause liver damage.

Do not use
- with any other product containing acetaminophen
- with any other product containing diphenhydramine, even one used on skin.
- in children under 12 years of age

Ask a doctor before use if you have
- a breathing problem such as emphysema or chronic bronchitis
- trouble urinating due to an enlarged prostate gland
- glaucoma

Ask a doctor or pharmacist before use if you are
- taking sedatives or tranquilizers.

When using this product
- drowsiness will occur
- avoid alcoholic drinks
- do not drive a motor vehicle or operate machinery

Stop use and ask a doctor if
- sleeplessness persists continuously for more than 2 weeks. Insomnia may be a symptom of serious underlying medical illness.
- new symptoms occur
- redness or swelling is present
- pain gets worse or lasts for more than 10 days
- fever gets worse or lasts for more than 3 days

If pregnant or breast-feeding, ask a health professional before use.

Keep out of reach of children.

Overdose warning: Taking more than the recommended dose (overdose) may cause liver damage. In case of overdose, get medical help or contact a Poison Control Center right away. Quick medical attention is critical for adults as well as for children even if you do not notice any signs or symptoms.

Other information
- **do not use if carton is opened or neck wrap or foil inner seal imprinted with "Safety Seal®" is broken**
- Store between 20–25°C (68–77°F)

Professional Information:
Overdosage Information:
For overdosage information, please refer to pgs. 679–680

Inactive Ingredients:
Caplets: carnauba wax, cellulose, cornstarch, FD&C Blue #1, FD&C Blue #2, hypromellose, magnesium stearate, polyethylene glycol, polysorbate 80, sodium citrate, sodium starch glycolate, titanium dioxide.
Geltabs/Gelcaps: Benzyl Alcohol, Butylparaben, Castor Oil, Cellulose, Corn Starch, D&C Red #28, Edetate Calcium Disodium, FD&C Blue #1, Gelatin, hypromellose, Magnesium Stearate, Methylparaben, Propylparaben, Sodium Citrate, Sodium Lauryl Sulfate, Sodium Propionate, Sodium Starch Glycolate, Titanium Dioxide, iron oxide.

How Supplied:
Caplets (colored light blue imprinted "Tylenol PM") tamperevident bottles of 24, 50, 100, and 150 and 225.
Gelcaps (colored blue and white imprinted "TYLENOL PM") tamper-evident bottles of 24 and 50.
Geltabs (colored blue and white imprinted "TYLENOL PM") tamper-evident bottles of 24, 50, and 100 and 150.

Shown in Product Identification Guide, page 514

Continued on next page

**Maximum Strength
TYLENOL® Sinus Day
Non-Drowsy
Geltabs, Gelcaps and Caplets**

**Maximum Strength
TYLENOL® Sinus
Night Time Caplets**

**TYLENOL® Sinus Severe
Congestion Caplets**

Product information for all dosage forms of TYLENOL Sinus have been combined under this heading.

Description: Each *Maximum Strength TYLENOL® Sinus Day Non-Drowsy Geltab, Gelcap, or Caplet* contains acetaminophen 500 mg and pseudoephedrine HCl 30 mg. Each *Maximum Strength TYLENOL® Sinus Night Time Caplet* contains acetaminophen 500 mg, doxylamine succinate 6.25 mg and pseudoephedrine HCl 30 mg. Each *Tylenol Sinus Severe Congestion Caplet* contains acetaminophen 325 mg, guaifenesin 200 mg, and pseudoephedrine HCl 30 mg.

Actions:

Maximum Strength TYLENOL® Sinus Day Non-Drowsy contains a clinically proven analgesic-antipyretic and a decongestant. Maximum allowable non-prescription levels of acetaminophen and pseudoephedrine provide temporary relief of sinus pain and headache and congestion. Acetaminophen is equal to aspirin in analgesic and antipyretic effectiveness and it is unlikely to produce many of the side effects associated with aspirin and aspirin-containing products. Acetaminophen produces analgesia by elevation of the pain threshold and antipyresis through action on the hypothalamic heat regulating center. Pseudoephedrine hydrochloride is a sympathomimetic amine which promotes sinus cavity drainage by reducing nasopharyngeal mucosal congestion.

Maximum Strength TYLENOL® Sinus Night Time Caplets contain, in addition to the above ingredients, an antihistamine which provides temporary relief of runny nose and itching of the nose or throat.

Tylenol Sinus Severe Congestion contains a clinically proven analgesic-antipyretic, an expectorant, and a decongestant. Maximum allowable non-prescription levels of acetaminophen, guaifenesin, and pseudoephedrine HCl provide temporary relief of sinus pain, headache, and congestion. Acetaminophen is equal to aspirin in analgesic and antipyretic effectiveness and its unlikely to produce many of the side effects associated with aspirin and aspirin-containing products. Acetaminophen produces analgesia by elevation of the pain threshold and antipyresis through action on the hypothalamic heat regulating center. Guaifenesin is an expectorant which helps loosen phlgm (mucus) and

thin bronchial secretions to make coughs more productive. Pseudoephedrine hydrochloride is a sympathomimetic amine which promotes sinus cavity drainage by reducing nasopharyngeal mucosal congestion.

Uses:

Maximum Strength TYLENOL® Sinus Day Non-Drowsy: temporarily relieves:
• sinus pain • headache • nasal and sinus congestion

Maximum Strength TYLENOL® Sinus Night Time: temporarily relieves:
• nasal congestion • sinus pressure • sinus pain • headache • runny nose • sneezing • itchy, watery eyes • itching of the nose or throat

Tylenol Sinus Severe Congestion temporarily relieves:
• minor aches and pains
• sinus headache
• temporarily relieves nasal congestion associated with sinusitis
• promotes nasal and/or sinus drainage
• helps loosen phlegm (mucus) and thin bronchial secretions to make coughs more productive

Directions:

Maximum Strength TYLENOL® Sinus Day Non-Drowsy:
• **do not take more than directed (see overdose warning)**

adults and children 12 years and over	• take 2 every 4–6 hours as needed • do not take more than 8 in 24 hours
children under 12 years	• do not use this adult product in children under 12 years of age; this will provide more than the recommended dose (overdose) and may cause liver damage.

Maximum Strength TYLENOL® Sinus Night Time:
• **do not take more than directed (see overdose warning)**

adults and children 12 years and over	• take 2 caplets every 4–6 hours as needed • do not take more than 8 caplets in 24 hours
children under 12 years	• do not use this adult product in children under 12 years of age; this will provide more than the recommended dose (overdose) and may cause liver damage.

Tylenol Sinus Severe Congestion
• **Do not exceed recommended dosage**

adults and children 12 years and over	• take 2 caplets every 4–6 hours as needed • do not take more than 8 caplets in 24 hours
children under 12 years	• not intended for use in children under 12. Ask your doctor.

Warnings:

Alcohol warning: If you consume 3 or more alcoholic drinks every day, ask your doctor whether you should take acetaminophen or other pain relievers/fever reducers. Acetaminophen may cause liver damage.

Do not use
• if you are now taking a prescription monamine oxidase inhibitor (MAOI) (certain drugs for depression, psychiatric or emotional conditions or Parkinson's disease), or for 2 weeks after stopping the MAOI drug. If you do not know if your prescription drug contains an MAOI, ask a doctor or pharmacist before taking this product
• with any other product containing acetaminophen

Stop use and ask a doctor if
• new symptoms occur
• redness or swelling is present
• pains gets worse or last for more than 7 days
• fever gets worse or lasts for more than 3 days
• you get nervous, dizzy or sleepless

Tylenol Sinus Severe Congestion

Stop use and ask a doctor if
• new symptoms occur
• redness or swelling is present
• pain, nasal congestion, or cough gets worse or lasts for more than 7 days
• you get nervous, dizzy or sleepless
• cough comes back or occurs with rash or headache that lasts. These could be signs of a serious condition.

If pregnant or breast feeding, ask a health professional before use.

Keep out of reach of children.

Overdose warning: Taking more than the recommended dose (overdose) may cause liver damage. In case of overdose get medical help or contact a Poison Control Center right away. Quick medical attention is critical for adults as well as for children even if you do not notice any signs or symptoms.

Maximum Strength TYLENOL® Sinus Day Non-Drowsy Geltabs, Gelcaps and Caplets

Ask a doctor if you have
• heart disease • high blood pressure
• thyroid disease • diabetes
• trouble urinating due to an enlarged prostate gland

When using this product
• do not exceed recommend dosage

Maximum Strength TYLENOL® Sinus Night Time Caplets

Ask a doctor before use if you have
• heart disease • glaucoma • diabetes
• thyroid disease • high blood pressure

- trouble urinating due to an enlarged prostate gland • a breathing problem such as emphysema or chronic bronchitis

When using this product
- do not exceed recommended dosage
- marked drowsiness may occur
- avoid alcoholic drinks
- alcohol, sedatives and tranquilizers may increase drowsiness
- be careful when driving a motor vehicle or operating machinery
- excitability may occur, especially in children

Ask a doctor or pharmacist before use if you are taking sedatives or tranquilizers

Tylenol Sinus Severe Congestion Caplets

Ask a doctor before use if you have
- heart disease • diabetes • thyroid disease • cough that occurs with too much phlegm (mucus) • high blood pressure • trouble urinating due to an enlarged prostate gland • chronic cough that lasts or occurs with smoking, asthma, chronic bronchitis or emphysema

Other Information:
- do not use if carton is opened or if blister unit is broken

Maximum Strength TYLENOL® Sinus Geltabs and Gelcaps
- store at room temperature; avoid high humidity and excessive heat 40°C (104°F)

Maximum Strength TYLENOL® Sinus Caplets and Maximum Strength TYLENOL® Sinus Night Time Caplets
- store at room temperature

Tylenol Sinus Severe Congestion
- Store at 20–25 degrees Celsius (68–77 degrees Farhenheit)

Professional Information:
Overdosage Information

For overdosage information, please refer to pgs. 679–680

Inactive Ingredients:

Maximum Strength TYLENOL® Sinus Day Non-Drowsy Formula: **Caplets:** carnauba wax, cellulose, corn starch, D&C Yellow #10, FD&C Blue #1, FD&C Red #40, hypromellose, iron oxide, magnesium stearate, polyethylene glycol, polysorbate 80, sodium starch glycolate, titanium dioxide.

Gelcaps and Geltabs: benzyl alcohol, butylparaben, castor oil, cellulose, corn starch, D&C Yellow #10, edetate calcium disodium, FD&C Blue #1, gelatin, hypromellose, iron oxide, magnesium stearate, methylparaben, propylparaben, sodium lauryl sulfate, sodium propionate, sodium starch glycolate, titanium dioxide.

Maximum Strength TYLENOL® Sinus Night Time Caplets: black iron oxide, carnauba wax, cellulose, corn starch, FD&C Blue #1, FD&C Blue #2, hypromellose, propylene glycol, silicon dioxide, sodium starch glycolate, stearic acid, titanium dioxide, triacetin, yellow iron oxide.

Tylenol Sinus Severe Congestion: cellulose, corn starch, croscarmellose sodium, D&C yellow #10, FD&C blue #1, FD&C Red #40, flavor, iron oxide, mannitol,

polyethylene glycol, polyvinyl alcohol, povidone, silicon dioxide, stearic acid, sucralose, talc, titanium dioxide.

How Supplied:
Maximum Strength TYLENOL® Sinus Day Non-Drowsy Formula:
Caplets: Light green-colored, imprinted with "TYLENOL Sinus" in green ink—blister packs of 24 and 48.
Gelcaps: Green- and white-colored, imprinted with "TYLENOL Sinus" in dark green ink—blister packs of 24 and 48.
Geltabs: Green-colored on one side and white-colored on opposite side, imprinted with "TYLENOL Sinus" in gray ink—blister packs of 24 and 48.
Maximum Strength TYLENOL® Sinus Night Time Caplets: Green-colored, imprinted with "Tylenol Sinus NT"—blister packs of 24.
These products are also available in a convenience pack containing Maximum Strength TYLENOL® Sinus Day Non-Drowsy (pack of 12) and Maximum Strength TYLENOL® Sinus Night Time (pack of 12).
Tylenol Sinus Severe Congestion are light green-colored caplets printed with "Tylenol Sinus SC" in black ink and are available in blister packs of 12, 24, and 48.

Shown in Product Identification Guide, page 514

**Maximum Strength TYLENOL®
Sore Throat Adult Liquid**

Description: *Maximum Strength TYLENOL® Sore Throat Liquid* is available in Honey Lemon Flavor or Wild Cherry Flavor and contains acetaminophen 1000 mg in each 30 mL (2 Tablespoonsful).

Actions: Acetaminophen is a clinically proven analgesic/antipyretic. Acetaminophen produces analgesia by elevation of the pain threshold and antipyresis through action on the hypothalamic heat regulating center. Acetaminophen is equal to aspirin in analgesic and antipyretic effectiveness and it is unlikely to produce many of the side effects associated with aspirin and aspirin-containing products.

Uses:
temporarily relieves minor aches and pains due to:
- sore throat • headache • muscular aches • the common cold
- temporarily reduces fever

Directions:
- do not take more than directed (see overdose Warning)

adults and children 12 years and over	• take 2 tablespoons (tbsp) in dose cup provided every 4 to 6 hours as needed • do not take more than 8 tablespoons in 24 hours
children under 12 years	do not use this adult product in children under 12 years of age; this will provide more than the recommended dose (overdose) of TYLENOL® and may cause liver damage.

Precautions: If a rare sensitivity reaction occurs, the drug should be discontinued.

Warnings:
Alcohol warning: If you consume 3 or more alcoholic drinks every day, ask your doctor whether you should take acetaminophen or other pain relievers/fever reducers. Acetaminophen may cause liver damage.
Sore throat warning: If sore throat is severe, persists for more than 2 days, is accompanied or followed by fever, headache, rash, nausea or vomiting, consult a doctor promptly.
Do not use
- with any other product containing acetaminophen
Stop use and ask a doctor if
- new symptoms occur
- redness or swelling is present
- pain gets worse or lasts for more than 10 days
- fever gets worse or lasts for more than 3 days
If pregnant or breast-feeding, ask a health professional before use.
Keep out of the reach of children.
Overdose warning: Taking more than the recommended dose (overdose) may cause liver damage. In case of overdose, get medical help or contact a Poison Control Center right away. Quick medical attention is critical for adults as well as for children even if you do not notice any signs or symptoms.
Other Information
- Do not use if carton is opened or if bottle wrap or foil inner seal imprinted "Safety Seal®" is broken or missing
- store at room temperature

Professional Information:
Overdosage Information
For overdosage information, please refer to pgs. 679–680

Inactive Ingredients: *Maximum Strength TYLENOL® Sore Throat Honey-Lemon-Flavored Adult Liquid:* caramel color, citric acid, flavor, high fructose corn syrup, polyethylene glycol, propylene glycol, purified water, saccharin sodium, sodium benzoate, sorbitol
Maximum Strength TYLENOL® Sore Throat Wild Cherry-Flavored Adult Liquid: citric acid, D&C Red # 33, FD&C Red # 40, flavor, high fructose corn syrup, polyethylene glycol, propylene glycol, purified water, saccharin sodium, sodium benzoate, sorbitol

Continued on next page

Tylenol Sore Throat Liq.—Cont.

How Supplied:
Honey lemon-flavored or wild cherry-flavored liquid in child-resistant tamper-evident bottles of 8 fl. oz.

Shown in Product Identification Guide, page 515

WOMEN'S TYLENOL®
Menstrual Relief Pain Reliever/ Diuretic Caplets

Description: Each *Women's Tylenol® Menstrual Relief Caplet* contains acetaminophen 500 mg and pamabrom 25 mg.

Actions: *Women's TYLENOL® Menstrual Relief Caplets* contain a clinically proven analgesic-antipyretic and a diuretic. Maximum allowable non-prescription levels of acetaminophen and pamabrom provide temporary relief of minor aches and pains due to cramps, headache, and backache and water retention, weight gain, bloating, swelling and full feeling associated with the premenstrual and menstrual periods. Acetaminophen is equal to aspirin in analgesic and antipyretic effectiveness and it is unlikely to produce many of the side effects associated with aspirin containing products. Acetaminophen produces analgesia by elevation of the pain threshold. Pamabrom is a diuretic which relieves water retention.

Uses:
- temporarily relieves minor aches and pains due to:
  - cramps • headache • backache
- temporarily relieves water-weight gain, bloating, swelling and full feeling associated with the premenstrual and menstrual periods

Directions:
- **do not take more than directed**
adults and children 12 years and over: take 2 caplets every 4 to 6 hours; do not take more than 8 caplets in 24 hours, or as directed by a doctor
children under 12 years: do not use this adult product in children under 12 years of age; this will provide more than the recommended dose (overdose) and may cause liver damage

Precautions: If a rare sensitivity reaction occurs, the drug should be discontinued.

Warnings:
Alcohol warning: If you consume 3 or more alcoholic drinks every day, ask your doctor whether you should take acetaminophen or other pain relievers/ fever reducers. Acetaminophen may cause liver damage.
Do not use
- with any other product containing acetaminophen
Stop use and ask a doctor if
- new symptoms occur
- redness or swelling is present
- pain gets worse or lasts for more than 10 days

If pregnant or breast-feeding, ask a health professional before use.
Keep out of reach of children.
Overdose Warning: Taking more than the recommended dose (overdose) may cause liver damage. In case of overdose, get medical help or contact a Poison Control Center right away. Prompt medical attention is critical for adults as well as for children even if you do not notice any signs or symptoms.
Other Information:
- **do not use if carton is opened, or if neck wrap or foil inner seal imprinted "Safety Seal®" is broken or missing**
- store at room temperature, avoid excessive heat 104°F (40°C)

Professional Information:
Overdosage Information
For overdosage information, please refer to pgs. 679–680

Inactive Ingredients
cellulose, corn starch, hypromellose, magnesium stearate, polydextrose, polyethylene glycol, sodium starch glycolate, titanium dioxide, triacetin.

How Supplied:
White capsule shaped caplets with TYME printed on one side in tamper-evident bottles of 24.

Shown in Product Identification Guide, page 515

Concentrated TYLENOL®
acetaminophen Infants' Drops

Children's TYLENOL®
acetaminophen Suspension Liquid and Soft Chews Chewable Tablets

Junior Strength TYLENOL®
acetaminophen Soft Chews Chewable Tablets

Product information for all dosages of Children's TYLENOL have been combined under this heading

Description: *Concentrated TYLENOL® Infants' Drops* are stable, alcohol-free, grape-flavored and purple in color or cherry-flavored and red in color. Each 1.6 mL contains 160 mg acetaminophen. *Concentrated TYLENOL® Infants' Drops* features the SAFE-TY-LOCK™ Bottle. The SAFE-TY-LOCK™ Bottle has a unique safety barrier inside the bottle which helps make administration easier. The integrated dropper promotes proper administration. The innovative design eliminates excess product on dropper. The star-shaped barrier inside the bottle minimizes spills and discourages pouring into a spoon. *Children's TYLENOL® Suspension Liquid* is stable, alcohol-free, cherry-flavored and red in color, or bubble gum-flavored and pink in color, grape-flavored and purple in color, or very berry strawberry-flavored and red in color. Each 5 mL (one teaspoonful) contains 160 mg acetaminophen. Each *Children's TYLENOL® Soft Chews Chewable Tablet* contains 80 mg acetaminophen in a grape, bubble gum, or

fruit flavor. *Each Junior Strength TYLENOL® Soft Chews Chewable Tablet* contains 160 mg acetaminophen in a grape or fruit-flavored chewable tablet.

Actions: Acetaminophen is a clinically proven analgesic/antipyretic. Acetaminophen produces analgesia by elevation of the pain threshold and antipyresis through action on the hypothalamic heat-regulating center. Acetaminophen is equal to aspirin in analgesic and antipyretic effectiveness and it is unlikely to produce many of the side effects associated with aspirin and aspirin-containing products.

Uses:
Concentrated TYLENOL® Infants' Drops: temporarily:
- reduces fever
- relieves minor aches and pains due to:
  - the common cold • flu • headaches • sore throat • immunizations • toothaches
Children's TYLENOL® Suspension Liquid and Children's TYLENOL® Soft Chews Chewable Tablets: temporarily relieves minor aches and pains due to: the common cold • flu • headaches • sore throat • immunizations • toothaches
- temporarily reduces fever
Junior Strength TYLENOL® Soft Chews Chewable Tablets: temporarily relieves minor aches and pains due to: • the common cold • flu • headache • muscle aches • sprains • overexertion
- temporarily reduces fever

Directions: See Table 1: Children's Tylenol Dosing Chart on pgs. 692–694

Precautions: If a rare sensitivity reaction occurs, the drug should be discontinued.

Warnings:
Sore throat warning: if sore throat is severe, persists for more than 2 days, is accompanied or followed by fever, headache, rash, nausea, or vomiting, consult a doctor promptly (excluding *Junior Strength TYLENOL® Soft Chews Chewable Tablets*).
Do not use
- with any other product containing acetaminophen
When using this product
- **do not exceed recommended dose (see overdose warning)**
Stop use and ask a doctor if
- new symptoms occur
- redness or swelling is present
- pain gets worse or lasts for more than 5 days
- fever gets worse or lasts for more than 3 days
Keep out of the reach of children.
Overdose warning: Taking more than the recommended dose (overdose) may cause liver damage. In case of overdose, get medical help or contact a Poison Control Center right away. Quick medical attention is critical even if you do not notice any signs or symptoms.

Other Information:
Concentrated TYLENOL® Infants' Drops:
• **Do not use if plastic carton wrap or bottle wrap imprinted "Safety Seal®" is broken or missing.**
• Store at room temperature
Children's TYLENOL® Suspension Liquid:
•**Do not use if bottle wrap, or foil inner seal imprinted "Safety Seal®" is broken or missing**
• Store at room temperature
Children's TYLENOL® Soft Chews Chewable Tablets:
• phenylketonurics: fruit and grape contain phenylalanine 3 mg per tablet, bubble gum contains phenylalanine 6 mg per tablet
• **Do not use if carton is opened or if neck wrap or foil inner seal imprinted "Safety Seal®" is broken or missing.**
Store at room temperature (Grape: Keep product away from direct light) *Junior Strength TYLENOL® Soft Chews Chewable Tablets:*
• Phenylketonurics: contains phenylalanine 6 mg per tablet
• **Do not use if carton is opened or if blister unit is broken**
• Store at room temperature (Grape: Keep product away from direct light)

Professional Information:
Overdosage Information for all Infants', Children's & Junior Strength Tylenol® Products

ACETAMINOPHEN: Acetaminophen in massive overdosage may cause hepatic toxicity in some patients. In adults and adolescents ($\geq$ 12 years of age), hepatic toxicity may occur following ingestion of greater than 7.5 to 10 grams over a period of 8 hours or less. Fatalities are infrequent (less than 3–4% of untreated cases) and have rarely been reported with overdoses of less than 15 grams. In children (<12 years of age), an acute overdosage of less than 150 mg/kg has not been associated with hepatic toxicity. Early symptoms following a potentially hepatotoxic overdose may include: nausea, vomiting, diaphoresis and general malaise. Clinical and laboratory evidence of hepatic toxicity may not be apparent until 48 to 72 hours postingestion. In adults and adolescents, any individual presenting with an unknown amount of acetaminophen ingested or with a questionable or unreliable history about the time of ingestion should have a plasma acetaminophen level drawn and be treated with N-acetylcysteine. For full prescribing information, refer to the N-acetylcysteine package insert. Do not await results of assays for plasma acetaminophen levels before initiating treatment with N-acetylcysteine. The following additional procedures are recommended: Promptly initiate gastric decontamination of the stomach. A plasma acetaminophen assay should be obtained as early as possible, but no sooner than four hours following ingestion. If an acetaminophen *extended release* product is involved, it may be appropriate to obtain an additional plasma acetaminophen level 4–6 hours following the initial acetaminophen level. If either acetaminophen level plots above the treatment line on the acetaminophen overdose nomogram, N-acetylcysteine treatment should be continued for a full course of therapy. Liver function studies should be obtained initially and repeated at 24-hour intervals. Serious toxicity or fatalities have been extremely infrequent following an acute acetaminophen overdose in young children, possibly because of differences in the way they metabolize acetaminophen. In children, the maximum potential amount ingested can be more easily estimated. If more than 150 mg/kg or an unknown amount was ingested, obtain a plasma acetaminophen level as soon as possible, but no sooner than 4 hours following ingestion. If an acetaminophen *extended release* product is involved, it may be appropriate to obtain an additional plasma acetaminophen level 4–6 hours following the initial acetaminophen level. If either acetaminophen level plots above the treatment line on the acetaminophen overdose nomogram, N-acetylcysteine treatment should be initiated and continued for a full course of therapy. If an assay cannot be obtained and the estimated acetaminophen ingestion exceeds 150 mg/kg, dosing with N-acetylcysteine should be initiated and continued for a full course of therapy. For additional emergency information, call your regional poison center or call the Rocky Mountain Poison Center toll-free, (1-800-525-6115).

Our pediatric Tylenol® combination products contain active ingredients in addition to acetaminophen. The following is basic overdose information regarding those ingredients.

CHLORPHENIRAMINE: Chlorpheniramine toxicity should be treated as you would an antihihistamine/anticholinergic overdose and is likely to be present within a few hours after acute ingestion.

DEXTROMETHORPHAN: Acute dextromethorphan overdose usually does not result in serious signs and symptoms unless massive amounts have been ingested. Signs and symptoms of a substantial overdose may include nausea and vomiting, visual disturbances, CNS disturbances and urinary retention.

DIPHENHYDRAMINE: Diphenhydramine toxicity should be treated as you would an antihistamine/anticholinergic overdose and is likely to be present within a few hours after acute ingestion.

PSEUDOEPHEDRINE: Symptoms from pseudoephedrine overdose consist most often of mild anxiety, tachycardia and/or mild hypertension. Symptoms usually appear within 4 to 8 hours of ingestion and are transient, usually requiring no treatment.

For additional emergency information, please contact your local poison control center.

Inactive Ingredients:
Concentrated TYLENOL® Infants' Drops: **Cherry-Flavored:** butylparaben, cellulose, citric acid, corn syrup, FD&C Red #40, flavors, glycerin, propylene glycol, purified water, sodium benzoate, sorbitol, xanthan gum. **Grape-Flavored:** butylparaben, cellulose, citric acid, corn syrup, D&C Red #33, FD&C Blue #1, flavors, glycerin, propylene glycol, purified water, sodium benzoate, sorbitol, xanthan gum.
Children's TYLENOL® Suspension Liquid: butylparaben, cellulose, citric acid, corn syrup, flavors, glycerin, propylene glycol, purified water, sodium benzoate, sorbitol, xanthan gum. In addition to the above ingredients cherry-flavored suspension contains FD&C Red #40, bubble gum-flavored suspension contains D&C Red #33 and FD&C Red #40, grape-flavored suspension contains D&C Red #33 and FD&C Blue #1 and very berry strawberry-flavored suspension contains FD&C Red #10.
Children's TYLENOL® Soft Chews Chewable Tablets: **Fruit-Flavored:** aspartame, cellulose, cellulose acetate citric acid, D&C Red #7, flavors, magnesium stearate, mannitol, povidone. **Grape-Flavored:** aspartame, cellulose, cellulose acetate, citric acid, D&C Red #7, D&C Red #30, FD&C Blue #1, flavors, magnesium stearate, mannitol, povidone. **Bubble Gum-Flavored:** aspartame, cellulose, cellulose acetate, D&C Red #7, flavors, magnesium stearate, mannitol, povidone.
Junior Strength TYLENOL® Soft Chews Chewable Tablets: **Fruit-Flavored:** aspartame, cellulose, citric acid, D&C Red #7, flavors, magnesium stearate, mannitol, povidone. **Grape-Flavored:** aspartame, cellulose, citric acid, D&C Red #7, D&C Red #30, FD&C Blue #1, flavors, magnesium stearate, mannitol, povidone.

How Supplied:
Concentrated TYLENOL® Infants' Drops: (purple-colored grape): bottles of ½ oz (15 mL) and 1 oz (30 mL); (red-colored cherry): bottles of ½ oz and 1 oz, each with calibrated plastic dropper.
Children's TYLENOL® Suspension Liquid: (red-colored cherry): bottles of 2 and 4 fl oz. (pink-colored bubble gum and purple-colored grape): bottles of 4 fl. oz.
Children's TYLENOL® Soft Chews Chewable Tablets: (pink-colored fruit, purple-colored grape, pink-colored bubble gum, scored, imprinted "TY80"). Bottles of 30 and also blister packaged 60's and 96's (fruit).
Junior Strength TYLENOL® Soft Chews Chewable Tablets: (purple-colored grape or pink-colored fruit, imprinted "TY 160") Package of 24. All packages listed above are safety sealed and use child-resistant safety caps or blisters.

Shown in Product Identification Guide, page 512 & 513

Continued on next page

CHILDREN'S TYLENOL® Plus Allergy

Description: *Children's TYLENOL® Plus Allergy* is Bubble Gum flavored and contains no alcohol or aspirin. Each teaspoon (5 mL) contains acetaminophen 160 mg, diphenhydramine HCl 12.5 mg and pseudoephedrine HCl 15 mg.

Actions: *Children's TYLENOL® Plus Allergy* combines the analgesic-antipyretic acetaminophen with the antihistamine diphenhydramine hydrochloride and the decongestant pseudoephedrine hydrochloride to provide fast, effective, temporary relief of all your child's symptoms associated with hay fever and other respiratory allergies including sneezing, sore throat, itchy throat, itchy/watery eyes, runny nose, stuffy nose and nasal congestion. Acetaminophen is equal to aspirin in analgesic and antipyretic effectiveness and it is unlikely to produce the side effects often associated with aspirin or aspirin-containing products.

Uses: temporarily relieves these hay fever and upper respiratory allergy symptoms:
- nasal congestion • sore throat
- runny nose • sneezing
- stuffy nose • minor aches and pains
- itchy, watery eyes
- temporarily reduces fever

Directions:
See Table 1: Children's Tylenol Dosing Chart on pgs. 692–694

Precautions: If a rare sensitivity reaction occurs, the drug should be discontinued.

Warnings:
Sore throat warning: If sore throat is severe, persists for more than 2 days, is accompanied or followed by fever, headache, rash, nausea or vomiting, consult a doctor promptly.

Do not use
- in a child who is taking a prescription monoamine oxidase inhibitor (MAOI) (certain drugs for depression, psychiatric, or emotional conditions, or Parkinson's disease) or for 2 weeks after stopping the MAOI drug. If you do not know if your child's prescription drug contains an MAOI, ask a doctor or pharmacist before giving this product.
- with any other product containing acetaminophen.
- with any other product containing diphenhydramine, even one used on skin

Ask a doctor before use if the child has
- heart disease • high blood pressure
- thyroid disease • diabetes
- glaucoma • a breathing problem such as chronic bronchitis

When using this product
- **do not exceed recommended dosage (see overdose warning)**
- marked drowsiness may occur
- excitability may occur, especially in children

Stop use and ask a doctor if
- new symptoms occur
- redness or swelling is present
- pain gets worse or lasts for more than 5 days
- fever gets worse or lasts for more than 3 days

- nervousness, dizziness or sleeplessness occurs

Keep out of reach of children.

Overdose Warning: Taking more than the recommended dose (overdose) may cause liver damage. In case of overdose, get medical help or contact a Poison Control Center right away. Quick medical attention is critical even if you do not notice any signs or symptoms

Other Information:
- **do not use if plastic carton wrap, bottle wrap, or foil inner seal imprinted "Safety Seal®" is broken or missing.**
- store at room temperature

Professional Information:
Overdosage Information:
For overdosage information, please refer to pg. 689

Inactive Ingredients: benzoic acid, citric acid, corn syrup, D&C Red #33, FD&C Red #40, flavors, polyethylene glycol, propylene glycol, purified water, sodium benzoate, sorbitol.

How Supplied: Pink-colored, Bubble Gum flavored liquid in child resistant tamper-evident bottles of 4 fl. oz.
Shown in Product Identification Guide, page 512

Concentrated TYLENOL® Infants' Drops Plus Cold Nasal Decongestant, Fever Reducer & Pain Reliever

Concentrated TYLENOL® Infants' Drops Plus Cold & Cough Nasal Decongestant, Fever Reducer & Pain Reliever

Children's TYLENOL® Plus Cold Suspension Liquid and Chewable Tablets

Children's TYLENOL® Plus Cold & Cough Suspension Liquid and Chewable Tablets

Description: *Concentrated TYLENOL® Infants' Drops Plus Cold* are alcohol-free, aspirin-free, BubbleGum-flavored and red in color. Each 1.6 mL contains acetaminophen 160 mg and pseudoephedrine HCl 15 mg. *Concentrated TYLENOL® Infants' Drops Plus Cold & Cough* are alcohol-free, aspirin-free, Cherry-flavored and red in color. Each 1.6 mL contains acetaminophen 160 mg, dextromethorphan HBr 5 mg, and pseudoephedrine HCl 15 mg. *Children's TYLENOL® Plus Cold Suspension Liquid* is Grape-flavored and contains no alcohol or aspirin. Each teaspoon (5 mL) contains acetaminophen 160 mg, chlorpheniramine maleate 1 mg and pseudoephedrine HCl 15 mg. *Children's TYLENOL® Plus Cold Chewable Tablets* are Grape-flavored and each tablet contains acetaminophen 80 mg, chlorpheniramine maleate 0.5 mg and pseudoephedrine HCl 7.5 mg. *Children's TYLENOL® Plus Cold & Cough Suspension Liquid* is Cherry-flavored

and contains no alcohol or aspirin. Each teaspoonful (5 mL) contains acetaminophen 160 mg, chlorpheniramine maleate 1 mg, dextromethorphan HBr 5 mg and pseudoephedrine HCl 15 mg. *Children's TYLENOL® Plus Cold & Cough Chewable Tablets* are Cherry-flavored and each tablet contains acetaminophen 80 mg, chlorpheniramine maleate 0.5 mg, dextromethorphan HBr 2.5 mg, and pseudoephedrine HCl 7.5 mg.

Actions: Acetaminophen is a clinically proven analgesic/antipyretic. Acetaminophen produces analgesia by elevation of the pain threshold and antipyresis through action on the hypothalamic heat-regulating center. Acetaminophen is equal to aspirin in analgesic and antipyretic effectiveness and it is unlikely to produce many of the side effects associated with aspirin and aspirin-containing products.
Pseudoephedrine hydrochloride is a sympathomimetic amine which provides temporary relief of nasal congestion. Chlorpheniramine maleate is an antihistamine that provides temporary relief of runny nose, sneezing and watery and itchy eyes.
Dextromethorphan hydrobromide is a cough suppressant which helps relieve coughs.

Uses:
Concentrated TYLENOL® Infants' Drops Plus Cold, temporarily relieves these cold symptoms:
- minor aches and pains
- nasal congestion • headaches
- temporarily reduces fever

Concentrated TYLENOL® Infants' Drops Plus Cold & Cough, temporarily relieves these cold symptoms:
- coughs • nasal congestion
- minor aches and pains
- sore throat • headaches
- temporarily reduces fever

Children's TYLENOL® Plus Cold Suspension Liquid and *Chewable Tablets:* temporarily relieves these cold symptoms:
- nasal congestion • sore throat • runny nose • sneezing • headache • minor aches and pains
- temporarily reduces fever

Children's TYLENOL® Plus Cold & Cough Suspension Liquid and *Chewable Tablets:* temporarily relieves these cold symptoms:
- nasal congestion • sore throat • runny nose • sneezing • headache • minor aches and pains • coughs
temporarily reduces fever

Directions: See Table 1: Children's Tylenol Dosing Chart on pgs. 692–694

Precautions: If a rare sensitivity reaction occurs, the drug should be discontinued.

Warnings:
Sore throat warning: If sore throat is severe, persists for more than 2 days, is accompanied by or followed by fever, headache, rash, nausea or vomiting, con-

sult a doctor promptly (does not apply to *Concentrated TYLENOL® Infants' Drops Plus Cold*)

Do not use
- in a child who is taking a prescription monoamine oxidase inhibitor (MAOI) (certain drugs for depression, psychiatric or emotional conditions, or Parkinson's disease), or for 2 weeks after stopping the MAOI drug. If you do not know if your child's prescription drug contains an MAOI, ask a doctor or pharmacist before giving this product.
- with any other products containing acetaminophen

Keep out of reach of children.

Overdose Warning: Taking more than the recommended dose (overdose) may cause liver damage. In case of overdose, get medical help or contact a Poison Control Center right away. Quick medical attention is critical even if you do not notice any signs or symptoms.

Stop use and ask a doctor if
- new symptoms occur
- redness or swelling is present
- pain gets worse or lasts for more than 5 days
- fever gets worse or lasts for more than 3 days
- nervousness, dizziness or sleeplessness occurs
- cough lasts for more than 7 days, comes back or occurs with fever, rash or headache that lasts. These could be signs of a serious condition. (*Concentrated TYLENOL® Infants' Drops Plus Cold & Cough and Children's TYLENOL® Plus Cold & Cough Products* only)

Concentrated TYLENOL® Infants' Drops Plus Cold,

Ask a doctor before use if the child has
- heart disease • high blood pressure
- thyroid disease • diabetes

When using this product
- do not exceed recommended dosage (see overdose warning)

Concentrated TYLENOL® Infants' Drops Plus Cold & Cough

Ask a doctor before use if the child has
- heart disease • high blood pressure
- cough that occurs with too much phlegm (mucus) • thyroid disease • diabetes • chronic cough that lasts as occurs with asthma

When using this product
- do not exceed recommended dosage (see Overdose warning)

Children's TYLENOL® Plus Cold Suspension Liquid and Chewable Tablets

Ask a doctor before use if the child has
- heart disease • thyroid disease • glaucoma • high blood pressure • diabetes
- a breathing problem such as chronic bronchitis

When using this product
- do not exceed recommended dosage (see overdose warning)
- drowsiness may occur
- excitability may occur, especially in children

Children's TYLENOL® Plus Cold & Cough Suspension Liquid and Chewable Tablets

Ask a doctor before use if the child has
- heart disease • thyroid disease • glaucoma • high blood pressure • diabetes

cough that occurs with too much phlegm (mucus) • chronic cough that lasts as occurs with asthma

When using this product
- do not exceed recommended dosage (see overdose warning)
- drowsiness may occur
- excitability may occur, especially in children

Other Information
Concentrated TYLENOL® Infants' Drops Plus Cold, Concentrated TYLENOL® Infants' Drops Plus Cold & Cough
- do not use if plastic carton wrap or bottle wrap imprinted "Safety Seal®" is broken or missing
- store at room temperature

Children's TYLENOL® Plus Cold & Cough Suspension Liquid, Children's TYLENOL® Plus Cold Suspension Liquid
- do not use if bottle wrap or foil inner seal imprinted "Safety Seal®" is broken or missing
- store at room temperature

Children's TYLENOL® Plus Cold Chewable Tablets
- phenylketonurics: contains phenylalanine 6 mg per tablet
- do not use if carton is opened or if blister unit is broken
- store at room temperature

Children's TYLENOL® Plus Cold & Cough Chewable Tablets
- phenylketonurics: contains phenylalanine 4 mg per tablet
- do not use if carton is opened or if blister unit is broken
- store at room temperature

Professional Information:
Overdosage Information: For overdosage information, please refer to pg. 689

Inactive Ingredients:
Concentrated TYLENOL® Infants' Drops Plus Cold: citric acid, corn syrup, FD&C Red #40, flavors, polyethylene glycol, propylene glycol, sodium benzoate, sodium saccharin.
Concentrated TYLENOL® Infants' Drops Plus Cold & Cough: acesulfame potassium, citric acid, corn syrup, FD&C Red #40, flavors, polyethylene glycol, propylene glycol, sodium benzoate.
Children's TYLENOL® Plus Cold: Suspension Liquid: acesulfame potassium, butylparaben, cellulose, citric acid, corn syrup, D&C Red #33, FD&C Blue #1, FD&C Red #40, flavors, glycerin, propylene glycol, purified water, sodium benzoate, sorbitol, xanthan gum. **Chewable Tablets:** aspartame, basic polymethacrylate, cellulose, cellulose acetate, citric acid, D&C Red #7, FD&C Blue #1, flavors, hypromellose, magnesium stearate, mannitol.
Children's TYLENOL® Plus Cold & Cough: Suspension Liquid: acesulfame potassium, cellulose, citric acid, corn syrup, D&C Red #33, FD&C Red #40, flavors, glycerin, sodium benzoate, sorbitol, xanthan gum. **Chewable Tablets:** aspartame, basic polymethacrylate, cellulose, cellulose acetate, D&C Red #7, flavors, hypromellose, magnesium stearate, mannitol.

How Supplied:
Concentrated TYLENOL® Infants' Drops Plus Cold: Red colored, Bubble Gum flavored drops in child resistant tamper-evident bottles of $1/2$ fl. oz.
Concentrated TYLENOL® Infants' Drops Plus Cold & Cough: Red colored, Cherry Flavored drops in Child resistant tamper evident bottles of $1/2$ fl. oz.
Children's TYLENOL® Plus Cold: Suspension Liquid: Purple-colored-bottles of 4 fl. oz. Store at room temperature. Chewable Tablets: Purple-colored, imprinted "TYLENOL COLD" on one side and "TC" on opposite side- blisters of 24.
Children's TYLENOL® Plus Cold & Cough: Suspension Liquid: Red colored, Cherry flavored liquid in child resistant tamper-evident bottles of 4 fl. oz.
Chewable Tablets: Red-colored, imprinted TYLENOL C/C" on one side and "TC/C" on the opposite side- blisters of 24.
Check cold bottle color – clear or white (opaque)

Shown in Product Identification Guide, page 513

**Children's
TYLENOL® Plus Flu**

Description: *Children's TYLENOL® Plus Flu* Suspension Liquid is Bubble Gum flavored and contains no alcohol or aspirin. Each teaspoon (5 mL) contains acetaminophen 160 mg, chlorpheniramine maleate 1 mg, dextromethorphan HBr 7.5 mg and pseudoephedrine HCl 15 mg.

Actions: *Children's TYLENOL® Plus Flu* Suspension Liquid combines the analgesic-antipyretic acetaminophen with the decongestant pseudoephedrine hydrochloride, the cough suppressant dextromethorphan hydrobromide and the antihistamine chlorpheniramine maleate to provide fast, effective, temporary relief of all your child's symptoms associated with flu including fever, body aches, headache, stuffy nose, runny nose, sore throat and coughs. Acetaminophen is equal to aspirin in analgesic and antipyretic effectiveness and it is unlikely to produce the side effects often associated with aspirin or aspirin-containing products.

Uses: temporarily relieves these cold and flu symptoms:
- nasal congestion • sore throat
- runny nose • sneezing
- headache • minor aches and pains
- coughs
- temporarily reduces fever

Directions: See Table 1: Children's Tylenol Dosing Chart on pgs. 692–694

Precautions: If a rare sensitivity reaction occurs, the drug should be discontinued.

Continued on next page

TABLE 1
Children's Tylenol® Dosing Chart

AGE GROUP	0–3 mos	4–11 mos	12–23 mos	2–3 yrs	4–5 yrs	6–8 yrs	9–10 yrs	11 yrs	12 yrs	Maximum doses/24 hrs
WEIGHT (if possible use weight to dose; otherwise use age)	6–11 lbs	12–17 lbs	18–23 lbs	24–35 lbs	36–47 lbs	48–59 lbs	60–71 lbs	72–95 lbs	96 lbs and over	
PRODUCT FORM **INGREDIENTS**	Dose to be administered based on weight or age†									
Infants' Drops in each (0.8 mL)										
Concentrated Tylenol Infants' Drops — Acetaminophen 80 mg	(0.4 mL)*	(0.8 mL)*	1.2 mL (0.8 + 0.4 mL)*	1.6 mL (0.8 + 0.8 mL)	—	—	—	—	—	5 times in 24 hrs
Concentrated Tylenol Infants' Drops Plus Cold — Acetaminophen 80 mg Pseudoephedrine HCl 7.5 mg	(0.4 mL)*	(0.8 mL)*	1.2 mL (0.8 + 0.4 mL)*	1.6 mL (0.8 + 0.8 mL)	—	—	—	—	—	4 times in 24 hrs
Concentrated Tylenol Infants' Drops Plus Cold & Cough — Acetaminophen 80 mg Dextromethorphan HBr 2.5 mg Pseudoephedrine HCl 7.5 mg	(0.4 mL)*	(0.8 mL)*	1.2 mL (0.8 + 0.4 mL)*	1.6 mL (0.8 + 0.8 mL)	—	—	—	—	—	4 times in 24 hrs
Children's Liquids Per 5 mL teaspoonful (TSP)										
Children's Tylenol Suspension Liquid — Acetaminophen 160 mg	—	½ TSP*	¾ TSP*	1 TSP	1 ½ TSP	2 TSP	2 ½ TSP	3 TSP	—	5 times in 24 hrs
Children's Tylenol Plus Cold Suspension Liquid — Acetaminophen 160 mg Chlorpheniramine Maleate 1 mg Pseudoephedrine HCl 15 mg	—	½ TSP**	¾ TSP**	1 TSP**	1 ½ TSP**	2 TSP	2 ½ TSP	3 TSP	—	4 times in 24 hrs

Product	Active Ingredients										
Children's Tylenol Plus Cold & Cough Suspension Liquid	Acetaminophen 160 mg Chlorpheniramine Maleate 1 mg Dextromethorphan HBr 5 mg Pseudoephedrine HCl 15 mg	—	$^{1}/_{2}$ TSP**	$^{3}/_{4}$ TSP**	1 TSP**	1 $^{1}/_{2}$ TSP**	2 TSP	2 $^{1}/_{2}$ TSP	3 TSP	—	4 times in 24 hrs
Children's Tylenol Plus Flu Suspension Liquid†	Acetaminophen 160 mg Chlorpheniramine Maleate 1 mg Dextromethorphan HBr 7.5 mg Pseudoephedrine HCl 15 mg	—	$^{1}/_{2}$ TSP**	$^{3}/_{4}$ TSP**	1 TSP**	1 $^{1}/_{2}$ TSP**	2 TSP	2 $^{1}/_{2}$ TSP	3 TSP	—	4 times in 24 hrs
Children's Tylenol Plus Sinus Suspension Liquid	Acetaminophen 160 mg Pseudoephedrine HCl 15 mg	—	$^{1}/_{2}$ TSP*	$^{3}/_{4}$ TSP*	1 TSP	1 $^{1}/_{2}$ TSP	2 TSP	2 $^{1}/_{2}$ TSP	3 TSP	—	4 times in 24 hrs
Children's Tylenol Plus Allergy Liquid	Acetaminophen 160 mg Diphenhydramine HCl 12.5 mg Pseudoephedrine HCl 15 mg	—	$^{1}/_{2}$ TSP**	$^{3}/_{4}$ TSP**	1 TSP**	1 $^{1}/_{2}$ TSP**	2 TSP	2 $^{1}/_{2}$ TSP	3 TSP	—	4 times in 24 hrs
Children's Tablets	**Per tablet**										
Children's Tylenol Soft Chews Chewable Tablets	Acetaminophen 80 mg	—	—	—	2 tablets	3 tablets	4 tablets	5 tablets	6 tablets	—	5 times in 24 hrs
Children's Tylenol Plus Cold Chewable Tablets	Acetaminophen 80 mg Chlorpheniramine Maleate 0.5 mg Pseudoephedrine HCl 7.5 mg	—	—	—	2 tablets**	3 tablets**	4 tablets	5 tablets	6 tablets	—	4 times in 24 hrs

(Table continued on next page)

(Continued from previous page)

Product	Active Ingredients									Maximum Dosage
Children's Tylenol Plus Cold & Cough Chewable Tablets	Acetaminophen 80 mg Chlorpheniramine Maleate 0.5 mg Dextromethorphan HBr 2.5 mg Pseudoephedrine HCl 7.5 mg	—	—	2 tablets**	3 tablets**	4 tablets	5 tablets	6 tablets	—	4 times in 24 hrs
Junior Strength Tylenol Soft Chews Chewable Tablets	Acetaminophen 160 mg	—	—	—	—	2 tablets	2¹/₂ tablets	3 tablets	4 tablets	5 times in 24 hrs
Simply Stuffy Liquid	pseudoephedrine HCl 15 mg	¹/₂ tsp.	³/₄ tsp.	1 tsp	1¹/₂ tsp	2 tsp	2¹/₂ tsp	3 tsp	—	4 times in 24 hours
Simply Cough Liquid	dextromethorphan HBr 5 mg	¹/₂ tsp	³/₄ tsp	1 tsp	1¹/₂ tsp	2 tsp	2¹/₂ tsp	3 tsp	—	4 times in 24 hrs

†All products may be dosed every 4 hours, if needed; except for Children's Tylenol Flu which is dosed every 6–8 hrs, if needed.
*Under 2 years (under 24 lbs), consult a doctor.
**Under 6 years (under 48 lbs), consult a doctor.
• Infants' Tylenol Drops are more concentrated than Children's Tylenol Liquids. The Infants' Concentrated Drops have been specifically designed for use only with enclosed dropper. Do not use any other dosing device with this product.
• Children's Tylenol Liquids are less concentrated than Infants' Tylenol Concentrated Drops. The Children's Tylenol Liquids have been specifically designed for use with the enclosed measuring cup. Use only enclosed measuring cup to dose this product.
• Children's Tylenol Soft Chews Chewable Tablets are not the same concentration as Junior Strength Tylenol Soft Chews Chewable Tablets.
• Junior Strength Tylenol Soft Chews Chewable Tablets and Caplets contain twice as much medicine as Children's Tylenol Soft Chews Chewable Tablets.

Warnings:

Sore throat warning: If sore throat is severe, persists for more than 2 days, is accompanied or followed by fever, headache, rash, nausea or vomiting, consult a doctor promptly.

Do not use

- in a child who is taking a monoamine oxidase inhibitor (MAOI) (certain drugs for depression, psychiatric or emotional conditions, or Parkinson's disease), or for 2 weeks after stopping the MAOI drug. If you do not know if your child's prescription drug contains an MAOI, ask a doctor or pharmacist before giving this product.
- with any other product containing acetaminophen.

Ask a doctor before use if the child has

- heart disease • thyroid disease
- glaucoma • high blood pressure
- diabetes • cough that occurs with too much phlegm (mucus)
- chronic cough that lasts as occurs with asthma

When using this product

- **do not exceed recommended dosage (see overdose warning)**
- drowsiness may occur
- excitability may occur, especially in children

Stop use and ask a doctor if

- new symptoms occur
- redness or swelling is present
- pain gets worse or lasts for more than 5 days
- fever gets worse or lasts for more than 3 days
- nervousness, dizziness or sleeplessness occurs
- cough lasts more than 7 days, comes back or occurs with fever, rash or headache that lasts. These could be signs of a serious condition.

Keep out of reach of children.

Overdose Warning: Taking more than the recommended dose (overdose) may cause liver damage. In case of overdose, get medical help or contact a Poison Control Center right away. Quick medical attention is critical even if you do not notice any signs or symptoms.

Other Information:

- **do not use if bottle wrap or foil inner seal imprinted "Safety Seal®" is broken or missing**
- store at room temperature

Professional Information:

Overdosage Information: For overdosage information, please refer to pg. 689

Inactive Ingredients: acesulfame potassium, cellulose, citric acid, corn syrup, D&C Red #33, FD&C Red #40, flavors, glycerin, purified water, sodium benzoate, sorbitol, xanthan gum.

How Supplied: Pink colored, Bubble Gum flavored liquid in child resistant tamper-evident bottle of 4 fl. oz.

Shown in Product Identification Guide, page 513

CHILDREN'S TYLENOL® Plus Sinus

Description: *Children's TYLENOL® Plus Sinus* Suspension Liquid is Fruit Burst-flavored and contains no alcohol or aspirin. Each teaspoon (5 mL) contains acetaminophen 160 mg and pseudoephedrine HCl 15 mg.

Actions: *Children's TYLENOL® Plus Sinus* Suspension Liquid combines the analgesic-antipyretic acetaminophen with the decongestant pseudoephedrine hydrochloride to provide fast, effective, temporary relief of all your child's sinus symptoms including stuffy nose, sinus headache, sinus pressure, sinus pain, and nasal congestion. Acetaminophen is equal to aspirin in analgesic and antipyretic effectiveness and is unlikely to produce the side effects often associated with aspirin or aspirin-containing products.

Uses:

temporarily relieves:
• sinus congestion • stuffy nose • sinus pressure • minor aches, pains and headache • temporarily reduces fever

Directions:

See Table 1: Children's Tylenol Dosing Chart on pgs. 692–694

Precautions: If a rare sensitivity reaction occurs, the drug should be discontinued.

Warnings:

Do not use

- in a child who is taking a prescription monoamine oxidase inhibitor (MAOI) (certain drugs for depression, psychiatric, or emotional conditions, or Parkinson's disease), or for 2 weeks after stopping the MAOI drug. If you do not know if your child's prescription drug contains an MAOI, ask a doctor or pharmacist before giving this product.
- with any products containing acetaminophen

Ask a doctor before use if the child has

- heart disease • high blood pressure
- thyroid disease • diabetes

When using this product

- **do not exceed recommended dosage (see overdose warning)**

Stop use and ask a doctor if

- new symptoms occur
- redness or swelling is present
- pain gets worse or lasts for more than 5 days
- fever gets worse or lasts for more than 3 days
- nervousness, dizziness or sleeplessness occurs

Keep out of reach of children.

Overdose Warning: Taking more than the recommended dose (overdose) may cause liver damage. In case of overdose, get medical help or contact a Poison Control Center right away. Quick medical attention is critical even if you do not notice any signs or symptoms.

Other Information:

- **do not use if plastic carton wrap, bottle wrap, or foil inner seal imprinted "Safety Seal®" is broken or missing**
- store at room temperature

Professional Information:

Overdosage Information:
For overdosage information, please refer to pg. 689

Inactive Ingredients: acesulfame potassium, cellulose, citric acid, corn syrup, D&C Red #33, FD&C Red #40, flavors, glycerin, purified water, sodium benzoate, sorbitol, xanthan gum.

How Supplied: Red-colored, Fruit flavored liquid in child resistant tamper-evident bottles of 4 fl. oz.

Shown in Product Identification Guide, page 513

Children's TYLENOL® Dosing Chart

[See table on pages 692 through 694]

Mission Pharmacal Company

10999 IH 10 WEST
SUITE 1000
SAN ANTONIO, TX 78230-1355

Direct Inquiries to:
PO Box 786099
San Antonio, TX 78278-6099
TOLL FREE: (800) 292-7364
(210) 696-8400
FAX: (210) 696-6010
For Medical Information Contact:
In Emergencies:
Mary Ann Walter

THERA-GESIC®

[thĕr'ə-jē-zik]
TOPICAL ANALGESIC CREME

Active Ingredients:

	Purpose:
Menthol 1%	Analgesic
Methyl Salicylate 15%	Counterirritant

Use: Temporary relief of minor aches and pains of muscles and joints associated with: Arthritis, simple backaches, strains, bruises, sprains.

Warnings:

For external use only. Use only as directed. Avoid contact with eyes or mucous membranes.

Do not bandage tightly Do not bandage, wrap or cover until after washing the areas where THERA-GESIC has been applied.

Do not use

- immediately after shower or bath
- if skin is sensitive to oil of wintergreen (methyl salicylate)
- on wounds or damaged skin

Ask a doctor before use

- for children under 2 and through 12 years of age
- if prone or sensitive to allergic reactions from aspirin or salicylate

Continued on next page

Thera-Gesic—Cont.

When using this product
• discontinue use if skin irritation develops, or redness is present
• do not swallow
• do not use a heating pad after application of THERA-GESIC

Stop use and ask a doctor if condition worsens, or if symptoms persist for more than 7 days or clear up and occur again within a few days.

If pregnant or breast-feeding, ask a health professional before use.

Keep out of reach of children to avoid accidental poisoning. If swallowed, get medical help or contact a Poison Control Center right away.

Directions: Adults and children 12 or more years of age: Apply thin layers of creme into and around the sore or painful area, not more than 3 to 4 times daily. The number of thin layers controls the intensity of the action of THERA-GESIC. One thin layer provides a mild effect, two thin layers provide a strong effect and three thin layers provide a very strong effect. SEE WARNINGS.

Other Information: Once THERA-GESIC has penetrated the skin, the area may be washed, leaving it dry, clean and fragrance-free without decreasing the effectiveness of the product. Avoid contact with clothing or other surfaces. Store at 20–25° C (68–77° F).

Inactive Ingredients: Carbomer 934, Dimethicone, Glycerine, Methylparaben, Propylparaben, Sodium Lauryl Sulfate, Trolamine, Water.

How Supplied:
NDC 0178-0320-03   3 oz. tube
NDC 0178-0320-05   5 oz. tube

THERA-GESIC® PLUS
[thĕr ə-jē-zĭk]
TOPICAL ANALGESIC CREME

Active Ingredients: .... **Purpose:**
Methyl Salicylate
    25% .... Topical Analgesic
Menthol 4% .... Topical Analgesic

Use: Temporary relief of minor aches and pains of muscles and joints associated with: arthritis, simple backaches, strains, bruises, sprains.

Warnings:
For external use only. Use only as directed. Avoid contact with eyes or mucous membranes.

Do not bandage tightly. Do not bandage, wrap or cover until after washing the areas where THERA-GESIC® PLUS has been applied.

Do not use
• immediately after shower or bath
• if skin is sensitive to oil of wintergreen (methyl salicylate)
• on wounds or damaged skin

Ask a doctor before use
• for children under 2 and through 12 years of age
• if prone or sensitive to allergic reactions from aspirin or salicylate

When using this product
• discontinue use if skin irritation develops, or redness is present
• do not swallow
• do not use a heating pad after application of THERA-GESIC® PLUS

Stop use and ask a doctor if condition worsens, or if symptoms persist for more than 7 days or clear up and occur again within a few days.

If pregnant or breast-feeding, ask a health professional before use.

Keep out of reach of children to avoid accidental posoning. If swallowed, get medical help or contact a Poison Control Center right away.

Directions: Adults and children 12 or more years of age: Apply thin layers of creme into and around the sore or painful area, not more than 3 to 4 times daily. The number of thin layers controls the intensity of the action of THERA-GESIC® PLUS. One thin layer provides a mild effect, two thin layers provide a strong effect and three thin layers provide a very strong effect. SEE WARNINGS.

Other Information: Once THERA-GESIC® PLUS has penetrated the skin, the area may be washed, leaving it dry, clean and fragrance-free without decreasing the effectiveness of the product. Avoid contact with clothing or other surfaces. Store at 20–25°C (68–77°F).

Inactive Ingredients: Aloe Vera, Carbomer 980, Dimethicone, Glycerine, Methylparaben, Propylparaben, Sodium Lauryl Sulfate, Trolamine, Water.

How Supplied:
NDC 0178-0350-03   3 oz. tube
NDC 0178-0350-05   5 oz. tube

Novartis Consumer Health, Inc.

**200 KIMBALL DRIVE
PARSIPPANY, NJ 07054-0622**

Direct Product Inquiries to:
Consumer & Professional Affairs
(800) 452-0051
Fax: (800) 635-2801

Or write to above address.

DESENEX® ANTIFUNGALS
All products are Prescription Strength
Shake Powder
Liquid Spray
Spray Powder
Jock Itch Spray Powder

Drug Facts

Active Ingredient: **Purpose:**
Miconazole nitrate 2% .... Antifungal

Uses: Shake Powder, Liquid Spray, and Spray Powder
• cures most athlete's foot (tinea pedis) and ringworm (tinea corporis) • relieves itching, scaling, burning, and discomfort that can accompany athlete's foot
Jock Itch Spray Powder
• cures most jock itch (tinea cruris) • relieves itching, scaling, burning and discomfort that can accompany jock itch

Warnings: Liquid Spray, Spray Powder, Jock Itch Spray Powder
For external use only
Flammability Warning: For Spray Powder, Spray Liquid, and Jock Itch Spray Powder Contents under pressure. Do not puncture or incinerate. Flammable mixture; do not use near fire or flame, or expose to heat or temperatures above 49°C (120°F). Use only as directed. Intentional misuse by deliberately concentrating and inhaling the contents can be harmful or fatal.
Do not use • in or near the mouth or the eyes • for nail or scalp infections
When using this product • do not get into the eyes or mouth
Stop use and ask a doctor if • irritation occurs or gets worse • no improvement within 4 weeks for athlete's foot and ringworm, or no improvement within 2 weeks for jock itch.
Keep out of reach of children. If swallowed, get medical help or contact a poison control center right away.

Directions:
• adults and children 2 years and older
• wash the affected area with soap and water and dry completely before applying
Shake Powder
• apply a thin layer over affected area twice a day (morning and night) or as directed by a doctor
• pay special attention to the spaces between the toes. Wear well-fitting, ventilated shoes and change shoes and socks at least once a day.
• use every day for 4 weeks
• supervise children in the use of this product
• children under 2 years of age: ask a doctor
Liquid Spray and Spray Powder
• shake can well, hold 4″ to 6″ from skin
• spray a thin layer over affected area twice a day (morning and night) or as directed by a doctor
• for athlete's foot pay special attention to the spaces between the toes. Wear well-fitting, ventilated shoes and change shoes and socks at least once a day.
• use daily for 4 weeks
Jock Itch Spray Powder
• shake can well, hold 4″ to 6″ from skin
• spray a thin layer over affected area twice a day (morning and night) or as directed by a doctor
• use daily for 2 weeks
Other Information: • store at controlled room temperature 20-25°C (68-77°F) • see bottom of can for lot number and expiration date
Liquid Spray, Spray Powder and Jock Itch Spray Powder
• if clogging occurs, remove button and clean nozzle with a pin

Inactive Ingredients: Shake Powder—corn starch, corn starch/acrylamide/sodium acrylate polymer, fragrance, talc Liquid Spray—polyethylene glycol 300, polysorbate 20, SD alcohol 40-B (15%w/w) Propellant: dimethyl ether Spray Powder, Jock Itch Spray Powder—aloe vera gel, aluminum starch octenyl succinate, isopropyl myristate, propylene carbonate, SD alcohol 40-B (10% w/w), sorbitan monooleate, stearalkonium hectorite Propellant: isobutane/propane

How Supplied: Shake Powder-1.5 oz, 3 oz, 4 oz plastic bottles.
Spray Powder-3 oz, 4 oz cans
Liquid Spray-3.5 oz, 4.6 oz cans
Jock Itch Spray Powder-3 oz and 4 oz cans
Novartis Consumer Health, Inc.
Parsippany, NJ 07054-0622 ©2004
Shown in Product Identification Guide, page 515

EX•LAX®
Chocolated Laxative Pieces

Active Ingredient: Sennosides, USP, 15mg

Use: For Relief of
• OCCASIONAL CONSTIPATION (IRREGULARITY). This product generally produces bowel movement in 6 to 12 hours.

Directions: Adults and children 12 years of age and over: chew 2 chocolated pieces once or twice daily. Children 6 to under 12 years of age: chew 1 chocolated piece once or twice daily. Children under 6 years of age: consult a doctor.

Warnings:
• as with any drug, if you are pregnant or nursing a baby, seek the advice of a health professional before using this product.
Unless directed by a doctor, do not use
• laxative products when abdominal pain, nausea, or vomiting is present.
• laxative products for a period longer than 1 week.
Consult a doctor before using a laxative if
• you have noticed a sudden change in bowel habits that persists over a period of 2 weeks.
Consult a doctor and stop using a laxative if
• rectal bleeding occurs or you fail to have a bowel movement after use because this may indicate a serious condition.
Keep this and all drugs out of the reach of children
In case of accidental overdose, seek professional assistance or contact a poison control center immediately.

Inactive Ingredients: cocoa, confectioners sugar, hydrogenated palm kernel oil, lecithin, non-fat dry milk, vanillin. Store at controlled room temperature 20–25°C (68–77°F)

How Supplied: Available in boxes of 18 ct. and 48 ct. chewable chocolated pieces.
Novartis Consumer Health, Inc.
Parsippany, NJ 07054-0622 ©2003
Shown in Product Identification Guide, page 516

EX•LAX® Laxative Pills
Regular Strength Ex•Lax® Laxative Pills
Maximum Strength Ex•Lax® Laxative Pills

Active Ingredients: *Regular Strength Ex•Lax Laxative Pills:* Sennosides, USP, 15 mg. *Maximum Relief Formula Ex•Lax Laxative Pills:* Sennosides, USP, 25 mg.

Use: For Relief of
• OCCASIONAL CONSTIPATION (IRREGULARITY). This product generally produces bowel movement in 6 to 12 hours.

Warnings:
• as with any drug, if you are pregnant or nursing a baby, seek the advice of a health professional before using this product.
Unless directed by a doctor, do not use:
• laxative products when abdominal pain, nausea, or vomiting is present.
• laxative products for a period longer than 1 week.
Consult a doctor before using a laxative if:
• you have noticed a sudden change in bowel habits that persists over a period of 2 weeks.
Consult a doctor and stop using a laxative if:
• rectal bleeding occurs or you fail to have a bowel movement after use because this may indicate a serious condition.
Keep this and all drugs out of the reach of children. In case of accidental overdose, seek professional assistance or contact a poison control center immediately.

Dosage and Administration: *Regular Strength Ex•Lax Laxative Pills, and Maximum Strength Ex•Lax Laxative Pills*—Adults and children 12 years of age and over: take 2 pills once or twice daily with a glass of water. Children 6 to under 12 years of age: take 1 pill once or twice daily with a glass of water. Children under 6 years of age: consult a doctor.

Inactive Ingredients: *Regular Strength Ex•Lax Laxative Pills*—acacia, alginic acid, carnauba wax, colloidal silicon dioxide, dibasic calcium phosphate, iron oxides, magnesium stearate, microcrystalline cellulose, sodium benzoate, sodium lauryl sulfate, starch, stearic acid, sucrose, talc, titanium dioxide. Sodium-free. *Maximum Strength Ex•Lax Laxative Pills:* acacia, alginic acid, FD&C Blue No. 1 aluminum lake, carnauba wax, colloidal silicon dioxide, dibasic calcium phosphate, magnesium stearate, microcrystalline cellulose, povidone, sodium benzoate, sodium lauryl sulfate, starch, stearic acid, sucrose, talc, titanium dioxide. Very low sodium.
Store at controlled room temperature 20–25°C (68–77°F)

How Supplied: *Regular Strength Ex•Lax Laxative Pills*—Available in boxes of 8 ct. and 30 ct. pills. *Maximum Strength Ex•Lax Laxative Pills*—Available in boxes of 24 ct., 48 ct., and 90 ct. pills.
Novartis Consumer Health, Inc.
Parsippany, NJ 07054-0622 ©2003
Shown in Product Identification Guide, page 515

EX•LAX® MILK OF MAGNESIA STIMULANT FREE Liquid: Laxative/Antacid, Chocolate Creme, Mint, Raspberry Creme

Active Ingredient: Magnesium hydroxide – 400 mg per teaspoon (5 ml)

Uses: As a Laxative: To relieve occasional constipation (irregularity). This saline laxative product generally produces bowel movement in ½ to 6 hours.
As an Antacid: To relieve acid indigestion, sour stomach and heartburn and upset stomach due to these symptoms.

Warnings:
Laxative Warnings: Do not take any laxative if abdominal pain, nausea, vomiting or kidney disease are present unless directed by a doctor. If you have noticed a sudden change in bowel habits persisting for over 2 weeks, consult a doctor before using a laxative. Laxative products should not be used for a period longer than 1 week, unless directed by a doctor. Rectal bleeding or failure to have a bowel movement after use of a laxative may indicate a serious condition. Discontinue use and consult your doctor. Ask a doctor or pharmacist before use if you are taking any other drug. Take this product 2 or more hours before or after other drugs. Laxatives may affect how other drugs work.

Antacid Warnings: Do not take more than the maximum recommended daily dosage in a 24 hour period (See Directions), or use the maximum dosage of this product for more than two weeks, or use this product if you have kidney disease, except under the advice and super-

Continued on next page

Information on Novartis Consumer Health, Inc. products appearing on these pages is effective as of November 2003.

Ex-Lax M.O.M.—Cont.

vision of a doctor. May have laxative effect. Ask a doctor or pharmacist before use if you are taking a prescription drug. Antacids may interact with certain prescription drugs.

Laxative and Antacid Warnings: As with any drug, if you are pregnant or nursing a baby, seek the advice of a health professional before using this product. Keep out of reach of children. In case of overdose, get medical help or contact a poison control center right away.

Directions: Shake well before using.
For Laxative Use: Adults/Children – 12 years and older: 2–4 tablespoonsful (TBSP) at bedtime or upon arising, followed by a full glass (8 oz.) of liquid.
Children: – 6–11 years: 1–2 tablespoonsful (TBSP), followed by a full glass (8 oz.) of liquid.
Children 2–5 years: DO NOT USE DOSAGE CUP 1–3 teaspoonsful, followed by a full glass (8 oz.) of liquid.
Under 2 years: Consult a doctor.
FOR ANTACID USE: DO NOT USE DOSAGE CUP – Adults/Children - 12 years and older: 1–3 teaspoonsful, up to four times a day or as directed by a doctor.

Inactive Ingredients:
Chocolate Creme: carboxymethylcellulose sodium, flavors, glycerin, hypromellose, microcrystalline cellulose, purified water, saccharin sodium, simethicone, sorbitol.
Mint: carboxymethylcellulose sodium, flavors, glycerin, hypromellose, microcrystalline cellulose, purified water, saccharin sodium, simethicone, sorbitol.
Raspberry Creme: carboxymethylcellulose sodium, flavors, glycerin, hypromellose, microcrystalline cellulose, purified water, saccharin sodium, simethicone, sorbitol.

How Supplied: EX•LAX MILK OF MAGNESIA is available in chocolate creme, mint and raspberry creme flavors and comes in 12 oz. (355 ml) bottles.
Store at controlled room temperature 20–25°C (68–77°F). Keep tightly closed and avoid freezing.
Distributed by:
Novartis Consumer Health, Inc.
Parsippany, NJ 07054-0622 ©2003
Shown in Product Identification Guide, page 515 & 516

EX•LAX® ULTRA
Stimulant Laxative

Drug Facts:

Active Ingredient
(in each tablet):   **Purpose:**
Bisacodyl, 5 mg .... Stimulant laxative

Uses: • relieves occasional constipation • generally produces bowel movement in 6 to 12 hours

Warnings:
Do not use laxative products when abdominal pain, nausea, or vomiting are present
Ask a doctor before use if you
• want to administer to a child under 6 years of age
• have noticed a sudden change in bowel habits that persists over a period of 2 weeks
• cannot swallow without chewing
• are taking any other drug. Take this product 2 or more hours before or after other drugs.
Laxatives may affect how other drugs work.
When using this product
• do not chew or crush tablets
• do not take within 1 hour of taking an antacid or milk
• do not use for a period longer than 1 week
• it may cause abdominal discomfort, faintness and cramps
Stop use and ask a doctor if
• rectal bleeding or failure to have a bowel movement occur after use of a laxative.
These may be signs of a serious condition.
If pregnant or breast-feeding, ask a health care professional before use.
Keep out of reach of children. In case of overdose, get medical help or contact a Poison Control Center right away.

Directions: • take with a glass of water

Adults and children 12 years of age and over	take one tablet daily. If necessary, take up to a maximum of three tablets in a single dose once daily.
Children 6 to under 12 years of age	take one tablet
Children under 6 years of age	consult a doctor

Other Information: each tablet contains: sodium 0.1mg
• store at controlled room temperature 20–25°C (68–77°F)

Inactive Ingredients: ammonium hydroxide, butyl alcohol, colloidal silicon dioxide, croscarmellose sodium, FD&C yellow 6, iron oxide black, isopropyl alcohol, lactose, magnesium stearate, methacrylic acid, methanol, methylparaben, microcrystalline cellulose, PEG 3350, polyvinyl alcohol, propylene glycol, SD-45 alcohol, shellac, silica, sodium bicarbonate, sodium lauryl sulfate, talc, titanium dioxide, triethyl citrate.

How Supplied: Available in boxes of 24 ct. and 48 ct. cartons.
Tamper Evident Feature: Ex•Lax® Pills are sealed in blister packets. Use only if the individual seal is unbroken.
Questions? call **1-800-452-0051** 24 hours a day, 7 days a week.

Tablets Non-USP (Disintegration)
Novartis Consumer Health, Inc.
Parsippany, NJ 07054-0622 ©2003
Shown in Product Identification Guide, page 516

GAS–X® REGULAR STRENGTH
Antigas Chewable Tablets
GAS–X® EXTRA STRENGTH
Antigas Softgels and Chewable Tablets
GAS–X® MAXIMUM STRENGTH
Antigas Softgels
GAS–X® WITH MAALOX®
Antigas/Antacid Softgels and Chewable Tablets

Active Ingredients:
Regular Strength—Each chewable tablet contains simethicone 80 mg.
Extra Strength—Each chewable tablet and swallowable softgel contains simethicone, 125 mg.
Maximum Strength—Each Swallowable softgel contains simethicone, 166 mg.
Gas-X with Maalox Tablets—Each extra strength chewable tablet contains simethicone 125 mg and calcium carbonate 500 mg.
Gas-X with Maalox Softgels—Each swallowable softgel contains simethicone 62.5 mg and calcium carbonate 250 mg.

Inactive Ingredients:
Regular Strength Peppermint Creme: calcium carbonate, dextrose, flavors, maltodextrin, starch
Regular Strength Cherry Creme: calcium carbonate, D&C Red 30 aluminum lake, dextrose, flavors, maltodextrin, propylene glycol, soy protein isolate
Extra Strength Peppermint Creme: calcium phosphate tribasic, colloidal silicon dioxide, D&C Yellow 10 aluminum lake, D&C Red 30 aluminum lake, dextrose, flavors, maltodextrin, starch
Extra Strength Cherry Creme: calcium phosphate tribasic, colloidal silicon dioxide, D&C Red 30 aluminum lake, dextrose, flavors, maltodextrin, propylene glycol, soy protein isolate, starch
Extra Strength Softgels: D&C Yellow 10, FD&C Blue 1, FD&C Red 40, gelatin, glycerin, peppermint oil, purified water, sorbitol, titanium dioxide
Maximum Strength Softgels: FD&C Blue 1, FD&C Red 40, gelatin, glycerin, peppermint oil, purified water, sorbitol
Gas-X With Maalox Wildberry Tablets: colloidal silicon dioxide, D&C Red 30, dextrose, flavors, maltodextrin, mannitol, pregelatinized starch, talc, tribasic calcium phosphate
Gas-X With Maalox Orange Tablets: colloidal silicon dioxide, dextrose, FD&C yellow 6 aluminum lake, flavors, maltodextrin, mannitol, pregelatinized starch, talc, tribasic calcium phosphate

Gas-X® With Maalox® Softgels:
D&C Red 28, FD&C Blue 1, gelatin, glycerin, polyethylene glycol, polysorbate 80, silicon dioxide, sorbitol, titanium dioxide, purified water

Use:
Gas-X: For the relief of pressure and bloating commonly referred to as gas.
Gas-X with Maalox: Relief of the concurrent symptoms of gas associated with heartburn, sour stomach or acid indigestion.

Warning: Keep out of reach of children.

Gas-X
Drug Interaction Precautions: No known drug interaction.
Gax-X® with Maalox® Tablets and Softgels
Warnings:
Ask a doctor or pharmacist before use if you are now taking a prescription drug. Antacids may interact with certain prescription drugs.

Gas-X
Dosage and Administration: For Chewable Tablets: Adults: Chew one or two tablets as needed after meals or at bedtime. Do not exceed six Regular Strength chewable tablets or four Extra Strength chewable tablets in 24 hours except under the advice and supervision of a physician.
For Extra Strength Softgels: Adults: Swallow with water 1 or 2 softgels as needed after meals or at bedtime. Do not exceed 4 softgels in 24 hours except under the advice and supervision of a physician.
For Maximum Strength Softgels: Adults: Swallow with water 1 or 2 softgels as needed after meals or at bedtime. Do not exceed 3 softgels in 24 hours except under the advice and supervision of a physician.
For Gas-X with Maalox Tablets: Chew 1 to 2 tablets as symptoms occur or as directed by a physician. Do not take more than 4 tablets in a 24-hour period or use the maximum dosage for more than 2 weeks except under the advice and supervision of a physician.
For Gas-X® with Maalox® Softgels: Adults: Swallow with water 2 to 4 softgels as symptoms occur or as directed by a physician. Do not exceed 8 softgels in a 24 hour period or use the maximum dosage for more than 2 weeks except under the advice and supervision of a physician.

Professional Labeling: Gas-X may be used in the alleviation of postoperative bloating/pressure, and for use in endoscopic examination.

How Supplied:
Regular Strength Chewable tablets are available in peppermint creme and cherry creme flavored, chewable, scored tablets in boxes of 36 tablets.
Extra Strength Chewable tablets are available in peppermint creme and cherry creme flavored, chewable, scored tablets in boxes of 18 tablets.
Easy-to-swallow, tasteless/Extra Strength Softgels are available in boxes of 10 pills, 30 pills, 50 pills and 60 pills.

Easy-to-swallow, tasteless/Maximum Strength Softgels are available in boxes of 50 pills.
Gas-X With Maalox Tablets are available in orange and wild berry flavored, chewable tablets in boxes of 8 tablets and 24 tablets
Easy-to-swallow, tasteless/Gax-X with Maalox Softgels are available in boxes of 24 pills and 48 pills.

Shown in Product Identification Guide, page 516

LAMISIL ᴬᵀ® CREAM

Active Ingredient:	**Purpose:**

Terbinafine
  hydrochloride 1% .... Antifungal

Uses:
• **cures most athlete's foot (tinea pedis)**
• **cures most jock itch (tinea cruris) and ringworm (tinea corporis)**
• **relieves itching, burning, cracking and scaling which accompany these conditions**

Warnings:
For external use only
Do not use • on nails or scalp
• in or near the mouth or the eyes
• for vaginal yeast infections
When using this product do not get into the eyes. If eye contact occurs, rinse thoroughly with water.
Stop use and ask a doctor if too much irritation occurs or gets worse.
Keep out of reach of children. If swallowed, get medical help or contact a poison control center right away.

Directions:
• adults and children 12 years and over
  • use the tip of the cap to break the seal and open the tube
  • wash the affected skin with soap and water and dry completely before applying
  • **for athlete's foot** wear well-fitting, ventilated shoes. Change shoes and socks at least once daily.
  • **between the toes only:** apply twice a day (morning and night) for **1 week** or as directed by a doctor.

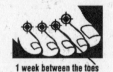

1 week between the toes

• **on the bottom or sides of the foot:** apply twice a day (morning and night) for **2 weeks** or as directed by a doctor.

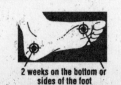

2 weeks on the bottom or sides of the foot

• **for jock itch and ringworm:** apply once a day (morning **or** night) for **1 week** or as directed by a doctor.
• wash hands after each use
• children under 12 years: ask a doctor
Other Information: • do not use if seal on tube is broken or is not visible
• store at controlled room temperature 20–25°C (68–77°F)

Inactive Ingredients: benzyl alcohol, cetyl alcohol, cetyl palmitate, isopropyl myristate, polysorbate 60, purified water, sodium hydroxide, sorbitan monostearate, stearyl alcohol.

How Supplied: Athlete's Foot — Net wt. 12g (.42 oz.) tube and 24g (.85 oz.) tube, Jock Itch — Net wt. 12g (.42 oz.) tube.

Questions? call **1-800-452-0051** 24 hours a day, 7 days a week.
Novartis Consumer Health, Inc.
Parsippany, NJ 07054-0622 ©2002
Shown in Product Identification Guide, page 516

MAALOX MAX® MAXIMUM STRENGTH ANTACID/ANTI-GAS Liquid
Oral Suspension Antacid/Anti-Gas

Liquids
☐ **Lemon**
☐ **Cherry**
☐ **Mint**
☐ **Vanilla Crème**
☐ **Wild Berry**

Drug Facts:
[See table at top of next page]

Uses: For the relief of
• acid indigestion
• heartburn
• sour stomach
• upset stomach associated with these symptoms
• bloating and pressure commonly referred to as gas

Warnings:
Ask a doctor before use if you have kidney disease.
Ask a doctor or pharmacist before use if you are taking a prescription drug. Antacids may interact with certain prescription drugs.
Stop use and ask a doctor if symptoms last for more than 2 weeks
Keep out of reach of children.

Directions:
• shake well before using
• Adults/children 12 years and older: take 2 to 4 teaspoons four times a day or as directed by a physician

Continued on next page

Information on Novartis Consumer Health, Inc. products appearing on these pages is effective as of November 2003.

Maalox Antacid/Anti-Gas—Cont.

- do not take more than 12 teaspoonsful in 24 hours or use the maximum dosage for more than 2 weeks.
- Children under 12 years: consult a physician

To aid in establishing proper dosage schedules, the following information is provided:

MAALOX Max® Maximum Strength Antacid/Anti-Gas	Per 2 Tsp. (10 mL) (Minimum Recommended Dosage)
Acid neutralizing capacity	38.8 mEq

Inactive Ingredients: butylparaben, carboxymethylcellulose sodium, D&C yellow #10 (lemon flavor only), flavor, hypromellose, microcrystalline cellulose, potassium citrate, propylparaben, purified water, saccharin sodium, sorbitol.

Professional Labeling

Indications: As an antacid for symptomatic relief of hyperacidity associated with the diagnosis of peptic ulcer, gastritis, peptic esophagitis, gastric hyperacidity, or hiatal hernia. As an antiflatulent to alleviate the symptoms of gas, including postoperative gas pain.

Warnings: Prolonged use of aluminum-containing antacids in patients with renal failure may result in or worsen dialysis osteomalacia. Elevated tissue aluminum levels contribute to the development of the dialysis encephalopathy and osteomalacia syndromes. Small amounts of aluminum are absorbed from the gastrointestinal tract and renal excretion of aluminum is impaired in renal failure. Aluminum is not well removed by dialysis because it is bound to albumin and transferrin, which do not cross dialysis membranes. As a result, aluminum is deposited in bone, and dialysis osteomalacia may develop when large amounts of aluminum are ingested orally by patients with impaired renal function.

Aluminum forms insoluble complexes with phosphate in the gastrointestinal tract, thus decreasing phosphate absorption. Prolonged use of aluminum-containing antacids by normophosphatemic patients may result in hypophosphatemia if phosphate intake is not adequate. In its more severe forms, hypophosphatemia can lead to anorexia, malaise, muscle weakness, and osteomalacia.

Advantages: In addition to the fast acting antacid ingredients, Aluminum Hydroxide and Magnesium Hydroxide, MAALOX® Max™ Maximum Strength Antacid/Antigas contains the powerful

	Maalox Max® Maximum Strength Antacid/Anti-Gas	
Active Ingredients	Per Tsp. (5 mL)	Purpose
Aluminum Hydroxide (equivalent to dried gel, USP)	400 mg	antacid
Magnesium Hydroxide	400 mg	antacid
Simethicone	40 mg	antigas

antigas ingredient, simethicone, to provide concurrent fast relief from discomfort associated with gas.

How Supplied:
MAALOX MAX® MAXIMUM STRENGTH ANTACID/ANTI-GAS Liquid Oral Suspension Antacid/Anti-Gas
Lemon is available in plastic bottles of 12 fl. oz. (355 mL), and 26 fl. oz. (769 mL).
Cherry is available in plastic bottles of 12 fl. oz. (355 mL) and 26 fl. oz. (769 mL).
Mint is available in plastic bottles of 12 fl. oz. (355 mL) and.
Vanilla Crème is available in Plastic Bottles of 12 fl. oz. (355 mL).
Wild Berry is available in Plastic Bottles of 12 fl. oz. (355 mL).
Novartis Consumer Health, Inc.
Parsippany, NJ 07054-0622 ©2003

Shown in Product Identification Guide, page 517

MAALOX®
Regular Strength
Liquid Antacid/Anti-Gas

Liquids
- Cooling Mint
- Smooth Cherry
[See table below]

Uses: For the relief of
- acid indigestion
- heartburn
- sour stomach
- upset stomach associated with these symptoms
- bloating and pressure commonly referred to as gas

Warnings:
Ask a doctor before use if you have kidney disease

Ask a doctor or pharmacist before use if you are taking a prescription drug. Antacids may interact with certain prescription drugs.
Stop use and ask a doctor if symptoms last for more than 2 weeks
Keep out of reach of children.

Directions:
- shake well before using
- Adults/children 12 years and older: take 2 to 4 teaspoons four times a day or as directed by a physician
- do not take more than 16 teaspoonsful in 24 hours or use the maximum dosage for more than 2 weeks.
- Children under 12 years: consult a physician

Inactive Ingredients: butylparaben, carboxymethylcellulose sodium, flavor, hypromellose, microcrystalline cellulose, propylparaben, purified water, saccharin sodium, sorbitol.

Maalox Suspension Per 2 Tsp. (10 mL) (Minimum Recommended Dosage)	
Acid neutralizing capacity	19.4 mEq

Professional Labeling
Indications: As an antacid for symptomatic relief of hyperacidity associated with the diagnosis of peptic ulcer, gastritis, peptic esophagitis, gastric hyperacidity, or hiatal hernia. As an antiflatulent to alleviate the symptoms of gas, including postoperative gas pain.

Warnings: Prolonged use of aluminum-containing antacids in patients with renal failure may result in or worsen dialysis osteomalacia. Elevated tissue aluminum levels contribute to the

Drug Facts

Active Ingredients	Maalox Suspension 5 mL teaspoon	Purpose
Aluminum Hydroxide (equivalent to dried gel, USP)	200 mg	Antacid
Magnesium Hydroxide	200 mg	Antacid
Simethicone	20 mg	Antigas

development of the dialysis encephalopathy and osteomalacia syndromes. Small amounts of aluminum are absorbed from the gastrointestinal tract and renal excretion of aluminum is impaired in renal failure. Aluminum is not well removed by dialysis because it is bound to albumin and transferrin, which do not cross dialysis membranes. As a result, aluminum is deposited in bone, and dialysis osteomalacia may develop when large amounts of aluminum are ingested orally by patients with impaired renal function. Aluminum forms insoluble complexes with phosphate in the gastrointestinal tract, thus decreasing phosphate absorption. Prolonged use of aluminum-containing antacids by normophosphatemic patients may result in hypophosphatemia if phosphate intake is not adequate. In its more severe forms, hypophosphatemia can lead to anorexia, malaise, muscle weakness, and osteomalacia.

Advantages: In addition to the fast acting antacid ingredients, Aluminum Hydroxide and Magnesium Hydroxide, MAALOX® Regular Strength Antacid/Antigas contains the powerful antigas ingredient, simethicone, to provide concurrent fast relief from discomfort associated with gas.

How Supplied:
Maalox® Cooling Mint Suspension is available in plastic bottles of 5 oz. (148 mL), 12 oz. (355 mL) and 26 oz. (769 mL)
Maalox® Smooth Cherry Suspension is available in plastic bottles of 12 oz. (355 mL)
Novartis Consumer Health, Inc.
Parsippany, NJ 07054-0622 ©2003
Shown in Product Identification Guide, page 516

MAXIMUM STRENGTH MAALOX® TOTAL Stomach Relief™
Bismuth Subsalicylate/Upset Stomach Reliever
Peppermint

Drug Facts

Active Ingredient: **Purpose:**
(in each 15 mL*)
Bismuth subsalicylate
    525 mg .... Upset stomach reliever

---
*15 mL = 1 tablespoon

Uses: • upset stomach • heartburn • nausea • fullness • indigestion

Warnings:
Reye's syndrome: Children and teenagers who have or are recovering from chicken pox or flu-like symptoms should not use this product. When using this product, if changes in behavior with nausea and vomiting occur, consult a doctor because these symptoms could be an early sign of Reye's syndrome, a rare but serious illness.

Allergy alert: Do not take this product if you are allergic to salicylates (including aspirin) unless directed by a doctor.
Ask a doctor or pharmacist before use if you are taking a prescription drug for anticoagulation (blood thinning), diabetes, gout, or arthritis
Stop use and ask a doctor if
• symptoms last more than 2 days
• ringing in the ears or a loss of hearing occurs if taken with other salicylates-containing preparations (such as aspirin)
If pregnant or breast-feeding, ask a health care professional before use.
Keep out of reach of children. In case of overdose, get medical help or contact a poison control center right away.

Directions: • shake well before using
• adults and children 12 years of age and older: 2 tablespoons (30 mL) every 1/2 hour to 1 hour, as required, not to exceed 8 tablespoons (120 mL) in 24 hours.
• children under 12 years of age: ask a doctor
Other Information:
• **each tablespoon contains:** sodium 3.3 mg
• each tablespoon contains: salicylate 232 mg
• store at controlled room temperature 20–25°C (68–77°F)
• keep tightly closed and avoid freezing

Inactive Ingredients: carboxymethylcellulose sodium, ethyl alcohol, flavor, methylparaben, microcrystalline cellulose, propylene glycol, propylparaben, purified water, salicylic acid, sodium salicylate, sorbitol, sucralose, xanthan gum
Questions? call **1-800-452-0051** 24 hours a day, 7 days a week.
U.S. Patent No. 5,904,973
Novartis Consumer Health, Inc.
Parsippany, NJ 07054-0622   ©2004
Made in Canada

MAXIMUM STRENGTH MAALOX® TOTAL Stomach Relief™
Bismuth Subsalicylate/Upset Stomach Reliever
Strawberry

Drug Facts

Active Ingredient: **Purpose:**
(in each 15 mL*)
Bismuth subsalicylate
    525 mg .... Upset stomach reliever

---
* 15 mL = 1 tablespoon

Uses: • upset stomach • heartburn • nausea • fullness • indigestion

Warnings:
Reye's syndrome: Children and teenagers who have or are recovering from chicken pox or flu-like symptoms should not use this product. When using this product, if changes in behavior with nausea and vomiting occur, consult a doctor

because these symptoms could be an early sign of Reye's syndrome, a rare but serious illness.
Allergy alert: Do not take this product if you are allergic to salicylates (including aspirin) unless directed by a doctor.
Ask a doctor or pharmacist before use if you are taking a prescription drug for anticoagulation (blood thinning), diabetes, gout, or arthritis
Stop use and ask a doctor if
• symptoms last more than 2 days
• ringing in the ears or a loss of hearing occurs if taken with other salicylates-containing preparations (such as aspirin)
If pregnant or breast-feeding, ask a health care professional before use.
Keep out of reach of children. In case of overdose, get medical help or contact a poison control center right away.

Directions: • shake well before using
• adults and children 12 years of age and older: 2 tablespoons (30 mL) every ½ hour to 1 hour, as required, not to exceed 8 tablespoons (120 mL) in 24 hours
• children under 12 years of age: ask a doctor
Other Information:
• **each tablespoon contains:** sodium 3.3 mg
• each tablespoon contains: salicylate 232 mg
• store at controlled room temperature 20–25°C (68–77°F)
• keep tightly closed and avoid freezing

Inactive Ingredients: carboxymethylcellulose sodium, flavor, methylparaben, microcrystalline cellulose, propylene glycol, propylparaben, purified water, salicylic acid, sodium salicylate, sorbitol, sucralose, xanthan gum
Questions? call **1-800-452-0051** 24 hours a day, 7 days a week.
U.S. Patent No. 5,904,973
Novartis Consumer Health, Inc.
Parsippany, NJ 07054-0622 ©2004
Made in Canada
Shown in Product Identification Guide, page 516

Quick Dissolve
MAALOX® Regular Strength Antacid.
Calcium Carbonate
Chewable Tablets
Lemon and Wild Berry flavors. Quick Dissolving Tablets

MAALOX® Regular Strength
Drug Facts

Active Ingredient: **Purpose:**
(in each tablet)
Calcium carbonate
    600 mg .... Antacid

Continued on next page

Information on Novartis Consumer Health, Inc. *products appearing on these pages is effective as of November 2003.*

Maalox Quick Dissolve—Cont.

Uses: For the relief of
- acid indigestion
- heartburn
- sour stomach
- upset stomach associated with these symptoms

Warnings:
Ask a doctor or pharmacist before use if you are: presently taking a prescription drug. Antacids may interact with certain prescription drugs
Stop use and ask a doctor if symptoms last for more than 2 weeks.
Keep out of reach of children.

Directions:
- Chew 1 to 2 tablets as symptoms occur or as directed by a physician
- do not take more than 12 tablets in a 24-hour period or use the maximum dosage for more than 2 weeks except under the advice and supervision of a physician

Other Information:
- Phenylketonurics: Contains Phenylalanine, .5 mg per tablet
- store at controlled room temperature 20–25°C (68–77°F)
- keep tightly closed and dry
- Acid neutralizing capacity (per 2 tablets) is 21.6 mEq.

Inactive Ingredients: aspartame, colloidal silicon dioxide, croscarmellose sodium, D&C Red #30 aluminum lake, D&C Yellow #10 aluminum lake, dextrose, FD&C Blue #1 aluminum lake, flavors, magnesium stearate, maltodextrin, mannitol, pregelatinized starch.

How Supplied:
Lemon — Plastic Bottles of 85 ct. Tablets.
Wild Berry — Plastic Bottles of 45 ct. Tablets.
Questions? call 1-800-452-0051 24 hours a day, 7 days a week.
Novartis Consumer Health, Inc.
Parisppany, NJ 07054-0622 ©2003
Shown in Product Identification Guide, page 516

Quick Dissolve
MAALOX Max® Maximum Strength
Antacid/Antigas.
Calcium Carbonate and Simethicone Chewable Tablets
Assorted, Lemon and Wild Berry Flavors. Quick Dissolving Tablets

Drug Facts:
MAALOX Max® Maximum Strength

Active Ingredients:
(in each tablet)	Purpose:
Calcium carbonate 1000 mg	Antacid
Simethicone 60 mg	Antigas

Uses: For the relief of
- acid indigestion
- heartburn
- sour stomach
- upset stomach associated with these symptoms

- bloating and pressure commonly referred to as gas

Warnings:
Allergy Alert: contains FD&C Yellow #5 aluminum lake (tartrazine) as a color additive
Ask a doctor or pharmacist before use if you are: presently taking a prescription drug. Antacids may interact with certain prescription drugs.
Stop use and ask a doctor if: symptoms last for more than 2 weeks.
Keep out of reach of children.

Directions:
- Chew 1 to 2 tablets as symptoms occur or as directed by a physician
- do not take more than 8 tablets in a 24-hour period or use the maximum dosage for more than 2 weeks except under the advice and supervision of a physician

Other Information:
- store at controlled room temperature 20–25°C (68–77°F)
- keep tightly closed and dry
- Acid neutralizing capacity (per 2 tablets) is 34mEq.

Inactive Ingredients: acesulfame K, colloidal silicon dioxide, croscarmellose sodium, dextrose, FD&C Red #40 aluminum lake, FD&C Yellow #5 aluminum lake, FD&C Yellow #6 aluminum lake, flavors, magnesium stearate, maltodextrin, mannitol, pregelatinized starch.

How Supplied:
Lemon — Plastic Bottles of 35 and 65 Tablets.
Wild Berry — Plastic Bottles of 35 and 65 Tablets.
Assorted — Plastic Bottles of 35, 65 and 90 Tablets.
Questions? call 1-800-452-0051 24 hours a day, 7 days a week.
Novartis Consumer Health, Inc.
Parsippany, NJ 07054-0622 ©2003
Shown in Product Identification Guide, page 517

THERAFLU® Severe Cold Caplets
Pain Reliever-Fever Reducer (Acetaminophen)/Antihistamine (Chlorpheniramine) Cough Suppressant (Dextromethorphan)/Nasal Decongestant (Pseudoephedrine)

Drug Facts
Active Ingredients:
(in each caplet)	Purpose:
Acetaminophen 500 mg	Pain reliever/ Fever reducer
Chlorpheniramine maleate 2 mg	Antihistamine
Dextromethorphan HBr 15 mg	Cough suppressant
Pseudoephedrine HCl 30 mg	Nasal decongestant

Uses: temporarily relieves these symptoms:
- headache • minor aches and pains
- runny nose • sneezing • itchy nose or throat • itchy, watery eyes • fever • minor sore throat pain • nasal and sinus congestion • cough due to minor throat and bronchial irritation

Warnings:
Alcohol Warning: If you consume 3 or more alcoholic drinks every day, ask your doctor whether you should take acetaminophen or any other pain relievers/ fever reducers. Acetaminophen may cause liver damage.
Do not use • if you are now taking a prescription monamine oxidase inhibitor (MAOI) (certain drugs for depression), psychiatric, or emotional conditions, or Parkinson's disease), or for 2 weeks after stopping the MAOI drug. If you do not know if your prescription drug contains an MAOI, ask a doctor or pharmacist before taking this product.
• with any other product containing acetaminophen **(see Overdose Warning)**
Ask a doctor before use if you have
- heart disease • high blood pressure
- thyroid disease • diabetes • glaucoma
- a breathing problem such as emphysema, asthma, or chronic bronchitis
- trouble urinating due to an enlarged prostate gland
- cough that occurs with smoking, too much phlegm (mucus) or chronic cough that lasts
Ask a doctor or pharmacist before use if you are taking sedatives or tranquilizers.
When using this product • do not use more than directed • avoid alcoholic drinks
- marked drowsiness may occur
- alcohol, sedatives, and tranquilizers may increase drowsiness
- be careful when driving a motor vehicle or operating machinery
- excitability may occur, especially in children
Stop use and ask a doctor if • nervousness, dizziness, or sleeplessness occurs
- symptoms do not improve for 7 days or occur with a fever
- cough persists for more than 7 days, comes back, or occurs with a fever, rash, or persistent headache
- symptoms do not improve for 10 days (pain) or for 3 days (fever)
- sore throat persists for more than 2 days, and occurs with a fever, headache, rash, nausea, or vomiting. These could be signs of a serious condition.
If pregnant or breast-feeding, ask a health care professional before use.
Keep out of reach of children.
Overdose Warning: Taking more than the recommended dose can cause serious health problems, including serious liver damage. In case of overdose, get medical help or contact a poison control center right away. Prompt medical attention is critical for adults as well as for children even if you do not notice any signs or symptoms.

Directions:
- do not use more than directed **(see Overdose Warning)**
- take every 6 hours; not more than 8 caplets in 24 hours
- adults and children 12 years of age and over: 2 caplets every 6 hours

- children under 12 years of age: consult a doctor

Other Information: • each caplet contains: **sodium 6 mg** • store at controlled room temperature 20–25°C (68–77°F)

Inactive Ingredients: colloidal silicon dioxide, croscarmellose sodium, D&C Yellow 10 aluminum lake, FD&C Blue 1 aluminum lake, FD&C Yellow 6 aluminum lake, gelatin, hydroxypropyl cellulose, hypromellose, lactose, magnesium stearate, methylparaben, polydextrose, polyethylene glycol, pregelatinized starch, titanium dioxide, triacetin

How Supplied: 24 coated caplets
Novartis Consumer Health, Inc.
Parsippany, NJ 07054-0622
©2003

Shown in Product Identification Guide, page 517

THERAFLU® Severe Cold Non-Drowsy Caplets
Pain Reliever-Fever Reducer
(Acetaminophen)/Cough
Suppressant (Dextromethorphan)
Nasal Decongestant
(Pseudoephedrine)

Drug Facts

Active Ingredients:
(in each caplet)   **Purpose:**
Acetaminophen 500 mg ... Pain reliever/
                                        Fever reducer
Dextromethorphan
    HBr 15 mg .... Cough suppressant
Pseudoephedrine
    HCl 30 mg .... Nasal decongestant

Uses: temporarily relieves these symptoms:
- minor aches and pains • minor sore throat pain • nasal and sinus congestion • cough due to minor throat and bronchial irritation

Warnings:
Alcohol Warning: If you consume 3 or more alcoholic drinks every day, ask your doctor whether you should take acetaminophen or any other pain relievers/fever reducers. Acetaminophen may cause liver damage.

Do not use • if you are now taking a prescription monoamine oxidase inhibitor (MAOI) (certain drugs for depression, psychiatric, or emotional conditions, or Parkinson's disease), or for 2 weeks after stopping the MAOI drug. If you do not know if your prescription drug contains an MAOI, ask a doctor or pharmacist before taking this product.
• with any other product containing acetaminophen (**see Overdose Warning**)

Ask a doctor before use if you have
- heart disease • high blood pressure
- thyroid disease • diabetes
- trouble urinating due to an enlarged prostate gland • glaucoma
- persistent or chronic cough as occurs with emphysema, asthma, or chronic bronchitis

- cough that occurs with smoking, too much phlegm (mucus) or chronic cough that lasts

When using this product • do not use more than directed

Stop use and ask a doctor if • nervousness, dizziness, or sleeplessness occurs
- symptoms do not improve for 7 days or occur with a fever
- cough persists for more than 7 days, comes back, or occurs with a fever, rash, or persistent headache
- symptoms do not improve for 10 days (pain) or for 3 days (fever)
- sore throat persists for more than 2 days, and occurs with a fever, headache, rash, nausea, or vomiting. These could be signs of a serious condition.

If pregnant or breast-feeding, ask a health care professional before use.

Keep out of reach of children.

Overdose Warning: Taking more than the recommended dose can cause serious health problems, including serious liver damage. In case of overdose, get medical help or contact a poison control center right away. Prompt medical attention is critical for adults as well as for children even if you do not notice any signs or symptoms.

Directions:
- do not use more than directed (**see Overdose Warning**)
- take every 6 hours; not more than 8 caplets in 24 hours
- adults and children 12 years of age and over: 2 caplets every 6 hours
- children under 12 years of age: consult a doctor

Other Information: • each caplet contains: **sodium 6 mg**
- store at controlled room temperature 20 25°C (68 77°F)

Inactive Ingredients: colloidal silicon dioxide, croscarmellose sodium, D&C Yellow 10 aluminum lake, FD&C Red 40 aluminum lake, FD&C Yellow 6 aluminum lake, gelatin, hydroxypropyl cellulose, hypromellose, lactose, magnesium stearate, methylparaben, polydextrose, polyethylene glycol, pregelatinized starch, titanium dioxide, triacetin

How Supplied: 12 coated caplets
Novartis Consumer Health, Inc.
Parsippany, NJ 07054-0622
©2003

Shown in Product Identification Guide, page 517

THERAFLU® Cold & Cough
Pain Reliever-Fever Reducer
(Acetaminophen)
Antihistamine (Chlorpheniramine)
Cough Suppressant
(Dextromethorphan)
Nasal Decongestant
(Pseudoephedrine)

Drug Facts

Active Ingredients
(in each packet):   **Purpose:**
Acetaminophen
    650 mg ..... Pain reliever/Fever reducer
Chlorpheniramine maleate
    4 mg .... Antihistamine
Dextromethorphan HBr
    20 mg .... Cough suppressant
Pseudoephedrine HCl
    60 mg .... Nasal decongestant

Uses: temporarily relieves these symptoms: • headache • sneezing • runny nose • fever • minor aches and pains • itchy nose or throat • itchy, watery eyes • minor sore throat pain • nasal and sinus congestion • cough due to minor throat and bronchial irritation

Warnings:
Alcohol Warning: If you consume 3 or more alcoholic drinks every day, ask your doctor whether you should take acetaminophen or other pain relievers/fever reducers. Acetaminophen may cause liver damage.

Do not use • if you are now taking a prescription monoamine oxidase inhibitor (MAOI) (certain drugs for depression, psychiatric, or emotional conditions, or Parkinson's disease), or for 2 weeks after stopping the MAOI drug. If you do not know if your prescription drug contains an MAOI, ask a doctor or pharmacist before taking this product.
• with any other product containing acetaminophen (**see Overdose Warning**)

Ask a doctor before use if you have
heart disease • high blood pressure • thyroid disease • diabetes • glaucoma • a breathing problem such as emphysema, asthma, or chronic bronchitis • trouble urinating due to an enlarged prostate gland • cough that occurs with smoking, too much phlegm (mucus) or chronic cough that lasts

Ask a doctor or pharmacist before use if you are taking sedatives or tranquilizers.

When using this product • do not use more than directed • avoid alcoholic drinks • marked drowsiness may occur • alcohol, sedatives, and tranquilizers may increase drowsiness • be careful when driving a motor vehicle or operating machinery • excitability may occur, especially in children

Stop use and ask a doctor if • nervousness, dizziness, or sleeplessness occurs
- symptoms do not improve for 7 days or occur with a fever
- cough persists for more than 7 days, comes back, or occurs with a fever, rash, or persistent headache
- symptoms do not improve for 10 days (pain) or for 3 days (fever)
- sore throat persists for more than 2 days, and occurs with a fever, headache, rash, nausea, or vomiting. These could be signs of a serious condition.

If pregnant or breast-feeding, ask a health care professional before use.

Keep out of reach of children.

Continued on next page

Information* on Novartis Consumer Health, Inc. *products appearing on these pages is effective as of November 2003.

Theraflu Cold & Cough—Cont.

Overdose Warning: Taking more than the recommended dose can cause serious health problems, including serious liver damage. In case of overdose, get medical help or contact a poison control center right away. Prompt medical attention is critical for adults as well as for children even if you do not notice any signs or symptoms.

Directions:
• do not use more than directed **(see Overdose Warning)**
• take every 4 to 6 hours; not to exceed 4 packets in 24 hours or as directed by a doctor.
• adults and children 12 years of age and over: dissolve contents of one packet into 6 oz. hot water; sip while hot
• children under 12 years of age: consult a doctor
Sweeten to taste if desired.

Microwave heating directions
• add contents of one packet and 6 oz. cool water to a microwave-safe cup and stir briskly. Microwave on high 1 1/2 minutes or until hot. Do not boil water or overheat, and remember to stir liquid between reheatings.

Other Information:
• each packet contains: **sodium 19 mg**
• Phenylketonurics: Contains Phenylalanine 13 mg per adult dose
• store at controlled room temperature 20-25°C (68-77°F)

How Supplied: 6 packets

Inactive Ingredients: acesulfame K, aspartame, citric acid, D&C yellow 10, flavors, maltodextrin, silicon dioxide, sodium citrate, sucrose, tribasic calcium phosphate
Questions? call **1-800-452-0051** 24 hours a day, 7 days a week.
Distributed by:
Novartis Consumer Health, Inc.
Parsippany, NJ 07054-0622
©2003   Made in Canada

THERAFLU® Cold & Sore Throat
Pain Reliever-Fever Reducer
(Acetaminophen)
Antihistamine (Chlorpheniramine)
Nasal Decongestant
(Pseudoephedrine)

Drug Facts

**Active Ingredients
(in each packet):**   **Purpose:**
Acetaminophen
   650 mg .... Pain reliever/
                      Fever reducer
Chlorpheniramine maleate
   4 mg .... Antihistamine
Pseudoephedrine HCl
   60 mg .... Nasal decongestant

Uses: temporarily relieves these symptoms: • headache • minor aches and pains • runny nose • itchy nose or throat • fever • minor sore throat pain • sneezing • nasal and sinus congestion • itchy, watery eyes

Warnings:
Alcohol Warning: If you consume 3 or more alcoholic drinks every day, ask your doctor whether you should take acetaminophen or other pain relievers/fever reducers. Acetaminophen may cause liver damage.
Do not use • if you are now taking a prescription monoamine oxidase inhibitor (MAOI) (certain drugs for depression, psychiatric, or emotional conditions, or Parkinson's disease), or for 2 weeks after stopping the MAOI drug. If you do not know if your prescription drug contains an MAOI, ask a doctor or pharmacist before taking this product.
• with any other product containing acetaminophen **(see Overdose Warning)**
Ask a doctor before use if you have
• heart disease • high blood pressure
• thyroid disease • diabetes • glaucoma
• a breathing problem such as emphysema or chronic bronchitis
• trouble urinating due to an enlarged prostate gland
Ask a doctor or pharmacist before use if you are taking sedatives or tranquilizers.
When using this product • do not use more than directed • avoid alcoholic drinks • drowsiness may occur • alcohol, sedatives, and tranquilizers may increase drowsiness • be careful when driving a motor vehicle or operating machinery • excitability may occur, especially in children
Stop use and ask a doctor if • nervousness, dizziness, or sleeplessness occurs • symptoms do not improve for 7 days or occur with a fever • symptoms do not improve for 10 days (pain) or for 3 days (fever) • sore throat persists for more than 2 days, and occurs with a fever, headache, rash, nausea, or vomiting. These could be signs of a serious condition.
If pregnant or breast-feeding, ask a health care professional before use.
Keep out of reach of children.
Overdose Warning: Taking more than the recommended dose can cause serious health problems, including serious liver damage. In case of overdose, get medical help or contact a poison control center right away. Prompt medical attention is critical for adults as well as for children even if you do not notice any signs or symptoms.

Directions:
• do not use more than directed **(see Overdose Warning)**
• take every 4 to 6 hours; not to exceed 4 packets in 24 hours or as directed by a doctor.
• adults and children 12 years of age and over: dissolve contents of one packet into 6 oz. hot water, sip while hot
• children under 12 years of age: consult a doctor
Sweeten to taste if desired.

Microwave heating directions
• add contents of one packet and 6 oz. cool water to a microwave-safe cup and stir briskly. Microwave on high 1 1/2 minutes or until hot. Do not boil water or overheat, and remember to stir liquid between reheatings.

Other Information:
• each packet contains: **sodium 19 mg**
• Phenylketonurics: Contains Phenylalanine 11 mg per adult dose
• store at controlled room temperature 20-25°C (68-77°F)

How Supplied: 6 Packets

Inactive Ingredients: acesulfame K, aspartame, citric acid, D&C Yellow 10, flavors, maltodextrin, silicon dioxide, sodium citrate, sucrose, tribasic calcium phosphate
Questions? call **1-800-452-0051**
24 hours a day, 7 days a week.
Distributed by:
Novartis Consumer Health, Inc.
Parsippany, NJ 07054-0622
©2003   Made in Canada

THERAFLU®
Flu & Chest Congestion
Pain Reliever-Fever Reducer
(Acetaminophen)
Cough Suppressant)
(Dextromethorphan)
Expectorant (Guaifenesin)
Nasal Decongestant
(Pseudoephedrine)

Drug Facts

**Active Ingredients
(in each packet):**   **Purpose:**
Acetaminophen
   1000 mg .... Pain reliever/
                      Fever reducer
Dextromethorphan HBr
   30 mg .... Cough suppressant
Guaifenesin
   400 mg .... Expectorant
Pseudoephedrine HCl
   60 mg .... Nasal decongestant

Uses: temporarily relieves these symptoms:
• fever • minor aches and pains • headache and sore throat • nasal congestion • chest congestion by loosening phlegm to help clear bronchial passageways

Warnings: Alcohol Warning: If you consume 3 or more alcoholic drinks every day, ask your doctor whether you should take acetaminophen or other pain relievers/fever reducers. Acetaminophen may cause liver damage.
Do not use • if you are now taking a prescription monoamine oxidase inhibitor (MAOI) (certain drugs for depression, psychiatric, or emotional conditions, or Parkinson's disease), or for 2 weeks after stopping the MAOI drug. If you do not know if your prescription drug contains an MAOI, ask a doctor or pharmacist before taking this product.
• with any other product containing acetaminophen **(see Overdose Warning)**
Ask a doctor before use if you have
• heart disease • high blood pressure
• thyroid disease • diabetes • a breathing problem such as emphysema or chronic bronchitis
• trouble urinating due to an enlarged prostate gland

• cough that occurs with too much pheglm (mucus)
• chronic cough that lasts or as occurs with smoking, asthma, emphysema, or chronic bronchitis

When using this product • do not use more than directed

Stop use and ask a doctor if • nervousness, dizziness, or sleeplessness occurs
• symptoms do not improve for 7 days or occur with a fever
• cough persists for more than 7 days, comes back, or occurs with a fever, rash, or persistent headache
• symptoms do not improve for 10 days (pain) or for 3 days (fever)
• sore throat persists for more than 2 days, and occurs with a fever, headache, rash, nausea, or vomiting. These could be signs of a serious condition.

If pregnant or breast-feeding, ask a health care professional before use.

Keep out of reach of children.

Overdose Warning: Taking more than the recommended dose can cause serious health problems, including serious liver damage. In case of overdose, get medical help or contact a poison control center right away. Prompt medical attention is critical for adults as well as for children even if you do not notice any signs or symptoms.

Directions:
• do not use more than directed **(see Overdose Warning)**
• take every 6 hours; not to exceed 4 packets in 24 hours or as directed by a doctor.
• adults and children 12 years of age and over: dissolve contents of one packet into 6 oz. hot water; sip while hot
• children under 12 years of age: consult a doctor

Sweeten to taste if desired.

Microwave heating directions
• add contents of one packet and 6 oz. cool water to a microwave-safe cup and stir briskly. Microwave on high 1 1/2 minutes or until hot. Do not boil water or overheat, and remember to stir liquid between reheatings.

Other Information:
• each packet contains: **sodium 15 mg**
• Phenylketonurics: Contains Phenylalanine 24 mg per adult dose
• store at controlled room temperature 20-25°C (68-77°F)

How Supplied: 6 Packets

Inactive Ingredients: acesulfame K, aspartame, calcium phosphate, citric acid, D&C Yellow 10, FD&C Red 40, flavors, maltodextrin, silicon dioxide, sodium citrate, sucrose

Questions? call **1-800-452-0051**

24 hours a day, 7 days a week.

Distributed by:

Novartis Consumer Health, Inc.

Parsippany, NJ 07054-0622

©2003   Made in Canada

THERAFLU® Flu & Sore Throat
Pain Reliever-Fever Reducer (Acetaminophen)
Antihistamine (Chlorpheniramine)
Nasal Decongestant (Pseudoephedrine)

Drug Facts

Active Ingredients
(in each packet):   **Purpose:**
Acetaminophen
    1000 mg .... Pain reliever/
                                    Fever reducer
Chlorpheniramine maleate
    4 mg .... Antihistamine
Pseudoephedrine
    HCl 60 mg .... Nasal decongestant

Uses: temporarily relieves these symptoms:
• headache • minor aches and pains
• runny nose • itchy nose or throat
• fever
• minor sore throat pain • sneezing
• nasal and sinus congestion • itchy, watery eyes

Warnings:
Alcohol Warning: If you consume 3 or more alcoholic drinks every day, ask your doctor whether you should take acetaminophen or other pain relievers/fever reducers. Acetaminophen may cause liver damage.

Do not use • if you are now taking a prescription monoamine oxidase inhibitor (MAOI) (certain drugs for depression, psychiatric, or emotional conditions, or Parkinson's disease), or for 2 weeks after stopping the MAOI drug. If you do not know if your prescription drug contains an MAOI, ask a doctor or pharmacist before taking this product.
• with any other product containing acetaminophen **(see Overdose Warning)**

Ask a doctor before use if you have
• heart disease • high blood pressure
• thyroid disease • diabetes • glaucoma
• a breathing problem such as emphysema or chronic bronchitis
• trouble urinating due to an enlarged prostate gland
• cough that occurs with too much phlegm (mucus) or chronic cough that lasts

Ask a doctor or pharmacist before use if you are taking sedatives or tranquilizers.

When using this product • do not use more than directed • avoid alcoholic drinks • drowsiness may occur • alcohol, sedatives, and tranquilizers may increase drowsiness • be careful when driving a motor vehicle or operating machinery • excitability may occur, especially in children

Stop use and ask a doctor if • nervousness, dizziness, or sleeplessness occurs
• symptoms do not improve for 7 days or occur with a fever
• symptoms do not improve for 10 days (pain) or for 3 days (fever)
• sore throat persists for more than 2 days, and occurs with a fever, headache, rash, nausea, or vomiting. These could be signs of a serious condition.

If pregnant or breast-feeding, ask a health care professional before use.

Keep out of reach of children.

Overdose Warning: Taking more than the recommended dose can cause serious health problems, including serious liver damage. In case of overdose, get medical help or contact a poison control center right away. Prompt medical attention is critical for adults as well as for children even if you do not notice any signs or symptoms.

Directions:
• do not use more than directed **(see Overdose Warning)**
• take every 6 hours; not to exceed 4 packets in 24 hours or as directed by a doctor
• adults and children 12 years of age and over: dissolve contents of one packet into 6 oz. hot water; sip while hot.
• children under 12 years of age: consult a doctor
Sweeten to taste if desired.

Microwave heating directions
• add contents of one packet and 6 oz. cool water to a microwave-safe cup and stir briskly. Microwave on high 1 1/2 minutes or until hot. Do not boil water or overheat, and remember to stir liquid between reheatings.

Other Information:
• each packet contains: **sodium 12 mg**
• Phenylketonurics: Contains Phenylalanine 22 mg per adult dose
• store at controlled room temperature 20-25°C (68-77°F)

How Supplied: 6 Packets

Inactive Ingredients: acesulfame K, aspartame, citric acid, D&C Yellow 10, FD&C Blue 1, FD&C Red 40, flavors, maltodextrin, silicon dioxide, sodium citrate, sucrose, tribasic calcium phosphate
Questions? call **1-800-452-0051**
24 hours a day, 7 days a week.
Distributed by:
Novartis Consumer Health, Inc.
Parsippany, NJ 07054-0622
©2003   Made in Canada

_____

THERAFLU ® Severe Cold
Pain Reliever-Fever Reducer (Acetaminophen)
Antihistamine (Chlorpheniramine)
Cough Suppressant (Dextromethorphan)
Nasal Decongestant (Pseudoephedrine)

Drug Facts

Active Ingredients
(in each packet):   **Purpose:**
Acetaminophen
    1000 mg .... Pain reliever/
                                    Fever reducer
Chlorpheniramine maleate
    4 mg .... Antihistamine

Continued on next page

_____

Information on Novartis Consumer Health, Inc. products appearing on these pages is effective as of November 2003.

Theraflu Severe Cold—Cont.

Dextromethorphan HBr
  30 mg .... Cough suppressant
Pseudoephedrine HCl
  60 mg .... Nasal decongestant

Uses: temporarily relieves these symptoms: • headache • minor aches and pains • runny nose • sneezing • itchy nose or throat • fever • itchy, watery eyes • minor sore throat pain • nasal and sinus congestion • cough due to minor throat and bronchial irritation

Warnings:
Alcohol Warning: If you consume 3 or more alcoholic drinks every day, ask your doctor whether you should take acetaminophen or other pain relievers/fever reducers. Acetaminophen may cause liver damage.

Do not use • if you are now taking a prescription monoamine oxidase inhibitor (MAOI) (certain drugs for depression, psychiatric, or emotional conditions, or Parkinson's disease), or for 2 weeks after stopping the MAOI drug. If you do not know if your prescription drug contains an MAOI, ask a doctor or pharmacist before taking this product.
• with any other product containing acetaminophen (**see Overdose Warning**)
Ask a doctor before use if you have
• heart disease • high blood pressure
• thyroid disease • diabetes • glaucoma
• a breathing problem such as emphysema, asthma, or chronic bronchitis
• trouble urinating due to an enlarged prostate gland
• cough that occurs with smoking, too much phlegm (mucus) or chronic cough that lasts
Ask a doctor or pharmacist before use if you are taking sedatives or tranquilizers.

When using this product • do not use more than directed • avoid alcoholic drinks
• marked drowsiness may occur • alcohol, sedatives, and tranquilizers may increase drowsiness
• be careful when driving a motor vehicle or operating machinery
• excitability may occur, especially in children
Stop use and ask a doctor if • nervousness, dizziness, or sleeplessness occurs
• symptoms do not improve for 7 days or occur with a fever
• cough persists for more than 7 days, comes back, or occurs with a fever, rash, or persistent headache
• symptoms do not improve for 10 days (pain) or for 3 days (fever)
• sore throat persists for more than 2 days, and occurs with a fever, headache, rash, nausea, or vomiting. These could be signs of a serious condition.
If pregnant or breast-feeding, ask a health care professional before use.
Keep out of reach of children.
Overdose Warning: Taking more than the recommended dose can cause serious health problems, including serious liver damage. In case of overdose, get medical help or contact a poison control center right away. Prompt medical atten-

tion is critical for adults as well as for children even if you do not notice any signs or symptoms.

Directions:
• do not use more than directed (**see Overdose Warning**)
• take every 6 hours; not to exceed 4 packets in 24 hours or as directed by a doctor
• adults and children 12 years of age and over: dissolve contents of one packet into 6 oz. hot water; sip while hot
• children under 12 years of age: consult a doctor
Sweeten to taste if desired.
Microwave heating directions
• add contents of one packet and 6 oz. cool water to a microwave-safe cup and stir briskly. Microwave on high 1 1/2 minutes or until hot. Do not boil water or overheat, and remember to stir liquid between reheatings.
Other Information:
• each packet contains: **sodium 19 mg**
• Phenylketonurics: Contains Phenylalanine 17 mg per adult dose
• store at controlled room temperature 20-25°C (68-77°F)

How Supplied: 6 Packets

Inactive Ingredients: acesulfame K, aspartame, citric acid, D&C yellow 10, flavors, maltodextrin, silicon dioxide, sodium citrate, sucrose, tribasic calcium phosphate
Questions? call **1-800-452-0051** 24 hours a day, 7 days a week.
Distributed by:
Novartis Consumer Health, Inc.
Parsippany, NJ 07054-0622
©2003   Made in Canada
Shown in Product Identification Guide, page 517

THERAFLU® Severe Cold Non-Drowsy
**Pain Reliever-Fever Reducer (Acetaminophen)
Cough Suppressant (Dextromethorphan)
Nasal Decongestant (Pseudoephedrine)**

Drug Facts

Active Ingredients
(in each packet):   **Purpose:**
Acetaminophen
  1000 mg .... Pain reliever/
                       Fever reducer
Dextromethorphan HBr
  30 mg .... Cough suppressant
Pseudoephedrine HCl
  60 mg .... Nasal decongestant

Uses: temporarily relieves these symptoms: • minor aches and pains
• minor sore throat pain • nasal and sinus congestion
• cough due to minor throat and bronchial irritation

Warnings:
Alcohol Warning: If you consume 3 or more alcoholic drinks every day, ask your doctor whether you should take acetaminophen or any other pain relievers/fever reducers. Acetaminophen may cause liver damage.

Do not use • if you are now taking a prescription monoamine oxidase inhibitor (MAOI) (certain drugs for depression, psychiatric, or emotional conditions, or Parkinson's disease), or for 2 weeks after stopping the MAOI drug. If you do not know if your prescription drug contains an MAOI, ask a doctor or pharmacist before taking this product.
• with any other product containing acetaminophen (**see Overdose Warning**)
Ask a doctor before use if you have
• heart disease • high blood pressure
• thyroid disease • diabetes • glaucoma
• persistent or chronic cough as occurs with emphysema, asthma, or chronic bronchitis
• trouble urinating due to an enlarged prostate gland
• cough that occurs with smoking, too much phlegm (mucus) or chronic cough that lasts
When using this product • do not use more than directed
Stop use and ask a doctor if • nervousness, dizziness, or sleeplessness occurs
• symptoms do not improve for 7 days or occur with a fever
• cough persists for more than 7 days, comes back, or occurs with a fever, rash, or persistent headache
• symptoms do not improve for 10 days (pain) or for 3 days (fever)
• sore throat persists for more than 2 days, and occurs with a fever, headache, rash, nausea, or vomiting. These could be signs of a serious condition.
If pregnant or breast-feeding, ask a health care professional before use.
Keep out of reach of children.
Overdose Warning: Taking more than the recommended dose can cause serious health problems, including serious liver damage. In case of overdose, get medical help or contact a poison control center right away. Prompt medical attention is critical for adults as well as for children even if you do not notice any signs or symptoms.

Directions:
• do not use more than directed (**see Overdose Warning**)
• take every 6 hours; not to exceed 4 packets in 24 hours or as directed by a doctor
• adults and children 12 years of age and over: dissolve contents of one packet into 6 oz. hot water; sip while hot
• children under 12 years of age: consult a doctor
Sweeten to taste if desired.
Microwave heating directions
• add contents of one packet and 6 oz. cool water to a microwave-safe cup and stir briskly. Microwave on high 1 1/2 minutes or until hot. Do not boil water or overheat, and remember to stir liquid between reheatings.
Other Information:
• each packet contains: **sodium 19 mg**
• Phenylketonurics: Contains Phenylalanine 17 mg per adult dose
• store at controlled room temperature 20-25°C (68-77°F)

How Supplied: 6 Packets

Inactive Ingredients: acesulfame K, aspartame, citric acid, D&C yellow 10, flavors, maltodextrin, silicon dioxide, sodium citrate, sucrose, tribasic calcium phosphate

Questions? call 1-800-452-0051 24 hours a day, 7 days a week.

Distributed by:
Novartis Consumer Health, Inc.
Parsippany, NJ 07054-0622
©2003   Made in Canada
Shown in Product Identification
Guide, page 517

THERAFLU® Severe Cold & Cough
Pain Reliever/Fever Reducer (Acetaminophen)
Antihistamine (Chlorpheniramine)
Cough Suppressant (Dextromethorphan)
Nasal Decongestant (Pseudoephedrine)

Drug Facts

Active Ingredients
(in each packet):   **Purpose:**
Acetaminophen
    1000 mg .... Pain reliever/
                                    Fever reducer
Chlorpheniramine maleate
    4 mg .... Antihistamine
Dextromethorphan HBr
    30 mg .... Cough suppressant
Pseudoephedrine HCl
    60 mg .... Nasal decongestant

Uses: temporarily relieves these symptoms:
• headache • minor aches and pains
• runny nose • sneezing • itchy nose or throat
• itchy, watery eyes • fever • minor sore throat pain
• nasal and sinus congestion • cough due to minor throat and bronchial irritation

Warnings:
Alcohol Warning: If you consume 3 or more alcoholic drinks every day, ask your doctor whether you should take acetaminophen or other pain relievers/fever reducers. Acetaminophen may cause liver damage.

Do not use • if you are now taking a prescription monoamine oxidase inhibitor (MAOI) (certain drugs for depression, psychiatric, or emotional conditions, or Parkinson's disease), or for 2 weeks after stopping the MAOI drug. If you do not know if your prescription drug contains an MAOI, ask a doctor or pharmacist before taking this product.
• with any other product containing acetaminophen (see **Overdose Warning**)

Ask a doctor before use if you have
• heart disease • high blood pressure
• thyroid disease • diabetes • glaucoma
• a breathing problem such as emphysema, asthma, or chronic bronchitis
• trouble urinating due to an enlarged prostate gland
• cough that occurs with smoking, too much phlegm (mucus) or chronic cough that lasts

Ask a doctor or pharmacist before use if you are taking sedatives or tranquilizers.

When using this product • do not use more than directed • avoid alcoholic drinks

• marked drowsiness may occur • alcohol, sedatives, and tranquilizers may increase drowsiness
• be careful when driving a motor vehicle or operating machinery
• excitability may occur, especially in children

Stop use and ask a doctor if • nervousness, dizziness, or sleeplessness occurs
• symptoms do not improve for 7 days or occur with a fever
• cough persists for more than 7 days, comes back, or occurs with a fever, rash, or persistent headache
• symptoms do not improve for 10 days (pain) or for 3 days (fever)
• sore throat persists for more than 2 days, and occurs with a fever, headache, rash, nausea, or vomiting. These could be signs of a serious condition.

If pregnant or breast-feeding, ask a health care professional before use.

Keep out of reach of children.

Overdose Warning: Taking more than the recommended dose can cause serious health problems, including serious liver damage. In case of overdose, get medical help or contact a poison control center right away. Prompt medical attention is critical for adults as well as for children even if you do not notice any signs or symptoms.

Directions:
• do not use more than directed **(see Overdose Warning)**
• take every 6 hours; not to exceed 4 packets in 24 hours or as directed by a doctor
• adults and children 12 years of age and over: dissolve contents of one packet into 6 oz. hot water; sip while hot
• children under 12 years of age: consult a doctor
Sweeten to taste if desired.

Microwave heating directions
• add contents of one packet and 6 oz. cool water to a microwave-safe cup and stir briskly. Microwave on high 1 1/2 minutes or until hot. Do not boil water or overheat, and remember to stir liquid between reheatings.

Other Information:
• each packet contains: **sodium 14 mg**
• Phenylketonurics: Contains Phenylalanine 27 mg per adult dose
• store at controlled room temperature 20-25°C (68-77°F)

How Supplied: 6 packets

Inactive Ingredients: acesulfame K, aspartame, citric acid, FD&C Blue 1, FD& C Red 40, flavors, maltodextrin, silicon dioxide, sodium citrate, sucrose, tribasic calcium phosphate

Questions? call 1-800-452-0051 24 hours a day, 7 days a week.

Distributed by:
Novartis Consumer Health, Inc.
Parsippany, NJ 07054-0622
©2003   Made in Canada

TRIAMINIC® ALLERCHEWS™
Orally Disintegrating Tablets
24 Hour Non-Drowsy†
Allergy

Active Ingredient
(in each tablet):   **Purpose:**
Loratadine 10 mg .... Antihistamine

Uses: temporarily relieves these symptoms due to hay fever or other upper respiratory allergies: • runny nose • sneezing • itchy, watery eyes • itching of the nose or throat

Warnings:
Do not use if you have ever had an allergic reaction to this product or any of its ingredients.

Ask a doctor before use if you have liver or kidney disease.

Your doctor should determine if you need a different dose.

When using this product do not take more than directed.

Taking more than directed may cause drowsiness.

Stop use and ask a doctor if an allergic reaction to this product occurs. Seek medical help right away.

If pregnant or breast-feeding, ask a health professional before use.

Keep out of reach of children. In case of overdose, get medical help or contact a Poison Control Center right away.

Directions: Place one tablet on tongue; tablet disintegrates, with or without water.

adults and children 6 years of age and over	1 tablet daily; not more than 1 tablet in 24 hours
children under 6 years of age	ask a doctor
consumers with liver or kidney disease	ask a doctor

Other Information:
• store between 20 and 25°C (68 and 77°F)
• keep in a dry place
• use tablet immediately after opening individual blister

How Supplied: 8 and 24 Tablets

Inactive Ingredients: croscarmellose sodium, crospovidone, hypromellose, magnesium stearate, mannitol, microcrystalline cellulose

Questions? call   1-800-452-0051 24 hours a day, 7 days a week.

Distributed by:
Novartis Consumer Health, Inc.
Parsippany, NJ 07054-0622 ©2004

---

†When used as directed
Shown in Product Identification
Guide, page 517

Continued on next page

Information on Novartis Consumer Health, Inc. *products appearing on these pages is effective as of* November 2003.

TRIAMINIC® Chest & Nasal Congestion (Expectorant, Nasal Decongestant)
Citrus Flavor

Drug Facts

Active Ingredients:
(in each 5 mL, 1 teaspoon):   Purpose:
Guaifenesin,
USP, 50 mg .... Expectorant
Pseudoephedrine HCl,
USP, 15 mg .... Nasal decongestant

Uses: temporarily relieves these symptoms:
• chest congestion by loosening phlegm (mucus) to help clear bronchial passageways • nasal and sinus congestion

Warnings:
Do not use in a child who is taking a prescription monoamine oxidase inhibitor (MAOI) (certain drugs for depression, psychiatric or emotional conditions, or Parkinson's disease), or for 2 weeks after stopping the MAOI drug. If you do not know if the child's prescription drug contains an MAOI, ask a doctor or pharmacist before giving this product.
Ask a doctor before use if the child has
• heart disease • high blood pressure
• thyroid disease • diabetes • glaucoma
• cough that occurs with too much phlegm (mucus) • chronic cough that lasts or a breathing problem such as asthma or chronic bronchitis
When using this product
• do not use more than directed
Stop use and ask a doctor if
• nervousness, dizziness, or sleeplessness occur • symptoms do not improve within 7 days or occur with a fever
• cough persists for more than 7 days, comes back, or occurs with a fever, rash, or persistent headache. These could be signs of a serious condition.
Keep out of reach of children. In case of overdose, get medical help or contact a poison control center right away.

Directions:
• take every 4 to 6 hours; not more than 4 doses in 24 hours or as directed by a doctor

children 6 to under 12 years of age	2 teaspoons
children 2 to under 6 years of age	1 teaspoon
children under 2 years of age	ask a doctor

Other Information:
• each teaspoon contains: **sodium 2 mg**
• contains no aspirin
• store at controlled room temperature 20–25°C (68–77°F)

Inactive Ingredients: benzoic acid, D&C Yellow 10, edetate disodium, FD&C Yellow 6, flavors, glycerin, polyethylene glycol, propylene glycol, purified water, sorbitol, sucrose
Questions? Call toll-free **1-800-452-0051** 24 hours a day, 7 days a week.

For more information plus helpful tips visit www.triaminic.com
Novartis Consumer Health, Inc.
Parsippany, NJ 07054-0622 ©2004

How Supplied: 4 fl oz (118 mL)
Shown in Product Identification Guide, page 518

TRIAMINIC® Cold & Allergy
Antihistamine, Nasal Decongestant-
Orange Flavor
TRIAMINIC® Cold & Cough
Antihistamine, Cough Suppressant, Nasal Decongestant-
Cherry Flavor
TRIAMINIC® Flu, Cough & Fever
Antihistamine, Cough Suppressant, Fever Reducer/Pain Reliever, Nasal Decongestant-
Bubble Gum Flavor
TRIAMINIC® Night Time Cough & Cold
Antihistamine, Cough Suppressant, Nasal Decongestant-
Grape Flavor

Drug Facts:
Active Ingredients:
(in each 5 mL, 1 teaspoon)
TRIAMINIC® Cold & Allergy
Orange Flavor
Chlorpheniramine maleate,
USP, 1 mg .... Antihistamine
Pseudoephedrine HCl,
USP, 15 mg .... Nasal decongestant
TRIAMINIC® Cold & Cough
Cherry Flavor
Chlorpheniramine maleate,
USP, 1 mg .... Antihistamine
Dextromethorphan HBr,
USP, 5 mg .... Cough suppressant
Pseudoephedrine HCl,
USP, 15 mg .... Nasal decongestant
TRIAMINIC® Flu, Cough & Fever
Bubble Gum Flavor
Acetaminophen,
USP, 160 mg .... Fever reducer/Pain reliever
Chlorpheniramine maleate,
USP, 1 mg .... Antihistamine
Dextromethorphan HBr,
USP, 7.5 mg .... Cough suppressant
Pseudoephedrine HCl,
USP, 15 mg .... Nasal decongestant
TRIAMINIC® Night Time Cough & Cold
Grape Flavor
Chlorpheniramine maleate,
USP, 1 mg .... Antihistamine
Dextromethorphan HBr,
USP, 7.5 mg .... Cough suppressant
Pseudoephedrine HCl,
USP, 15 mg .... Nasal decongestant

Uses: temporarily relieves these symptoms:
TRIAMINIC® Cold & Allergy
Antihistamine, Nasal Decongestant-
Orange Flavor
• itchy, watery eyes • runny nose • itchy nose or throat • sneezing • nasal and sinus congestion

TRIAMINIC® Cold & Cough
Antihistamine, Cough Suppressant, Nasal Decongestant-
Cherry Flavor
• cough due to minor throat and bronchial irritation • runny nose • nasal and sinus congestion • sneezing • itchy nose or throat • itchy, watery eyes

TRIAMINIC® Flu, Cough & Fever
Antihistamine, Cough Suppressant, Fever Reducer/Pain Reliever, Nasal Decongestant-
Bubble Gum Flavor
• fever • minor aches and pains • headache and sore throat • cough due to minor throat and bronchial irritation • nasal and sinus congestion • sneezing • itchy nose or throat • itchy, watery eyes

TRIAMINIC® Night Time Cough & Cold
Antihistamine, Cough Suppressant, Nasal Decongestant-
Grape Flavor
• cough due to minor throat and bronchial irritation • runny nose • nasal and sinus congestion • sneezing • itchy nose or throat • itchy, watery eyes

Warnings:
Do not use • in a child who is taking a prescription monoamine oxidase inhibitor (MAOI) (certain drugs for depression, psychiatric or emotional conditions, or Parkinson's disease), or for 2 weeks after stopping the MAOI drug. If you do not know if the child's prescription drug contains an MAOI, ask a doctor or pharmacist before giving this product.
Specific to Flu, Cough & Fever: with any another product containing acetaminophen
• **(see Overdose Warning)**
Ask a doctor before use if the child has
• heart disease • high blood pressure
• thyroid disease • diabetes • glaucoma
• cough that occurs with too much phlegm (mucus) **(does not apply to Cold & Allergy)** • a breathing problem such as asthma or chronic bronchitis • chronic cough that lasts **(does not apply to Cold & Allergy)**
Ask a doctor or pharmacist before use if the child is taking sedatives or tranquilizers.
When using this product
• do not use more than directed • excitability may occur, especially in children • marked drowsiness may occur **(does not apply to Cold & Allergy)** • sedatives and tranquilizers may increase drowsiness
Stop use and ask a doctor if
• nervousness, dizziness, or sleeplessness occur
• symptoms do not improve within 7 days or occur with a fever **(does not apply to Flu, Cough, Fever)**
• cough persists for more than 7 days, comes back, or occurs with fever, rash, or persistent headache. These could be signs of a serious condition.
Specific only to Flu, Cough & Fever:
• symptoms do not improve within 5 days (pain) or 3 days (fever).

- sore throat persists for more than 2 days or occurs with headache, fever, rash, nausea or vomiting

These could be signs of a serious condition.

Keep out of reach of children. In case of overdose, get medical help or contact a poison control center right away.

Pertains only to Flu, Cough & Fever:
Overdose Warning: Taking more than the recommended dose can cause serious health problems, including serious liver damage. In case of overdose, get medical help or contact a poison control center right away.

Prompt medical attention is critical even if you do not notice any signs or symptoms.

Directions:
TRIAMINIC® Cold & Allergy
Antihistamine, Nasal Decongestant-Orange Flavor (see below Triaminic® Cold & Cough) and (see table on next page or below)

TRIAMINIC® Cold & Cough
Antihistamine, Cough Suppressant, Nasal Decongestant-Cherry Flavor
Take every 4 to 6 hours; not more than 4 doses in 24 hours or as directed by a doctor.

| children 6 to under 12 years of age | 2 teaspoons |
| children under 6 years of age | ask a doctor |

TRIAMINIC® Flu, Cough & Fever
Antihistamine, Cough Suppressant, Fever Reducer/Pain Reliever, Nasal Decongestant-
Bubble Gum Flavor (see below Triaminic® Cold & Night Time Cough)

TRIAMINIC® Night Time Cough & Cold
Antihistamine, Cough Suppressant, Nasal Decongestant-
Grape Flavor
Take every 6 hours; not more than 4 doses in 24 hours or as directed by a doctor.

| children 6 to under 12 years of age | 2 teaspoons |
| children under 6 years of age | ask a doctor |

Other Information:
TRIAMINIC® Cold & Allergy
Antihistamine, Nasal Decongestant-Orange Flavor
- contains no aspirin
- store at controlled room temperature 20–25°C (68–77°F).

TRIAMINIC® Cold & Cough
Antihistamine, Cough Suppressant, Nasal Decongestant-
Cherry Flavor
- each teaspoon contains: **sodium 10 mg**
- contains no aspirin
- store at controlled room temperature 20–25°C (68–77°F).

TRIAMINIC® Flu, Cough & Fever
Antihistamine, Cough Suppressant, Fever Reducer/Pain Reliever, Nasal Decongestant-

Bubble Gum Flavor
- each teaspoon contains: **sodium 3 mg**
- contains no aspirin
- protect from light
- store at controlled room temperature 20–25°C (68–77°F).

TRIAMINIC® Night Time Cough & Cold
Antihistamine, Cough Suppressant, Nasal Decongestant-
Grape Flavor
- each teaspoon contains: **sodium 7.5 mg**
- contains no aspirin
- store at controlled room temperature 20–25°C (68–77°F).

Inactive Ingredients:
TRIAMINIC® Cold & Allergy
Antihistamine, Nasal Decongestant-Orange Flavor

benzoic acid, edetate disodium, FD&C Yellow 6, flavors, purified water, sorbitol, sucrose

TRIAMINIC® Cold & Cough
Antihistamine, Cough Suppressant, Nasal Decongestant-
Cherry Flavor

benzoic acid, FD&C Red 40, flavors, propylene glycol, purified water, sodium chloride, sorbitol, sucrose

TRIAMINIC® Flu, Cough & Fever
Antihistamine, Cough Suppressant, Fever Reducer/Pain Reliever, Nasal Decongestant-
Bubble Gum Flavor

acesulfame K, benzoic acid, citric acid, D&C Red 33, dibasic potassium phosphate, disodium edetate, FD&C Red 40, flavors, glycerin, polyethylene glycol, potassium chloride, propylene glycol, purified water, sucrose, other ingredients

TRIAMINIC® Night Time Cough & Cold
Antihistamine, Cough Suppressant, Nasal Decongestant
Grape Flavor

benzoic acid, citric acid, dibasic sodium phosphate, edetate disodium, FD&C Blue 1, FD&C Red 40, flavors, propylene glycol, purified water, sorbitol, sucrose

How Supplied:
TRIAMINIC® Cold & Cough
TRIAMINIC® Night Time Cough & Cold
Bottles of 4 fl. oz. (118 mL) and 8 fl.oz. (236 mL)

TRIAMINIC® Cold & Allergy
TRIAMINIC® Flu, Cough & Fever
Bottle of 4 fl. oz. (118 mL)

Questions: call **1-800-452-0051** 24 hours a day, 7 days a week.

For more information about Triaminic® visit our website at www.triaminic.com

Novartis Consumer Health, Inc.
Parsippany, NJ 07054-0622 ©2004

Shown in Product Identification Guide, page 518

TRIAMINIC® Cough
Cough Suppressant, Nasal Decongestant-Berry Flavor

TRIAMINIC® Cough & Nasal Congestion
Cough Suppressant, Nasal Decongestant-Orange
Strawberry Flavor

TRIAMINIC® Cough & Sore Throat
Cough Suppressant, Nasal Decongestant, Pain Reliever/Fever Reducer-Grape Flavor

Drug Facts:
Active Ingredients:
(in each 5 mL, 1 teaspoon)
TRIAMINIC® Cough
Berry Flavor
Dextromethorphan HBr, USP 5 mg .... Cough suppressant
Pseudoephedrine, HCl, USP, 15 mg .... Nasal decongestant

TRIAMINIC® Cough & Nasal Congestion
Orange Strawberry Flavor
Dextromethorphan HBr, USP, 7.5 mg .... Cough suppressant
Pseudoephedrine, HCl, USP, 15 mg .... Nasal decongestant

TRIAMINIC® Cough & Sore Throat
Grape Flavor
Acetaminophen, USP, 160 mg ...... Fever reducer/Pain reliever
Dextromethorphan HBr, USP, 7.5 mg .... Cough suppressant
Pseudoephedrine HCl, USP, 15 mg .... Nasal decongestant

Uses: Temporarily relieves these symptoms:
TRIAMINIC® Cough
Cough Suppressant, Nasal Decongestant- (see Cough & Nasal Congestion)
Berry Flavor

TRIAMINIC® Cough & Nasal Congestion
Cough Suppressant, Nasal Decongestant-Orange Strawberry Flavor
- cough due to minor throat and bronchial irritation • nasal and sinus congestion

TRIAMINIC® Cough & Sore Throat
Cough Suppressant, Nasal Decongestant, Pain Reliever/Fever Reducer
Grape Flavor
- sore throat pain • minor aches and pains • cough due to minor throat and bronchial irritation • fever • nasal and sinus congestion

Warnings:
Do not use • in a child who is taking a prescription monoamine oxidase inhibi-

Continued on next page

Information on Novartis Consumer Health, Inc. *products appearing on these pages is effective as of November 2003.*

Triaminic Cough—Cont.

tor (MAOI) (certain drugs for depression, psychiatric or emotional conditions, or Parkinson's disease), or for 2 weeks after stopping the MAOI drug. If you do not know if the child's prescription drug contains an MAOI, ask a doctor or pharmacist before giving this product.

Specific to Cough & Sore Throat: with any another product containing acetaminophen

(see Overdose Warning)

Ask a doctor before use if the child has
• heart disease • high blood pressure • thyroid disease • diabetes • glaucoma • cough that occurs with too much phlegm (mucus) • chronic cough that lasts or a breathing problem such as asthma or chronic bronchitis

Ask a doctor or pharmacist before use if the child is taking sedatives or tranquilizers.

When using this product
• do not use more than directed

Stop use and ask a doctor if
• nervousness, dizziness, or sleeplessness occurs • symptoms do not improve within 7 days or occur with a fever • cough persists for more than 7 days, comes back, or occurs with fever, rash, or persistent headache. These could be signs of a serious condition.

Specific to Cough & Sore Throat:
• sore throat persists for more than 2 days, or occurs with headache, fever, rash, nausea, or vomiting. These could be signs of a serious condition. • symptoms do not improve for 5 days (pain) or 3 days (fever)

Keep out of reach of children. In case of overdose, get medical help or contact a poison control center right away. **Pertains only to cough & sore throat:** Prompt medical attention is critical for adults as well as for children even if you do not notice any signs or symptoms.

Overdose Warning: Taking more than the recommended dose can cause serious health problems, including serious liver damage. In case of overdose, get medical help or contact a poison control center right away.

Prompt medical attention is critical even if you do not notice any signs or symptoms.

Directions:

Triaminic® Cough
• take every 4 to 6 hours; not more than 4 doses in 24 hours or as directed by a doctor (also see table below)

Triaminic® Cough & Nasal Congestion
• take every 6 hours; not more than 4 doses in 24 hours or as directed by a doctor (also see table below)

Triaminic® Cough & Sore Throat
• do not use more than directed **(see Overdose Warning)**
• take every 6 hours; not more than 4 doses in 24 hours or as directed by a doctor

children 6 to under 12 years of age	2 teaspoons
children 2 to under 6 years of age	1 teaspoon
children under 2 years of age	ask a doctor

Other Information:

TRIAMINIC® Cough
Cough Suppressant, Nasal Decongestant
Berry Flavor
• each teaspoon contains: **sodium 20 mg**
• contains no aspirin
• store at controlled room temperature 20–25°C (68–77°F)

TRIAMINIC® Cough & Nasal Congestion
Cough Suppressant, Nasal Decongestant
Orange Strawberry Flavor
• each teaspoon contains: **sodium 7 mg**
• contains no aspirin
• store at controlled room temperature 20–25°C (68–77°F)

TRIAMINIC® Cough & Sore Throat
Cough Suppressant, Nasal Decongestant, Pain Reliever/Fever Reducer
Grape Flavor
• each teaspoon contains: **sodium 5 mg**
• contains no aspirin
• store at controlled room temperature 20–25°C (68–77°F)

Inactive Ingredients:

TRIAMINIC® Cough
Cough Suppressant, Nasal Decongestant
Berry Flavor
benzoic acid, FD&C Blue 1, FD&C Red 40, flavors, propylene glycol, purified water, sodium chloride, sorbitol, sucrose

TRIAMINIC® Cough & Nasal Congestion
Cough Suppressant, Nasal Decongestant
Orange Strawberry Flavor
benzoic acid, citric acid, dibasic sodium phosphate, edetate disodium, flavors, propylene glycol, purified water, sorbitol, sucrose

TRIAMINIC® Cough & Sore Throat
Cough suppressant, Nasal Decongestant, Pain Reliever/Fever Reducer
Grape Flavor
citric acid, edetate disodium, FD&C Blue 1, FD&C Red 40, flavors, glycerin, polyethylene glycol, propylene glycol, purified water, sodium benzoate, sodium citrate, sorbitol, sucrose

How Supplied:
Triaminic® Cough
Triaminic® Cough & Nasal Congestion
  Bottles of 4 fl. oz. (118 mL)
Triaminic® Cough & Sore Throat
  Bottles of 4 fl. oz. (118 mL)
Questions: call **1-800-452-0051** 24 hours a day, 7 days a week.
For more information about Triaminic® visit our website at www.triaminic.com

Novartis Consumer Health, Inc.
Parsippany, NJ 07054-0622 ©2004
Shown in Product Identification Guide, page 518

TRIAMINIC® Softchews® Allergy
Runny Nose & Congestion
Orange Flavor
Antihistamine, Nasal Decongestant

Drug Facts

Active Ingredients
(in each tablet):   **Purpose:**
Chlorpheniramine maleate, USP,
1 mg .... Antihistamine
Pseudoephedrine HCl, USP,
15 mg .... Nasal decongestant

Uses: temporarily relieves these symptoms: • nasal and sinus congestion • runny nose • sneezing • itchy nose or throat • itchy, watery eyes

Warnings:
Do not use • in a child who is taking a prescription monoamine oxidase inhibitor (MAOI) (certain drugs for depression, psychiatric or emotional conditions, or Parkinson's disease), or for 2 weeks after stopping the MAOI drug. If you do not know if the child's prescription drug contains an MAOI, ask a doctor or pharmacist before giving this product.

Ask a doctor before use if the child has
• heart disease • high blood pressure • thyroid disease • diabetes • glaucoma • a breathing problem such as chronic bronchitis

Ask a doctor or pharmacist before use if the child is taking sedatives or tranquilizers.

When using this product • do not use more than directed • drowsiness may occur • sedatives and tranquilizers may increase drowsiness • excitability may occur, especially in children

Stop use and ask a doctor if • nervousness, dizziness, or sleeplessness occur • symptoms do not improve within 7 days, or occur with fever, rash, or persistent headache. These could be signs of a serious condition.

Keep out of reach of children. In case of overdose, get medical help or contact a poison control center right away.

Directions:
• Let Softchews® tablet dissolve in mouth or chew Softchews® tablet before swallowing, whichever is preferred • take every 4 to 6 hours; not more than 4 doses in 24 hours or as directed by a doctor

| children 6 to under 12 years of age | 2 tablets every 4 to 6 hours |
| children under 6 years of age | ask a doctor |

Other Information:
• each Softchews® tablet contains: **sodium 5 mg**
• Phenylketonurics: Contains **Phenylalanine, 17.6 mg** per Softchews® tablet
• contains on aspirin
• store at controlled room temperature 20–25°C (68–77°F).

Inactive Ingredients: aspartame, carnauba wax, citric acid, crospovidone, ethylcellulose, FD&C Yellow 6 aluminum lake, flavors, fractionated coconut oil, hypromellose, magnesium stearate, mannitol, microcrystalline cellulose, mono- and di-glycerides, oleic acid, polyethylene glycol, silicon dioxide, sodium bicarbonate, sodium chloride, sorbitol, starch, sucrose, triethyl citrate

Questions? call **1-800-452-0051** 24 hours a day, 7 days a week.
For more information plus helpful tips visit www.triaminic.com

Distributed by:
Novartis Consumer Health, Inc.
Parsippany, NJ 07054-0622 ©2004
U.S. Pat. No. 5,178,878

How Supplied: 18 Softchews® Tablets
Shown in Product Identification Guide, page 517

TRIAMINIC® Softchews® Cold & Cough
Antihistamine, Cough Suppressant, Nasal Decongestant-
Cherry Flavor

Drug Facts:

Active Ingredients
(in each tablet): **Purpose:**
Chlorpheniramine maleate, USP,
1 mg .... Antihistamine
Dextromethorphan HBr, USP,
5 mg .... Cough suppressant
Pseudoephedrine HCl, USP,
15 mg .... Nasal decongestant

Uses: Temporarily relieves these symptoms:
• cough due to minor throat and bronchial irritation • runny nose • nasal and sinus congestion • sneezing • itchy nose or throat • itchy, watery eyes

Warnings:
Do not use • in a child who is taking a prescription monoamine oxidase inhibitor (MAOI) (certain drugs for depression, psychiatric, or emotional conditions, or Parkinson's disease), or for 2 weeks after stopping the MAOI drug. If you do not know if the child's prescription drug contains an MAOI, ask a doctor or pharmacist before giving this product.
Ask a doctor before use if the child has • heart disease • high blood pressure • thyroid disease • diabetes • glaucoma • cough that occurs with too much phlegm (mucus) or chronic cough that lasts • a breathing problem such as asthma or chronic bronchitis
Ask a doctor or pharmacist before use if the child is taking sedatives or tranquilizers.
When using this product • do not use more than directed • excitability may occur, especially in children • marked drowsiness may occur • sedatives and tranquilizers may increase drowsiness
Stop use and ask a doctor if • nervousness, dizziness, or sleeplessness occur • symptoms do not improve within 7 days or occur with fever • cough persists for more than 7 days, comes back or oc-

curs with fever, rash, or persistent headache. These could be signs of a serious condition.
Keep out of reach of children. In case of overdose, get medical help or contact a poison control center right away.

Directions: • Let Softchews® tablet dissolve in mouth or chew Softchews® tablet before swallowing, whichever is preferred
• take every 4 to 6 hours; not more than 4 doses in 24 hours or as directed by a doctor

children 6 to under 12 years of age	2 tablets every 4 to 6 hours
children under 6 years of age	ask a doctor

Other Information:
• each Softchews® tablet contains: **sodium 5 mg**
• Phenylketonurics: Contains **Phenylalanine, 17.7 mg** per Softchews® tablet
• contains no aspirin • store at controlled room temperature 20–25°C (68–77°F)

How Supplied: 18 Softchews® Tablets.

Inactive Ingredients: aspartame, carnauba wax, citric acid, crospovidone, D&C Red 27 aluminum lake, D&C Red 30 aluminum lake, ethylcellulose, FD&C Blue 2 aluminum lake, flavors, fractionated coconut oil, gum arabic, hypromellose, magnesium stearate, maltodextrin, mannitol, microcrystalline cellulose, mono- and di-glycerides, oleic acid, polyethylene glycol, povidone, silicon dioxide, sodium bicarbonate, sodium chloride, sorbitol, starch, sucrose, triethyl citrate
Questions? call toll-free **1-800-452-0051** 24 hours a day, 7 days a week.
For more information plus helpful tips visit www.triaminic.com

Distributed by:
Novartis Consumer Health, Inc.
Parsippany, NJ 07054-0622 ©2004
U.S. Pat. No. 5,178,878
Shown in Product Identification Guide, page 517

TRIAMINIC® Softchews® Cough & Sore Throat
Cough Suppressant, Nasal Decongestant, Pain Reliever/Fever Reducer
Grape Flavor

Drug Facts:

Active Ingredients:
(in each tablet): **Purpose:**
Acetaminophen, USP,
160 mg ...... Pain reliever/Fever reducer
Dextromethorphan HBr, USP,
5 mg .... Cough suppressant
Pseudoephedrine HCl, USP,
15 mg .... Nasal decongestant

Uses: temporarily relieves: • fever • minor aches and pains • headache and

sore throat • cough due to minor throat and bronchial irritation • nasal and sinus congestion

Warnings:
Do not use • in a child who is taking a prescription monoamine oxidase inhibitor (MAOI) (certain drugs for depression, psychiatric, or emotional conditions, or Parkinson's disease), or for 2 weeks after stopping the MAOI drug. If you do not know if the child's prescription drug contains an MAOI, ask a doctor or pharmacist before giving this product.
• with any other product containing acetaminophen (**see Overdose Warning**)
Ask a doctor before use if the child has • heart disease • high blood pressure • thyroid disease • diabetes • glaucoma • cough that occurs with too much phlegm (mucus) or chronic cough that lasts • a breathing problem such as asthma or chronic bronchitis
Ask a doctor or pharmacist before use if the child is taking sedatives or tranquilizers
When using this product • do not use more than directed
Stop use and ask a doctor if • nervousness, dizziness, or sleeplessness occur • symptoms do not improve for 5 days (pain) or 3 days (fever) • cough persists for more than 7 days, comes back or occurs with fever, rash, or headache • sore throat persists for more than 2 days, or occurs with persistent headache, fever, rash, nausea or vomiting. These could be signs of a serious condition.
Keep out of reach of children.
Overdose Warning: Taking more than the recommended dose can cause serious health problems, including serious liver damage. In case of overdose, get medical help or contact a poison control center right away. Prompt medical attention is critical for adults as well as for children even if you do not notice any signs or symptoms.

Directions:
• do not use more than directed (**see Overdose Warning**)
• Let Softchews® tablet dissolve in mouth or chew Softchews® tablet before swallowing, whichever is preferred
• take every 4 to 6 hours; not more than 4 doses in 24 hours or as directed by a doctor

children 6 to under 12 years of age	2 tablets every 4 to 6 hours
children 2 to under 6 years of age	1 tablet every 4 to 6 hours
children under 2 years of age	ask a doctor

Continued on next page

Information on **Novartis Consumer Health, Inc.** *products appearing on these pages is effective as of November 2003.*

Triaminic Softchews—Cont.

Other Information: • each Softchews® tablet contains: **sodium 8 mg**

• Phenylketonurics: Contains **Phenylalanine, 28.1 mg** per Softchews® tablet

• contains no aspirin

• store at controlled room temperature 20–25°C (68–77°F)

Inactive Ingredients: aspartame, citric acid, crospovidone, D&C Red 27 aluminum lake, dextrin, ethylcellulose, FD&C Blue 1 aluminum lake, flavors, fractionated coconut oil, hypromellose, magnesium stearate, maltodextrin, mannitol, microcrystalline cellulose, oleic acid, polyethylene glycol, povidone, sodium bicarbonate, sodium chloride, sorbitol, starch, sucrose, triethyl citrate

Questions? call **1-800-452-0051** 24 hours a day, 7 days a week.

For more information plus helpful tips visit www.triaminic.com

Distributed by:
Novartis Consumer Health, Inc.
Parsippany, NJ 07054-0622 ©2004
U.S. Pat. No. 5,178,878

How Supplied: 18 softchews® tablets
Shown in Product Identification Guide, page 517

TRIAMINIC™ SPRAY
Sore Throat
Grape Flavor

Active Ingredient: **Purpose:**
Phenol, 0.5% .... Anesthetic/Analgesic

Uses: temporarily relieves:
• sore mouth
• minor irritation or injury of the mouth and gums
• pain due to minor dental procedures, or orthodontic appliances
• pain associated with canker sores
• sore throat pain

Warnings:
When using this product
• do not use more than directed
Stop use and ask a doctor if
• sore throat is severe, persists for more than 2 days or is accompanied by difficulty in breathing.
• sore throat is accompanied or followed by fever, headache, rash, swelling, nausea or vomiting.
• sore mouth symptoms do not improve within 7 days or irritation, pain or redness persists or worsens. These could be signs of a serious condition.

Keep out of reach of children. In case of overdose, get medical help or contact a poison control center right away.

Directions: Triaminic Sore Throat Spray may be used every 2 hours or as directed by a dentist or physician.

Children 2 to under 12 years of age (with adult supervision):	For each application, spray up to 5 times into the throat or affected area.
Children under 2 years of age:	ask a physician or dentist.

Other Information:
• contains no aspirin, no alcohol or sugar
• store at controlled room temperature 20–25°C (68–77°F)

Inactive Ingredients: FD&C Blue 1, FD&C Red 40, flavors, glycerin, purified water, sodium saccharin, sorbitol
Questions? call **1-800-452-0051** 24 hours a day, 7 days a week.

Distributed by:
Novartis Consumer Health, Inc.
Parsippany, NJ 07054-0622 ©2004

How Supplied: 4 oz bottle
Shown in Product Identification Guide, page 517

TRIAMINIC® Vapor Patch® -Mentholated Cherry Scent Cough Suppressant
TRIAMINIC® Vapor Patch® -Menthol Scent Cough Suppressant

Active Ingredients
(in each patch):   **Purpose:**
Camphor 4.7% .... Cough suppressant
Menthol 2.6% .... Cough suppressant

Uses: temporarily relieves cough due to:
• a cold • minor throat and bronchial irritation to help you sleep

Warnings:
For external use only
Flammable: Keep away from fire or flame
Ask a doctor before use if the child has
• cough that occurs with too much phlegm (mucus)
• a persistent or chronic cough such as occurs with asthma
When using this product do not
• use more than directed • **heat** • **microwave** • **use near an open flame**
• **add to hot water or any container where heating water. May cause splattering and result in burns**
Additionally, do not
• **apply to eyes, wounds, sensitive, irritated or damaged skin**
• **take by mouth or place in nostrils**
Stop use and ask a doctor if • cough persists for more than 7 days, comes back, or occurs with fever, rash, or persistent headache. These could be signs of a serious condition. • too much skin irritation occurs or gets worse
Keep out of reach of children. If swallowed, get medical help or contact a poison control center right away.

Directions:
• **see important warnings under 'When using this product'**
• Children 2 to under 12 years of age:
 • Remove plastic backing
 • Apply patch to the throat or chest

• If the child has sensitive skin, the patch may be applied to the same area on clothing*
• Clothing should be loose about the throat and chest to help the vapors reach the nose and mouth
• Apply a new patch up to three times daily or as directed by a doctor
• May use with other cough suppressant products
• Children under 2 years of age: Ask a doctor
*The patch may not adhere to some types of polyester clothing

Other Information: † When used as directed, the product does not alter blood sugar levels
• store at controlled room temperature 20–25°C (68–77°F)
• protect from excessive heat

Inactive Ingredients: cherry scent: acrylic ester copolymer, aloe vera gel, eucalyptus oil, glycerin, karaya, propylene glycol, purified water, wild cherry fragrance
Menthol scent: acrylic ester copolymer, aloe vera gel, eucalyptus oil, glycerin, karaya, purified water, spirits of turpentine
Questions? call   **1-800-452-0051** 24 hours a day, 7 days a week.
      8040459001-7
      30127G
U.S. Patents 5536263, 5741510, 6090403, 6096333, 6096334, 6361790, other patents pending
For more information plus helpful tips visit www.triaminic.com

Distributed by:
Novartis Consumer Health, Inc.
Parsippany, NJ 07054-0622   ©2004

How Supplied: Ointment on a breathable patch
Shown in Product Identification Guide, page 517

Performance Health, Inc.
1017 BOYD ROAD
EXPORT, PA 15632-8997

Direct Inquiries to:
Phone - 724-733-9500
Fax - 724-733-4266
Email - PDR@Biofreeze.com

BIOFREEZE® PAIN RELIEVING GEL

Active Ingredient: Menthol 3.5%

Inactive Ingredients: Camphor (for scent), carbomer, FD&C blue #1, FD&C yellow #5, Glycerine, Herbal Extract (ILEX Paraguariensis), Isopropyl Alcohol, Methylparaben, Propylene Glycol, Silicon Dioxide, Triethanolamine, Water

Indications: Temporary relief from minor aches and pains of muscles and joints due to arthritis, backache, strains and sprains.

Warnings: Ask a doctor before use if you have sensitive skin. Keep away from excessive heat or open flame. Avoid contact with the eyes or mucous membranes. Do not apply to wounds or damaged skin. Do not use with other ointments, creams, sprays or liniments. Do not apply to irritated skin or if excessive irritation develops. Do not bandage. Wash hands after use. If pregnant or breast-feeding, ask a health professional before use. Keep out of reach of children. If accidentally ingested, get medical help or contact a Poison Control Center.

Directions: Adults and children 2 years of age and older: Apply to the affected areas not more than 3 to 4 times daily. Children under 2 years of age, consult physician.

How Supplied: 4 oz. tube, 3 oz. Roll-on and 5 gram packets for home use. 16 oz., 32 oz. and Gallon for professional use.

Pfizer Consumer Healthcare, Pfizer Inc.
201 TABOR ROAD MORRIS PLAINS, NJ 07950

Address Questions & Comments to:
Consumer Affairs, Pfizer Consumer Healthcare
182 Tabor Road
Morris Plains, NJ 07950
For Medical Emergencies/Information Contact:
1-(800)-223-0182
1-800-524-2624 (Spanish)
1-(800)-378-1783 (e.p.t.)
1-(800)-337-7266 (e.p.t.-Spanish)

BENADRYL® Allergy Kapseals® Capsules (also available in Ultratab™ Tablets)
[bĕ 'nă-drĭl]

Drug Facts:

Active Ingredient: **Purpose:**
(in each capsule)
Diphenhydramine HCl
25 mg .... Antihistamine

Uses:
• temporarily relieves these symptoms due to hay fever or other upper respiratory allergies:
  • runny nose
  • sneezing
  • itchy, watery eyes
  • itching of the nose or throat
• temporarily relieves these symptoms due to the common cold:
  • runny nose
  • sneezing

Warnings:

Do not use with any other product containing diphenhydramine, even one used on skin.

Ask a doctor before use if you have:
• glaucoma
• trouble urinating due to an enlarged prostate gland
• a breathing problem such as emphysema or chronic bronchitis
Ask a doctor or pharmacist before use if you are taking sedatives or tranquilizers
When using this product:
• marked drowsiness may occur
• avoid alcoholic drinks
• alcohol, sedatives, and tranquilizers may increase drowsiness
• be careful when driving a motor vehicle or operating machinery
• excitability may occur, especially in children
If pregnant or breast-feeding, ask a health professional before use.
Keep out of reach of children. In case of overdose, get medical help or contact a Poison Control Center right away.

Directions:
• take every 4 to 6 hours
• do not take more than 6 doses in 24 hours

adults and children 12 years of age and over	25 mg to 50 mg (1 to 2 capsules)
children 6 to under 12 years of age	12.5 mg** to 25 mg (1 capsule)
children under 6 years of age	ask a doctor

**12.5 mg dosage strength is not available in this package. Do not attempt to break capsules.

Other Information:
• store at 59° to 77°F in a dry place
• protect from light

Inactive Ingredients: Capsules: D&C red no. 28, FD&C blue no. 1, FD&C red no. 3, FD&C red no. 40, gelatin, glyceryl monooleate, lactose, magnesium stearate, and titanium dioxide. Printed with black edible ink.
Tablets: candelilla wax, crospovidone, dibasic calcium phosphate dihydrate, D&C red no. 27 aluminum lake, hypromellose, magnesium stearate, microcrystalline cellulose, polyethylene glycol, polysorbate 80, pregelatinized starch, stearic acid, and titanium dioxide.

Questions? call **1-800-524-2624** (English/Spanish), weekdays, 9 AM–5 PM EST

How Supplied: Benadryl tablets are supplied in boxes of 24 and 48, bottle of 100; capsules are supplied in boxes of 24 and 48.

Shown in Product Identification Guide, page 518

BENADRYL® Dye-Free Allergy Liqui-Gels® Softgels
[bĕ 'nă-drĭl]

Drug Facts:

Active Ingredient:
(in each softgel)   **Purpose:**
Diphenhydramine
HCl 25 mg .... Antihistamine

Uses:
• temporarily relieves these symptoms due to hay fever or other upper respiratory allergies:
  • runny nose
  • sneezing
  • itchy, watery eyes
  • itching of the nose or throat
• temporarily relieves these symptoms due to the common cold:
  • runny nose
  • sneezing

Warnings:

Do not use with any other product containing diphenhydramine, even one used on skin.

Ask a doctor before use if you have:
• glaucoma
• trouble urinating due to an enlarged prostate gland
• a breathing problem such as emphysema or chronic bronchitis
Ask a doctor or pharmacist before use if you are taking sedatives or tranquilizers
When using this product:
• marked drowsiness may occur
• avoid alcoholic drinks
• alcohol, sedatives, and tranquilizers may increase drowsiness
• be careful when driving a motor vehicle or operating machinery
• excitability may occur, especially in children
If pregnant or breast-feeding, ask a health professional before use.
Keep out of reach of children. In case of overdose, get medical help or contact a Poison Control Center right away.

Directions:
• take every 4 to 6 hours
• do not take more than 6 doses in 24 hours

Continued on next page

This product information was prepared in November 2003. On these and other Pfizer Consumer Healthcare Products, detailed information may be obtained by addressing Pfizer Consumer Healthcare, Pfizer, Inc., Morris Plains, NJ 07950

Benadryl Dye-Free—Cont.

adults and children 12 years of age and over	25 mg to 50 mg (1 to 2 softgels)
children 6 to under 12 years of age	12.5 mg** to 25 mg (1 softgel)
children under 6 years of age	ask a doctor

**12.5 mg dosage strength is not available in this package. Do not attempt to break softgels.

Other Information:
• store at 59° to 77°F in a dry place
• protect from heat, humidity, and light

Inactive Ingredients: Gelatin, glycerin, polyethylene glycol 400, and sorbitol. Softgels are imprinted with edible dye-free ink.

Questions? call **1-800-524-2624** (English/Spanish), weekdays, 9 AM–5 PM EST

How Supplied: Benadryl® Dye-Free Allergy Liqui-Gels® Softgels are supplied in boxes of 24.
Liqui-Gels is a registered trademark of R.P. Scherer Corporation.

Shown in Product Identification Guide, page 518

BENADRYL® Allergy & Sinus Tablets
(Formerly Benadryl Allergy/ Congestion)
[bĕ 'nă-drĭl]

Drug Facts:

Active Ingredients:
(in each tablet)　　　　　　**Purposes:**
Diphenhydramine HCl
　25 mg .... Antihistamine
Pseudoephedrine HCl
　60 mg .... Nasal decongestant

Uses:
• temporarily relieves these symptoms due to hay fever or other upper respiratory allergies:
　• runny nose
　• sneezing
　• itchy, watery eyes
　• nasal congestion
　• itching of the nose or throat
• temporarily relieves these symptoms due to the common cold:
　• runny nose
　• sneezing
　• nasal congestion

Warnings:
Do not use
• if you are now taking a prescription monoamine oxidase inhibitor (MAOI) (certain drugs for depression, psychiatric, or emotional conditions, or Parkinson's disease), or for 2 weeks after stopping the MAOI drug. If you do not know if your prescription drug contains an MAOI, ask a doctor or pharmacist before taking this product.

• with any other product containing diphenhydramine, even one used on skin.

Ask a doctor before use if you have:
• heart disease
• glaucoma
• thyroid disease
• diabetes
• high blood pressure
• trouble urinating due to an enlarged prostate gland
• a breathing problem such as emphysema or chronic bronchitis

Ask a doctor or pharmacist before use if you are taking sedatives or tranquilizers

When using this product:
• **do not use more than directed**
• marked drowsiness may occur
• avoid alcoholic drinks
• alcohol, sedatives, and tranquilizers may increase drowsiness
• be careful when driving a motor vehicle or operating machinery
• excitability may occur, especially in children

Stop use and ask a doctor if:
• you get nervous, dizzy, or sleepless
• symptoms do not improve within 7 days or are accompanied by fever

If pregnant or breast-feeding, ask a health professional before use.

Keep out of reach of children. In case of overdose, get medical help or contact a Poison Control Center right away.

Directions:
• adults and children 12 years of age and over: one (1) tablet
• take every 4 to 6 hours
• do not take more than 4 tablets in 24 hours
• children under 12 years of age: ask a doctor

Other Information:
• protect from light
• store at 59° to 77°F in a dry place

Inactive Ingredients: Croscarmellose sodium, dibasic calcium phosphate dihydrate, FD&C blue no. 1 aluminum lake, hypromellose, microcrystalline cellulose, polyethylene glycol, polysorbate 80, pregelatinized starch, stearic acid, titanium dioxide and zinc stearate. Printed with edible black ink.

Questions? call **1-800-524-2624** (English/Spanish), weekdays, 9 AM – 5 PM EST

How Supplied: Benadryl Allergy & Sinus Tablets are supplied in boxes of 24.
Shown in Product Identification Guide, page 518

BENADRYL® Allergy & Sinus Headache Caplets*
(also available in Gelcaps)
[bĕ 'nă-drĭl]
*Capsule Shaped Tablets

Drug Facts:

Active Ingredients:
(in each caplet)　　　　　　**Purposes:**
Acetaminophen 500 mg .... Pain reliever
Diphenhydramine HCl
　12.5 mg .... Antihistamine

Pseudoephedrine HCl
　30 mg .... Nasal decongestant

Uses:
• temporarily relieves these symptoms of hay fever and the common cold:
　• runny nose
　• sneezing
　• headache
　• minor aches and pains
　• nasal congestion
• temporarily relieves these additional symptoms of hay fever:
　• itching of the nose or throat
　• itchy, watery eyes

Warnings:
Alcohol warning: If you consume 3 or more alcoholic drinks every day, ask your doctor whether you should take acetaminophen or other pain relievers/ fever reducers. Acetaminophen may cause liver damage.

Do not use:
• with another product containing any of these active ingredients.
• if you are now taking a prescription monoamine oxidase inhibitor (MAOI) (certain drugs for depression, psychiatric, or emotional conditions, or Parkinson's disease), or for 2 weeks after stopping the MAOI drug. If you do not know if your prescription drug contains an MAOI, ask a doctor or pharmacist before taking this product.
• with any other product containing diphenhydramine, even one used on skin.

Ask a doctor before use if you have:
• heart disease
• glaucoma
• thyroid disease
• diabetes
• high blood pressure
• trouble urinating due to an enlarged prostate gland
• a breathing problem such as emphysema or chronic bronchitis

Ask a doctor or pharmacist before use if you are taking sedatives or tranquilizers

When using this product:
• **do not use more than directed**
• marked drowsiness may occur
• excitability may occur, especially in children
• avoid alcoholic drinks
• alcohol, sedatives, and tranquilizers may increase drowsiness
• be careful when driving a motor vehicle or operating machinery

Stop use and ask a doctor if:
• you get nervous, dizzy, or sleepless
• new symptoms occur
• symptoms do not get better
• you need to use more than 10 days
• fever occurs and lasts more than 3 days

If pregnant or breast-feeding, ask a health professional before use.

Keep out of reach of children.

Overdose warning: Taking more than the recommended dose may cause liver damage. In case of overdose, get medical help or contact a Poison Control Center right away. Quick medical attention is critical for adults as well as for children even if you do not notice any signs or symptoms.

Directions:
• do not use more than directed (see overdose warning)

- take every 6 hours while symptoms persist
- do not take more than 8 caplets in 24 hours or as directed by a doctor
- adults and children 12 years of age and over: 2 caplets
- children under 12 years of age: ask a doctor

Other Information:
- store at 59° to 77°F in a dry place

Inactive Ingredients: (Caplets): Candelilla wax, corn starch, croscarmellose sodium, D&C yellow no. 10 aluminum lake, FD&C blue no. 1 aluminum lake, FD&C yellow no. 6 aluminum lake, hydroxypropyl cellulose, hypromellose, microcrystalline cellulose, polyethylene glycol, polysorbate 80, pregelatinized starch, sodium starch glycolate, stearic acid, titanium dioxide, and zinc stearate (Gelcaps): Colloidal silicon dioxide, croscarmellose sodium, D&C yellow no. 10 Al lake, FD&C green no. 3 Al lake, gelatin, hypromellose, polysorbate 80, stearic acid and titanium dioxide.

Questions? call **1-800-524-2624** (English/Spanish), weekdays, 9 AM - 5 PM EST

How Supplied: Benadryl Allergy & Sinus Headache is available in boxes of 24 and 48 caplets, and boxes of 24, 48 and 72 gelcaps.

Shown in Product Identification Guide, page 518

BENADRYL® Maximum Strength Severe Allergy† & Sinus Headache Caplets*
[bĕ'nă-drĭl]
* Capsule Shaped Tablets
† Upper Respiratory Allergies Only

Drug Facts:

Active Ingredients:
(in each caplet)   **Purposes:**
Acetaminophen
   500 mg .... Pain reliever
Diphenhydramine
   HCl 25 mg .... Antihistamine
Pseudoephedrine
   HCl 30 mg .... Nasal decongestant

Uses:
- temporarily relieves these symptoms of hay fever and the common cold:
  - runny nose
  - headache
  - sneezing
  - minor aches and pains
  - nasal congestion
- temporarily relieves these additional symptoms of hay fever:
  - itching of the nose or throat
  - itchy, watery eyes

Warnings:
Alcohol warning: If you consume 3 or more alcoholic drinks every day, ask your doctor whether you should take acetaminophen or other pain relievers/fever reducers. Acetaminophen may cause liver damage.

Do not use:
- with another product containing any of these active ingredients
- if you are now taking a prescription monoamine oxidase inhibitor (MAOI) (certain drugs for depression, psychiatric, or emotional conditions, or Parkinson's disease), or for 2 weeks after stopping the MAOI drug. If you do not know if your prescription drug contains an MAOI, ask a doctor or pharmacist before taking this product.
- with any other product containing diphenhydramine, even one used on skin.

Ask a doctor before use if you have:
- heart disease
- glaucoma
- thyroid disease
- diabetes
- high blood pressure
- trouble urinating due to an enlarged prostate gland
- a breathing problem such as emphysema or chronic bronchitis

Ask a doctor or pharmacist before use if you are taking sedatives or tranquilizers

When using this product:
- **do not use more than directed**
- marked drowsiness may occur
- excitability may occur, especially in children
- avoid alcoholic drinks
- alcohol, sedatives, and tranquilizers may increase drowsiness
- be careful when driving a motor vehicle or operating machinery

Stop use and ask a doctor if:
- you get nervous, dizzy, or sleepless
- new symptoms occur
- symptoms do not get better
- you need to use more than 10 days
- fever occurs and lasts more than 3 days

If pregnant or breast-feeding, ask a health professional before use.

Keep out of reach of children.

Overdose warning: Taking more than the recommended dose may cause liver damage. In case of overdose, get medical help or contact a Poison Control Center right away. Quick medical attention is critical for adults as well as for children even if you do not notice any signs or symptoms.

Directions:
- do not use more than directed (see overdose warning)
- take every 6 hours while symptoms persist
- do not take more than 8 caplets in 24 hours or as directed by a doctor
- adults and children 12 years of age and over: 2 caplets
- children under 12 years of age: ask a doctor

Other Information:
- store at 59° to 77°F in a dry place

Inactive Ingredients: Carnauba wax, crospovidone, FD&C blue no. 1 aluminum lake, hypromellose, magnesium stearate, microcrystalline cellulose, polyethylene glycol, polysorbate 80, povidone, pregelatinized starch, sodium starch glycolate, stearic acid, and titanium dioxide

Questions? call **1-800-524-2624** (English/Spanish), weekdays, 9 AM – 5 PM EST

How Supplied: Available in 20 Caplets (capsule-shaped tablets).
Shown in Product Identification Guide, page 518

**Children's BENADRYL®
Allergy
Liquid Medication**
[bĕ'nă-drĭl]
Cherry Flavored

Drug Facts:

Active Ingredient: **Purpose:**
(in each 5 mL)
Diphenhydramine
   HCl 12.5 mg .... Antihistamine
5 mL = one teaspoonful

Uses:
- temporarily relieves these symptoms due to hay fever or other upper respiratory allergies:
  - runny nose
  - sneezing
  - itchy, watery eyes
  - itching of the nose or throat
- temporarily relieves these symptoms due to the common cold:
  - runny nose
  - sneezing

Warnings:
Do not use with any other product containing diphenhydramine, even one used on skin.

Ask a doctor before use if you have:
- glaucoma
- trouble urinating due to an enlarged prostate gland
- a breathing problem such as emphysema or chronic bronchitis

Ask a doctor or pharmacist before use if you are taking sedatives or tranquilizers

When using this product:
- marked drowsiness may occur
- avoid alcoholic drinks
- alcohol, sedatives, and tranquilizers may increase drowsiness
- be careful when driving a motor vehicle or operating machinery
- excitability may occur, especially in children

If pregnant or breast-feeding, ask a health professional before use.

Keep out of reach of children. In case of overdose, get medical help or contact a Poison Control Center right away.

Directions:
- take every 4 to 6 hours
- do not take more than 6 doses in 24 hours

Continued on next page

This product information was prepared in November 2003. On these and other Pfizer Consumer Healthcare Products, detailed information may be obtained by addressing Pfizer Consumer Healthcare, Pfizer, Inc., Morris Plains, NJ 07950

Children's Benadryl—Cont.

children under 6 years of age	ask a doctor
children 6 to under 12 years of age	1 to 2 teaspoonfuls (12.5 mg to 25 mg)
adults and children 12 years of age and over	2 to 4 teaspoonfuls (25 mg to 50 mg)

Other Information:
• store at 59° to 77°F

Inactive Ingredients: Citric acid, D&C red no. 33, FD&C red no. 40, flavors, glycerin, poloxamer 407, purified water, sodium benzoate, sodium chloride, sodium citrate, and sugar

Questions? call **1-800-524-2624** (English/Spanish), weekdays, 9 AM–5 PM EST

How Supplied: Children's Benadryl Allergy Liquid Medication is supplied in 4 and 8 fluid ounce bottles.
Shown in Product Identification Guide, page 518

Children's BENADRYL® Dye-Free Allergy Liquid Medication
[bĕ 'nă-drĭl]
Bubble Gum Flavored

Drug Facts:

Active Ingredient:
(in each 5 mL)   **Purpose:**
Diphenhydramine
HCl 12.5 mg .... Antihistamine
* 5 ml = one teaspoonful

Uses:
• temporarily relieves these symptoms due to hay fever or other upper respiratory allergies:
  • runny nose
  • sneezing
  • itchy, watery eyes
  • itching of the nose or throat
• temporarily relieves these symptoms due to the common cold:
  • runny nose
  • sneezing

Warnings:
Do not use with any other product containing diphenhydramine, even one used on skin.
Ask a doctor before use if you have
• glaucoma
• trouble urinating due to an enlarged prostate gland
• a breathing problem such as emphysema or chronic bronchitis
Ask a doctor or pharmacist before use if you are taking sedatives or tranquilizers
When using this product:
• marked drowsiness may occur
• avoid alcoholic drinks
• alcohol, sedatives, and tranquilizers may increase drowsiness
• be careful when driving a motor vehicle or operating machinery
• excitability may occur, especially in children
If pregnant or breast-feeding, ask a health professional before use.
Keep out of reach of children. In case of overdose, get medical help or contact a Poison Control Center right away.

Directions:
• take every 4 to 6 hours
• do not take more than 6 doses in 24 hours

children under 6 years of age	ask a doctor
children 6 to under 12 years of age	1 to 2 teaspoonfuls (12.5 mg to 25 mg)
adults and children 12 years of age and over	2 to 4 teaspoonfuls (25 mg to 50 mg)

Other Information:
• store at 59° to 77°F

Inactive Ingredients: Carboxymethylcellulose sodium, citric acid, flavor, glycerin, purified water, saccharin sodium, sodium benzoate, sodium citrate, and sorbitol solution

Questions? call **1-800-524-2624** (English/Spanish), weekdays, 9 AM – 5 PM EST

How Supplied: Children's Benadryl Dye-Free Allergy Liquid Medication is supplied in 4 fl. oz. bottles.
Shown in Product Identification Guide, page 518

Children's BENADRYL® Allergy/Cold

FASTMELT™
Dissolving Tablets
[bĕ 'nă-drĭl]
Cherry Flavored

Drug Facts:

Active Ingredients: **Purposes:**
(in each tablet)
Diphenhydramine citrate
19 mg* .... Antihistamine/cough
                                        suppressant
Pseudoephedrine HCl
30 mg .... Nasal decongestant

*equivalent to 12.5 mg of diphenhydramine HCl
Uses:
• temporarily relieves these symptoms of hay fever or the common cold:
  • runny nose
  • sneezing
  • nasal congestion
  • cough
• temporarily relieves these additional symptoms of hay fever:
  • itching of the nose or throat
  • itchy, watery eyes

Warnings:
Do not use
• if you are now taking a prescription monoamine oxidase inhibitor (MAOI) (certain drugs for depression, psychiatric, or emotional conditions, or Parkinson's disease), or for 2 weeks after stopping the MAOI drug. If you do not know if your prescription drug contains an MAOI, ask a doctor or pharmacist before taking this product.
• with any other product containing diphenhydramine, even one used on skin.

Ask a doctor before use if you have:
• heart disease
• high blood pressure
• thyroid disease
• trouble urinating due to an enlarged prostate gland
• diabetes
• cough accompanied by excessive phlegm (mucus)
• glaucoma
• a breathing problem such as emphysema or chronic bronchitis
• persistent or chronic cough such as occurs with smoking, asthma, or emphysema

Ask a doctor or pharmacist before use if you are taking sedatives or tranquilizers

When using this product:
• do not use more than directed
• marked drowsiness may occur
• excitability may occur, especially in children
• avoid alcoholic drinks
• alcohol, sedatives, and tranquilizers may increase drowsiness
• be careful when driving a motor vehicle or operating machinery

Stop use and ask a doctor if:
• you get nervous, dizzy, or sleepless
• symptoms do not improve within 7 days or are accompanied by fever
• cough persists for more than 1 week, tends to recur, or is accompanied by fever, rash, or persistent headache. These could be signs of a serious condition.

If pregnant or breast-feeding, ask a health professional before use.

Keep out of reach of children. In case of overdose, get medical help or contact a Poison Control Center right away.

Directions:
• place in mouth and allow to dissolve
• take every 4 hours

adults and children 12 years of age and over	2 tablets; do not take more than 8 tablets in 24 hours or as directed by a doctor
children 6 to under 12 years of age	1 tablet; do not take more than 4 tablets in 24 hours or as directed by a doctor
children under 6 years of age	ask a doctor

Other Information:
- **phenylketonurics:** contains phenylalanine 4.6 mg per tablet
- store at 59° to 77°F in a dry place

Inactive Ingredients: Aspartame, citric acid, D&C red no. 7 calcium lake, ethylcellulose, flavor, lactitol, magnesium stearate, mannitol, and stearic acid

Questions? call **1-800-524-2624** (English/Spanish), weekdays, 9 AM - 5 PM EST

How Supplied: Available in boxes of 20 dissolving tablets.

Shown in Product Identification Guide, page 518

BENADRYL® SINGLE INGREDIENT FASTMELT TABLETS FOR CHILDREN

[bĕ′nă-drĭl]

Drug Facts

**Active Ingredient
(in each tablet):**　　　**Purpose:**
Diphenhydramine citrate
19 mg* .... Antihistamine

*equivalent to 12.5 mg of diphenhydramine HCl

Uses:
- temporarily relieves these symptoms due to hay fever or other upper respiratory allergies:
  - runny nose • sneezing • itchy, watery eyes • itching of the nose or throat
- temporarily relieves these symptoms due to the common cold:
  - runny nose • sneezing

Warnings: **Do not use** with any other product containing diphenhydramine, even one used on skin

Ask a doctor before use if you have
- glaucoma • trouble urinating due to an enlarged prostate gland • a breathing problem such as emphysema or chronic bronchitis

Ask a doctor or pharmacist before use if you are taking sedatives or tranquilizers

When using this product
- marked drowsiness may occur • avoid alcoholic drinks • alcohol, sedatives, and tranquilizers may increase drowsiness • be careful when driving a motor vehicle or operating machinery • excitability may occur, especially in children

If pregnant or breast-feeding, ask a health professional before use.

Keep out of reach of children. In case of overdose, get medical help or contact a Poison Control Center right away.

Directions:
- take every 4 to 6 hours • do not take more than 6 doses in 24 hours

adults and children 12 years of age and over	2 to 4 tablets (38 mg to 76 mg)
children 6 to under 12 years of age	1 to 2 tablets (19 mg to 38 mg)
children under 6 years of age	ask a doctor

Other Information:
- **phenylketonurics:** contains phenylalanine 4.5 mg per tablet • store at 59° to 77°F in a dry place • protect from heat, humidity, and light

Inactive Ingredients: aspartame, citric acid, D&C red no. 7 calcium lake, ethylcellulose, flavors, lactitol monohydrate, magnesium stearate, mannitol, polyethylene, soy protein isolate, stearic acid
Questions? call **1-800-524-2624** (English/Spanish), weekdays, 9 AM – 5 PM EST

BENADRYL® Itch Relief Stick Extra Strength
Topical Analgesic/Skin Protectant
[bĕ′nă-drĭl]

Drug Facts:

Active Ingredients:　　　**Purposes:**
Diphenhydramine
　hydrochloride 2% .... Topical analgesic
Zinc
　acetate 0.1% .... Skin protectant

Uses:
- temporarily relieves pain and itching associated with
  - insect bites
  - minor burns
  - sunburn
  - minor skin irritations
  - minor cuts
  - scrapes
  - rashes due to poison ivy, poison oak, and poison sumac
- dries the oozing and weeping of poison ivy, poison oak and poison sumac

Warnings:
For external use only
Flammable. Keep away from fire or flame.
Do not use
- more often than directed
- on chicken pox or measles
- with any other product containing diphenhydramine, even one taken by mouth
- on large areas of the body, including large areas of poison ivy, sunburn, or broken, blistered or oozing skin
When using this product
- avoid contact with eyes
Stop use and ask a doctor if
- condition worsens or does not improve within 7 days
- symptoms persist for more than 7 days or clear up and occur again within a few days
Keep out of reach of children. If swallowed, get medical help or contact a Poison Control Center right away.

Directions:
- press tip of stick on affected skin area until liquid flows, then dab sparingly

- adults and children 6 years of age and older: apply to affected area not more than 3 to 4 times daily
- children under 6 years of age: ask a doctor

Other Information:
- store at 59 to 77° F

Inactive Ingredients: alcohol 73.5% v/v, glycerin, povidone, purified water, and tromethamine

Questions? call **1-800-524-2624** (English/Spanish), Monday to Friday, 9 AM - 5 PM EST

How Supplied: Benadryl® Itch Relief Stick is available in a .47 fl. oz (14 mL) dauber.

Shown in Product Identification Guide, page 518

BENADRYL® Itch Stopping Cream Original Strength
[bĕ′nă-drĭl]

Drug Facts
Active Ingredients:　　　**Purpose:**
Diphenhydramine　hydrochloride
1% .... Topical analgesic
Zinc acetate 0.1% .... Skin protectant

Uses:
- temporarily relieves pain and itching associated with:
- insect bites
- minor burns
- sunburn
- minor skin irritations
- minor cuts
- scrapes
- rashes due to poison ivy, poison oak, and poison sumac
- dries the oozing and weeping of poison ivy, poison oak, and poison sumac

Warnings:
For external use only
Do not use
- more often than directed
- on chicken pox or measles
- with any other product containing diphenhydramine, even one taken by mouth
- on large areas of the body, including large areas of poison ivy, sunburn, or broken, blistered or oozing skin
When using this product
- avoid contact with eyes
Stop use and ask a doctor if
- condition worsens or does not improve within 7 days
- symptoms persist for more than 7 days or clear up and occur again within a few days

Continued on next page

This product information was prepared in November 2003. On these and other Pfizer Consumer Healthcare Products, detailed information may be obtained by addressing Pfizer Consumer Healthcare, Pfizer, Inc., Morris Plains, NJ 07950

Benadryl Itch Cream—Cont.

Keep out of reach of children. If swallowed, get medical help or contact a Poison Control Center right away.

Directions:
- adults and children 2 years of age and older: apply to affected area not more than 3 to 4 times daily
- children under 2 years of age: ask a doctor

Other Information: • store at 59° to 77° F

Inactive Ingredients: cetyl alcohol, diazolidinyl urea, methylparaben, polyethylene glycol monostearate 1000, propylene glycol, propylparaben, and purified water

Questions? call **1-800-524-2624** (English/Spanish), Monday to Friday, 9 AM - 5 PM EST

How Supplied: Benadryl Itch Stopping Cream Original Strength is available in 1 oz (28.3 g).
Shown in Product Identification Guide, page 518

BENADRYL® Itch Stopping Cream Extra Strength
[bĕ 'nă-drĭl]

Drug Facts

Active Ingredients:	**Purpose:**

Diphenhydramine hydrochloride 2% .... Topical analgesic
Zinc acetate 0.1% .... Skin protectant

Uses:
- temporarily relieves pain and itching associated with:
  - insect bites
  - minor burns
  - sunburn
  - minor skin irritations
  - minor cuts
  - scrapes
  - rashes due to poison ivy, poison oak, and poison sumac
- dries the oozing and weeping of poison ivy, poison oak, and poison sumac

Warnings:
For external use only
Do not use
- more often than directed
- on chicken pox or measles
- with any other product containing diphenhydramine, even one taken by mouth
- on large areas of the body, including large areas of poison ivy, sunburn, or broken, blistered or oozing skin
When using this product
- avoid contact with eyes
Stop use and ask a doctor if
- condition worsens or does not improve within 7 days
- symptoms persist for more than 7 days or clear up and occur again within a few days
Keep out of reach of children. If swallowed, get medical help or contact a Poison Control Center right away.

Directions:
- adults and children 12 years of age and older: apply to affected area not more than 3 to 4 times daily
- children under 12 years of age: ask a doctor

Other Information: • store at 59° to 77° F

Inactive Ingredients: cetyl alcohol, diazolidinyl urea, methylparaben, polyethylene glycol monostearate 1000, propylene glycol, propylparaben, and purified water

Questions? call **1-800-524-2624** (English/Spanish), Monday to Friday, 9 AM - 5 PM EST

How Supplied: Benadryl Itch Stopping Cream Extra Strength is available in 1 oz (28.3 g) tubes.
Shown in Product Identification Guide, page 518

BENADRYL® Itch Stopping Gel Extra Strength
[bĕ 'nă-drĭl]

Drug Facts

Active Ingredient:	**Purpose:**

Diphenhydramine hydrochloride 2% .... Topical analgesic

Uses:
- temporarily relieves pain and itching associated with:
  - insect bites
  - minor burns
  - sunburn
  - minor skin irritations
  - minor cuts
  - scrapes
  - rashes due to poison ivy, poison oak, and poison sumac

Warnings:
For external use only
Do not use
- more often than directed
- on chicken pox or measles
- with any other product containing diphenhydramine, even one taken by mouth
- on large areas of the body, including large areas of poison ivy, sunburn, or broken, blistered or oozing skin
When using this product
- avoid contact with eyes
Stop use and ask a doctor if
- condition worsens
- symptoms persist for more than 7 days or clear up and occur again within a few days
Keep out of reach of children. If swallowed, get medical help or contact a Poison Control Center right away.

Directions:
- adults and children 12 years of age and older: apply to affected area not more than 3 to 4 times daily
- children under 12 years of age: ask a doctor

Other Information:
- store at 59° to 77° F

Inactive Ingredients: SD alcohol 38-B, camphor, citric acid, diazolidinyl urea, glycerin, hypromellose, methylparaben, propylene glycol, propylparaben, purified water, and sodium citrate

Questions? call **1-800-524-2624** (English/Spanish), Monday to Friday, 9 AM - 5 PM EST

How Supplied: Benadryl Itch Stopping Gel Extra Strength is supplied in 4 fl. oz. (118mL) bottles

---

BENADRYL® Itch Stopping Spray Extra Strength
[bĕ 'nă-drĭl]

Drug Facts

Active Ingredients:	**Purpose:**

Diphenhydramine hydrochloride 2% .... Topical analgesic
Zinc acetate 0.1% .... Skin protectant

Uses:
- temporarily relieves pain and itching associated with:
  - insect bites
  - minor burns
  - sunburn
  - minor skin irritations
  - minor cuts
  - scrapes
  - rashes due to poison ivy, poison oak, and poison sumac
- dries the oozing and weeping of poison ivy, poison oak, and poison sumac

Warnings:
For external use only
Flammable. Keep away from fire or flame
Do not use
- more often than directed
- on chicken pox or measles
- with any other product containing diphenhydramine, even one taken by mouth
- on large areas of the body, including large areas of poison ivy, sunburn, or broken, blistered or oozing skin
When using this product
- avoid contact with eyes
Stop use and ask a doctor if
- condition worsens or does not improve within 7 days
- symptoms persist for more than 7 days or clear up and occur again within a few days
Keep out of reach of children. If swallowed, get medical help or contact a Poison Control Center right away.

Directions:
- adults and children 12 years of age and older: apply to affected area not more than 3 to 4 times daily
- children under 12 years of age: ask a doctor

Other Information: • store at 59° to 77° F

Inactive Ingredients: alcohol 78% v/v, glycerin, povidone, purified water, and tris (hydroxymethyl) aminomethane

Questions? call **1-800-524-2624** (English/Spanish), Monday to Friday, 9 AM - 5 PM EST

How Supplied: Benadryl Itch Stopping Spray Extra Strength Spray is available in a 2 fl. oz. (59mL) pump spray bottle.
Shown in Product Identification Guide, page 518

BENGAY® External Analgesic Products

Description: BENGAY products contain menthol in an alcohol base gel, combinations of methyl salicylate and menthol in cream and ointment bases, as well as a combination of methyl salicylate, menthol and camphor in a non-greasy cream base; all suitable for topical application.

In addition to the Original Formula Pain Relieving Ointment (methyl salicylate, 18.3%; menthol, 16%), BENGAY is offered as BENGAY Greaseless Pain Relieving Cream (methyl salicylate, 15%; menthol, 10%), an Arthritis Formula NonGreasy Pain Relieving Cream (methyl salicylate, 30%; menthol, 8%), an Ultra Strength NonGreasy Pain Relieving Cream (methyl salicylate 30%; menthol 10%; camphor 4%), and Vanishing Scent NonGreasy Pain Relieving Gel (2.5% menthol).

Action and Uses: Methyl salicylate, menthol and camphor are external analgesics which stimulate sensory receptors of warmth and/or cold. This produces a counter-irritant response which provides temporary relief of minor aches and pains of muscles and joints associated with simple backache, arthritis, strains and sprains.

Several double-blind clinical studies of BENGAY products containing menthol-methyl salicylate have shown the effectiveness of this combination in counteracting minor pain of skeletal muscle stress and arthritis.

Three studies involving a total of 102 normal subjects in which muscle soreness was experimentally induced showed statistically significant beneficial results from use of the active product vs. placebo for lowered Muscle Action Potential (spasms), greater rise in threshold of muscular pain and greater reduction in perceived muscular pain.

Six clinical studies of a total of 207 subjects suffering from minor pain due to osteoarthritis and rheumatoid arthritis showed the active product to give statistically significant beneficial results vs. placebo for greater relief of perceived pain, increased range of motion of the affected joints and increased digital dexterity. In two studies designed to measure the effect of topically applied BENGAY vs. placebo on muscular endurance, discomfort, onset of exercise pain and fatigue, 30 subjects performed a submaximal three-hour run and another 30 subjects performed a maximal treadmill run. BENGAY was found to significantly decrease the discomfort during the submaximal and maximal runs, and increase the time before onset of fatigue during the maximal run.

Applied before workouts, BENGAY relaxes tight muscles and increases circulation to make exercising more comfortable, longer.

To help reduce muscle ache and soreness after exercise, BENGAY can be applied and allowed to work before taking a shower.

Directions: Apply to affected area not more than 3 to 4 times daily.

Warnings: For external use only. Use only as directed. Do not use with a heating pad. Keep away from children to avoid accidental ingestion. Do not swallow. If swallowed, get medical help or contact a Poison Control Center immediately. Do not bandage tightly. Keep away from eyes, mucous membranes, broken or irritated skin. If skin redness or excessive irritation develops, pain lasts for more than 10 days, or with arthritis—like conditions in children under 12, do not use and call a physician.
Shown in Product Identification Guide, page 518

BENGAY® Pain Relieving Patch
[bĕn-gā]

Drug Facts

Active Ingredient: **Purpose:**
Menthol 1.4% .... Topical analgesic (present as crystalline and natural forms)

Uses:
• temporarily relieves minor aches and pains of muscles and joints associated with:
  • simple backache • arthritis • strains
  • bruises • sprains

Warnings:
For external use only.
Do not use
• on wounds or damaged skin
• with a heating pad
• on a child under 12 years of age with arthritis-like conditions
Ask a doctor before use if you have
• redness over the affected area
When using this product
• avoid contact with eyes or mucous membranes
• do not bandage tightly
Stop use and ask a doctor if
• condition worsens or symptoms persist for more than 7 days
• symptoms clear up and occur again within a few days • excessive skin irritation occurs
Keep out of reach of children. If swallowed, get medical help or contact a Poison Control Center immediately.

Directions:
• open pouch and remove patch
• if desired, cut patch to size
• peel off protective backing and apply sticky side to affected area
• adults and children 12 years of age and older: apply to affected area not more than 3 to 4 times daily
• children under 12 years of age: consult a doctor
Other Information: • store at 20° to 25°C (68° to 77°F)

Inactive Ingredients: camphor, carboxymethylcellulose sodium, glycerin, kaolin, methyl acrylate/2-ethylhexyl acrylate copolymer, methyl salicylate, polyacrylic acid, polysorbate 80, sodium polyacrylate, tartaric acid, titanium dioxide, and water
Questions? call **1-800-223-0182**, weekdays, 9 AM – 5 PM EST
How Supplied: Bengay Pain Relieving Patch is available in cartons containing 5 individually sealed regular size patches and 4 individually sealed large size patches.
Shown in Product Identification Guide, page 518

CORTIZONE•5®
Ointment

Drug Facts

Active Ingredient: **Purpose:**
Hydrocortisone 0.5% .... Anti-itch

Uses:
• temporarily relieves itching of minor skin irritations, inflammation, and rashes due to:
  • eczema
  • insect bites
  • cosmetics
  • psoriasis
  • detergents
  • soaps
  • poison ivy, oak, sumac
  • jewelry
  • seborrheic dermatitis
  • and for external anal and genital itching
• other uses of this product should be only under the advice and supervision of a doctor

Warnings:
For external use only
Do not use
• for the treatment of diaper rash. Consult a doctor.
• in the genital area if you have a vaginal discharge. Consult a doctor.
When using this product
• avoid contact with the eyes
• do not exceed the recommended daily dosage unless directed by a doctor
• do not put directly in rectum by using fingers or any mechanical device
Stop use and ask a doctor if
• rectal bleeding occurs
• condition worsens, or if symptoms persist for more than 7 days or clear up and occur again within a few days, and do not begin use of any other hydrocortisone product unless you have asked a doctor
Keep out of reach of children. If swallowed, get medical help or contact a Poison Control Center right away.

Directions:
• adults and children 2 years of age and older:
  • apply to affected area not more than 3 to 4 times daily
  • children under 2 years of age: do not use, ask a doctor
• for external anal and genital itching, adults:

Continued on next page

This product information was prepared in November 2003. On these and other Pfizer Consumer Healthcare Products, detailed information may be obtained by addressing Pfizer Consumer Healthcare, Pfizer, Inc., Morris Plains, NJ 07950

Cortizone•5—Cont.

- when practical, clean the affected area with mild soap and warm water and rinse thoroughly
- gently dry by patting or blotting with toilet tissue or a soft cloth before applying
- apply to affected area not more than 3 to 4 times daily
- children under 12 years of age: ask a doctor

Other Information:
- store at 15° to 30°C (59° to 86°F)

Inactive Ingredients: aloe barbadensis extract and white petrolatum

Questions? call **1-800-223-0182,** Monday to Friday, 9 AM - 5 PM EST

How Supplied: CORTIZONE•5® ointment: 1 oz. tube.

CORTIZONE•10®
Creme

Drug Facts

Active Ingredient: **Purpose:**
Hydrocortisone 1% .... Anti-itch

Uses:
- temporarily relieves itching of minor skin irritations, inflammation, and rashes due to:
  - eczema
  - insect bites
  - cosmetics
  - psoriasis
  - detergents
  - soaps
  - poison ivy, oak, sumac
  - jewelry
  - seborrheic dermatitis
  - and for external anal and genital itching
- other uses of this product should be only under the advice and supervision of a doctor

Warnings:
For external use only
Do no use
- for the treatment of diaper rash. Consult a doctor.
- in the genital area if you have a vaginal discharge. Consult a doctor.

When using this product
- avoid contact with the eyes
- do not exceed the recommended daily dosage unless directed by a doctor
- do not put directly in rectum by using fingers or any mechanical device

Stop use and ask a doctor if
- rectal bleeding occurs
- condition worsens, or if symptoms persist for more than 7 days or clear up and occur again within a few days, and do not begin use of any other hydrocortisone product unless you have asked a doctor

Keep out of reach of children. If swallowed, get medical help or contact a Poison Control Center right away.

Directions:
- adults and children 2 years of age and older:

- apply to affected area not more than 3 to 4 times daily
- children under 2 years of age: do not use, ask a doctor
- for external anal and genital itching, adults:
  - when practical, clean the affected area with mild soap and warm water and rinse thoroughly
  - gently dry by patting or blotting with toilet tissue or a soft cloth before applying
  - apply to affected area not more than 3 to 4 times daily
  - children under 12 years of age: ask a doctor

Other Information: • store at 15° to 30°C (59° to 86°F)

Inactive Ingredients: aloe barbadensis gel, aluminum sulfate, calcium acetate, cetearyl alcohol, glycerin, light mineral oil, maltodextrin, methylparaben, potato dextrin, propylparaben, purified water, sodium cetearyl sulfate, sodium lauryl sulfate, white petrolatum, and white wax

Questions? call **1-800-223-0182,** Monday to Friday, 9 AM - 5 PM EST

How Supplied: CORTIZONE•10® creme: .5 oz., 1 oz. and 2 oz. tubes.
Shown in Product Identification Guide, page 519

CORTIZONE•10®
Ointment

Drug Facts
Active Ingredient: **Purpose:**
Hydrocortisone 1% .... Anti-itch

Uses:
- temporarily relieves itching of minor skin irritations, inflammation, and rashes due to:
  - eczema
  - insect bites
  - cosmetics
  - psoriasis
  - detergents
  - soaps
  - poison ivy, oak, sumac
  - jewelry
  - seborrheic dermatitis
  - and for external anal and genital itching
- other uses of this product should be only under the advice and supervision of a doctor

Warnings:
For external use only
Do not use
- for the treatment of diaper rash. Consult a doctor.
- in the genital area if you have a vaginal discharge. Consult a doctor.

When using this product
- avoid contact with the eyes
- do not exceed the recommended daily dosage unless directed by a doctor
- do not put directly in rectum by using fingers or any mechanical device

Stop use and ask a doctor if
- rectal bleeding occurs
- condition worsens, or if symptoms persist for more than 7 days or clear up and occur again within a few days, and do not begin use of any other hydrocortisone product unless you have asked a doctor

Keep out of reach of children. If swallowed, get medical help or contact a Poison Control Center right away.

Directions:
- adults and children 2 years of age and older:
  - apply to affected area not more than 3 to 4 times daily
  - children under 2 years of age: do not use, ask a doctor
- for external anal and genital itching, adults:
  - when practical, clean the affected area with mild soap and warm water and rinse thoroughly
  - gently dry by patting or blotting with toilet tissue or a soft cloth before applying
  - apply to affected area not more than 3 to 4 times daily
  - children under 12 years of age: ask a doctor

Other Information:
- store at 15° to 30°C (59° to 86°F)

Inactive Ingredients: white petrolatum
Questions? call **1-800-223-0182,** Monday to Friday, 9 AM - 5 PM EST

How Supplied: CORTIZONE•10® ointment: 1 oz. and 2 oz. tubes.
Shown in Product Identification Guide, page 519

CORTIZONE•10® Plus
Creme
Hydrocortisone Anti-Itch Cream

Drug Facts:
Active Ingredient: **Purpose:**
Hydrocortisone 1% .... Anti-itch

Uses:
- temporarily relieves itching of minor skin irritations, inflammation, and rashes due to:
  - eczema
  - insect bites
  - cosmetics
  - psoriasis
  - detergents
  - soaps
  - poison ivy, oak, sumac
  - jewelry
  - seborrheic dermatitis
  - and for external anal and genital itching
- other uses of this product should be only under the advice and supervision of a doctor

Warnings:
For external use only
Do not use
- for the treatment of diaper rash. Consult a doctor.
- in the genital area if you have a vaginal discharge. Consult a doctor.

When using this product
- avoid contact with the eyes
- do not exceed the recommended daily dosage unless directed by a doctor
- do not put directly in rectum by using fingers or any mechanical device

Stop use and ask a doctor if
- rectal bleeding occurs
- condition worsens, or if symptoms persist for more than 7 days or clear up and occur again within a few days, and do not begin use of any other hydrocortisone product unless you have asked a doctor

Keep out of reach of children. If swallowed, get medical help or contact a Poison Control Center right away.

Directions:
- adults and children 2 years of age and older:
  - apply to affected area not more than 3 to 4 times daily
  - children under 2 years of age: do not use, ask a doctor
- for external anal itching, adults:
  - when practical, clean the affected area with mild soap and warm water and rinse thoroughly
  - gently dry by patting or blotting with toilet tissue or a soft cloth before applying
  - children under 12 years of age: ask a doctor

Other Information: • store at 15° to 30°C (59° to 86°F)

Inactive Ingredients: aloe barbadensis gel, aluminum sulfate, calcium acetate, cetearyl alcohol, cetyl alcohol, corn oil, glycerin, isopropyl palmitate, light mineral oil, maltodextrin, methylparaben, potato dextrin, propylene glycol, propylparaben, purified water, sodium cetearyl sulfate, sodium lauryl sulfate, vitamin A palmitate, vitamin D, vitamin E, white petrolatum, and white wax

Questions? call **1-800-223-0182**, Monday to Friday, 9 AM - 5 PM EST

How Supplied: CORTIZONE•10® Plus creme: 1 oz. and 2 oz. tubes.
Shown in Product Identification Guide, page 519

CORTIZONE•10® MAXIMUM STRENGTH QUICK SHOT™ SPRAY

Drug Facts

Active Ingredient:　　**Purpose:**
Hydrocortisone 1% .... Anti-itch

Uses:
- temporarily relieves itching of minor skin irritations, inflammation, and rashes due to:
  - eczema
  - insect bites
  - cosmetics
  - psoriasis
  - detergents
  - soaps
  - poison ivy, oak, sumac
  - jewelry
  - seborrheic dermatitis
- other uses of this product should be only under the advice and supervision of a doctor

Warnings:
For external use only
Flammable - keep away from fire or flame
Do not use
- for the treatment of diaper rash. Consult a doctor.
When using this product
- avoid contact with the eyes
Stop use and ask a doctor if condition worsens, or if symptoms persist for more than 7 days or clear up and occur again within a few days, and do not begin use of any other hydrocortisone product unless you have asked a doctor

Keep out of reach of children. If swallowed, get medical help or contact a Poison Control Center right away.

Directions:
- adults and children 2 years of age and older: apply to affected area not more than 3 to 4 times daily
- children under 2 years of age: do not use; ask a doctor

Other Information:
- store at 15° to 30°C (59° to 86°F)
- store away from heat and protect from freezing

Inactive Ingredients: benzyl alcohol, propylene glycol, purified water, and SD alcohol 40-2 (60% v/v)

Questions? call **1-800-223-0182**, Monday to Friday, 9 AM - 5 PM EST

How Supplied: CORTIZONE•10® Quick Shot Spray: 1.5 oz. pump bottle
Shown in Product Identification Guide, page 519

DESITIN® CREAMY WITH ALOE and VITAMIN E
Zinc Oxide Diaper Rash Ointment

Drug Facts:

Active Ingredient:　　**Purpose:**
Zinc oxide 10% .... Skin protectant

Uses:
- helps treat and prevent diaper rash
- protects chafed skin due to diaper rash and helps seal out wetness

Warnings:
For external use only
When using this product
- avoid contact with the eyes
Stop use and ask a doctor if:
- condition worsens or does not improve within 7 days
Keep out of reach of children. If swallowed, get medical help or contact a Poison Control Center right away.

Directions:
- change wet and soiled diapers promptly
- cleanse the diaper area
- allow to dry
- apply ointment liberally as often as necessary, with each diaper change, especially at bedtime or any time when exposure to wet diapers may be prolonged

Other Information:
- store at 20° to 25°C (68° to 77°F)

Inactive Ingredients: aloe barbadensis gel, cyclomethicone, dimethicone, fragrance, methylparaben, microcrystalline wax, mineral oil, propylparaben, purified water, sodium borate, sorbitan sesquioleate, vitamin E, white petrolatum, and white wax

Questions? Call **1-800-223-0182**, Monday to Friday, 9 AM–5 PM EST

How Supplied: Desitin Creamy with Aloe and Vitamin E is available in 2 oz. (57g) and 4 oz. (113g) tubes.
Shown in Product Identification Guide, page 519

DESITIN® OINTMENT
Zinc Oxide Diaper Rash Ointment

Drug Facts:

Active Ingredient:　　**Purpose:**
Zinc oxide 40% .... Skin protectant

Uses:
- helps treat and prevent diaper rash
- protects chafed skin due to diaper rash and helps seal out wetness

Warnings:
For external use only.
When using this product
- avoid contact with the eyes
Stop use and ask a doctor if
- condition worsens or does not improve within 7 days
Keep out of reach of children. If swallowed, get medical help or contact a Poison Control Center right away.

Directions:
- change wet and soiled diapers promptly
- cleanse the diaper area
- allow to dry
- apply ointment liberally as often as necessary, with each diaper change, especially at bedtime or any time when exposure to wet diapers may be prolonged

Other Information:
- store at 15° to 30°C (59° to 86°F)

Inactive Ingredients: BHA, cod liver oil, fragrance, lanolin, methylparaben, petrolatum, talc, and water

Questions? call **1-800-223-0182**, Monday to Friday, 9 AM - 5 PM EST

How Supplied: Desitin Ointment is available in 1 ounce (28g), 2 ounce (57g), and 4 ounce (114g) tubes, and 9 ounce (255g) and 16 ounce (454g) jars.
Shown in Product Identification Guide, page 519

DRAMAMINE® Original Formula Tablets
DRAMAMINE® Chewable Formula Tablets
Antiemetic

Description: DRAMAMINE Original Formula Tablets and DRAMAMINE Chewable Formula Tablets contain dimenhydrinate, which is the chlorotheophylline salt of the antihistaminic agent diphenhydramine.

Active Ingredient: Dimenhydrinate 50 mg per tablet.

Continued on next page

This product information was prepared in November 2003. On these and other Pfizer Consumer Healthcare Products, detailed information may be obtained by addressing Pfizer Consumer Healthcare, Pfizer, Inc., Morris Plains, NJ 07950

Dramamine—Cont.

Indications: For prevention and treatment of the symptoms associated with motion sickness including nausea, vomiting, and dizziness

Directions: To prevent motion sickness, the first dose should be taken ½ to 1 hour before starting activity. To prevent or treat motion sickness, use the following dosing.

Adults and children 12 years and over: 1 to 2 tablets every 4–6 hours; not more than 8 tablets in 24 hours, or as directed by a doctor

Children 6 to under 12 years: ½ to 1 tablet every 6–8 hours: not more than 3 tablets in 24 hours, or as directed by a doctor

Children 2 to under 6 years: ¼ to ½ tablet every 6–8 hours; not more than 1 ½ tablets in 24 hours, or as directed by a doctor

Warnings:

Do not use in children under 2 years of age unless directed by a doctor.

Ask a doctor before use if you have

• a breathing problem such as emphysema or chronic bronchitis • glaucoma • difficulty in urination due to enlargement of the prostate gland

Ask a doctor or pharmacist before use if you are taking sedatives or tranquilizers

When using these products

• marked drowsiness may occur • avoid alcoholic drinks • alcohol, sedatives, and tranquilizers may increase drowsiness • be careful when driving a motor vehicle or operating machinery

If pregnant or breast-feeding, ask a health professional before use.

Keep out of reach of children.

In case of overdose, get medical help or contact a Poison Control Center right away.

Other Information:

Chewable Formula Tablets: Phenylketonurics: contains **phenylalanine** 1.5 mg per tablet. Also contains FD&C yellow No. 5 (tartrazine) as a color additive

Inactive Ingredients: DRAMAMINE Original Formula Tablets: colloidal silicon dioxide, croscarmellose sodium, lactose, magnesium stearate, microcrystalline cellulose

DRAMAMINE Chewable Formula Tablets: aspartame, citric acid, FD&C yellow no. 5, FD&C yellow no. 6, flavor, magnesium stearate, methacrylic acid copolymer, sorbitol

How Supplied: Original Formula Tablets: scored, white tablets, available in 12 ct. vials and 36 ct. packages

Chewable Formula Tablets: scored, orange tablets, available in 8 ct. and 24 ct. packages

Store at room temperature

DRAMAMINE® Less Drowsy Formula Tablets
Antiemetic

Description: DRAMAMINE Less Drowsy Formula contains meclizine hydrochloride.

Active Ingredient: Meclizine hydrochloride 25 mg per tablet

Indications: for prevention and treatment of the symptoms associated with motion sickness including nausea, vomiting, and dizziness

Directions: To prevent motion sickness, the first dose should be taken 1 hour before starting activity. To prevent or treat motion sickness, use the following dosing.

Adults and children 12 years and over: 1 to 2 tablets once daily, or as directed by a doctor

Warnings:

Do not use in children under 12 years of age unless directed by a doctor.

Ask a doctor before use if you have:

• a breathing problem such as emphysema or chronic bronchitis • glaucoma • difficulty in urination due to enlargement of the prostate gland

Ask a doctor or pharmacist before use if you are taking sedatives or tranquilizers

When using these products:

• drowsiness may occur • avoid alcoholic drinks • alcohol, sedatives, and tranquilizers may increase drowsiness • be careful when driving a motor vehicle or operating machinery

If pregnant or breast-feeding, ask a health professional before use.

Keep out of reach of children.

In case of overdose, get medical help or contact a Poison Control Center right away.

Inactive Ingredients: Colloidal silicon dioxide, corn starch, D&C yellow no. 10 (aluminum lake), lactose, magnesium stearate, microcrystalline cellulose

How Supplied: Yellow tablets in 8 ct. vials

Store at controlled room temperature 20°–25°C (68°–77°F)

e.p.t® PREGNANCY TEST
99% Accurate at detecting the pregnancy hormone. However, some pregnant women may not have detectable amounts of pregnancy hormone in their urine on the first day of the missed period or may have miscalculated the first day of their period

PLEASE READ INSTRUCTIONS CAREFULLY:

[See graphic below]

How to use: Remove the **e.p.t.** test stick from its foil packet just prior to use.

Remove the purple cap to expose the absorbent tip. Hold the test stick by its thumb grip. Point the absorbent tip downward. Place the absorbent tip in the urine flow for just 5 seconds, or dip the absorbent tip into a clean container of urine for just 5 seconds.

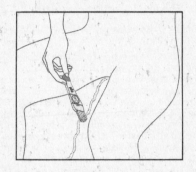

Place the test stick on a flat surface with the windows facing up for at least 3 minutes. (If you wish, replace the cap to cover the absorbent tip.) You may notice a light pink color moving across the windows.

Important: To avoid affecting the test result, wait at least 3 minutes before lifting the stick.

How to Read the Results:

Wait 3 minutes to read the result. A line will appear in the square window to show that the test is working properly. Be sure to read the result before 20 minutes have passed.

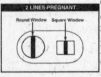

Two parallel lines, one in each window, indicate that you are **pregnant**. The lines can be different shades of pink and need not match the color in the illustration. Please see your doctor to discuss your pregnancy and the next steps. Early prenatal care is important to ensure the health of you and your baby.

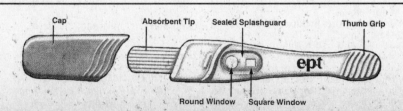

Cap   Absorbent Tip   Sealed Splashguard   Thumb Grip

ept

Round Window   Square Window

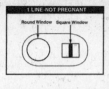

One line in the square window but none in the round window indicates that you are **not pregnant.** If your period does not start within a week, repeat the test. If you still get a negative result and your period has not started, please see your doctor.

Important: If no line appears in the square window, the test result is invalid. Do not read the result. Call our toll-free number 1-800-378-1783 (1-800-EPT-1STEP).

Questions? Call toll-free 1-800-378-1783 Registered nurses available 8:30 am - 5:00 pm EST weekdays, consumer specialists available until 8:00 pm, and recorded help available 24 hours, (including weekends).

Questions and Answers about e.p.t.® When can I use e.p.t?
e.p.t can be used any time of day as soon as you miss your period and any day thereafter.

How does e.p.t work?
e.p.t detects hCG (human Chorionic Gonadotropin), a hormone present in urine only during pregnancy. **e.p.t** can detect hCG in your urine as early as the first day your period is late.

What if the lines in the round and square windows are different shades of pink? As long as 2 parallel lines appear, one in each window, the result is positive, even if the two lines are different shades of pink.

What if I think the test result is incorrect? Following the instructions carefully should yield an accurate reading. If you think the result is incorrect, or if it is difficult to detect a line in the round window, repeat the test after 2–3 days with a new **e.p.t** stick.

Are there any factors that can affect the test result? Yes. Certain drugs which contain hCG or are used in combination with hCG (such as Humegon™, Pregnyl, Profasi, Pergonal, APL) and rare medical conditions. If you repeat the test and continue to get an unexpected result, contact your doctor.

Using **e.p.t** within 8 weeks of giving birth or having a miscarriage may cause a false positive result. The test may detect hCG still in your system from a previous pregnancy. You should ask your doctor for help in interpreting the result of your **e.p.t** test if you have recently been pregnant.

Factors which should <u>not</u> affect the test result include alcohol, analgesics (pain killers), antibiotics, birth control pills or hormone therapies containing clomiphene citrate (Clomid or Serophen). Store at room temperature 15°–30°C (59°–86°F). FOR IN-VITRO DIAGNOSTIC USE. (NOT FOR INTERNAL USE.) KEEP OUT OF THE REACH OF CHILDREN.

Please call our toll-free number 1-800-378-1783 with any questions about using e.p.t.
Shown in Product Identification Guide, page 519

KAOPECTATE® Anti-Diarrheal

Description: KAOPECTATE®, is a pleasant testing oral suspension for use in the control of diarrhea. Each 15 mL of KAOPECTATE® Anti-Diarrheal contains bismuth subsalicylate 262 mg, contributing 130 mg total salicylates. KAOPECTATE® Anti-Diarrheal is low sodium, with each 15 mL tablespoonful containing 10 mg sodium.

Active Ingredient: Bismuth subsalicylate.

Indication: Anti-diarrheal.

Warnings: Reye's syndrome: Children and teenagers who have or are recovering from chicken pox or flu-like symptoms should not use this product. When using this product, if changes in behavior with nausea and vomiting occur, consult a doctor because these symptoms could be an early sign of Reye's syndrome, a rare but serious illness.
Allergy Alert: Contains salicylate. Do not take if you are • allergic to salicylates (including aspirin) • taking other salicylate products
Do not use if you have • bloody or black stool • an ulcer • a bleeding problem
Ask a doctor before use if you have • fever • mucus in the stool **Ask a doctor or pharmacist before use if you are** taking any drug for • anticoagulation (thinning the blood) • diabetes • gout • arthritis **When using this product** a temporary, but harmless, darkening of the stool and/or tongue may occur **Stop use and ask a doctor if** • symptoms get worse • ringing in the ears or loss of hearing occurs • diarrhea lasts more than 2 days **If pregnant or breast-feeding,** ask a health professional before use. **Keep out of reach of children.** In case of overdose, get medical help or contact a Poison Control Center right away.

Directions: KAOPECTATE® Anti-Diarrheal • shake well immediately before each use • for accurate dosing, use convenient pre-measured dose cup • repeat dose every ½ hour to 1 hour as needed • do not exceed 8 doses in 24 hours • use until diarrhea stops but not more than 2 days • drink plenty of clear fluids to help prevent dehydration caused by diarrhea

Dosing Chart—Regular Strength KAOPECTATE®

Age	Dose
adults and children 12 years and over	30 mL or 2 tablespoonfuls

Inactive Ingredients:
KAOPECTATE® Anti-Diarrheal — Peppermint: caramel, carboxymethylcellulose sodium, FD&C red no. 40, flavor, microcrystalline cellulose, purified water, sodium salicylate, sorbic acid, sucrose, titanium dioxide, xanthan gum
KAOPECTATE® Anti-Diarrheal Regular Flavor (vanilla): caramel, carboxymethylcellulose sodium, flavor, microcrystalline cellulose, purified water, sodium salicylate, sorbic acid, sucrose, titanium dioxide, xanthan gum

How Supplied: KAOPECTATE® Anti-Diarrheal 262 mg Peppermint and 262 mg Regular Flavor (vanilla): available in 8 and 12 oz bottles; Store at room temperature 20° to 25C (68° to 77°F). Avoid excessive heat. **Do not use if inner seal is broken or missing.**

EXTRA STRENGTH KAOPECTATE® Anti-Diarrheal

Description: EXTRA STRENGTH KAOPECTATE® is a pleasant testing oral suspension for use in the control of diarrhea. Each 15 mL of EXTRA STRENGTH KAOPECTATE® Anti-Diarrheal contains bismuth subsalicylate 525 mg, contributing 236 mg total salicylates. EXTRA STRENGTH KAOPECTATE® is low sodium. Each 15 mL tablespoonful contains **sodium 11 mg**.

Active Ingredient: Bismuth subsalicylate.

Indication: Anti-diarrheal.

Warnings: Reye's syndrome: Children and teenagers who have or are recovering from chicken pox or flu-like symptoms should not use this product. When using this product, if changes in behavior with nausea and vomiting occur, consult a doctor because these symptoms could be an early sign of Reye's syndrome, a rare but serious illness.
Allergy Alert: Contains salicylate. Do not take if you are • allergic to salicylates (including aspirin) • taking other salicylate products
Do not use if you have • bloody or black stool • an ulcer • a bleeding problem
Ask a doctor before use if you have • fever • mucus in the stool **Ask a doctor or pharmacist before use if you are** taking any drug for • anticoagulation (thinning the blood) • diabetes • gout • arthritis **When using this product** a temporary, but harmless, darkening of

Continued on next page

This product information was prepared in November 2003. On these and other Pfizer Consumer Healthcare Products, detailed information may be obtained by addressing Pfizer Consumer Healthcare, Pfizer, Inc., Morris Plains, NJ 07950

Kaopectate—Cont.

the stool and/or tongue may occur **Stop use and ask a doctor if** • symptoms get worse • ringing in the ears or loss of hearing occurs • diarrhea lasts more than 2 days **If pregnant or breast-feeding,** ask a health professional before use. **Keep out of reach of children.** In case of overdose, get medical help or contact a Poison Control Center right away.

Directions: EXTRA STRENGTH KAOPECTATE® **Anti-Diarrheal** • **shake well** immediately before each use • for accurate dosing, use convenient pre-measured dose cup • repeat dose every hour as needed • do not exceed 4 doses in 24 hours • use until diarrhea stops but not more than 2 days • drink plenty of clear fluids to help prevent dehydration caused by diarrhea

Dosing Chart—Extra Strength KAOPECTATE®

Age	Dose
adults and children 12 years and over	30 mL or 2 tablespoonfuls

Inactive Ingredients: caramel, carboxymethylcellulose sodium, FD&C red no. 40, flavor, microcrystalline cellulose, purified water, sodium salicylate, sorbic acid, sucrose, titanium dioxide, xanthan gum

How Supplied: EXTRA STRENGTH KAOPECTATE® **Anti-Diarrheal 525 mg - Peppermint:** available in 8 oz bottles. Store at room temperature 20° to 25C (68° to 77°F). Avoid excessive heat. **Do not use if inner seal is broken or missing.**

Shown in Product Identification Guide, page 519

LISTERINE® Antiseptic
[lĭs 'tər en]

Active Ingredients: Thymol 0.064%, Eucalyptol 0.092%, Methyl Salicylate 0.060% and Menthol 0.042%.

Inactive Ingredients: Water, Alcohol 26.9%, Benzoic Acid, Poloxamer 407, Sodium Benzoate, and Caramel.

Indications: Use Listerine Antiseptic twice daily to help:
• Prevent & Reduce Plaque
• Prevent & Reduce Gingivitis
• Fight Bad Breath
• Kill Germs Between Teeth

Actions: Listerine Antiseptic has been shown to help prevent and reduce supragingival plaque accumulation and gingivitis when used in a conscientiously applied program of oral hygiene and regular professional care. Its effect on periodontitis has not been determined. Listerine is the only leading nonprescription mouthrinse that has received the American Dental Association's Council on Scientific Affairs Seal of Acceptance for helping to prevent and reduce plaque and gingivitis.

Directions: Rinse full strength for 30 seconds with 20 ml ($^2/_3$ fl. ounce or 4 teaspoonfuls) morning and night. If bad breath persists, see your dentist.

Warnings: Do not administer to children under twelve years of age. **Keep this and all drugs out of the reach of children.** Do not swallow. In case of accidental ingestion, seek professional assistance or contact a Poison Control Center immediately. Cold weather may cloud Listerine. Its antiseptic properties are not affected. Store at 59° to 77°F.

How Supplied: Listerine Antiseptic is supplied in 250 ml, 500 ml, 1.0 liter, 1.5 liter and 1.7 liter bottles, as well as 3 fl. oz. bottles. It is also available to professionals in 3 fl. oz. bottles and in gallon bottles.

Shown in Product Identification Guide, page 519

Natural Citrus LISTERINE® Antiseptic
[lĭs'tər en]

Drug Facts
Active Ingredients: **Purposes:**
Eucalyptol
  0.092% ...... Antiplaque/antigingivitis
Menthol
  0.042% ...... Antiplaque/antigingivitis
Methyl salicylate
  0.060% ...... Antiplaque/antigingivitis
Thymol
  0.064% ...... Antiplaque/antigingivitis

Uses: helps prevent and reduce:
• plaque • gingivitis

Warnings:
Do not use in children under 12 years of age
Keep out of reach of children. If more than used for rinsing is accidentally swallowed, get medical help or contact a Poison Control Center right away.

Directions:
• rinse full strength for 30 seconds with 20 ml (2/3 fluid ounce or 4 teaspoonfuls) morning and night
• do not swallow

Other Information: • store at 59° to 77°F
• cold weather may cloud this product. Its antiseptic properties are not affected.

Inactive Ingredients: water, alcohol (21.6%), sorbitol solution, natural flavoring, poloxamer 407, benzoic acid, sucrose, sodium benzoate, cochineal extract

Actions: Natural Citrus Listerine Antiseptic has been shown to help prevent and reduce supragingival plaque accumulation and gingivitis when used in a conscientiously applied program of oral hygiene and regular professional care. Its effect on periodontitis has not been determined.

Dosage and Administration: Rinse full strength for 30 seconds with 20 ml (2/3 fluid ounce or 4 teaspoonfuls) morning and night. Do not swallow.

How Supplied: Natural Citrus Listerine Antiseptic is supplied in 250 ml, 500 ml, 1.0 liter, and 1.5 liter bottles.

Shown in Product Identification Guide, page 519

COOL MINT LISTERINE® Antiseptic
[lĭs 'tər en]

Active Ingredients: Thymol 0.064%, Eucalyptol 0.092%, Methyl Salicylate 0.060% and Menthol 0.042%.

Inactive Ingredients: Water, Alcohol 21.6%, Sorbitol Solution, Flavoring, Poloxamer 407, Benzoic Acid, Sodium Saccharin, Sodium Benzoate, and FD&C Green #3.

Indications: Use Cool Mint Listerine Antiseptic twice daily to help:
• Prevent & Reduce Plaque
• Prevent & Reduce Gingivitis
• Fight Bad Breath
• Kills Germs Between Teeth.

Actions: Cool Mint Listerine Antiseptic has been shown to help prevent and reduce supragingival plaque accumulation and gingivitis when used in a conscientiously applied program of oral hygiene and regular professional care. Its effect on periodontitis has not been determined. Listerine is the only leading nonprescription mouthrinse that has received the American Dental Association's Council on Scientific Affairs Seal of Acceptance for helping to prevent and reduce plaque and gingivitis.

Directions: Rinse full strength for 30 seconds with 20 ml ($^2/_3$ fl. ounce or 4 teaspoonfuls) morning and night. If bad breath persists, see your dentist.

Warnings: Do not administer to children under twelve years of age. **Keep this and all drugs out of the reach of children.** Do not swallow. In case of accidental ingestion, seek professional assistance or contact a Poison Control Center immediately. Cold weather may cloud Cool Mint Listerine. Its antiseptic properties are not affected. Store at 59° to 77°F.

How Supplied: Cool Mint Listerine Antiseptic is supplied in 250 ml, 500 ml, 1.0 liter, 1.5 liter bottles and 1.7 liter bottles, as well as 3 fl. oz. bottles. It is also available to professionals in 3 fl. oz. bottles and in gallon bottles.

Shown in Product Identification Guide, page 519

FRESHBURST® LISTERINE® Antiseptic
[lĭs 'tər en]

Active Ingredients: Thymol 0.064%, Eucalyptol 0.092%, Methyl Salicylate 0.060% and Menthol 0.042%.

Inactive Ingredients: Water, Alcohol 21.6%, Sorbitol Solution, Flavoring, Poloxamer 407, Benzoic Acid, Sodium Saccharin, Sodium Benzoate, D&C Yellow #10, and FD&C Green #3.

Indications: Use FreshBurst Listerine Antiseptic twice daily to help:
• Prevent & Reduce Plaque
• Prevent & Reduce Gingivitis
• Fight Bad Breath
• Kill Germs Between Teeth

Actions: FreshBurst Listerine Antiseptic has been shown to help prevent and reduce supragingival plaque accumulation and gingivitis when used in a conscientiously applied program of oral hygiene and regular professional care. Its effect on periodontitis has not been determined. Listerine is the only leading nonprescription mouthrinse that has received the American Dental Association's Council on Scientific Affairs Seal of Acceptance for helping to prevent and reduce plaque and gingivitis.

Directions: Rinse full strength for 30 seconds with 20 ml ($^2/_3$ fl. ounce or 4 teaspoonfuls) morning and night. If bad breath persists, see your dentist.

Warnings: Do not administer to children under twelve years of age. **Keep this and all drugs out of the reach of children.** Do not swallow. In case of accidental ingestion, seek professional assistance or contact a Poison Control Center immediately. Cold weather may cloud FreshBurst Listerine. Its antiseptic properties are not affected. Store at 59° to 77°F.

How Supplied: FreshBurst Listerine Antiseptic is supplied in 250 ml, 500 ml, 1.0 liter, 1.5 liter bottles and 1.7 liter bottles, as well as 3 fl. oz. bottles. It is also available to professionals in 3 fl. oz. bottles and in gallon bottles.
Shown in Product Identification Guide, page 519

**TARTAR CONTROL LISTERINE®
Antiseptic**
[*ls'tərĕn*]

Active Ingredients: Thymol 0.064%, Eucalyptol 0.092%, Methyl Salicylate 0.060%, and Menthol 0.042%.

Inactive Ingredients: Water, Alcohol 21.6%, Sorbitol Solution, Flavoring, Poloxamer 407, Sodium Saccharin, Benzoic Acid, Zinc Chloride, Sodium Benzoate, and FD&C Blue #1.

Indications: Use Tartar Control Listerine Antiseptic twice daily to help:
• Prevent & Fight Tartar Build-up
• Prevent & Reduce Plaque
• Prevent & Reduce Gingivitis
• Fight Bad Breath
• Kill Germs Between Teeth

Actions: Tartar Control Listerine Antiseptic has been shown to help prevent and reduce supragingival plaque accumulation and gingivitis when used in a conscientiously applied program of oral

hygiene and regular professional care. It has also been shown to help reduce the formation of tartar above the gumline. Its effect on periodontitis has not been determined. Listerine is the only leading nonprescription mouthrinse that has received the American Dental Association's Council on Scientific Affairs Seal of Acceptance for helping to prevent and reduce plaque and gingivitis.

Directions: Rinse full strength for 30 seconds with 20ml (2/3 fluid ounce or 4 teaspoonfuls) morning and night. If bad breath persists, see your dentist.

Warnings: Do not administer to children under twelve years of age. **Keep this and all drugs out of the reach of children.** Do not swallow. In case of accidental overdose, seek professional assistance or contact a Poison Control Center immediately. Cold weather may cloud Tartar Control Listerine. Its antiseptic properties are not affected. Store at 59° to 77°F.

How Supplied: Tartar Control Listerine Antiseptic is supplied in 250 ml, 500 ml, 1.0 liter and 1.5 liter bottles.
Shown in Product Identification Guide, page 519

**LUBRIDERM® Advanced Therapy
Creamy Lotion**
[*lū brĭ dĕrm*]

Ingredients: Water, Cetyl Alcohol, Glycerin, Mineral Oil, Cyclomethicone, Propylene Glycol Dicaprylate/Dicaprate, PEG-40 Stearate, Isopropyl Isostearate, Emulsifying Wax, Lecithin, Carbomer 940, Diazolidinyl Urea, Titanium Dioxide, Sodium Benzoate, BHT, Tri(PPG-3 Myristyl Ether) Citrate, Disodium EDTA, Retinyl Palmitate, Tocopheryl Acetate, Sodium Pyruvate, Iodopropynyl Butylcarbamate, Fragrance, Sodium Hydroxide, Xanthan Gum.

Uses: Lubriderm Advanced Therapy's nourishing, rich and creamy formula helps heal extra-dry skin. Its unique combination of nutrient-enriched moisturizers penetrate dry skin leaving you with soft, smooth and comfortable skin. This non-greasy feeling lotion absorbs quickly and is non-comedogenic.

Directions: Smooth Lubriderm on hands and body every day.
For external use only.

How Supplied: Available in 6, 10, 16, and 19.6 fl. oz plastic bottles and a 3.3 fl. oz. tube.
Shown in Product Identification Guide, page 519

LUBRIDERM® DAILY UV SPF 15
[*lū brĭ dĕrm*]
For Normal to Dry Skin

Developed by dermatologists for healthier skin, Lubriderm Daily UV hydrates

and helps protect your skin. Its unique formula combines essential moisturizing elements with dermatologist-recommended SPF 15 sun protection. This clean, non-greasy feeling lotion is perfect to use every day for smoother, healthier, skin.
• Broad spectrum sunscreen provides protection against damaging UVA and UVB rays (SPF 15)
• A light, non-greasy feeling lotion that's ideal for everyday use
• Mild formula is PABA-free and dye-free

Sun alert:
Limiting sun exposure, wearing protective clothing, and using sunscreens may reduce the risks of skin aging, skin cancer, and other harmful effects of the sun.

Drug Facts:

Active Ingredients:	Purpose:
Octinoxate 7.5%	Sunscreen
Octisalate 4%	Sunscreen
Oxybenzone 3%	Sunscreen

Uses:
• helps prevent sunburn
• higher SPF gives more sunburn protection

Warnings:
For external use only.
When using this product keep out of eyes. Rinse with water to remove.
Stop use and ask a doctor if rash or irritation develops and lasts
Keep out of reach of children. If swallowed, get medical help or contact a Poison Control Center right away.

Directions:
• apply liberally before sun exposure and as needed
• children under 6 months of age: ask a doctor

Other Information:
• store at 20° to 25°C (68° to 77°F)

Inactive Ingredients: purified water, C 12-15 alkyl benzoate, ceteraryl alcohol (and) ceteareth-20, cetyl alcohol, glyceryl monostearate, propylene glycol, white petrolatum, diazolidinyl urea, trolamine, edetate disodium, xanthan gum, acrylates/C 10-30 alkyl acrylate crosspolymer, vitamin E, iodopropynyl butylcarbamate, fragrance, carbomer
Questions? call **1-800-223-0182,** weekdays, 9 AM–5 PM EST

How Supplied: Available in 6, 10, 16 fl. oz plastic bottles and a 3.3 fl. oz. tube.
Shown in Product Identification Guide, page 519

Continued on next page

This product information was prepared in November 2003. On these and other Pfizer Consumer Healthcare Products, detailed information may be obtained by addressing Pfizer Consumer Healthcare, Pfizer, Inc., Morris Plains, NJ 07950

LUBRIDERM®
Seriously Sensitive® Lotion
[lū brĭ dĕrm]

Ingredients: Water, Butylene Glycol, Mineral Oil, Petrolatum, Glycerin, Cetyl Alcohol, Propylene Glycol Dicaprylate/Dicaprate, PEG-40 Stearate, C11-13 Isoparaffin, Glyceryl Stearate, Tri (PPG-3 Myristyl Ether) Citrate, Emulsifying Wax, Dimethicone, DMDM Hydantoin, Methylparaben, Carbomer 940, Ethylparaben, Propylparaben, Titanium Dioxide, Disodium EDTA, Sodium Hydroxide, Butylparaben, Xanthan Gum.

Uses: Lubriderm Seriously Sensitive Lotion's unique combination of emollients provides sensitive dry skin with the moisture it needs while helping to create a protective layer. It is non-comedogenic, 100% lanolin free, fragrance free, and dye free so its appropriate for skin that is sensitive to these ingredients. It is nongreasy feeling and absorbs quickly.

Directions: Smooth on hands and body everyday. Particularly effective when used after showering or bathing. For external use only.

How Supplied: Available in 1, 6, 10, and 16 fl. oz. plastic bottles and 3.3 fl. oz. tube.

Shown in Product Identification Guide, page 519

LUBRIDERM®
Skin Therapy Moisturizing Lotion
[lū brĭ dĕrm]

Ingredients: Scented—Water, Mineral Oil, Petrolatum, Sorbitol Solution, Stearic Acid, Lanolin, Lanolin Alcohol, Cetyl Alcohol, Glyceryl Stearate/PEG-100 Stearate, Triethanolamine, Dimethicone, Propylene Glycol, Microcrystalline Wax, Tri(PPG-3 Myristyl Ether) Citrate, Disodium EDTA, Methylparaben, Ethylparaben, Propylparaben, Fragrance, Xanthan Gum, Butylparaben, Methyldibromo Glutaronitrile.

Fragrance Free—Contains Water, Mineral Oil, Petrolatum, Sorbitol Solution, Stearic Acid, Lanolin, Lanolin Alcohol, Cetyl Alcohol, Glyceryl Stearate/PEG-100 Stearate, Triethanolamine, Dimethicone, Propylene Glycol, Microcrystalline Wax, Tri(PPG-3 Myristyl Ether) Citrate, Disodium EDTA, Methylparaben, Ethylparaben, Propylparaben, Xanthan Gum, Butylparaben, Methyldibromo Glutaronitrile.

Uses: Lubriderm provides the essential moisturizing elements that contribute to healthy skin. Its unique combination of emollients penetrate dry skin to effectively moisturize without leaving a greasy feel. Lubriderm helps heal and protect skin from dryness, absorbs rapidly for a clean, natural feel and is non-comedogenic so it won't clog pores.

Directions: Smooth on hands and body every day. Particularly effective when used after showering or bathing. For external use only.

How Supplied:
Scented: Available in 6, 10, 16 and 19.6 oz fl. oz. plastic bottles.
Fragrance Free: Available in 6, 10 and 16 fl. oz. plastic bottles and 3.3 fl. oz. tube.

Shown in Product Identification Guide, page 520

NASALCROM® Nasal Spray
Nasal Allergy Symptom Controller

Description: NASALCROM Nasal Spray contains a liquid formulation of cromolyn sodium that stabilizes mast cells that release histamine. NASALCROM is neither an antihistamine nor a decongestant nor a corticosteroid. In addition to treating nasal allergy symptoms, it decreases the allergic reaction by reducing the release of histamine, the trigger of allergy symptoms, from mast cells. NASALCROM has no known drug interactions and is safe to use with medications including other allergy medications.

Active Ingredient: (per spray) Cromolyn sodium 5.2mg

Indications: To prevent and relieve nasal symptoms of hay fever and other nasal allergies.
• runny/itchy nose • sneezing • allergic stuffy nose

Directions:
• parent or care provider must supervise the use of this product by young children. Adults and children 2 years and older:
• spray once into each nostril. Repeat 3–4 times a day (every 4–6 hours). If needed, may be used up to 6 times a day.
• use every day while in contact with the cause of your allergies (pollen, molds, pets, and dust)
• to **prevent** nasal allergy symptoms, use before contact with the cause of your allergies. For best results, start using up to one week before contact.
• if desired, you can use this product with other medications, including other allergy medications.
• children under 2 years: Do not use unless directed by a doctor

Warnings:
Do not use • if you are allergic to any of the ingredients
Ask a doctor before use if you have
• fever • discolored nasal discharge • sinus pain • wheezing
When using this product • it may take several days of use to notice an effect. Your best effect may not be seen for 1 to 2 weeks • brief stinging or sneezing may occur right after use • do not use to treat sinus infection, asthma, or cold symptoms • do not share this bottle with anyone else as this may spread germs

Stop use and ask a doctor if
• shortness of breath, wheezing, or chest tightness occurs • hives or swelling of the mouth or throat occurs • your symptoms worsen • you have new symptoms • your symptoms do not begin to improve within two weeks
• you need to use more than 12 weeks
If pregnant or breast feeding ask a health professional before use.
Keep out of reach of children. If swallowed, get medical help or contact a Poison Control Center right away.

Inactive Ingredients: benzalkonium chloride, edetate disodium, purified water

How Supplied: NASALCROM Nasal Spray is available in 13mL (100 metered sprays) and 26mL (200 metered sprays) sizes
Store between 20°–25°C (68°–77°F). Keep away from light.

NEOSPORIN® Ointment
[nē "uh-spō' rŭn]

Drug Facts

Active Ingredients

(in each gram):	Purpose:
Bacitracin	
400 units	First aid antibiotic
Neomycin 3.5 mg	First aid antibiotic
Polymyxin B	
5,000 units	First aid antibiotic

Use: first aid to help prevent infection in minor:
• cuts • scrapes • burns

Warnings:
For external use only.
Do not use
• if you are allergic to any of the ingredients
• in the eyes
• over large areas of the body
Ask a doctor before use if you have
• deep or puncture wounds
• animal bites
• serious burns
Stop use and ask a doctor if
• you need to use longer than 1 week
• condition persists or gets worse
• rash or other allergic reaction develops
Keep out of reach of children. If swallowed, get medical help or contact a Poison Control Center right away.

Directions:
• clean the affected area
• apply a small amount of this product (an amount equal to the surface area of the tip of a finger) on the area 1 to 3 times daily
• may be covered with a sterile bandage

Other Information:
• store at 20° to 25°C (68° to 77° F)

Inactive Ingredients: cocoa butter, cottonseed oil, olive oil, sodium pyruvate, vitamin E, and white petrolatum

Questions? call **1-800-223-0182**, weekdays, 9 AM - 5 PM EST

How Supplied: Tubes, $^1/_2$ oz (14.2 g), 1 oz (28.3 g), $^1/_{32}$ oz (0.9 g) foil packets packed 10 per box (Neo To Go®) or 144 per box.

Shown in Product Identification Guide, page 519

NEOSPORIN® SCAR SOLUTION™

[*nē"uh-spō'run*]

Silicone Scar Sheets

Uses: • Significantly improves the appearance of existing scars • Helps prevent the formation of scars on newly healed wounds

What is Neosporin® Scar Solution™?
Neosporin Scar Solution contains 28 silicone scar sheets that are indicated for use on raised and discolored scars. Silicone sheet technology is clinically proven to significantly improve the appearance of scars and has been used by burn centers and plastic surgeons for years. Each sheet is thin, self-adhesive and fabric-backed, which makes Neosporin Scar Solution convenient to wear under clothing.

How does Neosporin Scar Solution work?
Neosporin Scar Solution sheets use patented Silon® technology, and are believed to mimic the natural barrier function of normal skin... improving the appearance of scars, both new and old. Silicone sheets have been shown to improve the appearance of scars, even those that are years old.
One package (28 sheets) of Neosporin Scar Solution provides the full, 12-week supply recommended to improve the appearance of scars.

What types of scars does Neosporin Scar Solution work on?
Neosporin Scar Solution sheets are effective on keloids and hypertrophic scars, which are distinguished by a raised and discolored appearance. These scars may result from burns, surgical procedures and minor skin injuries.

Are Neosporin Scar Solution sheets effective on both existing and new scars?
Neosporin Scar Solution sheets are effective on existing scars and may help prevent the formation of scars on newly closed, dry wounds.

Can Neosporin Scar Solution sheets be used anywhere on the body?
When used as directed, Neosporin Scar Solution sheets can be used on any part of the body.

Can I wear Neosporin Scar Solution sheets at the gym or in the shower?
Although Neosporin Scar Solution sheets may be worn while exercising or bathing, it is recommended that sheets be removed.

Can Neosporin Scar Solution sheets be used for various sizes of scars?
Yes, Neosporin Scar Solution sheets can be used for various sizes of scars; however, the sheet should extend completely around the scarred area.

How do I apply Neosporin Scar Solution?

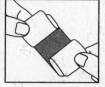

Step 1
Wash and dry existing scar or newly healed wound area. Do not use on open wounds.

Step 2
Tear open packet and peel off liner from adhesive side of sheet.

Step 3
Apply sheet with adhesive side directly on scar. Sheet should cover beyond the scarred area on all sides.

Step 4
Remove and wash sheet daily. Each sheet can be used for up to 4 days. After 3-4 days, discard old sheet in trash and replace with new one.

Usage Tips
• Each sheet should be worn for a minimum of 12 hours per day.
• Gradual improvements may be seen in 4–8 weeks.
• For best results, product should be used for at least 8 weeks.
• Sheets can be cut to fit the size of smaller scars, or applied side by side for larger ones. Trim sheet prior to removing from liner.
• Wash and dry individual sheet with mild soap and water to improve adhesion between wearing. To dry, pat fabric side of sheet. If sheets do not properly adhere to skin, medical tape may be used to hold sheets in place.

Cautions
• This product is not sterile and does not contain antibiotics.
• Do not use on open wounds or unhealed skin.
• If a rash or other allergic reaction occurs, stop use and consult a doctor.
• Keep out of reach of children under age 3 and pets, as sheets may present a choking hazard.
• Do not place adhesive side of sheet on fabrics or furniture.

Questions or Comments?
Call **1-800-223-0182**. Information is available 24 hours a day, 7 days a week.

Dist: **PFIZER CONSUMER HEALTHCARE**

Morris Plains, NJ 07950 USA

© 2003 Pfizer www.prodhelp.com

Licensed under U.S. Patent #4,832,009

Silon® is a registered trademark of Bio Med Sciences, Inc

07-0654-01

How Supplied: Neosporin Scar Solution contains 28 sheets per carton.

Shown in Product Identification Guide, page 519

NEOSPORIN® + PAIN RELIEF
MAXIMUM STRENGTH Cream

[*nē"uh-spō'rŭn*]

Drug Facts

Active Ingredients

(in each gram):	Purpose:
Neomycin 3.5 mg	First aid antibiotic
Polymyxin B 10,000 units	First aid antibiotic
Pramoxine HCl 10 mg	External analgesic

Uses: first aid to help prevent infection and for temporary relief of pain or discomfort in minor:

• cuts • scrapes • burns

Warnings:

For external use only.

Do not use
• if you are allergic to any of the ingredients
• in the eyes
• over large areas of the body

Ask a doctor before use if you have
• deep or puncture wounds
• animal bites • serious burns

Stop use and ask a doctor if
• you need to use longer than 1 week
• condition persists or gets worse
• symptoms persist for more than 1 week, or clear up and occur again within a few days
• rash or other allergic reaction develops

Keep out of reach of children. If swallowed, get medical help or contact a Poison Control Center right away.

Directions:
• adults and children 2 years of age and older
  • clean the affected area
  • apply a small amount of this product (an amount equal to the surface area of the tip of a finger) on the area 1 to 3 times daily
  • may be covered with a sterile bandage
• children under 2 years of age: ask a doctor

Other Information:
• store at 20° to 25°C (68° to 77° F)

Inactive Ingredients: emulsifying wax, methylparaben, mineral oil, propylene glycol, purified water, and white petrolatum

Continued on next page

This product information was prepared in November 2003. On these and other Pfizer Consumer Healthcare Products, detailed information may be obtained by addressing Pfizer Consumer Healthcare, Pfizer, Inc., Morris Plains, NJ 07950

Neosporin + Cream—Cont.

Questions? call **1-800-223-0182**, weekdays, 9 AM–5 PM EST

How Supplied: ½ oz (14.2 g) tubes

NEOSPORIN® + PAIN RELIEF MAXIMUM STRENGTH Ointment
[nē "uh-spō 'rŭn]

Drug Facts

Active Ingredients
(in each gram): Purpose:
Bacitracin
500 units .... First aid antibiotic
Neomycin 3.5 mg ..... First aid antibiotic
Polymyxin B
10,000 units .... First aid antibiotic
Pramoxine HCl
10 mg .... External analgesic

Uses: first aid to help prevent infection and for temporary relief of pain or discomfort in minor:
• cuts • scrapes • burns

Warnings:
For external use only.
Do not use
• if you are allergic to any of the ingredients
• in the eyes
• over large areas of the body
Ask a doctor before use if you have
• deep or puncture wounds
• animal bites
• serious burns
Stop use and ask a doctor if
• you need to use longer than 1 week
• condition persists or gets worse
• symptoms persist for more than 1 week, or clear up and occur again within a few days
• rash or other allergic reaction develops
Keep out of reach of children. If swallowed, get medical help or contact a Poison Control Center right away.

Directions:
• adults and children 2 years of age and older
  • clean the affected area
  • apply a small amount of this product (an amount equal to the surface area of the tip of a finger) on the area 1 to 3 times daily
  • may be covered with a sterile bandage
• children under 2 years of age: ask a doctor

Other Information:
• store at 20° to 25°C (68° to 77° F)

Inactive Ingredient: white petrolatum

Questions? call **1-800-223-0182**, weekdays, 9 AM - 5 PM EST

How Supplied: ¹/₂ oz (14.2 g) and 1 oz (28.3 g) tubes

Shown in Product Identification Guide, page 519

PEDIACARE® Multi-Symptom Cold-Liquid
PEDIACARE® Multi-Symptom Cold-Chewable
PEDIACARE® NightRest-Cough & Cold Liquid
PEDIACARE® Cold & Allergy-Liquid
PEDIACARE® Long-Acting Cough-Plus Cold Liquid
PEDIACARE® Long-Acting Cough-Plus Cold Chewable
PEDIACARE® Infants' Drops-Decongestant
PEDIACARE® Infants' Drops-Decongestant & Cough

Description: PEDIACARE products are available in eight different formulas, allowing you to select the ideal product to temporarily relieve your patient's symptoms. **PEDIACARE® Multi-Symptom Cold Liquid** and **PEDIACARE® Multi-Symptom Cold Chewable** contain an antihistamine, chlorpheniramine maleate, a nasal decongestant, pseudoephedrine HCl, and a cough suppressant, dextromethorphan hydrobromide, to provide temporary relief of nasal congestion, runny nose, sneezing and coughing due to the common cold, hay fever or other upper respiratory allergies. **PEDIACARE® NightRest Cough & Cold Liquid** contains a decongestant, pseudoephedrine hydrochloride, an antihistamine, chlorpheniramine maleate, and a cough suppressant, dextromethorphan hydrobromide, to provide temporary relief of coughs, nasal congestion, runny nose and sneezing due to the common cold, hayfever or other upper respiratory allergies. **PEDIACARE® Cold & Allergy Liquid** contains a decongestant, pseudoephedrine hydrochloride, and an antihistamine, chlorpheniramine maleate, to provide temporary relief of nasal congestion, runny nose and sneezing due to the common cold, hayfever or other respiratory allergies. **PEDIACARE® Long-Acting Cough Plus Cold Liquid** and **PEDIACARE® Long-Acting Cough Plus Cold Chewable** contain a decongestant, pseudoephedrine hydrochloride, and a cough suppressant, dextromethorphan hydrobromide, to provide temporary relief of nasal congestion and coughing due to the common cold, hayfever or other respiratory allergies. **PEDIACARE® Infants' Drops Decongestant** contains a decongestant, pseudoephedrine hydrochloride, to provide temporary relief of nasal congestion due to the common cold, hay fever or other upper respiratory allergies. **PEDIACARE® Infants' Drops Decongestant & Cough** contains a decongestant, pseudoephedrine hydrochloride, and a cough suppressant, dextromethorphan hydrobromide, to provide temporary relief of nasal congestion and coughing due to common cold, hay fever or other upper respiratory allergies.

Active Ingredients: Each 5 mL of **PEDIACARE® Multi-Symptom Cold** Liquid contains pseudoephedrine hydrochloride 15 mg, chlorpheniramine maleate 1 mg and dextromethorphan hydrobromide 5 mg. Each chewable tablet of **PEDIACARE® Multi-Symptom Cold Chewable** contains pseudoephedrine hydrochloride 15mg, chlorpheniramine maleate 1mg and dextromethorphan hydrobromide 5 mg. Each 0.8 mL oral dropper of **PEDIACARE® Infants' Drops Decongestant** contains pseudoephedrine hydrochloride 7.5 mg. Each 0.8 mL of **PEDIACARE® Infants' Drops Decongestant & Cough** contains pseudoephedrine hydrochloride 7.5 mg and dextromethorphan hydrobromide 2.5 mg. Each 5 mL of **PEDIACARE® NightRest Cough & Cold Liquid** contains pseudoephedrine hydrochloride 15 mg, chlorpheniramine maleate 1 mg and dextromethorphan hydrobromide 7.5 mg. Each 5mL of **PEDIACARE® Cold & Allergy Liquid** contains pseudoephedrine hydrochloride 15mg and chlorpheniramine maleate 1mg. Each 5mL of **PEDIACARE® Long-Acting Cough Plus Cold Liquid** contains pseudoephedrine hydrochloride 15mg and dextromethorphan hydrobromide 7.5mg. Each chewable tablet of **PEDIACARE® Long-Acting Cough Plus Cold Chewable** contains pseudoephedrine hydrochloride 15mg and dextromethorphan hydrobromide 7.5mg. **PEDIACARE® Multi-Symptom Cold Liquid** and **NightRest Cough & Cold Liquid** are cherry flavored, alcohol free and red in color. **PEDIACARE® Cold & Allergy Liquid** is bubblegum flavored, alcohol free and pink in color. **PEDIACARE® Long-Acting Cough Plus Cold Liquid** is grape flavored, alcohol free and purple in color. **PEDIACARE® Multi-Symptom Cold Chewable tablets** are cherry flavored, pink in color with PC3 imprinting. **PEDIACARE® Long-Acting Cough Plus Cold Chewable tablets** are grape flavored, purple in color with PC2 imprinting. **PEDIACARE® Infants' Drops Decongestant** is fruit flavored, alcohol free and clear, non-staining in color. **PEDIACARE® Infants' Drops Decongestant & Cough** is cherry flavored, alcohol free and clear, non-staining in color.

Professional Dosage: A calibrated dosage cup is provided for accurate dosing of the **PEDIACARE** Liquid formulas. A calibrated oral dropper is provided for accurate dosing of **PEDIACARE® Infants' Drops.** All doses of **PEDIACARE® Multi-Symptom Cold, Cold & Allergy Liquid,** as well as **PEDIACARE® Infants' Drops** may be repeated every 4–6 hours, not to exceed 4 doses in 24 hours. **PEDIACARE® NightRest Cough & Cold Liquid** and **Long-Acting Cough Plus Cold Liquid** may be repeated every 6–8 hrs, not to exceed 4 doses in 24 hours.
[See table at top of next page]

Warnings: Keep this and all medication out of the reach of children.

Age Group	0–3 mos	4–11 mos	12–23 mos	2–3 yrs	4–5 yrs	6–8 yrs	9–10 yrs	11 yrs	Dosage
Weight (lbs)	6–11 lbs	12–17 lbs	18–23 lbs	24–35 lbs	36–47 lbs	48–59 lbs	60–71 lbs	72–95 lbs	
PEDIACARE® Infants' Drops Decongestant*	¹/₂ dropper (0.4 mL)	1 dropper (0.8 mL)	1¹/₂ droppers (1.2 mL)	2 droppers (1.6 mL)					q4–6h
PEDIACARE® Infants' Drops Decongestant & Cough*	¹/₂ dropper (0.4 mL)	1 dropper (0.8 mL)	1¹/₂ droppers (1.2 mL)	2 droppers (1.6 mL)					q4–6h
PEDIACARE® Long-Acting Cough Plus Cold Liquid*			¹/₂ tsp	1 tsp	1¹/₂ tsp	2 tsp	2¹/₂ tsp	3 tsp	q6–8h
PEDIACARE® Multi-Symptom Cold Liquid**				1 tsp	1¹/₂ tsp	2 tsp	2¹/₂ tsp	3 tsp	q4–6h
PEDIACARE® NightRest Cough & Cold Liquid**				1 tsp	1¹/₂ tsp	2 tsp	2¹/₂ tsp	3 tsp	q6–8h
PEDIACARE® Cold & Allergy Liquid**				1 tsp	1¹/₂tsp	2 tsp	2¹/₂ tsp	3 tsp	q4–6h
PEDIACARE® Long-Acting Cough Plus Cold Chewable*				1 tablet	1 tablet	2 tablets	2 tablets	3 tablets	q6–8h
PEDIACARE® Multi-Symptom Cold Chewable**				1 tablet	1 tablet	2 tablets	2 tablets	3 tablets	q4–6h

*Administer to children under 2 years only on the advice of a physician.
**Administer to children under 6 years only on the advice of a physician.

In case of accidental overdosage, contact a physician or poison control center immediately.

The following information appears on the appropriate package labels:
PEDIACARE® Multi-Symptom Cold Liquid, NightRest Cough & Cold Liquid, Cold & Allergy Liquid and **PEDIACARE® Multi-Symptom Cold Chewable:** Do not exceed recommended dosage. If nervousness, dizziness or sleeplessness occur, discontinue use and consult a doctor. If symptoms do not improve within 7 days or are accompanied by fever, consult a doctor. A persistent cough may be a sign of a serious condition. If cough persists for more than one week, tends to recur or is accompanied by fever, rash, or persistent headache, consult a doctor. Do not give this product for persistent or chronic cough such as occurs with asthma or if cough is accompanied by excessive phlegm (mucus) unless directed by a doctor. May cause excitability especially in children. May cause drowsiness. Sedatives and tranquilizers may increase the drowsiness effect. Do not give this product to children who are taking sedatives or tranquilizers without first consulting the child's doctor. Do not give this product to children who have a breathing problem such as chronic bron-

chitis, or who have glaucoma, heart disease, high blood pressure, thyroid disease or diabetes, without first consulting the child's doctor.
PEDIACARE® Long-Acting Cough Plus Cold Liquid and **PEDIACARE® Long-Acting Cough Plus Cold Chewable:** Do not exceed recommended dosage. If nervousness, dizziness, or sleeplessness occur, discontinue use and consult a doctor. If symptoms do not improve within 7 days or are accompanied by fever, consult a doctor. A persistent cough may be a sign of a serious condition. If cough persists for more than one week, tends to recur or is accompanied by fever, rash, or persistent headache, consult a doctor. Do not give this product for persistent or chronic cough such as occurs with asthma or if cough is accompanied by excessive phlegm (mucus) unless directed by a doctor. Do not give this product to a child who has heart disease, high blood pressure, thyroid disease or diabetes unless directed by a doctor. Take by mouth only.
PEDIACARE® Infants' Drops Decongestant: Do not exceed the recommended dosage. If nervousness, dizziness or sleeplessness occur, discontinue use and consult a doctor. If symptoms do not improve within 7 days or are accompanied

by fever, consult a physician. Do not give this product to a child who has heart disease, high blood pressure, thyroid disease or diabetes unless directed by a doctor. Take by mouth only. Not for nasal use.
PEDIACARE® Infants' Drops Decongestant & Cough: Do not exceed recommended dosage. If nervousness, dizziness, or sleeplessness occur, discontinue use and consult a doctor. If symptoms do not improve within 7 days or are accompanied by fever, consult a doctor. A persistent cough may be a sign of a serious condition. If cough persists for more than one week, tends to recur or is accompanied by fever, rash, or persistent headache, consult a doctor. Do not give this product for persistent or chronic cough

Continued on next page

This product information was prepared in November 2003. On these and other Pfizer Consumer Healthcare Products, detailed information may be obtained by addressing Pfizer Consumer Healthcare, Pfizer, Inc., Morris Plains, NJ 07950

Pediacare—Cont.

such as occurs with asthma or if cough is accompanied by excessive phlegm (mucus) unless directed by a doctor. Do not give this product to a child who has heart disease, high blood pressure, thyroid disease or diabetes unless directed by a doctor. Take by mouth only. Not for nasal use.

Drug Interaction Precaution: Do not give this product to a child who is taking a prescription monoamine oxidase inhibitor (MAOI) (certain drugs for depression, psychiatric or emotional conditions), or for 2 weeks after stopping the MAOI drug. If you are uncertain whether your child's prescription drug contains an MAOI, consult a health professional before giving this product.

Overdosage: Acute dextromethorphan overdose usually does not result in serious signs and symptoms unless massive amounts have been ingested. Signs and symptoms of a substantial overdose may include nausea and vomiting, visual disturbances, CNS disturbances, and urinary retention. Symptoms from pseudoephedrine overdose consist most often of mild anxiety, tachycardia and/or mild hypertension. Symptoms usually appear within 4 to 8 hours of ingestion and are transient, usually requiring no treatment. Chlorpheniramine toxicity should be treated as you would an antihistamine/anticholinergic overdose and is likely to be present within a few hours after acute ingestion.

Inactive Ingredients: PEDIACARE® Multi-Symptom Cold Liquid: citric acid, corn syrup, FD&C red no. 40, flavor, glycerin, propylene glycol, purified water, sodium benzoate, sorbitol.

PEDIACARE® Multi-Symptom Cold Chewable: aspartame, carnauba wax, citric acid, colloidal silicon dioxide, crospovidone, D&C red no. 27 aluminum lake, ethylcellulose, flavors, hypromellose, magnesium stearate, mannitol, microcrystalline cellulose, mono & diglycerides, povidone, silcon dioxide, sucrose

PEDIACARE® NightRest Cough & Cold: citric acid, corn syrup, FD&C red no. 40, flavors, glycerin, propylene glycol, purified water, sodium benzoate, sodium carboxymethylcellulose, sorbitol.

PEDIACARE® Cold & Allergy Liquid: citric acid, corn syrup, FD&C red no. 40, flavors, glycerin, propylene glycol, purified water, sodium benzoate, sorbitol.

PEDIACARE® Long-Acting Cough Plus Cold Liquid: citric acid, corn syrup, FD&C blue no. 1, FD&C red no. 40, flavors, glycerin, propylene glycol, purified water, sodium benzoate, sorbitol.

PEDIACARE® Long-Acting Cough Plus Cold Chewable: aspartame, citric acid, colloidal silicon dioxide, crospovidone, D&C red no. 27 aluminum lake, ethylcellulose, FD&C blue no. 1 aluminum lake, flavor, magnesium stearate, mannitol, microcrystalline cellulose, povidone, sucrose

PEDIACARE® Infants' Drops Decongestant: benzoic acid, citric acid, FD&C red no. 40, flavors, glycerin, polyethylene glycol, propylene glycol, purified water, sodium benzoate, sorbitol, sucrose.

PEDIACARE® Infants' Drops Decongestant & Cough: citric acid, flavors, glycerin, purified water, sodium benzoate, sorbitol.

How Supplied: PEDIACARE® Multi-Symptom Cold Liquid, Night-Rest Cough & Cold Liquid (color red), **Cold & Allergy** (color pink), and **Long-Acting Cough Plus Cold** (color purple)-bottles of 4 fl. oz. (120 mL) with child-resistant safety cap and calibrated dosage cup. **Multi-Symptom Cold Chewable Tablets** (color pink, imprinted PC3), and **Long-Acting Cough Plus Cold Chewable Tablets** (color purple, imprinted PC2)-individually sealed blister packaging in boxes of 18. **PEDIACARE® Infants' Drops Decongestant** (color red) and **PEDIACARE® Infants' Drops Decongestant & Cough** (clear)—bottles of ½ fl. oz. (15 mL) with calibrated dropper. Store bottled product in original outer carton until depleted.
Shown in Product Identification Guide, page 519 & 520

POLYSPORIN® Ointment
[pŏl 'ē-spō 'rŭn]

Drug Facts

Active Ingredients
(in each gram): | **Purpose:**
Bacitracin
500 units .... First aid antibiotic
Polymyxin B
10,000 units .... First aid antibiotic

Use: first aid to help prevent infection in minor:
• cuts • scrapes • burns

Warnings:
For external use only.
Do not use
• if you are allergic to any of the ingredients
• in the eyes
• over large areas of the body
Ask a doctor before use if you have
• deep or puncture wounds
• animal bites
• serious burns
Stop use and ask a doctor if
• you need to use longer than 1 week
• condition persists or gets worse
• rash or other allergic reaction develops
Keep out of reach of children. If swallowed, get medical help or contact a Poison Control Center right away.

Directions:
• clean the affected area
• apply a small amount of this product (an amount equal to the surface area of the tip of a finger) on the area 1 to 3 times daily
• may be covered with a sterile bandage
Other Information:
• store at 20° to 25°C (68° to 77° F)
Inactive Ingredient: white petrolatum base

Questions? call **1-800-223-0182**, weekdays, 9 AM - 5 PM EST

How Supplied: Tubes, ½ oz (14.2 g), 1 oz (28.3 g); ¹⁄₃₂ oz (0.9 g) foil packets packed in cartons of 144.
Shown in Product Identification Guide, page 520

POLYSPORIN® Powder
[pŏl 'ē-spō 'rŭn]

Drug Facts

Active Ingredients
(in each gram): | **Purpose:**
Bacitracin
500 units .... First aid antibiotic
Polymyxin B
10,000 units .... First aid antibiotic

Use: first aid to help prevent infection in minor:
• cuts • scrapes • burns

Warnings:
For external use only.
Do not use
• if you are allergic to any of the ingredients
• in the eyes
• over large areas of the body
Ask a doctor before use if you have
• deep or puncture wounds
• animal bites
• serious burns
Stop use and ask a doctor if
• you need to use longer than 1 week
• condition persists or gets worse
• rash or other allergic reaction develops
Keep out of reach of children. If swallowed, get medical help or contact a Poison Control Center right away.

Directions:
• clean the affected area
• apply a light dusting of the powder on the area 1 to 3 times daily
• may be covered with a sterile bandage

Other Information:
• store at 20° to 25°C (68° to 77° F)
• do not refrigerate

Inactive Ingredient: lactose base
Questions? call **1-800-223-0182**, weekdays, 9 AM - 5 PM EST

How Supplied: 0.35 oz (10 g) shaker-vial.
Shown in Product Identification Guide, page 520

MEN'S ROGAINE® EXTRA STRENGTH
(5% Minoxidil Topical Solution)
Hair Regrowth Treatment

Description: Men's ROGAINE Extra Strength is a colorless solution for use only on the scalp to help regrow hair in men.

Active Ingredient: Minoxidil 5% w/v

Use: to regrow hair on the top of the scalp (vertex only)

Warnings:

For external use only. For use by men only.

Flammable: Keep away from fire or flame

Do not use if:

- you are a woman
- your amount of hair loss is different than that shown on the side of the product carton or your hair loss is on the front of the scalp. 5% minoxidil topical solution is not intended for frontal baldness or receding hairline.
- you have no family history of hair loss
- your hair loss is sudden and/or patchy
- you do not know the reason for your hair loss
- you are under 18 years of age. Do not use on babies and children.
- your scalp is red, inflamed, infected, irritated, or painful
- you are using other medicines on the scalp

Ask a doctor before use if you have heart disease

When using this product:

- do not apply on other parts of the body
- avoid contact with the eyes. In case of accidental contact, rinse eyes with large amounts of cool tap water.
- some people have experienced changes in hair color and/or texture
- it takes time to regrow hair. Results may occur at 2 months with twice a day usage. For some men, you may need to use this product for at least 4 months before you see results.
- the amount of hair regrowth is different for each person. This product will not work for all men.

Stop use and ask a doctor if:

- chest pain, rapid heartbeat, faintness, or dizziness occurs
- sudden, unexplained weight gain occurs
- your hands or feet swell
- scalp irritation or redness occurs
- unwanted facial hair growth occurs
- you do not see hair regrowth in 4 months

May be harmful if used when pregnant or breast-feeding.

Keep out of reach of children. If swallowed, get medical help or contact a Poison Control Center right away.

Directions: See inner product carton and enclosed booklet for complete directions. Part your hair and apply one ml 2 times a day directly onto the scalp in the area of hair thinning/loss. Spread the liquid evenly over the hair loss area. If you use your fingers, wash hands with soap and warm water immediately. Using more or more often will not improve results. Continued use is necessary to increase and keep your hair regrowth, or hair loss will begin again. **After each use of the dauber applicator, replace overcap to make child-resistant.**

Other Information: See hair loss pictures on side of product carton. Before use, read all information on product carton and enclosed booklet. Keep the product carton. It contains important information. Hair regrowth has not been shown to last longer than 48 weeks in large clinical trials with continuous treatment with 5% minoxidil topical solution for men. In clinical studies with mostly white men aged 18–49 years with moderate degrees of hair loss, 5% minoxidil topical solution for men provided more hair regrowth than 2% minoxidil topical solution. Store at controlled room temperature 20° to 25°C (68° to 77° F)

Inactive Ingredients: Alcohol (30% v/v), propylene glycol (50% v/v), and purified water.

How Supplied: Men's ROGAINE Extra Strength is available in packs of one, three, or four 60 mL bottles. (One 60 mL bottle is a one-month supply.)

Shown in Product Identification Guide, page 520

WOMEN'S ROGAINE®
(2% Minoxidil Topical Solution) Hair Regrowth Treatment

Description: ROGAINE is a colorless liquid medication for use on the scalp to help regrow hair.

Active Ingredient: Minoxidil 2% w/v

Use: to regrow hair on the scalp

Warnings:

For external use only

Flammable: Keep away from fire or flame

Do not use if

- your degree of hair loss is more than that shown on the side of the product carton, because this product may not work for you
- you have no family history of hair loss
- your hair loss is sudden and/or patchy
- your hair loss is associated with childbirth
- you do not know the reason for your hair loss
- you are under 18 years of age. Do not use on babies and children.
- your scalp is red, inflamed, infected, irritated, or painful
- you use other medicines on the scalp

Ask a doctor before use if you have heart disease

When using this product

- do not apply on other parts of the body
- avoid contact with the eyes. In case of accidental contact, rinse eyes with large amounts of cool tap water.
- some people have experienced changes in hair color and/or texture
- it takes time to regrow hair. You may need to use this product 2 times a day for at least 4 months before you see results.
- the amount of hair regrowth is different for each person. This product will not work for everyone

Stop use and ask a doctor if

- chest pain, rapid heartbeat, faintness, or dizziness occurs
- sudden, unexplained weight gain occurs
- your hands or feet swell
- scalp irritation or redness occurs
- unwanted facial hair growth occurs
- you do not see hair regrowth in 4 months

If pregnant or breast-feeding ask a health professional before use.

Keep out of reach of children. If swallowed, get medical help or contact a Poison Control Center right away.

Directions: See inner product carton and enclosed booklet for complete directions. Part your hair and apply one ml 2 times a day directly onto the scalp in the area of hair thinning/loss. Spread the liquid evenly over the hair loss area. If you use your fingers, wash hands with soap and warm water immediately. Using more or more often will not improve results. Continued use is necessary to increase and keep your hair regrowth, or hair loss will begin again. **After each use of the dauber applicator, replace overcap to make child-resistant.**

Other Information: See hair loss pictures on side of product carton. Before use, read all information on product carton and enclosed booklet. Keep the product carton. It contains important information. In clinical studies of mostly white women aged 18–45 years with mild to moderate degrees of hair loss, the following response to 2% minoxidil topical solution was reported: 19% of women reported moderate hair regrowth after using 2% minoxidil topical solution for 8 months (19% had moderate regrowth; 40% had minimal regrowth). This compares with 7% of women reporting moderate hair regrowth after using the placebo, the liquid without minoxidil in it, for 8 months (7% had moderate regrowth; 33% had minimal regrowth). Store at controlled room temperature 20° to 25°C (68° to 77° F)

Inactive Ingredients: Alcohol (60% v/v), propylene glycol (20% v/v), and purified water.

How Supplied: Women's ROGAINE is available in packs of one, three, or four 60 mL bottles. (One 60 mL bottle is a one-month supply.)

Shown in Product Identification Guide, page 520

ROLAIDS® Antacid Tablets
Original Peppermint, Spearmint, and Cherry

Drug Facts:

Active Ingredients (in each tablet):   **Purpose:**

Calcium carbonate 550 mg   Antacid
Magnesium hydroxide 110 mg   Antacid

Uses: relieves: • heartburn • sour stomach • acid indigestion • upset stomach due to these symptoms

Continued on next page

This product information was prepared in November 2003. On these and other Pfizer Consumer Healthcare Products, detailed information may be obtained by addressing Pfizer Consumer Healthcare, Pfizer, Inc., Morris Plains, NJ 07950

Rolaids—Cont.

Warnings:
Ask a doctor or pharmacist before use if you are
- presently taking a prescription drug. Antacids may interact with certain prescription drugs.
- do not take more than 12 tablets in a 24-hour period, or use the maximum dosage for more than 2 weeks, except under the advice and supervision of a physician.

Keep out of reach of children.

Directions
- chew 2 to 4 tablets, hourly if needed

Other Information:
- each tablet contains: calcium 220 mg and magnesium 45 mg
- store at 59° to 77°F in a dry place

Inactive Ingredients: Peppermint and Spearmint Flavors: dextrose, flavoring, magnesium stearate, polyethylene glycol, pregelatinized starch and sucrose
Cherry Flavor: dextrose, flavoring, magnesium stearate, polyethylene glycol, pregelatinized starch, D&C red no. 27 aluminum lake, and sucrose

Actions: Rolaids® provides rapid neutralization of stomach acid. Each tablet has an acid-neutralizing capacity of 14.7 mEq and the ability to maintain the pH of stomach contents at 3.5 or greater for a significant period of time.

Dosage and Administration: Chew 2 to 4 tablets as symptoms occur. Repeat hourly if symptoms return, or as directed by a physician.

How Supplied: Rolaids® is available in 12-tablet rolls, 3-packs containing three 12-tablet rolls and in bottles containing 150 or 300 tablets.
Shown in Product Identification Guide, page 520

EXTRA STRENGTH ROLAIDS®
Antacid Tablets
Freshmint, Fruit, Cool Strawberry, and Tropical Punch Flavors

Drug Facts:

Active Ingredients:
(in each tablet):	Purpose:
Calcium carbonate 675 mg	Antacid
Magnesium hydroxide 135 mg	Antacid

Uses: relieves: • heartburn • sour stomach • acid indigestion • upset stomach due to these symptoms

Warnings: Ask a doctor or pharmacist before use if you are
- presently taking a prescription drug. Antacids may interact with certain prescription drugs.
- do not take more than 10 tablets in a 24-hour period, or use the maximum dosage for more than 2 weeks, except under the advice and supervision of a physician.

Keep out of reach of children.

Directions:
- chew 2 to 4 tablets, hourly if needed

Other Information:
- each tablet contains: calcium 271 mg and magnesium 56 mg
- store at 59° to 77° F in a dry place

Inactive Ingredients: Freshmint Flavor: dextrose, flavoring, magnesium stearate, polyethylene glycol, pregelatinized starch and sucrose
Fruit Flavor: dextrose, flavoring, magnesium stearate, polyethylene glycol, pregelatinized starch, sucrose and FD&C yellow no. 5 aluminum lake (tartrazine)
Cool Strawberry and Tropical Punch: carmine, dextrose, flavoring, magnesium stearate, polyethylene glycol, pregelatinized starch and sucrose

Actions: Extra Strength Rolaids® provides rapid neutralization of stomach acid. Each tablet has an acid-neutralizing capacity of 18.2 mEq and the ability to maintain the pH of stomach contents at 3.5 or greater for a significant period of time.

Dosage and Administration: Chew 2 to 4 tablets as symptoms occur. Repeat hourly if symptoms return, or as directed by a physician.

How Supplied: Extra Strength Rolaids® is available in 10-tablet rolls, 3-packs containing three 10-tablet rolls and in bottles containing 100 tablets.
Shown in Product Identification Guide, page 520

ROLAIDS MULTI-SYMPTOM® ANTACID & ANTIGAS TABLETS
[rō-lāds]
Berry, Cool Mint

Drug Facts

Active Ingredients
(in each tablet):	Purpose:
Calcium carbonate 675 mg	Antacid
Magnesium hydroxide 135 mg	Antacid
Simethicone 60 mg	Antigas

Uses: relieves: • heartburn • acid indigestion • pressure, bloating and discomfort commonly referred to as gas

Warnings:
Ask a doctor or pharmacist before use if you are presently taking a prescription drug. Antacids may interact with certain prescription drugs.
Do not take more than 8 tablets in a 24-hour period, or use the maximum dosage for more than 2 weeks, except under the advice and supervision of a physician.
Keep out of reach of children.

Directions: chew 2 to 4 tablets, hourly if needed

Other Information:
- each tablet contains: calcium 271 mg and magnesium 56 mg
- store at 59° to 77°F in a dry place

Inactive Ingredients: Berry Flavor: corn starch, dextrose, FD&C blue #1, FD&C red #3, flavoring, magnesium stearate, polyethylene glycol, pregelatinized starch, and sucrose

Inactive Ingredients: Cool Mint Flavor: corn starch, dextrose, FD&C blue #1, flavoring, magnesium stearate, polyethylene glycol, pregelatinized starch, and sucrose

Actions: Rolaids Multi-Symptom provides rapid neutralization of stomach acid and also facilitates the release of trapped air, typically referred to as gas, in the digestive tract. Each tablet has an acid-neutralization capacity of 18.2 mEq and the ability to maintain the pH of stomach contents at 3.5 greater for a significant period of time.

Dosage and Administration: Chew 2 to 4 tablets as symptoms occur. Repeat hourly if symptoms return, or as directed by a physician.

How Supplied: Rolaids Multi-Symptom is available in 10-tablet rolls, 3-packs containing three 10-tablet rolls and in bottles containing 100 tablets.
Shown in Product Identification Guide, page 520

SUDAFED® Non-Drowsy 12 Hour Nasal Decongestant Tablets
[sū 'duh-fĕd]
*Capsule-shaped Tablets

Drug Facts:

Active Ingredient:
(in each tablet)	Purpose:
Pseudoephedrine HCl 120 mg	Nasal decongestant

Uses:
- temporarily relieves nasal congestion due to the common cold, hay fever or other upper respiratory allergies, and nasal congestion associated with sinusitis
- temporarily relieves sinus congestion and pressure

Warnings:
Do not use if you are now taking a prescription monoamine oxidase inhibitor (MAOI) (certain drugs for depression, psychiatric, or emotional conditions, or Parkinson's disease), or for 2 weeks after stopping the MAOI drug. If you do not know if your prescription drug contains an MAOI, ask a doctor or pharmacist before taking this product.
Ask a doctor before use if you have:
- heart disease
- high blood pressure
- thyroid disease
- diabetes
- trouble urinating due to an enlarged prostate gland

When using this product:
- do not use more than directed

Stop use and ask a doctor if:
- you get nervous, dizzy, or sleepless
- symptoms do not improve within 7 days or are accompanied by fever

If pregnant or breast-feeding, ask a health professional before use.

Keep out of reach of children. In case of overdose, get medical help or contact a Poison Control Center right away.

Directions:
- adults and children 12 years of age and over: one tablet every 12 hours not to exceed two tablets in 24 hours
- children under 12 years of age: use of product not recommended

Other Information:
- store at 59° to 77°F in a dry place
- protect from light

Inactive Ingredients: hypromellose, magnesium stearate, microcrystalline cellulose, polyethylene glycol, povidone, and titanium dioxide. May also contain: candelilla wax or carnauba wax. Printed with edible blue ink.

Questions? call **1-800-524-2624** (English/Spanish), weekdays, 9 AM–5 PM EST

How Supplied: Boxes of 10 and 20.
Shown in Product Identification Guide, page 520

SUDAFED® Non-Drowsy 24 Hour Nasal Decongestant Tablets
[sū 'duh-fěd]

Drug Facts:

Active Ingredient:
(in each tablet)　　　　　**Purpose:**
Pseudoephedrine
　HCl 240 mg .... Nasal decongestant

Uses:
- temporarily relieves nasal congestion due to the common cold, hay fever or other upper respiratory allergies, and nasal congestion associated with sinusitis
- reduces swelling of nasal passages
- relieves sinus pressure

Warnings:
Do not use if you are now taking a prescription monoamine oxidase inhibitor (MAOI) (certain drugs for depression, psychiatric, or emotional conditions, or Parkinson's disease), or for 2 weeks after stopping the MAOI drug. If you do not know if your prescription drug contains an MAOI, ask a doctor or pharmacist before taking this product.
Ask a doctor before use if you have:
- heart disease
- high blood pressure
- thyroid disease
- trouble urinating due to an enlarged prostate gland
- diabetes
- had obstruction or narrowing of the bowel. Rarely, tablets of this kind may cause bowel obstruction (blockage), usually in people with severe narrowing of the bowel (esophagus, stomach or intestine).
When using this product:
- do not use more than directed
Stop use and ask a doctor if:
- you get nervous, dizzy, or sleepless
- symptoms do not improve within 7 days or are accompanied by fever
- you experience persistent abdominal pain or vomiting
If pregnant or breast-feeding, ask a health professional before use.

Keep out of reach of children. In case of overdose, get medical help or contact a Poison Control Center right away.

Directions:
- adults and children 12 years of age and over: **swallow one** whole tablet with fluid every 24 hours
- **do not exceed one tablet in 24 hours**
- **do not divide, crush, chew or dissolve the tablet**
- the tablet does not completely dissolve and may be seen in the stool (this is normal)
- not for use in children under 12 years of age

Other Information:
- store at 59° to 77°F in a dry place

Inactive Ingredients: Cellulose, cellulose acetate, hydroxypropyl cellulose, hypromellose, magnesium stearate, polyethylene glycol, polysorbate 80, povidone, sodium chloride, and titanium dioxide

Questions? call **1-800-524-2624** (English/Spanish), weekdays, 9 AM – 5 PM EST

How Supplied: Box of 5 tablets and 10 tablets. **BLISTER PACKAGED FOR YOUR PROTECTION. DO NOT USE IF INDIVIDUAL SEALS ARE BROKEN.**
Shown in Product Identification Guide, page 521

SUDAFED® Non-Drowsy Nasal Decongestant 30-mg Tablets
[sū 'duh-fěd]

Drug Facts:

Active Ingredient:
(in each tablet)　　　　　**Purpose:**
Pseudoephedrine HCl
　30 mg .... Nasal decongestant

Uses:
- temporarily relieves nasal congestion due to the common cold, hay fever or other upper respiratory allergies, and nasal congestion associated with sinusitis
- temporarily relieves sinus congestion and pressure

Warnings:
Do not use if you are now taking a prescription monoamine oxidase inhibitor (MAOI) (certain drugs for depression, psychiatric, or emotional conditions, or Parkinson's disease), or for 2 weeks after stopping the MAOI drug. If you do not know if your prescription drug contains an MAOI, ask a doctor or pharmacist before taking this product.
Ask a doctor before use if you have:
- heart disease
- high blood pressure
- thyroid disease
- diabetes
- trouble urinating due to an enlarged prostate gland
When using this product:
- do not use more than directed
Stop use and ask a doctor if:
- you get nervous, dizzy, or sleepless
- symptoms do not improve within 7 days or are accompanied by fever
If pregnant or breast-feeding, ask a health professional before use.

Keep out of reach of children. In case of overdose, get medical help or contact a Poison Control Center right away.

Directions:
- take every 4 to 6 hours
- do not take more than 4 doses in 24 hours

adults and children 12 years of age and over	2 tablets
children 6 to under 12 years of age	1 tablet
children under 6 years of age	ask a doctor

Other Information:
- store at 59° to 77°F in a dry place

Inactive Ingredients: Acacia, candelilla wax, corn starch, FD&C red no. 40 aluminum lake, FD&C yellow no. 6 aluminum lake, hypromellose, lactose monohydrate, magnesium stearate, pharmaceutical glaze, poloxamer 407, polyethylene glycol, polyethylene oxide, polysorbate 60, povidone, sodium benzoate, sodium lauryl sulfate, stearic acid, sucrose, talc, and titanium dioxide. Printed with edible black ink.

Questions? call **1-800-524-2624** (English/Spanish), weekdays, 9 AM – 5 PM EST

How Supplied: Boxes of 24, 48 and 96.
Shown in Product Identification Guide, page 520

SUDAFED® NON-DROWSY NON-DRYING SINUS, LIQUID CAPS
[sū 'duh-fěd]

Drug Facts:

Active Ingredients:　　　　　**Purposes:**
(in each liquid cap)
Guaifenesin 200 mg .... Expectorant
Pseudoephedrine
　HCl 30 mg .... Nasal decongestant

Uses:
- temporarily relieves nasal congestion associated with sinusitis
- promotes nasal and/or sinus drainage
- temporarily relieves sinus congestion and pressure
- helps loosen phlegm (mucus) and thin bronchial secretions to rid the bronchial passageways of bothersome mucus and make coughs more productive

Continued on next page

This product information was prepared in November 2003. On these and other Pfizer Consumer Healthcare Products, detailed information may be obtained by addressing Pfizer Consumer Healthcare, Pfizer, Inc., Morris Plains, NJ 07950

Sudafed Non-Drying—Cont.

Warnings:
Do not use if you are now taking a prescription monoamine oxidase inhibitor (MAOI) (certain drugs for depression, psychiatric, or emotional conditions, or Parkinson's disease), or for 2 weeks after stopping the MAOI drug. If you do not know if your prescription drug contains an MAOI, ask a doctor or pharmacist before taking this product.

Ask a doctor before use if you have:
- heart disease
- high blood pressure
- thyroid disease
- diabetes
- trouble urinating due to an enlarged prostate gland
- cough that occurs with too much phlegm (mucus)
- persistent or chronic cough such as occurs with smoking, asthma, chronic bronchitis, or emphysema

When using this product:
- **do not use more than directed**

Stop use and ask a doctor if:
- you get nervous, dizzy, or sleepless
- symptoms do not improve within 7 days or are accompanied by fever
- cough persists for more than 1 week, tends to recur, or is accompanied by a fever, rash, or persistent headache. These could be signs of a serious condition.

If pregnant or breast-feeding, ask a health professional before use.

Keep out of reach of children. In case of overdose, get medical help or contact a Poison Control Center right away.

Directions:
- adults and children 12 years of age and over: swallow 2 liquid caps
- take every 4 hours
- do not exceed 8 liquid caps in 24 hours
- children under 12 years of age: ask a doctor

Other Information:
- store at 59° to 77°F
- protect from heat, humidity, and light

Inactive Ingredients: FD&C blue no. 1, gelatin, glycerin, polyethylene glycol 400, povidone, propylene glycol, and sorbitol. Printed with edible white ink.

Questions? call **1-800-524-2624** (English/Spanish), weekdays, 9 AM - 5 PM EST

How Supplied: Sudafed Non-Drying Sinus is supplied in boxes of 24 liquid caps.

Shown in Product Identification Guide, page 520

SUDAFED® Non-drowsy Severe Cold Caplets
(Formerly Sudafed Severe Cold Formula)
[sū 'duh-fĕd]

Drug Facts:

Active Ingredients: **Purpose:**
(in each caplet)
Acetaminophen
    500 mg ...... Pain reliever/fever reducer

Dextromethorphan HBr
    15 mg .... Antitussive
Pseudoephedrine HCl
    30 mg .... Nasal decongestant

Uses:
- temporarily relieves these symptoms due to the common cold:
  - nasal congestion
  - headache
  - minor aches and pains
  - muscular aches
  - cough
  - sore throat
  - fever

Warnings:
Alcohol warning: If you consume 3 or more alcoholic drinks every day, ask your doctor whether you should take acetaminophen or other pain relievers/fever reducers. Acetaminophen may cause liver damage.

Do not use:
- with another product containing any of these active ingredients
- if you are now taking a prescription monoamine oxidase inhibitor (MAOI) (certain drugs for depression, psychiatric, or emotional conditions, or Parkinson's disease), or for 2 weeks after stopping the MAOI drug. If you do not know if your prescription drug contains an MAOI, ask a doctor or pharmacist before taking this product.

Ask a doctor before use if you have:
- heart disease
- thyroid disease
- diabetes
- high blood pressure
- trouble urinating due to an enlarged prostate gland
- cough accompanied by excessive phlegm (mucus)
- persistent or chronic cough as occurs with smoking, asthma, or emphysema

When using this product:
- **do not use more than directed**

Stop use and ask a doctor if:
- new symptoms occur
- sore throat is severe
- you get nervous, dizzy, or sleepless
- symptoms do not get better
- you need to use more than 10 days
- redness or swelling is present
- fever gets worse or lasts more than 3 days
- cough persists for more than 7 days, tends to recur, or is accompanied by rash, or persistent headache. These could be signs of a serious condition.
- sore throat lasts for more than 2 days, is accompanied or followed by fever, headache, rash, swelling, nausea, or vomiting

If pregnant or breast-feeding, ask a health professional before use.

Keep out of reach of children.

Overdose warning: Taking more than the recommended dose may cause liver damage. In case of overdose, get medical help or contact a Poison Control Center right away. Quick medical attention is critical for adults as well as for children even if you do not notice any signs or symptoms.

Directions:
- do not use more than directed (see overdose warning)
- adults and children 12 years of age and over: 2 caplets

- children under 12 years of age: ask a doctor
- take every 6 hours while symptoms persist
- do not take more than 8 caplets in 24 hours or as directed by a doctor

Other Information:
- store at 59° to 77°F in a dry place

Inactive Ingredients: candelilla wax, crospovidone, hypromellose, magnesium stearate, microcrystalline cellulose poloxamer 407, polyethylene glycol, polyethylene oxide, povidone, pregelatinized starch, silicon dioxide, sodium lauryl sulfate, stearic acid, and titanium dioxide

Questions? call toll free **1-800-524-2624**, Monday to Friday, 9 AM – 5 PM EST

How Supplied: Boxes of 12 and 24 caplets; boxes of 12 tablets.
Shown in Product Identification Guide, page 520

SUDAFED® Sinus & Allergy Tablets
(Formerly Sudafed Cold & Allergy)
[sū 'duh-fĕd]

Drug Facts:

Active Ingredients: **Purposes:**
(in each tablet)
Chlorpheniramine maleate
    4 mg .... Antihistamine
Pseudoephedrine HCl
    60 mg .... Nasal decongestant

Uses:
- temporarily relieves these symptoms due to hay fever (allergic rhinitis) or other upper respiratory allergies:
  - runny nose
  - sneezing
  - itchy, watery eyes
  - nasal congestion
  - itching of the nose or throat
- temporarily relieves these symptoms due to the common cold:
  - runny nose
  - sneezing
  - nasal congestion

Warnings:
Do not use if you are now taking a prescription monoamine oxidase inhibitor (MAOI) (certain drugs for depression, psychiatric, or emotional conditions, or Parkinson's disease), or for 2 weeks after stopping the MAOI drug. If you do not know if your prescription drug contains an MAOI, ask a doctor or pharmacist before taking this product.

Ask a doctor before use if you have:
- high blood pressure
- thyroid disease
- heart disease
- glaucoma
- diabetes
- trouble urinating due to an enlarged prostate gland
- a breathing problem such as emphysema or chronic bronchitis

Ask a doctor or pharmacist before use if you are taking sedatives or tranquilizers

When using this product:
- **do not use more than directed**
- drowsiness may occur

- excitability may occur, especially in children
- avoid alcoholic drinks
- alcohol, sedatives, and tranquilizers may increase drowsiness
- be careful when driving a motor vehicle or operating machinery

Stop use and ask a doctor if:
- you get nervous, dizzy, or sleepless
- symptoms do not improve within 7 days or are accompanied by fever

If pregnant or breast-feeding, ask a health professional before use.
Keep out of reach of children. In case of overdose, get medical help or contact a Poison Control Center right away.

Directions:
- take every 4 to 6 hours
- do not take more than 4 doses in 24 hours

adults and children 12 years of age and over	1 tablet
children 6 to under 12 years of age	½ tablet
children under 6 years of age	ask a doctor

Other Information:
- store at 59° to 77°F in a dry place

Inactive Ingredients: Lactose, magnesium stearate, potato starch, and povidone

Questions? call **1-800-524-2624** (English/Spanish), weekdays, 9 AM–5 PM EST

How Supplied: Boxes of 24 tablets.
Shown in Product Identification Guide, page 520

SUDAFED® Non-drowsy Sinus Headache Caplets and Tablets (Formerly Sudafed Sinus)
[sū 'duh-fĕd]

Drug Facts:

Active Ingredients:
(in each caplet)   **Purposes:**
Acetaminophen 500 mg .... Pain reliever
Pseudoephedrine
   HCl 30 mg .... Nasal decongestant

Uses:
- temporarily relieves nasal congestion associated with sinusitis
- temporarily relieves headache, minor aches, and pains

Warnings:
Alcohol warning: If you consume 3 or more alcoholic drinks every day, ask your doctor whether you should take acetaminophen or other pain relievers/fever reducers. Acetaminophen may cause liver damage.
Do not use:
- with another product containing any of these active ingredients.
- if you are now taking a prescription monoamine oxidase inhibitor (MAOI) (certain drugs for depression, psychiatric, or emotional conditions, or Parkinson's disease), or for 2 weeks after

stopping the MAOI drug. If you do not know if your prescription drug contains an MAOI, ask a doctor or pharmacist before taking this product.
Ask a doctor before use if you have:
- heart disease
- thyroid disease
- diabetes
- high blood pressure
- trouble urinating due to an enlarged prostate gland

When using this product:
- do not use more than directed
Stop use and ask a doctor if:
- you get nervous, dizzy, or sleepless
- new symptoms occur
- symptoms do not get better
- you need to use more than 10 days
- fever occurs and lasts for more than 3 days

If pregnant or breast-feeding, ask a health professional before use.
Keep out of reach of children.
Overdose warning: Taking more than the recommended dose may cause liver damage. In case of overdose, get medical help or contact a Poison Control Center right away. Quick medical attention is critical for adults as well as for children even if you do not notice any signs or symptoms.

Directions:
- do not use more than directed (see overdose warning)
- children under 12 years of age: ask a doctor
- adults and children 12 years of age and over: 2 caplets every 6 hours while symptoms persist
- do not take more than 8 caplets in 24 hours or as directed by a doctor

Other Information:
- store at 59° to 77°F in a dry place

Inactive Ingredients: calcium stearate, candelilla wax, croscarmellose sodium, crospovidone, FD&C yellow no. 6 aluminum lake, hypromellose, microcrystalline cellulose, polyethylene glycol, polysorbate 80, povidone, pregelatinized starch, stearic acid and titanium dioxide.

Questions? call **1-800-524-2624** (English/Spanish), weekdays, 9 AM–5 PM EST

How Supplied: Boxes of 24 and 48 caplets; boxes of 24 tablets.
Shown in Product Identification Guide, page 520

MAXIMUM STRENGTH UNISOM SLEEPGELS®
Nighttime Sleep Aid

Drug Facts

Active Ingredient
(in each softgel):   **Purpose:**
Diphenhydramine HCl
   50 mg .... Nighttime sleep-aid

Use:
- helps to reduce difficulty falling asleep

Warnings:
Do not use
- for children under 12 years of age
- with any other product containing diphenhydramine, even one used on skin.

Ask a doctor before use if you have
- a breathing problem such as emphysema or chronic bronchitis
- glaucoma
- trouble urinating due to an enlarged prostate gland

Ask a doctor or pharmacist before use if you are taking sedatives or tranquilizers
When using this product avoid alcoholic drinks

Stop use and ask a doctor if sleeplessness persists continuously for more than 2 weeks. Insomnia may be a symptom of serious underlying medical illness.
If pregnant or breast-feeding, ask a health professional before use.
Keep out of reach of children. In case of overdose, get medical help or contact a Poison Control Center right away.

Directions:
- adults and children 12 years of age and over: 1 softgel (50 mg) at bedtime if needed, or as directed by a doctor

Other Information:
- store at 59° to 86°F (15° to 30°C)

Inactive Ingredients: FD&C blue no. 1, gelatin, glycerin, polyethylene glycol, polyvinyl acetate phthalate, propylene glycol, purified water, sorbitol, and titanium dioxide

Questions? call **1-800-223-0182**, weekdays, 9 AM – 5 PM EST

How Supplied: Boxes of 16 liquid filled softgels in child resistant blisters and boxes of 8 with non-child resistant packaging. Also in a 32 count easy to open child resistant bottle.
Shown in Product Identification Guide, page 520

UNISOM® SleepTabs™
[yu 'na-som]
Nighttime Sleep Aid
(doxylamine succinate)

Drug Facts

Active Ingredient: **Purpose:**
(in each tablet)
Doxylamine succinate
   25 mg .... Nighttime sleep-aid

Use:
- helps to reduce difficulty in falling asleep

Warnings:
Ask a doctor before use if you have
- a breathing problem such as asthma, emphysema or chronic bronchitis
- glaucoma
- trouble urinating due to an enlarged prostate gland

Continued on next page

This product information was prepared in November 2003. On these and other Pfizer Consumer Healthcare Products, detailed information may be obtained by addressing Pfizer Consumer Healthcare, Pfizer, Inc., Morris Plains, NJ 07950

Unisom—Cont.

Ask a doctor or pharmacist before use if you are taking any other drugs
When using this product
- avoid alcoholic beverages
- take only at bedtime

Stop use and ask a doctor if sleeplessness persists continuously for more than two weeks. Insomnia may be a symptom of serious underlying medical illness.

If pregnant or breast-feeding, ask a health professional before use.

Keep out of reach of children. In case of overdose, get medical help or contact a Poison Control Center right away.

Directions:
- adults: take one tablet 30 minutes before going to bed; take once daily or as directed by a doctor
- do not give to children under 12 years of age

Other Information:
- store at 59° to 86°F (15° to 30°C)

Inactive Ingredients: dibasic calcium phosphate, FD&C blue no. 1 aluminum lake, magnesium stearate, microcrystalline cellulose, and sodium starch glycolate

Questions?
call **1-800-223-0182**, Monday to Friday, 9 AM - 5 PM EST

How Supplied: Boxes of 8, 32 and 48 tablets in child resistant packaging. Boxes of 16 tablets in non-child resistant packaging.

Shown in Product Identification Guide, page 521

VISINE® ORIGINAL
Redness Reliever Eye Drops

Description: Visine Original is a redness reliever eye drop that gives fast relief of redness of the eye due to minor eye irritation caused by conditions such as smoke, dust, other airborne pollutants and swimming.
Visine Original is a sterile, isotonic, buffered ophthalmic solution containing tetrahydrozoline hydrochloride. The effectiveness of Visine in relieving conjunctival hyperemia has been demonstrated by numerous clinicals, including several double-blind studies, involving more than 2,000 subjects suffering from acute or chronic hyperemia induced by a variety of conditions. Visine was found to be efficacious in providing relief from conjunctival hyperemia.

Active Ingredient: **Purpose:**
Tetrahydrozoline
  HCl 0.05% .... Redness reliever

Use:
- for the relief of redness of the eye due to minor eye irritations

Warnings:
Ask a doctor before use if you have narrow angle glaucoma
When using this product
- pupils may become enlarged temporarily

- overuse may cause more eye redness
- remove contact lenses before using
- do not use if this solution changes color or becomes cloudy
- do not touch tip of container to any surface to avoid contamination
- replace cap after each use

Stop use and ask a doctor if
- you feel eye pain
- changes in vision occur
- redness or irritation of the eye lasts
- condition worsens or lasts more than 72 hours

If pregnant or breast-feeding, ask a health professional before use.

Keep out of reach of children. If swallowed, get medical help or contact a Poison Control Center right away.

Directions:
- put 1 to 2 drops in the affected eye(s) up to 4 times daily
- children under 6 years of age: ask a doctor

Other Information:
- store at 15° to 30°C (59° to 86°F)

Inactive Ingredients: benzalkonium chloride, boric acid, edetate disodium, purified water, sodium borate, and sodium chloride
Questions? call **1-800-223-0182**, Monday to Friday, 9 AM – 5 PM EST

Caution: Do not use if Visine-imprinted neckband on bottle is broken or missing.

How Supplied: In 0.5 fl. oz. and 1.0 fl. oz. plastic dispenser bottle and 0.5 fl. oz. plastic bottle with eye dropper.

Shown in Product Identification Guide, page 521

VISINE-A®
Antihistamine & Redness Reliever Eye Drops

Drug Facts:

Active Ingredients: **Purpose:**
Naphazoline hydrochloride
  0.025% .... Redness reliever
Pheniramine maleate
  0.3% .... Antihistamine

Uses: Temporarily relieves itchy, red eyes due to:
- pollen
- ragweed
- grass
- animal hair and dander

Warnings:
Do not use
- if you are sensitive to any ingredient in this product
Ask a doctor before use if you have:
- heart disease
- high blood pressure
- narrow angle glaucoma
- trouble urinating due to an enlarged prostate gland
When using this product:
- pupils may become enlarged temporarily
- do not touch tip of container to any surface to avoid contamination
- replace cap after each use

- remove contact lenses before using
- do not use if this solution changes color or becomes cloudy
- overuse may cause more eye redness

Stop use and ask a doctor if:
- you feel eye pain
- changes in vision occur
- redness or irritation of the eye lasts
- condition worsens or lasts more than 72 hours

Keep out of reach of children. If swallowed, get medical help or contact a Poison Control Center right away. Accidental swallowing by infants and children may lead to coma and marked reduction in body temperature.

Directions:
- adults and children 6 years of age and over: put 1 or 2 drops in the affected eye(s) up to 4 times a day
- children under 6 years of age: consult a doctor

Other Information:
- some users may experience a brief tingling sensation
- store between 15° and 25°C (59° and 77°F)

Inactive Ingredients: boric acid and sodium borate buffer system preserved with benzalkonium chloride (0.01%) and edetate disodium (0.1%), sodium hydroxide and/or hydrochloric acid (to adjust pH), and purified water

Questions? call **1-800-223-0182**, Monday to Friday, 9 AM – 5 PM EST

Caution: Do not use if Visine imprinted neckband on bottle is broken or missing.

How Supplied: In 0.5 fl. oz. plastic dispenser bottle.

Shown in Product Identification Guide, page 521

VISINE A.C.®
Astringent/Redness Reliever Eye Drops

Drug Facts:

Active Ingredients: **Purposes:**
Tetrahydrozoline
  HCl 0.05% .... Redness reliever
Zinc sulfate 0.25% .... Astringent

Use:
- for temporary relief of discomfort and redness of the eye due to minor eye irritations

Warnings:
Ask a doctor before use if you have narrow angle glaucoma
When using this product:
- pupils may become enlarged temporarily
- overuse may cause more eye redness
- remove contact lenses before using
- do not use if this solution changes color or becomes cloudy
- do not touch tip of container to any surface to avoid contamination
- replace cap after each use

Stop use and ask a doctor if:
- you feel eye pain
- changes in vision occur
- redness or irritation of the eye lasts

- condition worsens or lasts more than 72 hours

If pregnant or breast-feeding, ask a health professional before use.

Keep out of reach of children. If swallowed, get medical help or contact a Poison Control Center right away.

Directions:
- put 1 to 2 drops in the affected eye(s) up to 4 times daily
- children under 6 years of age: ask a doctor

Other Information:
- some users may experience a brief tingling sensation
- store at 15° to 30°C (59° to 86°F)

Inactive Ingredients: benzalkonium chloride, boric acid, edetate disodium, purified water, sodium chloride, and sodium citrate

Questions? call **1-800-223-0182,** Monday to Friday, 9 AM – 5 PM EST

Caution: Do not use if Visine-imprinted neckband on bottle is broken or missing.

How Supplied: In 0.5 fl. oz. and 1.0 fl. oz. plastic dispenser bottle.

VISINE ADVANCED RELIEF®
Lubricant/Redness Reliever Eye Drops

Drug Facts:

Active Ingredients:	Purposes:
Dextran 70 0.1%	Lubricant
Polyethylene glycol 400 1%	Lubricant
Povidone 1%	Lubricant
Tetrahydrozoline HCl 0.05%	Redness reliever

Uses:
- for the relief of redness of the eye due to minor eye irritations
- for use as a protectant against further irritation or to relieve dryness of the eye

Warnings:

Ask a doctor before use if you have narrow angle glaucoma

When using this product:
- pupils may become enlarged temporarily
- overuse may cause more eye redness
- remove contact lenses before using
- do not use if this solution changes color or becomes cloudy
- do not touch tip of container to any surface to avoid contamination
- replace cap after each use

Stop use and ask a doctor if:
- you feel eye pain
- changes in vision occur
- redness or irritation of the eye lasts
- condition worsens or lasts more than 72 hours

If pregnant or breast-feeding, ask a health professional before use.

Keep out of reach of children. If swallowed, get medical help or contact a Poison Control Center right away.

Directions:
- put 1 or 2 drops in the affected eye(s) up to 4 times daily
- children under 6 years of age: ask a doctor

Other Information:
- store at 15° to 30°C (59° to 86°F)

Inactive Ingredients: benzalkonium chloride, boric acid, edetate disodium, purified water, sodium borate, and sodium chloride

Questions? call **1-800-223-0182,** Monday to Friday, 9 AM – 5 PM EST

Caution: Do not use if Visine-imprinted neckband on bottle is broken or missing.

How Supplied: In 0.5 fl. oz. and 1.0 fl. oz. plastic dispenser bottle.

Shown in Product Identification Guide, page 521

VISINE L.R.®
Redness Reliever Eye Drops

Drug Facts:

Active Ingredient:	Purpose:
Oxymetazoline HCl 0.025%	Redness reliever

Use:
- for the relief of redness of the eye due to minor eye irritations

Warnings:

Ask a doctor before use if you have narrow angle glaucoma

When using this product:
- overuse may cause more eye redness
- remove contact lenses before using
- do not use if this solution changes color or becomes cloudy
- do not touch tip of container to any surface to avoid contamination
- replace cap after each use

Stop use and ask a doctor if:
- you feel eye pain
- changes in vision occur
- redness or irritation of the eye lasts
- condition worsens or lasts more than 72 hours

If pregnant or breast-feeding, ask a health professional before use.

Keep out of reach of children. If swallowed, get medical help or contact a Poison Control Center right away.

Directions:
- adults and children 6 years of age and over: put 1 or 2 drops in the affected eye(s)
- this may be repeated as needed every 6 hours or as directed by a doctor
- children under 6 years of age: ask a doctor

Other Information:
- store at 15° to 30°C (59° to 86°F)

Inactive Ingredients: benzalkonium chloride, boric acid, edetate disodium, purified water, sodium borate, and sodium chloride

Questions? call **1-800-223-0182,** Monday to Friday, 9 AM – 5 PM EST

Caution: Do not use if Visine-imprinted neckband on bottle is broken or missing.

How Supplied: In 0.5 fl. oz. and 1 fl. oz. plastic dispenser bottle.

VISINE TEARS®
Lubricant Eye Drops

Description: Visine Tears® Lubricant Eye Drops cools and comforts your dry, scratchy, irritated eyes, and helps them feel their best. It relieves the dryness caused by computer use, reading, wind, heat and air conditioning, while it protects your eyes from further irritation. Visine Tears is safe to use as often as needed.

Active Ingredients:	Purpose:
Glycerin 0.2%	Lubricant
Hypromellose 0.2%	Lubricant
Polyethylene glycol 400 1%	Lubricant

Uses:
- for the temporary relief of burning and irritation due to dryness of the eye
- for protection against further irritation

Warnings:

When using this product
- remove contact lenses before using
- do not use if this solution changes color or becomes cloudy
- do not touch tip of container to any surface to avoid contamination
- replace cap after each use

Stop use and ask a doctor if
- you feel eye pain
- changes in vision occur
- redness or irritation of the eye lasts
- condition worsens or lasts more than 72 hours

If pregnant or breast-feeding, ask a health professional before use.

Keep out of reach of children. If swallowed, get medical help or contact a Poison Control Center right away.

Directions:
- put 1 or 2 drops in the affected eye(s) as needed
- children under 6 years of age: ask a doctor

Other Information:
- store at 15° to 30°C (59° to 86°F)

Inactive Ingredients: ascorbic acid, benzalkonium chloride, boric acid, dextrose, disodium phosphate, glycine, magnesium chloride, potassium chloride, purified water, sodium borate, sodium chloride, sodium citrate, and sodium lactate

Continued on next page

This product information was prepared in November 2003. On these and other Pfizer Consumer Healthcare Products, detailed information may be obtained by addressing Pfizer Consumer Healthcare, Pfizer, Inc., Morris Plains, NJ 07950

Visine Tears—Cont.

Questions? call **1-800-223-0182**, Monday to Friday, 9 AM – 5 PM EST

Caution: Do not use if Visine-imprinted neckband on bottle is broken or missing.

How Supplied: In 0.5 fl. oz. and 1 fl. oz. plastic dispenser bottle.
Shown in Product Identification Guide, page 521

VISINE TEARS®

Preservative Free, Single-Use Containers

Lubricant Eye Drops

Drug Facts:

Active Ingredients:	**Purpose:**
Glycerin 0.2%	Lubricant
Hypromellose 0.2%	Lubricant
Polyethylene glycol 400 1%	Lubricant

Uses:
• for the temporary relief of burning and irritation due to dryness of the eye
• for protection against further irritation

Warnings:
When using this product
• remove contact lenses before using
• do not use if this solution changes color or becomes cloudy
• do not touch tip of container to any surface to avoid contamination
• do not reuse; once opened, discard
Stop use and ask a doctor if:
• you feel eye pain
• changes in vision occur
• redness or irritation of the eye lasts
• condition worsens or lasts more than 72 hours
If pregnant or breast-feeding, ask a health professional before use.
Keep out of reach of children. If swallowed, get medical help or contact a Poison Control Center right away.

Directions:
• put 1 or 2 drops in the affected eye(s) as needed
• children under 6 years of age: ask a doctor

Other Information:
• store at 15° to 30°C (59° to 86°F)

Inactive Ingredients: ascorbic acid, dextrose, disodium phosphate, glycine, magnesium chloride, potassium chloride, purified water, sodium chloride, sodium citrate, sodium lactate, and sodium phosphate

Questions? call **1-800-223-0182**, Monday to Friday, 9 AM - 5 PM EST

Caution: Use only if unit dose container is intact.

How Supplied: 1 box contains 28 single-use containers, 0.01 fl. oz. (0.4 mL) each
Shown in Product Identification Guide, page 521

ZANTAC 75®
Ranitidine Tablets 75 mg
Acid Reducer

[*zan ' tak*]

Drug Facts:

Active Ingredient:
(in each tablet)   **Purpose:**
Ranitidine 75 mg
(as ranitidine
hydrochloride 84 mg) .... Acid reducer

Uses:
• relieves heartburn associated with acid indigestion and sour stomach
• prevents heartburn associated with acid indigestion and sour stomach brought on by certain foods and beverages

Warnings:
Allergy alert: Do not use if you are allergic to ranitidine or other acid reducers
Do not use:
• if you have trouble swallowing
• with other acid reducers
Stop use and ask a doctor if:
• stomach pain continues
• you need to take this product for more than 14 days
If pregnant or breast-feeding, ask a health professional before use.

Keep out of reach of children. In case of overdose, get medical help or contact a Poison Control Center right away.

Directions:
• adults and children 12 years and over:
  • to **relieve** symptoms, swallow 1 tablet with a glass of water
  • to **prevent** symptoms, swallow 1 tablet with a glass of water **30 to 60 minutes before** eating food or drinking beverages that cause heartburn
  • can be used up to twice daily (up to 2 tablets in 24 hours)
• children under 12 years: ask a doctor

Other Information:
• do not use if foil under bottle cap or individual blister unit is open or torn
• store at 20°–25°C (68°–77°F)
• avoid excessive heat or humidity
• this product is sodium and sugar free

Inactive Ingredients: hypromellose, magnesium stearate, microcrystalline cellulose, synthetic red iron oxide, titanium dioxide, triacetin

Read the Label: Read the directions, consumer information leaflet and warnings before use. Keep the carton. It contains important information.

Questions? call **1-800-223-0182**. Information is available 24 hours a day, 7 days a week.

How Supplied: Zantac 75 is available in convenient blister packs in boxes of 4, 10, 20 and 30 tablets, and in bottles of 60, 80 and 124 count.
Shown in Product Identification Guide, page 521

Pharmacia Consumer Healthcare

(See Pfizer Consumer Healthcare, Pfizer Inc.)

The Procter & Gamble Company
**P. O. BOX 599
CINCINNATI, OH 45201**

Direct Inquiries to:
Consumer Relations
(800) 832–3064

HEAD & SHOULDERS CLASSIC CLEAN DANDRUFF SHAMPOO

Head & Shoulders Classic Clean Dandruff Shampoo for normal/oily hair offers effective control of persistent dandruff and beautiful hair from a pleasant-to-use formula. Double-blind, expert-graded testing have proven that it reduces dandruff very effectively. It is also gentle enough to use every day for clean, manageable hair.
The formula ingredients below are for Classic Clean version. Head & Shoulders is also available in a Classic Clean 2-in-1 version for increased manageability and hair damage prevention. The key formula difference is increased dimethicone conditioner and substitution of Polyquaternium-10 polymer instead of Guar Hydroxypropyltrimonium Chloride.

Drug Facts

Active Ingredient: **Purpose:**
Pyrithione zinc 1%   Anti-dandruff

Uses: helps prevent recurrence of flaking and itching associated with dandruff

Warnings:
For external use only
When using this product
• avoid contact with eyes. If contact occurs, rinse eyes thoroughly with water.
Stop use and ask a doctor if
• condition worsens or does not improve after regular use of this product as directed.
Keep this and all drugs out of reach of children. If swallowed, get medical help or contact a Poison Control Center right away.

Directions:
• for maximum dandruff control, use every time you shampoo.
• wet hair.
• massage onto scalp
• rinse.

- repeat if desired.
- for best results use <u>at least</u> twice a week or as directed by a doctor.

Inactive Ingredients: Water, Ammonium laureth sulfate, Ammonium lauryl sulfate, Glycol distearate, Dimethicone, Cetyl alcohol, Cocamide MEA, Fragrance, Sodium chloride, Guar hydroxypropyltrimonium chloride, Hydrogenated polydecene, Sodium citrate, Sodium benzoate, Trimethylolpropane tricaprylate/tricaprate, Citric acid, Benzyl alcohol, Methylchloroisothiazolinone, Methylisothiazolinone, Ext. D&C violet no. 2, FD&C blue no. 1, Ammonium xylenesulfonate

How Supplied: Head & Shoulders Classic Clean Dandruff Shampoo is available in 2.0 FL, 6.8 FL OZ, 13.5 FL OZ, 25.4 FL OZ, 33.9 FL OZ unbreakable plastic bottles.

Questions [or comments]? **1-800-723-9569**

HEAD & SHOULDERS DRY SCALP CARE DANDRUFF SHAMPOO

Head & Shoulders Dry Scalp Care Dandruff Shampoo offers effective control of persistent dandruff and beautiful hair from a pleasant-to-use formula. Double-blind, expert-graded testing have proven that it reduces dandruff very effectively. It is also gentle enough to use every day for clean, manageable hair.

The formula ingredients below are for Dry Scalp version. Head & Shoulders is also available in a conditioning Smooth & Silky 2-in-1 version whose primary formula difference is a lower level of the moisturizing and protective conditioning ingredient Dimethicone and substitution of Polyquarternium-10 polymer for a portion of the Guar Hydroxypropyltrimonium Chloride.

Drug Facts

Active Ingredient: **Purpose:**
Pyrithione zinc 1%   Anti-dandruff

Uses: Helps prevent recurrence of flaking and itching associated with dandruff

Warnings:

For external use only

When using this product
- avoid contact with eyes. If contact occurs, rinse eyes thoroughly with water.

Stop use and ask a doctor if
- condition worsens or does not improve after regular use of this product as directed.

Keep this and all drugs out of reach of children. If swallowed, get medical help or contact a Poison Control Center right away.

Directions:
- for maximum dandruff control, use every time you shampoo
- wet hair.

- massage onto scalp.
- rinse.
- repeat if desired.
- for best results use <u>at least</u> twice a week or as directed by a doctor.

Inactive Ingredients: Water, Ammonium laureth sulfate, Ammonium lauryl sulfate, Dimethicone, Glycol distearate, Cetyl alcohol, Cocamide MEA, Fragrance, Sodium chloride, Polyquaternium-10, Hydrogenated polydecene, Sodium citrate, Sodium benzoate, Trimethylolpropane tricaprylate/tricaprate, Citric acid, Benzyl alcohol, Methylchloroisothiazolinone, Methylisothiazolinone, Ext. D&C violet no. 2, FD&C blue no. 1, Ammonium xylenesulfonate

How Supplied: Head & Shoulders Dry Scalp Care Dandruff Shampoo is available in 6.8 FL OZ, 13.5 FL OZ, 25.4 FL OZ, 33.9 FL OZ unbreakable plastic bottles.

Questions [or comments]? **1-800-723-9569**

HEAD & SHOULDERS® INTENSIVE TREATMENT DANDRUFF AND SEBORRHEIC DERMATITIS SHAMPOO

Head & Shoulders Intensive Treatment Dandruff and Seborrheic Dermatitis Shampoo offers effective control of persistent dandruff and beautiful hair from a pleasant-to-use formula. Double-blind, expert-graded testing have proven that it reduces dandruff very effectively. It is also gentle enough to use every day for clean, manageable hair.

Drug Facts

Active Ingredient: **Purpose:**
Selenium Sulfide 1%   Anti-dandruff
                               Anti-seborrheic dermatitis

Uses: Helps stop itching, flaking, scaling, irritation and redness associated with dandruff and seborrheic dermatitis.

Warnings:

For external use only

Ask a doctor before use if you have a condition that covers a large portion of the body.

When using this product
- avoid contact with eyes. If contact occurs, rinse eyes thoroughly with water.

Stop use and ask a doctor if
- condition worsens or does not improve after regular use of this product as directed.

Keep this and all drugs out of reach of children. If swallowed, get medical help or contact a Poison Control Center right away.

Directions:
- wet hair.
- massage onto scalp

- rinse thoroughly
- for best results use <u>at least</u> twice a week or as directed by a doctor.
- caution: if used on bleached, tinted, grey, or permed hair, rinse for 5 minutes
- for maximum dandruff control, use every time you shampoo

Inactive Ingredients: Water, Ammonium laureth sulfate, Ammonium lauryl sulfate, Glycol distearate, Cocamide MEA, Fragrance, Dimethicone, Tricetylmonium chloride, Ammonium xylenesulfonate, Cetyl alcohol, DMDM hydantoin, Sodium chloride, Stearyl alcohol, Hydroxypropyl methylcellulose, FD&C red no. 4

How Supplied: Head & Shoulders Intensive Treatment Dandruff and Seborrheic Dermatitis Shampoo is available in 13.5 FL OZ unbreakable plastic bottles.

Questions [or comments]? **1-800-723-9569**

METAMUCIL® FIBER LAXATIVE
[*met uh-mü sil*]
(psyllium husk)

Also see **Metamucil Dietary Fiber Supplement** *in PDR for Nonprescription Drugs*

Description: Metamucil contains psyllium husk (from the plant *Plantago ovata*), a bulk forming, natural therapeutic fiber for restoring and maintaining regularity when recommended by a physician. Metamucil contains no chemical stimulants and does not disrupt normal bowel function. Each dose of Metamucil powder and Metamucil Fiber Wafers contains approximately 3.4 grams of psyllium husk (or 2.4 grams of soluble fiber). Each dose of Metamucil capsules fiber laxative (5 capsules) contains approximately 2.6 grams of psyllium husk (or 2.0 grams of soluble fiber). Inactive ingredients, sodium, calcium, potassium, calories, carbohydrate, dietary fiber, and phenylalanine content are shown in the following table for all versions and flavors. Metamucil Smooth Texture Sugar-Free Regular Flavor and Metamucil capsules contains no sugar and no artificial sweeteners; Metamucil Smooth Texture Sugar-Free Orange Flavor contains aspartame (phenylalanine content per dose is 25 mg). Metamucil powdered products and Metamucil capsules are gluten-free. Metamucil Fiber Wafers contain gluten: Apple Crisp contains 0.7g/dose, Cinnamon Spice contains 0.5g/dose. Each two-wafer dose contains 5 grams of fat.

Actions: The active ingredient in Metamucil is psyllium husk, a natural fiber which promotes elimination due to its bulking effect in the colon. This bulking

Continued on next page

Metamucil—Cont.

effect is due to both the water-holding capacity of undigested fiber and the increased bacterial mass following partial fiber digestion. These actions result in enlargement of the lumen of the colon, and softer stool, thereby decreasing intraluminal pressure and straining, and speeding colonic transit in constipated patients.

Indications: Metamucil is indicated for the treatment of occasional constipation, and when recommended by a physician, for chronic constipation and constipation associated with irritable bowel syndrome, diverticulosis, hemorrhoids, convalescence, senility and pregnancy.

Pregnancy: Category B. If considering use of Metamucil as part of a cholesterol-lowering program, see **Metamucil Dietary Fiber Supplement** in Dietary Supplement Section.

Drug Facts

Active Ingredient:
(in each DOSE)   **Purpose:**
Psyllium husk
   approximately 3.4 g ..... Fiber therapy for regularity
For Metamucil capsules each dose of 5 capsules contains approximately 2.6 gm of psyllium husk.

Uses:
• effective in treating occasional constipation and restoring regularity

Warnings:

Choking: Taking this product without adequate fluid may cause it to swell and block your throat or esophagus and may cause choking. Do not take this product if you have difficulty in swallowing. If you experience chest pain, vomiting, or difficulty in swallowing or breathing after taking this product, seek immediate medical attention.

Ask a doctor before use if you have:
• a sudden change in bowel habits persisting for 2 weeks
• abdominal pain, nausea or vomiting

When using this product:
• may cause allergic reaction in people sensitive to inhaled or ingested psyllium

Metamucil Fiber Laxative/Dietary Fiber Supplement

Versions/Flavors	Ingredients (alphabetical order)	Sodium mg/dose	Calcium mg/dose	Potassium mg/dose	Calories kcal/dose	Total Carbohydrate g/dose	Dietary Fiber/(Soluble) g/dose	Dosage (Weight in gms)	How Supplied
Smooth Texture Orange Flavor Metamucil Powder	Citric Acid, FD&C Yellow #6, Natural and Artificial Flavor, Psyllium Husk, Sucrose	5	7	30	45	12	3 (2.4)	1 rounded tablespoon ~12g	Canisters: Doses: 48, 72, 114; Cartons: 30 single-dose packets.
Smooth Texture Sugar-Free Orange Flavor Metamucil Powder	Aspartame, Citric Acid, FD&C Yellow #6, Maltodextrin, Natural and Artificial Flavor, Psyllium Husk	5	7	30	20	5	3 (2.4)	1 rounded teaspoon ~5.8g	Canisters: Doses: 30, 48, 72, 114, 180; Cartons: 30 single-dose packets.
Smooth Texture Sugar-Free Regular Flavor Metamucil Powder	Citric Acid, Maltodextrin, Psyllium Husk	4	7	30	20	5	3 (2.4)	1 rounded teaspoon ~5.4g	Canisters: Doses: 48, 72 114.
Original Texture Regular Flavor Metamucil Powder	Psyllium Husk, Sucrose	3	6	30	25	7	3 (2.4)	1 rounded teaspoon ~7g	Canisters: Doses: 48, 72 114.
Original Texture Orange Flavor Metamucil Powder	Citric Acid, FD&C Yellow #6, Natural and Artificial Flavor, Psyllium Husk, Sucrose	5	6	30	40	11	3 (2.4)	1 rounded tablespoon ~11g	Canisters: Doses: 48,72 114.
Metamucil Capsules	Caramel color, FD&C Blue No. 1 Aluminum Lake, FD&C Red No. 40 Aluminum Lake, FD&C Yellow No. 6 Aluminum Lake, gelatin, polysorbate 80, psyllium husk	0	5	0	10	3	3 (2.4)	6 capsules 3.2g	Bottles: 100 ct, 160 ct, 300 ct
Fiber Laxative Wafers									
Apple Crisp Metamucil Wafers	(1)	20	14	60	120	17	6	2 wafers 24 g	Cartons: 12 doses
Cinnamon Spice Metamucil Wafers	(2)	20	14	60	120	17	6	2 wafers 24 g	Cartons: 12 doses

(1) ascorbic acid, brown sugar, cinnamon, corn oil, corn starch, fructose, lecithin, molasses, natural and artificial flavors, oat hull fiber, psyllium husk, sodium bicarbonate, sucrose, water, wheat flour
(2) ascorbic acid, cinnamon, corn oil, corn starch, fructose, lecithin, molasses, natural and artificial flavors, nutmeg, oat hull fiber, oats, psyllium husk, sodium bicarbonate, sucrose, water, wheat flour

Stop use and ask a doctor if:
• constipation lasts more than 7 days
• rectal bleeding occurs
These may be signs of a serious condition.

Keep out of reach of children. In case of overdose, get medical help or contact a Poison Control Center right away.

Directions: For Powders: Put one dose into an empty glass. Fill glass with at least 8 oz of water or your favorite beverage. Stir briskly and drink promptly. If mixture thickens, add more liquid and stir. Mix this product (child or adult dose) with at least 8 ounces (a full glass) of water or other fluid. For capsules: Take product with 8 oz of liquid (swallow 1 capsule at a time) up to 3 times daily. Take this product with at least 8 oz (a full glass) of liquid. For Wafers: Take this product (child or adult dose) with at least 8 ounces (a full glass) of liquid. Taking these products without enough liquid may cause choking. See choking warning.

Adults 12 yrs. & older	Powders: 1 dose in 8 oz of liquid. Capsules: 5 capsules with 8 oz of liquid (swallow one capsule at a time). Wafers: 1 dose with 8 oz of liquid. Take at the first sign of irregularity; can be taken up to 3 times daily. Generally produces effect in 12 – 72 hours.
6 – 11 yrs.	Powders: ½ adult dose in 8 oz of liquid. Wafers: 1 wafer with 8 oz of liquid. Can be taken up to 3 times daily. Capsules: consider use of powder or wafer products
Under 6 yrs.	consult a doctor

Laxatives, including bulk fibers, may affect how well other medicines work. If you are taking a prescription medicine by mouth, take this product at least 2 hours before or 2 hours after the prescribed medicine. As your body adjusts to increased fiber intake, you may experience changes in bowel habits or minor bloating. **New Users:** Start with 1 dose per day; gradually increase to 3 doses per day as necessary.

Other Information:
• **Each product contains:** sodium (See table for amount/dose)
• **PHENYLKETONURICS:** Smooth Texture Sugar Free Orange product contains phenylalanine 25 mg per dose
• Each product contains a 100% natural, therapeutic fiber

Inactive Ingredients: See table
Notice to Health Care Professionals: To minimize the potential for allergic reaction, health care professionals who frequently dispense powdered psyllium products should avoid inhaling airborne dust while dispensing these products.
Handling and Dispensing: To minimize generating airborne dust, spoon product from the canister into a glass according to label directions.

How Supplied: Powder: canisters and cartons of single-dose packets. Capsules: 100, 160 and 300 count bottles. Wafers: cartons of single dose packets. (See table) [See table at bottom of previous page]
Questions? 1-800-983-4237

Shown in Product Identification Guide, page 521

**PEPTO-BISMOL®
ORIGINAL LIQUID,
MAXIMUM STRENGTH LIQUID,
ORIGINAL AND CHERRY FLAVOR
CHEWABLE TABLETS
AND EASY-TO-SWALLOW CAPLETS
For upset stomach, indigestion, heartburn, nausea and diarrhea.**

Multi-symptom Pepto-Bismol® contains bismuth subsalicylate and is the only leading OTC stomach remedy clinically proven effective for both upper and lower GI symptoms. It has been clinically proven in double-blind placebo-controlled trials for relief of upset stomach symptoms and diarrhea.

Active Ingredient:
(per tablespoon/per tablet/per caplet)
Original Liquid/Tablets/Caplets
Bismuth subsalicylate 262 mg
Maximum Strength Liquid
Bismuth subsalicylate 525 mg

Inactive Ingredients:
[Original Liquid] benzoic acid, flavor, magnesium aluminum silicate, methylcellulose, red 22, red 28, saccharin sodium, salicylic acid, sodium salicylate, sorbic acid, water
[Maximum Strength Liquid] benzoic acid, flavor, magnesium aluminum silicate, methylcellulose, red 22, red 28, saccharin sodium, salicylic acid, sodium salicylate, sorbic acid, water
[Original Tablets] calcium carbonate, flavor, magnesium stearate, mannitol, povidone, red 27 aluminum lake, saccharin sodium, talc
[Cherry Tablets] adipic acid, calcium carbonate, flavor, magnesium stearate, mannitol, povidone, red 27 aluminum lake, red 40 aluminum lake, saccharin sodium, talc
[Caplets] calcium carbonate, magnesium stearate, mannitol, microcrystalline cellulose, polysorbate 80, povidone, red 27 aluminum lake, silicon dioxide, sodium starch glycolate.
Other Information:
Sodium Content
Original Liquid—each Tbsp contains: sodium 6 mg • low sodium
Maximum Strength Liquid—each Tbsp contains: sodium 6 mg • low sodium
Chewable Tablets—each Original or Cherry Flavor Tablet contains: sodium less than 1 mg • very low sodium
Caplets—each Caplet contains: sodium 2 mg • low sodium
Salicylate Content
Original Liquid—each Tbsp contains: salicylate 130 mg
Maximum Strength Liquid—each Tbsp contains: salicylate 236 mg
Chewable Tablets—each tablet contains: [original] salicylate 102 mg [cherry] salicylate 99 mg
Caplets—each caplet contains: salicylate 99 mg
All Forms are sugar free.

Indications:
• relieves upset stomach symptoms (i.e. indigestion, heartburn, nausea and fullness caused by over-indulgence in food and drink) without constipating; and,
• controls diarrhea.

Actions: For upset stomach symptoms, the active ingredient is believed to work via a topical effect on the stomach mucosa. For diarrhea, it is believed to work by several mechanisms in the gastrointestinal tract, including: 1) normalizing fluid movement via an antisecretory mechanism, 2) binding bacterial toxins and 3) antimicrobial activity.

Warnings:
Reye's syndrome: Children and teenagers who have or are recovering from chicken pox or flu-like symptoms should not use this product. When using this product, if changes in behavior with nausea and vomiting occur, consult a doctor because these symptoms could be an early sign of Reye's syndrome, a rare but serious illness.

Allergy alert: Contains salicylate. Do not take if you are
• allergic to salicylates (including aspirin)
• taking other salicylate products
Do not use if you have
• an ulcer
• a bleeding problem
• bloody or black stool
Ask a doctor before use if you have
• fever
• mucus in the stool
Ask a doctor or pharmacist before use if you are taking any drug for
• anticoagulation (thinning the blood)
• diabetes
• gout
• arthritis
When using this product a temporary, but harmless, darkening of the stool and/or tongue may occur

Stop use and ask a doctor if
• symptoms get worse

Continued on next page

Pepto-Bismol Original—Cont.

- ringing in the ears or loss of hearing occurs
- diarrhea lasts more than 2 days

If pregnant or breast feeding, ask a health professional before use.

Keep out of reach of children. In case of overdose, get medical help or contact a Poison Control Center right away.

Notes: May cause a temporary and harmless darkening of the tongue or stool. Stool darkening should not be confused with melena.

While no lead is intentionally added to Pepto-Bismol, this product contains certain ingredients that are mined from the ground and thus contain small amounts of naturally occurring lead. For example, bismuth, contained in the active ingredient of Pepto-Bismol, is mined and therefore contains some naturally occurring lead. The small amounts of naturally occurring lead in Pepto-Bismol are low in comparison to average daily lead exposure; this is for the information of healthcare professionals. Pepto-Bismol is indicated for treatment of acute upset stomach symptoms and diarrhea. It is not intended for chronic use.

Overdosage: In case of overdose, patients are advised to contact a physician or Poison Control Center. Emesis induced by ipecac syrup is indicated in large ingestions provided ipecac can be administered within one hour of ingestion. Activated charcoal should be administered after gastric emptying. Patients should be evaluated for signs and symptoms of salicylate toxicity.

Directions:

Pepto-Bismol® Original Liquid, Original & Cherry Flavor Chewable Tablets, and Caplets
[Original Liquid]
- shake well before using
- for accurate dosing, use dose cup
[Original Tablet, Cherry Tablets]
- chew or dissolve in mouth
[Caplets]
- swallow with water, do not chew

- adults and children 12 years and over: 1 dose (2 Tbsp or 30 ml; 2 tablets or 2 caplets) every 1/2 to 1 hour as needed
- do not exceed 8 doses (16 Tbsp or 240 ml; 16 tablets or capsules) in 24 hours
- use until diarrhea stops but not more than 2 days
- children under 12 years: ask a doctor
- drink plenty of clear fluids to help prevent dehydration caused by diarrhea

---

Pepto-Bismol® Maximum Strength Liquid
- shake well before use
- for accurate dosing, use dose cup
- adults and children 12 years and over: 1 dose (2 Tbsp 30 ml) every 1 hour as needed
- do not exceed 4 doses (8 Tbsp or 120 ml) in 24 hours
- use until diarrhea stops but not more than 2 days

- children under 12 years: ask a doctor
- drink plenty of clear fluids to help prevent dehydration caused by diarrhea

How Supplied: Pepto-Bismol® Original and Maximum Strength Liquids are pink. Pepto-Bismol® Original Liquid is available in: 4, 8, 12 and 16 fl oz bottles. Pepto-Bismol® Maximum Strength Liquid is available in: 4, 8 and 12 fl oz bottles. Pepto-Bismol® Original and Cherry Flavor Tablets are pink, round, chewable tablets imprinted with a debossed triangle and "Pepto-Bismol" on one side. Tablets are available in: boxes of 30 and 48. Pepto-Bismol® Caplets are pink and imprinted with "Pepto-Bismol" on one side. Caplets are available in bottles of 24 and 40.
- avoid excessive heat (over 104°F or 40°C)
- protect liquids from freezing

Questions: 1-800-717-3786
www.pepto-bismol.com

Shown in Product Identification Guide, page 521

PRILOSEC OTC™ TABLETS
[prī-lō-sĕk]

Drug Facts:

Active Ingredient:
(in each tablet)   **Purpose:**
Omeprazole magnesium delayed-release tablet 20.6 mg (equivalent to 20 mg omeprazole) .... Acid reducer

Use:
- treats frequent heartburn (occurs *2 or more* days a week)
- not intended for immediate relief of heartburn; this drug may take 1 to 4 days for full effect

Warnings:

Allergy alert: Do not use if you are allergic to omeprazole

Do not use if you have
- trouble or pain swallowing food
- vomiting with blood
- bloody or black stools

These may be signs of a serious condition. See your doctor.

Ask a doctor before use if you have
- had heartburn over 3 months. This may be a sign of a more serious condition.
- heartburn with **lightheadedness, sweating or dizziness**
- chest pain or shoulder pain with shortness of breath; sweating; pain spreading to arms, neck or shoulders; or lightheadedness
- frequent **chest pain**
- frequent wheezing, particularly with heartburn
- unexplained weight loss
- nausea or vomiting
- stomach pain

Ask a doctor or pharmacist before use if you are taking
- warfarin (blood-thinning medicine)
- prescription antifungal or anti-yeast medicines
- diazepam (anxiety medicine)
- digoxin (heart medicine)

Stop use and ask a doctor if
- your heartburn continues or worsens
- you need to take this product for more than 14 days
- you need to take more than 1 course of treatment every 4 months

If pregnant or breast-feeding, ask a health professional before use.

Keep out of reach of children. In case of overdose, get medical help or contact a Poison Control Center right away.

Directions:
- adults 18 years of age and older
- this product is to be used once a day (every 24 hours), every day for 14 days
- it may take 1 to 4 days for full effect, although some people get complete relief of symptoms within 24 hours

14-Day Course of Treatment
- swallow 1 tablet with a glass of water before eating in the morning
- take every day for 14 days
- do not take more than 1 tablet a day
- do not chew or crush the tablets
- do not crush tablets in food
- do not use for more than 14 days unless directed by your doctor

Repeated 14-Day Courses (if needed)
- you may repeat a 14-day course every 4 months
- **do not take for more than 14 days or more often than every 4 months unless directed by a doctor**
- children under 18 years of age: ask a doctor

Other Information:
- read the directions, warnings and package insert before use
- keep the carton and package insert. They contain important information.
- store at 20–25°C (68–77°F)
- keep product out of high heat and humidity
- protect product from moisture

How Prilosec OTC Works For Your Frequent Heartburn

Prilosec OTC works differently from other OTC heartburn products, such as antacids and other acid reducers. Prilosec OTC stops acid production at the source – the **acid pump** that produces stomach acid. Prilosec OTC is to be used once a day (every 24 hours), every day for 14 days.

What to Expect When Using Prilosec OTC

Prilosec OTC is a different type of medicine from antacids and other acid reducers. Prilosec OTC may take 1 to 4 days for full effect, although some people get complete relief of symptoms within 24 hours. Make sure you take the entire 14 days of dosing to treat your frequent heartburn.

Safety Record

For years, doctors have prescribed Prilosec to treat acid-related conditions in millions of people safely.

Who Should Take Prilosec OTC

This product is for adults (18 years and older) with **frequent heartburn**-when you have heartburn 2 or more days a week.

- Prilosec OTC is **not** intended for those who have heartburn infrequently, one episode of heartburn a week or less, or for those who want immediate relief of heartburn.

Tips for Managing Heartburn

- Do not lie flat or bend over soon after eating.
- Do not eat late at night or just before bedtime.
- Certain foods or drinks are more likely to cause heartburn, such as rich, spicy, fatty and fried foods, chocolate, caffeine, alcohol and even some fruits and vegetables.
- Eat slowly and do not eat big meals.
- If you are overweight, lose weight.
- If you smoke, quit smoking.
- Raise the head of your bed.
- Wear loose-fitting clothing around your stomach.

Inactive Ingredients: glyceryl monostearate, hydroxypropyl cellulose, hypromellose, iron oxide, magnesium stearate, methacrylic acid copolymer, microcrystalline cellulose, paraffin, polyethylene glycol 6000, polysorbate 80, polyvinylpyrrolidone, sodium stearyl fumarate, starch, sucrose, talc, titanium dioxide, triethyl citrate.

How Supplied: Prilosec OTC is available in 14 tablet, 28 tablet and 42 tablet sizes. These sizes contain one, two and three 14-day courses of treatment, respectively. Do not use for more than 14 days in a row unless directed by your doctor. For the 28 count (two 14-day courses) and the 42 count (three 14-day courses), you may repeat a 14-day course every 4 months.

Safety Feature – Do not use if tablet blister unit is open or torn.

Questions? 1-800-289-9181

Shown in Product Identification Guide, page 521

THERMACARE®

[thərm' ă-kār]

Therapeutic Heat Wraps with Air-Activated Heat Discs

Uses:

Back/Hip Wrap: Provides temporary relief of minor muscular and joint aches & pains associated with overexertion, strains, sprains, and arthritis.

Neck to Arm Wrap: Provides temporary relief of minor muscular and joint aches and pains associated with overexertion, strains, sprains and arthritis.

Menstrual Patch: Provides temporary relief of minor menstrual cramps and associated back ache.

Warnings:

Do not microwave or attempt to reheat this product to avoid risk of fire. This product has the potential to cause skin irritation or burns. Heat discs contain iron (~2 grams) which can be harmful if ingested. If ingested, rinse mouth with water and call a Poison Control Center right away. If the heat discs contents contact your skin or eyes, rinse right away with water.

Do not use:

- on broken or damaged skin
- with medicated lotions, creams, or ointments
- on areas of bruising or swelling that have occurred within 48 hours
- on people unable to remove the product, including children and infants
- on areas of the body where heat cannot be felt
- with other forms of heat

Ask a doctor before use if you have diabetes, poor circulation, rheumatoid arthritis or are pregnant.

When using this product: it is normal to experience temporary skin redness after removing the wrap. If your skin is still red after a few hours, stop using ThermaCare until the redness goes away completely. To reduce the risk of prolonged redness in the future, we recommend you: (a) wear for a shorter period of time, (b) wear looser clothing over wrap, (c) wear over a thin layer of clothing • Periodically check your skin: (a) if your skin is sensitive to heat, (b) if your tolerance to heat has decreased over the years, (c) when wearing a tight fitting belt or waistband • Consider wearing during the day before deciding to use during sleep.

Stop use and ask a doctor: if after 7 days (4 days for menstrual product) your pain gets worse or remains unchanged. This may be a sign of a more serious condition.

- if you experience any discomfort, swelling, rash or other changes on your skin that persist where the wrap is worn.

Keep out of reach of children and pets.

Directions: Tear open the pouch when ready to use. It may take up to 30 minutes for ThermaCare to reach its therapeutic temperature. Place on pain area on lower back or hip with darker discs toward skin. Attach firmly.

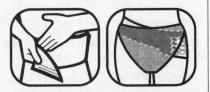

Peel away paper to reveal adhesive side. Place on pain area with adhesive side toward skin. Attach firmly.

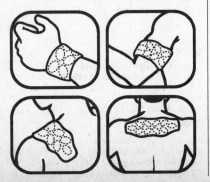

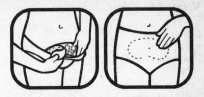

Peel away paper to reveal adhesive side. Place on pain area with adhesive side toward panties. Attach firmly.

For maximum effectiveness, we recommend you wear for 8 hours. Do <u>not</u> use for more than 8 hours in any 24 hour period.

DO NOT MICROWAVE

How Supplied:

Back/Hip Wrap: Available in trial size of 1 L/XL or in boxes of 2 S/M or L/XL wraps.

Neck to Arm: Available in boxes of 3 wraps.

Menstrual: Available in boxes of 3 patches.

Shown in Product Identification Guide, page 521

VICKS® 44® COUGH RELIEF
Dextromethorphan HBr/ Cough Suppressant
Alcohol 5%

- Maximum Strength
- Non-Drowsy
- For Adults & Children

Drug Facts:

Active Ingredient: (per 15 ml tablespoon)	Purpose:
Dextromethorphan HBr 30 mg	Cough suppressant

Uses: Temporarily relieves cough due to minor throat and bronchial irritation associated with a cold

Warnings:

Do not use if you are now taking a prescription monoamine oxidase inhibitor (MAOI) (certain drugs for depression, psychiatric or emotional conditions, or Parkinson's disease), or for 2 weeks after stopping the MAOI drug. If you do not know if your prescription drug contains an MAOI, ask a doctor or pharmacist before taking this product.

Ask a doctor before use if you have:
- cough that occurs with too much phlegm (mucus)
- persistent or chronic cough such as occurs with smoking, asthma, or emphysema

Stop use and ask a doctor if:
- cough lasts more than 7 days, comes back, or occurs with fever, rash, or headache that lasts. These could be signs of a serious condition.

If pregnant or breast feeding, ask a health professional before use.

Keep out of reach of children. In case of overdose, get medical help or contact a Poison Control Center right away.

Continued on next page

Vicks 44—Cont.

Directions:
- use teaspoon (tsp), tablespoon (TBSP) or dose cup
- do not exceed 4 doses per 24 hours
  Under 6 yrs. .... ask a doctor
  6–11 yrs. .... 1½ tsp (7½ ml)
  every 6-8 hours
  12 yrs. & older .... 1 TBSP (15 ml)
  every 6-8 hours

Other Information:
- **each tablespoon contains** sodium 31 mg
- store at room temperature

Inactive Ingredients: Alcohol, FD&C blue no.1, FD&C red 40, carboxymethylcellulose sodium, citric acid, flavor, high fructose corn syrup, polyethylene oxide, polyoxyl 40 stearate, propylene glycol, purified water, saccharin sodium, sodium benzoate, sodium citrate.

How Supplied: Available in 4 FL OZ (118 ml) 6 FL OZ (177 ml) plastic bottle. A calibrated dose cup accompanies each bottle.

TAMPER EVIDENT: Do not use if imprinted shrinkband is missing or broken.

Questions? 1-800-342-6844

Dist. by Procter & Gamble, Cincinnati, OH 45202.

US Pat 5,458,879   42434792

Shown in Product Identification Guide, page 521

VICKS® 44D®
Cough & Head Congestion Relief
Cough Suppressant/Nasal Decongestant
Alcohol 5%
- Maximum Strength
- Non-Drowsy
- For Adults & Children

Drug Facts:

Active Ingredients:
(per 15 ml tablespoon)   **Purpose:**
Dextromethorphan HBr
  30 mg .... Cough suppressant
Pseudoephedrine HCl
  60 mg .... Nasal decongestant

Uses: Temporarily relieves these cold symptoms
- cough
- nasal congestion

Warnings:
Failure to follow these warnings could result in serious consequences.

Do not use if you are now taking a prescription monoamine oxidase inhibitor (MAOI) (certain drugs for depression, psychiatric or emotional conditions, or Parkinson's disease), or for 2 weeks after stopping the MAOI drug. If you do not know if your prescription drug contains an MAOI, ask a doctor or pharmacist before taking this product.

Ask a doctor before use if you have:
- heart disease
- cough that lasts or is chronic such as occurs with smoking, asthma, or emphysema
- thyroid disease
- diabetes
- high blood pressure
- cough that occurs with too much phlegm (mucus)
- trouble urinating due to enlarged prostate gland

When using this product do not take more than directed.

Stop use and ask a doctor if:
- symptoms do not get better within 7 days or are accompanied by fever.
- you get nervous, dizzy or sleepless
- cough lasts more than 7 days, comes back, or occurs with fever, rash, or headache that lasts.
  These could be signs of a serious condition.

If pregnant or breast-feeding, ask a health professional before use.

Keep out of reach of children. In case of overdose, get medical help or contact a Poison Control Center right away.

Directions:
- use teaspoon (tsp), tablespoon (TBSP) or dose cup
- do not exceed 4 doses in a 24 hour period
  Under 6 yrs. .... ask a doctor
  6–11 yrs. .... 1½ tsp (7½ ml)
  every 6 hours
  12 yrs. & older .... 1 TBSP (15 ml)
  every 6 hours

Other Information:
- **each tablespoonful contains** sodium 31 mg
- store at room temperature

Inactive Ingredients: Alcohol, FD&C blue no. 1, carboxymethylcellulose sodium, citric acid, flavor, high fructose corn syrup, polyethylene oxide, polyoxyl 40 stearate, propylene glycol, purified water, FD&C red no. 40, saccharin sodium, sodium benzoate, sodium citrate.

How Supplied: Available in 1 FL OZ (30 ml) 4 FL OZ (118 ml) 6 FL OZ (177 ml) and 8 FL OZ (236 ml) plastic bottles. A calibrated dose cup accompanies each bottle.

TAMPER EVIDENT: Do not use if imprinted shrinkband is missing or broken.

Question? 1-800-342-6844

Dist. by Procter & Gamble, Cincinnati OH 45202.

US Pat 5,458,879   42434796

Shown in Product Identification Guide, page 521

VICKS® 44E®
Cough & Chest Congestion Relief
Cough Suppressant/Expectorant
Alcohol 5%
- Non-Drowsy
- For Adults & Children

Drug Facts:

Active Ingredients:
(per 15 ml tablespoon)   **Purpose:**
Dextromethorphan HBr
  20 mg .... Cough suppressant

Guaifenesin
  200 mg .... Expectorant

Uses:
- temporarily relieves cough due to the common cold
- helps loosen phlegm and thin bronchial secretions to rid the bronchial passageways of bothersome mucus

Warnings:

Do not use
- if you are now taking a prescription monoamine oxidase inhibitor (MAOI) (certain drugs for depression, psychiatric or emotional conditions, or Parkinson's disease), or for 2 weeks after stopping the MAOI drug. If you do not know if your prescription drug contains an MAOI, ask a doctor or pharmacist before taking this product.

Ask a doctor before use if you have:
- a sodium restricted diet
- persistent or chronic cough such as occurs with smoking, asthma, chronic bronchitis or emphysema
- cough that occurs with too much phlegm (mucus)

Stop use and ask a doctor if:
- cough lasts more than 7 days, comes back, or occurs with fever, rash, or headache that lasts. These could be signs of a serious condition.

If pregnant or breast-feeding, ask a health professional before use.

Keep out of reach of children. In case of overdose, get medical help or contact a Poison Control Center right away.

Directions:
- use teaspoon (tsp), tablespoon (TBSP) or dose cup
- do not exceed 6 doses per 24 hours
  Under 6 yrs. .... ask a doctor
  6–11 yrs. .... 1½ tsp (7½ ml)
  every 4 hours
  12 yrs. & older. .... 1 TBSP (15 ml)
  every 4 hours

Other Information:
- **each tablespoon contains** sodium 31 mg
- store at room temperature

Inactive Ingredients: Alcohol, FD&C blue 1, carboxymethylcellulose sodium, citric acid, flavor, high fructose corn syrup, polyethylene oxide, polyoxyl 40 stearate, propylene glycol, purified water, FD&C red no. 40, saccharin sodium, sodium benzoate, sodium citrate.

How Supplied: Available in 4 FL OZ (118 ml) 6 FL OZ (177 ml) and 8 FL OZ (236 ml) plastic bottles. A calibrated dose cup accompanies each bottle.

TAMPER EVIDENT: Do not use if imprinted shrinkband is missing or broken.

Questions? 1-800-342-6844

Dist. by Procter & Gamble, Cincinnati OH 45202.

US Pat 5,458,879   42434800

Shown in Product Identification Guide, page 521

**VICKS® 44M®
COUGH, COLD & FLU RELIEF**
Cough Suppressant/Nasal
Decongestant/Antihistamine/
Pain Reliever–Fever Reducer
Alcohol 10%

Maximum strength cough formula

Drug Facts:

Active Ingredients:
(per 5 ml teaspoon)   **Purpose:**
Acetaminophen
  162.5 mg ... Pain reliever/fever reducer
Chlorpheniramine maleate
  1 mg .... Antihistamine
Dextromethorphan HBr
  7.5 mg .... Cough suppressant
Pseudoephedrine HCl
  15 mg .... Nasal decongestant

Uses: Temporarily relieves cough/
cold/flu symptoms
• cough
• sneezing
• headache
• sore throat
• fever
• runny nose
• nasal congestion

Warnings:
**Failure to follow these warnings could
result in serious consequences.**
Alcohol warning If you consume 3 or
more alcoholic drinks every day, ask
your doctor whether you should take
acetaminophen or other pain relievers/
fever reducers. Acetaminophen may
cause liver damage.

Sore throat warning If sore throat is severe, persists more than two days, is accompanied or followed by a fever, headache, rash, nausea or vomiting, consult a
doctor promptly.

**Do not use • with other medicines con-
taining acetaminophen** if you are now
taking a prescription monoamine oxidase inhibitor (MAOI) (certain drugs for
depression, psychiatric or emotional conditions, or Parkinson's disease), or for 2
weeks after stopping the MAOI drug. If
you do not know if your prescription
drug contains an MAOI, ask a doctor or
pharmacist before taking this product.
Ask a doctor before use if you have:
• heart disease
• breathing problems or chronic cough
  such as occurs with smoking, asthma,
  chronic bronchitis or emphysema
• thyroid disease
• diabetes
• glaucoma
• high blood pressure
• cough that occurs with too much
  phlegm (mucus)
• trouble urinating due to enlarged prostate gland
**Ask a doctor or pharmacist before use if
you are** taking sedatives or tranquilizers.
When using this product:
• **do not use more than directed**
• excitability may occur, especially in
  children
• drowsiness may occur
• avoid alcoholic drinks
• be careful when driving a motor vehicle or operating machinery

• alcohol, sedatives, and tranquilizers
  may increase drowsiness
Stop use and ask a doctor if:
• you get nervous, dizzy or sleepless
• fever gets worse or lasts more than 3
  days
• new symptoms occur
• redness or swelling is present
• symptoms do not get better within 7
  days or are accompanied by fever
• cough lasts more than 7 days, comes
  back, or occurs with fever, rash, or
  headache that lasts.
  These could be signs of a serious condition.
If pregnant or breast-feeding, ask a
health professional before use.
Keep out of reach of children.
Overdose Warning: Taking more
than recommended dose can cause serious health problems. In case of overdose,
get medical help or contact a Poison Control Center right away. Quick medical attention is critical for adults as well as for
children even if you do not notice any
signs or symptoms.

Directions:
• take only as recommended—see **Overdose Warning**
• use teaspoon or dose cup
• do not exceed 4 doses per 24 hours
• children 12 and under: ask a doctor.
• 12 yrs. & older: take 4 teaspoons
  (20 ml) every 6 hours.

Other Information:
• **each teaspoon contains** sodium 8 mg
• store at room temperature

Inactive Ingredients: Alcohol, FD&C
blue 1, carboxymethylcellulose sodium,
citric acid, flavor, high fructose corn
syrup, polyethylene glycol, polyethylene
oxide, propylene glycol, purified water,
FD&C red 40, saccharin sodium, sodium
citrate.

How Supplied: Available in 4 FL OZ
(118 ml) 6 FL OZ (177 ml) and 8 FL OZ
(236 ml) plastic bottles. A calibrated dose
cup accompanies each bottle.

TAMPER EVIDENT: Do not use if imprinted shrinkband is missing or broken.

Not recommended for children.

Questions? 1-800-342-6844

Dist. by Procter & Gamble, Cincinnati
OH 45202.

US Pat 5,458,879   42434741

*Shown in Product Identification
Guide, page 521*

**CHILDREN'S VICKS® NYQUIL®
COLD/COUGH RELIEF**
Antihistamine/Nasal Decongestant/
Cough Suppressant

Children's NyQuil was specially formulated with three effective ingredients to
relieve nighttime cough, nasal congestion, and runny nose so children can
rest. Children's NyQuil® is alcohol free
and analgesic free and has a pleasant
cherry flavor.

Drug Facts:

Active Ingredients: **Purpose:**
(per tablespoon, 15 ml)
Chlorpheniramine maleate
  2 mg .... Antihistamine
Dextromethorphan HBr
  15 mg .... Cough suppressant
Pseudoephedrine HCl
  30 mg .... Nasal decongestant

Uses: Temporarily relieves cold symptoms:
• cough due to minor throat and bronchial irritation
• sneezing
• runny nose
• nasal congestion

Warnings:
**Failure to follow these warnings could
result in serious consequences.**
Do not use
• if you are now taking a prescription
  monoamine oxidase inhibitor (MAOI)
  (certain drugs for depression, psychiatric or emotional conditions, or Parkinson's disease), or for 2 weeks after
  stopping the MAOI durg. If you do not
  know if your prescription drug contains an MAOI, ask a doctor or pharmacist before taking this product.
Ask a doctor before use if you have:
• heart disease
• a breathing problem or chronic cough
  that lasts or as occurs with smoking,
  asthma, chronic bronchitis or emphysema
• thyroid disease
• diabetes
• glaucoma
• high blood pressure
• cough that occurs with too much
  phlegm (mucus)
• a sodium-restricted diet
• trouble urinating due to enlarged prostate gland
**Ask a doctor or pharmacist before use if
you are** taking sedatives or tranquilizers.
When using this product:
• **do not use more than directed**
• excitability may occur, especially in
  children
• drowsiness may occur
• avoid alcoholic drinks
• be careful when driving a motor vehicle or operating machinery
• alcohol, sedatives, and tranquilizers
  may increase drowsiness
Stop use and ask a doctor if:
• you get nervous, dizzy or sleepless
• symptoms do not get better within 7
  days or are accompanied by a fever
• cough lasts more than 7 days, comes
  back, or occurs with fever, rash, or
  headache that lasts.
  These could be signs of a serious condition.
If pregnant or breast-feeding, ask a
health professional before use.
Keep out of reach of children. In case of
overdose, get medical help or contact a
Poison Control Center right away. Quick
medical attention is critical for adults as
well as for children even if you do not notice any signs or symptoms.

Continued on next page

Vicks Children's Nyquil—Cont.

Directions:
- use tablespoon (TBSP) or dose cup
- do not exceed 4 doses per 24 hours
  under 6 yrs. .... ask a doctor
  6–11 yrs. .... 1 TBSP or 15 ml
  every 6 hours
  12 yrs. & older .... 2 TBSP or 30 ml
  every 6 hours

Other Information:
- **each tablespoon contains** sodium 71 mg
- store at room temperature

Inactive Ingredients: Citric acid, flavor, potassium sorbate, propylene glycol, purified water, FD&C red 40, sodium citrate, sucrose.

How Supplied: Available in 4 FL OZ (118 ml) 6 FL OZ (177 ml) plastic bottles with child-resistant, tamper-evident cap and a calibrated medicine cup.
Questions? 1-800-362-1683
Exp. Date: See Bottom.   42434744
Dist. by Procter & Gamble, Cincinnati OH 45202.

Shown in Product Identification Guide, page 522

VICKS® Cough Drops
Menthol Cough Suppressant/
Oral Anesthetic
Menthol and Cherry Flavors

CONSUMER INFORMATION: Vicks Cough Drops provide fast and effective relief. Each drop contains effective medicine to suppress your impulse to cough as it dissolves into a soothing syrup to relieve your sore throat.

Drug Facts:

Active Ingredient:
Menthol:

Active Ingredient: (per drop)	Purpose:
Menthol 3.3 mg ...... Cough suppressant/oral anesthetic

Cherry:

Active Ingredient: (per drop)	Purpose:
Menthol 1.7 mg ...... Cough suppressant/oral anesthetic

Uses: Temporarily relieves:
- sore throat
- coughs due to colds or inhaled irritants

Warnings:
Ask a doctor before use if you have:
- cough associated with excessive phlegm (mucus)
- persistent or chronic cough such as those caused by asthma, emphysema, or smoking
- a severe sore throat accompanied by difficulty in breathing or that lasts more than 2 days
- a sore throat accompanied or followed by fever, headache, rash, swelling, nausea or vomiting
Stop use and ask a doctor if:
- you need to use more than 7 days
- cough lasts more than 7 days, comes back, or occurs with fever, rash, or headache that lasts. These could be the signs of a serious condition.

If pregnant or breast-feeding, ask a health professional before use.
Keep out of reach of children.

Directions:
- under 5 yrs.: ask a doctor (menthol)
- adults & children 5 yrs & older: allow 2 drops to dissolve slowly in mouth (cherry)
- adults & children 5 yrs & older: allow 3 drops to dissolve slowly in mouth
Cough: may be repeated every hour.
Sore Throat: may be repeated every 2 hours.

Other Information:
- store at room temperature

Inactive Ingredients:
Menthol: Ascorbic acid, caramel, corn syrup, eucalyptus oil, sucrose.
Cherry: Ascorbic acid, citric acid, corn syrup, eucalyptus oil, FD&C blue 1, flavor, FD&C red 40, sucrose.

How Supplied: Vicks® Cough Drops are available in boxes of 20 triangular drops. Each red or green drop is debossed with "V."
Questions? 1-800-707-1709
Made in Mexico by Procter & Gamble Manufactura S. de R.I. de C.V. Dist. by Procter & Gamble
Cincinnati OH 45202
50144381

VICKS® DAYQUIL® LIQUID
VICKS® DAYQUIL® LIQUICAPS®
Multi-Symptom Cold/Flu Relief
Nasal Decongestant/
Pain Reliever/Cough
Suppressant/Fever Reducer
Non-drowsy

Drug Facts:

Active Ingredients:

LIQUID:

Active Ingredients: (per 15 ml tablespoon)	Purpose:
Acetaminophen
325 mg ...... Pain reliever/fever reducer
Dextromethorphan HBr
15 mg .... Cough suppressant
Pseudoephedrine HCl
30 mg .... Nasal decongestant

LIQUICAP®:

Active Ingredients: (per softgel)	Purpose:
Acetaminophen
325 mg ...... Pain reliever/fever reducer
Dextromethorphan HBr
15 mg .... Cough suppressant
Pseudoephedrine HCl
30 mg .... Nasal decongestant

Uses: Temporarily relieves common cold/flu symptoms:
- nasal congestion
- cough due to minor throat and bronchial irritation
- sore throat
- headache
- minor aches and pains
- fever

Warnings:
Failure to follow these warnings could result in serious consequences.
Alcohol warning: If you consume 3 or more alcoholic drinks every day, ask your doctor whether you should take acetaminophen or other pain relievers/fever reducers. Acetaminophen may cause liver damage.
Sore throat warning: If sore throat is severe, persists more than 2 days, is accompanied by fever, nausea, rash or vomiting, consult a doctor promptly.
**Do not use • with other medicines containing acetaminophen • if you are now taking a prescription monoamine oxidase inhibitor (MAOI) (certain drugs for depression, psychiatric or emotional conditions, or Parkinson's disease), or for 2 weeks after stopping the MAOI drug. If you do not know if your prescription drug contains an MAOI, ask a doctor or pharmacist before taking this product.
Ask a doctor before use if you have:
- heart disease
- thyroid disease
- diabetes
- persistent or chronic cough such as occurs with smoking, asthma, or emphysema
- high blood pressure
- cough that occurs with too much phlegm (mucus)
- trouble urinating due to enlarged prostate gland
- sodium-restricted diet (Specific to DayQuil Liquid only)
When using this product:
- do not use more than directed
Stop use and ask a doctor if:
- you get nervous, dizzy or sleepless
- fever gets worse or lasts more than 3 days
- new symptoms occur
- symptoms do not get better within 7 days or are accompanied by a fever
- redness or swelling is present
- cough lasts more than 7 days, comes back, or occurs with fever, rash, or headache that lasts. These could be the signs of a serious condition.
If pregnant or breast-feeding, ask a health professional before use.
Keep out of reach of children. Overdose warning: Taking more than the recommended dose can cause serious health problems. In case of overdose, get medical help or contact a Poison Control Center right away. Quick medical attention is critical for adults as well as for children even if you do not notice any signs or symptoms.

Directions:
- take only as recommended – see Overdose warning
LIQUID:
- use tablespoon (TBSP) or dose cup
- do not exceed 4 doses per 24 hours
  under 6 yrs. .... ask a doctor
  6–11 yrs. .... 1 TBSP or 15 ml
  every 6 hours
  12 yrs. & older .... 2 TBSP or 30 ml
  every 6 hours
- If taking NyQuil® and DayQuil, limit total to 4 doses per 24 hours.

LIQUICAP:
- take only as recommended – see **Over-dose Warning**
- do not exceed 4 doses per 24 hours
  under 6 yrs. .... ask a doctor
  6–11 yrs. .... 1 softgel with water
  every 6 hours
  12 yrs. & older .. 2 softgels with water
  every 6 hours
- If taking NyQuil® and DayQuil, limit total to 4 doses per 24 hours.

Other Information:
LIQUID:
- **each tablespoon contains** sodium 71 mg
- store at room temperature
LIQUICAP:
- store at room temperature

Inactive Ingredients:
LIQUID: Citric acid, FD&C yellow 6, flavor, glycerin, polyethylene glycol, propylene glycol, purified water, saccharin sodium, sodium citrate, sucrose.
LIQUICAP: FD&C red 40, FD&C yellow 6, gelatin, glycerin, polyethylene glycol, povidone, propylene glycol, purified water, sorbitol special, titanium dioxide.

How Supplied: Available in: **LIQUID** 6 FL OZ (177 ml) and 10 FL OZ (295 ml) plastic bottles with child-resistant, tamper-evident cap and a calibrated medicine cup.
LIQUICAP: in 2-count, 12-count and 36- 40- and 60-count child-resistant packages and 20- nonchild-resistant packages. Each softgel is imprinted: "DayQ."
LIQUID:
TAMPER EVIDENT: Do not use if imprinted shrinkband is missing or broken.
LIQUICAP, 12- and 36- 40- and 60-count:
TAMPER EVIDENT: This package is safety sealed and child resistant. Use only if blisters are intact. If difficult to open, use scissors.
LIQUICAP, 20-count:
This Package for households without young children.
TAMPER EVIDENT: Use only if blisters are intact. If difficult to open, use scissors.
Questions? 1-800-251-3374
Made in Canada
Dist. by Procter & Gamble
Cincinnati OH 45202
42435018
Shown in Product Identification Guide, page 521

VICKS® NYQUIL® COUGH
Antihistamine
Cough Suppressant
All Night Cough Relief
Cherry Flavor

alcohol 10%
Drug Facts:

Active Ingredients: **Purpose:**
(per 15 ml tablespoon)
Dextromethorphan HBr
15 mg .... Cough suppressant
Doxylamine succinate
6.25 mg .... Antihistamine

Uses:
Temporarily relieves cold symptoms
- cough
- runny nose and sneezing

Warnings:
Do not use if you are now taking a prescription monoamine oxidase inhibitor (MAOI) (certain drugs for depression, psychiatric or emotional conditions, or Parkinson's disease), or for 2 weeks after stopping the MAOI drug. If you do not know if your prescription drug contains an MAOI, ask a doctor or pharmacist before taking this product.

Ask a doctor before use if you have:
- asthma
- emphysema
- breathing problems
- excessive phlegm (mucus)
- glaucoma
- chronic bronchitis
- persistent or chronic cough
- cough associated with smoking
- trouble urinating due to enlarged prostate gland

Ask a doctor or pharmacist before use if you are:
taking sedatives or tranquilizers.

When using this product:
- **do not use more than directed**
- marked drowsiness may occur
- avoid alcoholic drinks
- excitability may occur, especially in children
- be careful when driving a motor vehicle or operating machinery
- alcohol, sedatives, and tranquilizers may increase drowsiness

Stop use and ask a doctor if:
- cough lasts more than 7 days, comes back, or occurs with fever, rash, or headache that lasts.
These could be signs of a serious condition.

If pregnant or breast-feeding, ask a health professional before use.

Keep out of reach of children. In case of overdose, get medical help or contact a Poison Control Center right away.

Directions: [1 oz bottle] use tablespoon (TBSP)
Use tablespoon (TBSP) or dose cup
- do not exceed 4 doses per 24 hours
Under 12 yrs. .... ask a doctor
12 yrs. and older .... 2 TBSP or 30 ml
every 6 hours
[6 & 10 oz bottle, twin, quad pack]
- if taking NyQuil and DayQuil®, limit total to 4 doses per day.
Other Information:
- **each tablespoon contains** sodium 17 mg
- store at room temperature

Inactive Ingredients: Alcohol, F&C blue no. 1, citric acid, flavor, high fructose corn syrup, polyethylene glycol, propylene glycol, purified water, FD&C red no. 40, saccharin sodium, sodium citrate

How Supplied: Available in 1 FL OZ (30 ml) 6 FL OZ (177 ml), 10 FL OZ (295 ml) plastic bottles with child-resistant, tamper-evident cap and calibrated Medicine cup.

TAMPER EVIDENT: Do not use if imprinted shrinkband is missing or broken.

Questions? 1-800-362-1683
Dist. by Procter & Gamble,
Cincinnati OH 45202. 42437885
Shown in Product Identification Guide, page 522

VICKS® NYQUIL® LIQUICAPS®
VICKS® NYQUIL® LIQUID
(Original and Cherry)
Multi-Symptom Cold/Flu Relief
Antihistamine/Cough
Suppressant/Pain Reliever/
Nasal Decongestant/
Fever Reducer

Liquid (Original and Cherry)—alcohol 10%

Drug Facts:

Active Ingredients:
LiquiCaps®:
Active Ingredients:	**Purpose:**
(per softgel)	

Acetaminophen
325 mg ...... Pain reliever/fever reducer
Dextromethorphan HBr
15 mg .... Cough suppressant
Doxylamine succinate
6.25 mg .... Antihistamine
Pseudoephedrine HCl
30 mg .... Nasal decongestant

Liquid (Original and Cherry):
Active Ingredients:	**Purpose:**
(per 15 ml tablespoon)	

Acetaminophen
500 mg ...... Pain reliever/fever reducer
Dextromethorphan HBr
15 mg .... Cough suppressant
Doxylamine succinate
6.25 mg .... Antihistamine
Pseudoephedrine HCl
30 mg .... Nasal decongestant

Uses:
LiquiCaps® Liquid (Original and Cherry):
Temporarily relieves these common cold/flu symptoms:
- nasal congestion
- cough due to minor throat & bronchial irritation
- sore throat
- headache
- minor aches and pains
- fever
- runny nose and sneezing

Warnings:
Failure to follow these warnings could result in serious consequences.
Alcohol warning If you consume 3 or more alcoholic drinks every day, ask your doctor whether you should take acetaminophen or other pain relievers/fever reducers. Acetaminophen may cause liver damage.
Sore throat warning If sore throat is severe, persists more than 2 days, is accompanied or followed by fever, rash, nausea, or vomiting, consult a doctor promptly.
Do not use • with other medications containing acetaminophen • if you are now taking a prescription monoamine

Continued on next page

Vicks Nyquil—Cont.

oxidase inhibitor (MAOI) (certain drugs for depression, psychiatric or emotional conditions, or Parkinson's disease), or for 2 weeks after stopping the MAOI drug. If you do not know if your prescription drug contains an MAOI, ask a doctor or pharmacist before taking this product.

Ask a doctor before use if you have:
- heart disease
- a breathing problem or chronic cough such as occurs with smoking, asthma, chronic bronchitis, or emphysema
- thyroid disease
- diabetes
- glaucoma
- high blood pressure
- cough that occurs with too much phlegm (mucus)
- chronic bronchitis

Ask a doctor or pharmacist before use if you are taking sedatives or tranquilizers.

When using this product
- **do not use more than directed**
- excitability may occur, especially in children
- marked drowsiness may occur
- avoid alcoholic drinks
- be careful when driving a motor vehicle or operating machinery
- alcohol, sedatives, and tranquilizers may increase drowsiness

Stop use and ask a doctor if:
- symptoms do not get better within 7 days or are accompanied by fever.
- you get nervous, dizzy or sleepless
- fever gets worse or lasts more than 3 days
- new symptoms occur
- swelling or redness is present.
- cough lasts more than 7 days, comes back, or occurs with fever, rash, or headache that lasts. These could be signs of a serious condition.

If pregnant or breast-feeding, ask a health professional before use.

Keep out of reach of children.

Overdose warning: Taking more than the recommended dose can cause serious health problems. In case of overdose, get medical help or contact a Poison Control Center right away. Quick medical attention is critical for adults as well as for children even if you do not notice any signs or symptoms.

Directions:
LiquiCaps®:
- take only as recommended – see **Overdose warning**
- children under 12 yrs.: ask a doctor.
- do not exceed 4 doses per 24 hours
- 12 yrs and older . . . . 2 softgels with water every 6 hours
- If taking NyQuil and DayQuil®, limit total to 4 doses per 24 hours.

Liquid (Original and cherry):

AGE	DOSAGE
take only as recommended – see **Overdose warning**	
use tablespoon (TBSP) or dose cup	
do not exceed 4 doses per 24 hours	
children under 12	ask a doctor

adults and children 12 years and over	2 TBSP (30 ml) every 6 hours

If taking NyQuil and DayQuil®, limit total to 4 doses per 24 hours.

Other Information:
LiquiCaps®:
- store at room temperature

Liquid (Original and Cherry):
- **each tablespoon contains** sodium 17 mg
- store at room temperature

Inactive Ingredients:
LiquiCaps®: FD&C Blue no. 1, gelatin, glycerin, polyethylene glycol, povidone, propylene glycol, purified water, sorbitol special, D&C Yellow no. 10, tilanium dioxide.

Liquid (Original): Alcohol, citric acid, flavor, FD&C Green no. 3, high fructose corn syrup, polyethylene glycol, propylene glycol, purified water, saccharin sodium, sodium citrate, yellow 6, D&C Yellow 10.

Liquid (Cherry): Alcohol, FD&C Blue 1, citric acid, flavor, high fructose corn syrup, polyethylene glycol, propylene glycol, purified water, FD&C Red 40, saccharin sodium, sodium citrate.

How Supplied:
LiquiCaps®: Available in 2-count 12- 20-, 40-, 60-count and 36-count child-resistant blister packages and 20-count nonchild resistant blister packages. Each softgel is imprinted: "NyQ".

Liquid: Available in 1 FL OZ (30 ml) 6 and 10 FL OZ (177 ml and 295 ml, respectively) 16 FL OZ (473 ml) plastic bottles with child-resistant, tamper-evident cap and calibrated medicine cup.

LiquiCaps®: 12- and 36-ct 20-, 40-, 60-count

TAMPER EVIDENT: This package is safety sealed and child resistant. Use only if blisters are intact. If difficult to open, use scissors.

Liquid (Original and cherry):

TAMPER EVIDENT: Do not use if imprinted shrinkband is missing or broken.

Questions? 1-800-362-1683

Liqui Caps®:
Made in Canada
Dist. by Procter & Gamble,
Cincinnati OH 45202.
©2001   42435017
Liquid (Original): Dist. by Procter & Gamble
Cincinnati OH 45202   42434786
Liquid (Cherry): Dist. by Procter & Gamble
Cincinnati OH 45202   42434789
Shown in Product Identification Guide, page 522

PEDIATRIC VICKS® 44e®
Cough & Chest Congestion Relief
Cough suppressant/Expectorant

- Non-drowsy
- Alcohol-free
- Aspirin-free

Drug Facts:

Active Ingredients:
(per 15 ml tablespoon)   **Purpose:**
Dextromethorphan
HBr 10 mg .... Cough suppressant
Guaifenesin 100mg .... Expectorant

Uses:
- temporarily relieves cough due to the common cold
- helps loosen phlegm and thin bronchial secretions to rid bronchial passageways of bothersome mucus

Warnings:
Do not use
- if you are now taking a prescription monoamine oxidase inhibitor (MAOI) (certain drugs for depression, psychiatric or emotional conditions, or Parkinson's disease), or for 2 weeks after stopping the MAOI drug. If you do not know if your prescription drug contains an MAOI, ask a doctor or pharmacist before taking this product.

Ask a doctor before use if you have:
- a sodium restricted diet
- cough that occurs with too much phlegm (mucus)
- persistent or chronic cough such as occurs with smoking, asthma, chronic bronchitis or emphysema

Stop use and ask a doctor if:
- cough lasts more than 7 days, comes back, or occurs with fever, rash, or headache that lasts. These could be signs of a serious condition.

If pregnant or breast-feeding, ask a health professional before use.

Keep out of reach of children. In case of overdose, get medical help or contact a Poison Control Center right away.

Directions:
- use tablespoon (TBSP) or dose cup
- do not exceed 6 doses per 24 hours

Under 2 yrs.	ask a doctor
2–5 yrs.	½ TBSP (7½ ml) every 4 hours
6–11 yrs.	1 TBSP (15 ml) every 4 hours
12 yrs.& older	2 TBSP (30 ml) every 4 hours

Other Information:
- **each tablespoon contains** sodium 30 mg
- store at room temperature

Inactive Ingredients: Carboxymethylcellulose sodium, citric acid, FD&C red no. 40, flavor, high fructose corn syrup, polyethylene oxide, polyoxyl 40 stearate, propylene glycol, purified water, saccharin sodium, sodium benzoate, sodium citrate.

How Supplied: 4 FL OZ (118 ml) plastic bottles. A calibrated dose cup accompanies each bottle.

TAMPER EVIDENT: Do not use if imprinted shrinkband is missing or broken.

Questions? 1-800-342-6844

Dist. by Procter & Gamble, Cincinnati OH 45202.
US Pat 5,458,879   42434802
Shown in Product Identification Guide, page 521

PEDIATRIC VICKS® 44m®
Cough & Cold Relief
Cough Suppressant/Nasal Decongestant/Antihistamine

- Alcohol-free
- Aspirin-free

Drug Facts:

Active Ingredients:
(per 15 ml tablespoon)   **Purpose:**
Chlorpheniramine maleate
  2 mg .... Antihistamine
Dextromethorphan HBr
  15 mg .... Cough suppressant
Pseudoephedrine HCl
  30 mg .... Nasal decongestant

Uses: Temporarily relieves cough/cold symptoms
- cough
- sneezing
- runny nose
- nasal congestion

Warnings:
Failure to follow these warnings could result in serious consequences.

Do not use:
- if you are now taking a prescription monoamine oxidase inhibitor (MAOI) (certain drugs for depression, psychiatric or emotional conditions, or Parkinson's disease), or for 2 weeks after stopping the MAOI drug. If you do not know if your prescription drug contains an MAOI, ask a doctor or pharmacist before taking this product.

Ask a doctor before use if you have:
- heart disease
- a sodium restricted diet
- a breathing problem or chronic cough that lasts or occurs with smoking, asthma, chronic bronchitis or emphysema
- thyroid disease
- diabetes
- glaucoma
- high blood pressure
- cough that occurs with too much phlegm (mucus)
- trouble urinating due to enlarged prostate gland

Ask a doctor or pharmicist before use if you are taking sedatives or tranquilizers.

When using this product:
- do not use more than directed
- excitability may occur, especially in children
- drowsiness may occur
- avoid alcoholic drinks
- be careful when driving a motor vehicle or operating machinery
- alcohol, sedatives, and tranquilizers may increase drowsiness

Stop use and ask a doctor if:
- you get nervous, dizzy or sleepless
- symptoms do not get better within 7 days or are accompanied by a fever.
- cough last more than 7 days, comes back, or occurs with fever, rash, or headache that lasts
  These could be signs of a serious condition.

If pregnant or breast-feeding, ask a health professional before use.

Keep out of reach of children. In case of overdose, get medical help or contact a Poison Control Center right away.

Directions:
- use tablespoon (TBSP) or dose cup
- do not exceed 4 doses per 24 hours
  Under 6 yrs. .... ask a doctor
  6–11 yrs. .... 1 TBSP (15 ml)
                                       every 6 hours
  12 yrs. & older .... 2 TBSP (30 ml)
                                       every 6 hours

Other Information:
- **each tablespoon contains** sodium 30 mg
- store at room temperature

Inactive Ingredients: Carboxymethylcellulose sodium, citric acid, FD&C red 40, flavor, high fructose corn syrup, polyethylene oxide, polyoxyl 40 stearate, propylene glycol, purified water, saccharin sodium, sodium benzoate, sodium citrate.

How Supplied: 4 FL OZ (118 ml) plastic bottles. A calibrated dose cup accompanies each bottle.
TAMPER EVIDENT: Do not use if imprinted shrinkband is missing or broken.
Questions? 1-800-342-6844
Dist. by Procter & Gamble, Cincinnati OH 45202.
US Pat 5,458,879   42434743
Shown in Product Identification Guide, page 521

VICKS® SINEX® [NASAL SPRAY]
[Ultra Fine Mist] for Sinus Relief
[sī ′něx]
Phenylephrine HCl Nasal Decongestant

Drug Facts:

Active Ingredients: **Purpose:**
Phenylephrine
  HCl 0.5% .... Nasal decongestant

Uses: Temporarily relieves sinus/nasal congestion due to
- colds
- hay fever
- upper respiratory allergies
- sinusitis

Warnings:
Ask a doctor before use if you have:
- heart disease
- thyroid disease
- diabetes
- high blood pressure
- trouble urinating due to enlarged prostate gland

When using this product:
- do not exceed recommended dosage
- use of this container by more than one person may cause infection
- temporary burning, stinging, sneezing, or increased nasal discharge may occur
- frequent or prolonged use may cause nasal congestion to recur or worsen

Stop use and ask a doctor if:
- symptoms persist for more than 3 days
If pregnant or breast-feeding, ask a health professional before use.

Keep out of reach of children. In case of accidental ingestion, get medical help or contact a poison control center right away.

Directions:
Nasal Spray:
- under 12 yrs. ask a doctor
- adults & children 12 yrs. & older: 2 or 3 sprays in each nostril without tilting your head, not more often than every 4 hours.
Ultra Fine Mist: Remove protective cap. Before using for the first time, prime the pump by firmly depressing its rim several times. Hold container with thumb at base and nozzle between first and second fingers. Without tilting your head, insert nozzle into nostril. Fully depress rim with a firm, even stroke and inhale deeply.
- under 12 yrs.: ask a doctor
- adults & children 12 yrs. & older: 2 or 3 sprays in each nostril, not more often than every 4 hours.

Other Information:
- store at room temperature

Inactive Ingredients: Benzalkonium chloride, camphor, chlorhexidine gluconate, citric acid, disodium EDTA, eucalyptol, menthol, purified water, tyloxapol

How Supplied: Available in $1/2$ FL OZ (14.7 ml) plastic squeeze bottle and $1/2$ FL OZ (14.7 ml) measured dose Ultra Fine mist pump. Note: This container is properly filled when approximately half full. Air space equal to one half of volume is necessary to propel the fine spray.
TAMPER EVIDENT:
Do not use if imprinted shrinkband is missing or broken.
Questions? 1-800-873-8276
Nasal Spray 42436771
Ultra Fine Mist 42436765
Dist. by Procter & Gamble
Cincinnati OH 45202

VICKS® SINEX®
[sī ′něx]
12-HOUR [Nasal Spray]
[Ultra Fine Mist] for Sinus Relief
Oxymetazoline HCl
Nasal Decongestant

Drug Facts:
Active Ingredients: **Purpose:**
Oxymetazoline HCl
  0.05% .... Nasal decongestant

Uses: Temporarily relieves sinus/nasal congestion due to
- colds
- hay fever
- upper respiratory allergies
- sinusitis

Warnings:
Ask a doctor before use if you have:
- heart disease
- thyroid disease
- diabetes
- high blood pressure
- trouble urinating due to enlarged prostate gland
When using this product:
- do not exceed recommended dosage
- temporary burning, stinging, sneezing, or increased nasal discharge may occur

Continued on next page

Vicks Sinex 12-Hour—Cont.

- frequent or prolonged use may cause nasal congestion to recur or worsen
- use of this container by more than one person may cause infection

Stop use and ask a doctor if:
- symptoms persist for more than 3 days

If pregnant or breast-feeding, ask a health professional before use.

Keep out of reach of children. In case of accidental ingestion, get medical help or contact a poison control center right away.

Directions:
Nasal Spray:
- under 6 yrs: ask a doctor
- adults & children 6 yrs. & older (with adult supervision): 2 or 3 sprays in each nostril without tilting your head, not more often than every 10 to 12 hours. Do not exceed 2 doses in 24 hours.

Ultra Fine Mist: Remove protective cap. Before using for the first time, prime the pump by firmly depressing its rim several times. Hold container with thumb at base and nozzle between first and second fingers. Without tilting your head, insert nozzle into nostril. Fully depress rim with a firm, even stroke and inhale deeply.
- under 6 yrs.: ask a doctor
- adults & children 6 yrs. & older (with adult supervision): 2 or 3 sprays in each nostril, not more often than every 10 to 12 hours. Do not exceed 2 doses in 24 hours.

Other Information:
- store at room temperature

Inactive Ingredients: Benzalkonium chloride, camphor, chlorhexidine gluconate, disodium EDTA, eucalyptol, menthol, potassium phosphate, purified water, sodium chloride, sodium phosphate, tyloxapol.

How Supplied: Available in ½ FL OZ (14.7 ml) plastic squeeze bottle and ½ FL OZ (14.7 ml) measured-dose Ultra Fine mist pump.

TAMPER EVIDENT: Do not use if imprinted shrinkband is missing or broken.
Nasal Spray 42436768
Ultra Fine Mist 42436763
Questions? 1-800-873-8276
Dist. by
Procter & Gamble,
Cincinnati OH 45202

VICKS® VAPOR INHALER
Levmetamfetamine/Nasal Decongestant

Drug Facts:

Active Ingredients: **Purpose:**
(per inhaler)
Levmetamfetamine
  50 mg .... Nasal decongestant

Uses: Temporarily relieves nasal congestion due to:
- a cold
- hay fever or other upper respiratory allergies
- sinusitis

Warnings:
When using this product:
- **do not exceed recommended dosage**
- temporary burning, stinging, sneezing, or increased nasal discharge may occur
- frequent or prolonged use may cause nasal congestion to recur or worsen
- do not use for more than 7 days
- do not use container by more than one person as it may spread infection
- use only as directed

Stop use and ask a doctor if:
- symptoms persist

If pregnant or breast-feeding, ask a health professional before use.

Keep out of reach of children. If swallowed, get medical help or contact a poison control center right away.

Directions:
The product delivers in each 800 ml air 0.04 to 0.15 mg of levmetamfetamine.
- do not use more often than every 2 hours
- under 6 yrs.: ask a doctor
- 6–11 yrs.: with adult supervision, 1 inhalation in each nostril
- 12 yrs. & older: 2 inhalation in each nostril.

Other Information:
- store at room temperature
- keep inhaler tightly closed.
- This inhaler is effective for a minimum of 3 months after first use.

Inactive Ingredients: Bornyl acetate, camphor, lavender oil, menthol, methy salicylate.

How Supplied: Available as a cylindrical plastic nasal inhaler.
Net weight: 0.007 OZ (204 mg).
TAMPER EVIDENT: Use only if imprinted wrap is intact.
Questions? 1-800-873-8276
Dist. by Procter & Gamble, Cincinnati OH 45202. ©2001 42438038

VICKS® VAPORUB®
VICKS® VAPORUB® CREAM
(greaseless)
[vā 'pō-rub]
Cough Suppressant/Topical Analgesic

Drug Facts:

Active Ingredients:
Vicks® VapoRub®:

Active Ingredients: **Purpose:**
Camphor 4.8% .... Cough suppressant, & topical analgesic
Eucalyptus oil 1.2% ...... Cough suppressant
Menthol 2.6% .... Cough suppressant, & topical analgesic
Vicks® VapoRub® Cream:
Active Ingredients: **Purpose:**
Camphor 5.2% .... Cough suppressant, & topical analgesic
Eucalyptus oil 1.2% ...... Cough suppressant
Menthol 2.8% .... Cough suppressant, & topical analgesic

Uses: • On chest & throat, temporarily relieves cough due to the common cold
- on aching muscles and joints, temporarily relieves minor aches & pains

Warnings:
Failure to follow these warnings could result in serious consequences.
For external use only; avoid contact with eyes.
Do not use:
- by mouth
- with tight bandages
- in nostrils
- on wounds or damaged skin

Ask a doctor before use if you have:
- cough that occurs with too much phlegm (mucus)
- persistent or chronic cough such as occurs with smoking, asthma or emphysema

When using this product do not:
- **heat**
- **microwave**
- **use near an open flame**
- **add to hot water or any container where heating water. May cause splattering and result in burns.**

Stop use and ask a doctor if:
- muscle aches/pains persist more than 7 days or come back
- cough lasts more than 7 days, comes back, or occurs with fever, rash, or headache that lasts.
  These could be signs of a serious condition.

If pregnant or breast-feeding, ask a health professional before use.

Keep out of reach of children. In case of accidental ingestion, get medical help or contact a Poison Control Center right away.

Directions: • **See important warnings under "When using this product"**
- under 2 yrs.: ask a doctor
- adults and children 2 yrs. & older: Rub a thick layer on chest & throat or rub on sore aching muscles. If desired, cover with a soft cloth. Keep clothing loose about throat/chest to help vapors reach the nose/mouth. Repeat up to three times per 24 hours or as directed by a doctor.

Other Information:
- store at room temperature

Inactive Ingredients:
Vicks® VapoRub®: Cedarleaf oil, nutmeg oil, special petrolatum, thymol, turpentine oil
Vicks® VapoRub® Cream: Carbomer 954, cedarleaf oil, cetyl alcohol, cetyl palmitate, cyclomethicone copolyol, dimethicone copolyol, dimethicone, EDTA, glycerin, imidazolidinyl urea, isopropyl palmitate, methylparaben, nutmeg oil, peg-100 stearate, propylparaben, purified water, sodium hydroxide, stearic acid, stearyl alcohol, thymol, titanium dioxide, turpentine oil

How Supplied:
Vicks VapoRub®: Available in 1.76 oz (50 g) 3.53 oz (100 g) and 6 oz (170 g) plastic jars 0.45 oz (12 g) tin.
Vicks® VapoRub® Cream: Available in 2 oz (60 g) 2.99 oz (85 g) tube ⅙ oz pouch.

Questions? 1-800-873-8276
www.vicks.com
Vicks® VapoRub® 50142932
Vicks® VapoRub® Cream 50117758
US Pat. 5,322,689
Made in Mexico by Procter & Gamble
Manufactura, S. de R.L. de C.V.
Dist. by Procter & Gamble,
Cincinnati OH 45202

VICKS® VAPOSTEAM®
[vā 'pō "stēm]
Liquid Medication for
Hot Steam Vaporizers.
Camphor/Cough
Suppressant

Drug Facts:

Active Ingredient: **Purpose:**
Camphor 6.2% .... Cough suppressant

Uses: Temporarily relieves cough associated with a cold.

Warnings:
Failure to follow these warnings could result in serious consequences.
For external use only
Flammable Keep away from fire or flame. For steam inhalation only at room temperature.
Ask a doctor before use if you have:
• a persistent or chronic cough such as occurs with smoking, emphysema or asthma
• cough that occurs with too much phlegm (mucus)
When using this product do not
• heat
• microwave
• use near an open flame
• take by mouth
• direct steam from the vaporizer too close to the face
• add to hot water or any container where heating water except when adding to cold water only in a hot steam vaporizer. May cause splattering and result in burns.
Stop use and ask a doctor if:
• cough lasts more than 7 days, comes back, or occurs with fever, rash, or headache that lasts.
These could be signs of a serious condition.
Keep out of reach of children. In case of eye exposure (flush eyes with water); or in case of accidental ingestion; seek medical help or contact a Poison Control Center right away.

Directions:
see important warnings under "When using this product"
• under 2 yrs.: ask a doctor
• adults & children 2 yrs. & older: use 1 tablespoon of solution for each quart of water or 1½ teaspoonsful of solution for each pint of water
• add solution directly to cold water only in a hot steam vaporizer
• follow manufacturer's directions for using vaporizer. Breathe in medicated vapors. May be repeated up to 3 times a day.

Inactive Ingredients: Alcohol 78%, cedarleaf oil, eucalyptus oil, laureth-7, menthol, nutmeg oil, poloxamer 124, silicone.

How Supplied: Available in 4 FL OZ (118 ml) and 8 FL OZ (235 ml) bottles.
Questions? 1-800-873-8276
Made in Mexico by Procter & Gamble
Manufactura S. de R.L. de C.V.
Dist. by Procter & Gamble
Cincinnati OH 45202
50144018

EDUCATIONAL MATERIAL

The Procter & Gamble Company offers to health care professionals a variety of journal reprints and patient education materials. For this information, please call **1-800-832-3064** or write:
Scientific Communications
The Procter & Gamble Company
P.O. Box 599
Cincinnati, OH 45201
Information is also available by visiting www.pg.com. Select the brand of interest from the *Product Help* section. Each brand site offers a *Contact Us* page in case of additional questions.

The Purdue Frederick Company
ONE STAMFORD FORUM
STAMFORD, CT 06901-3431

For Medical Information Contact:
Medical Department
(888) 726–7535

BETADINE® BRAND
First Aid Antibiotics +
Moisturizer Ointment

Actions: Topical broad-spectrum antibiotics polymyxin B sulfate and bacitracin zinc in a cholesterolized ointment* (moisturizer) base to help prevent infection. Formulated with a special blend of waxes and oils to help retain vital moisture needed to aid in healing.

Uses: First aid to help prevent infection in minor cuts, scrapes and burns.

Directions: Clean affected area. Apply small amount of this product (an amount equal to the surface area of the tip of the finger) on the area 1 to 3 times daily. May be covered with a sterile bandage.

Warnings: For External Use Only. Do not use in the eyes or apply over large areas of the body. In case of deep or puncture wounds, animal bites, or serious burns, consult a physician. Stop use and consult a physician if the condition persists or gets worse, or if a rash or other allergic reaction develops. Do not use this product if you are allergic to any of the ingredients. Do not use longer than 1 week unless directed by a physician.

Keep this and all medications out of the reach of children. In case of accidental ingestion, seek professional assistance or contact a Poison Control Center immediately.

Active Ingredients: Per gram: Polymyxin B Sulfate (10,000 IU) and Bacitracin Zinc (500 IU).

How Supplied: 1/2 oz. plastic tube with applicator tip. Store at room temperature.
* Formulated with Aquaphor®—a registered trademark of Beiersdorf AG.
Copyright 1998, 2003, The Purdue Frederick Company
Shown in Product Identification Guide, page 522

BETADINE® BRAND PLUS
First Aid Antibiotics + Pain Reliever
Ointment
[bā 'tăh-dīn"]

Actions: Topical broad-spectrum antibiotics polymyxin B sulfate and bacitracin zinc plus topical anesthetic in a cholesterolized ointment* (moisturizer) base to help prevent infection and relieve pain.

Uses: First aid to help prevent infection and provide temporary pain relief in minor cuts, scrapes and burns.

Directions: Clean affected area. Apply small amount of this product (an amount equal to the surface area of the tip of the finger) on the area 1 to 3 times daily. May be covered with a sterile bandage. Children under 2 years of age: Consult a physician.

Warnings: For External Use Only. Do not use in the eyes or apply over large areas of the body. In case of deep or puncture wounds, animal bites, or serious burns, consult a physician. Stop use and consult a physician if the condition persists or gets worse, or if a rash or other allergic reaction develops. Do not use this product if you are allergic to any of the ingredients. Do not use longer than 1 week unless directed by a physician. Keep this and all medications out of the reach of children. In case of accidental ingestion, seek professional assistance or contact a Poison Control Center immediately.

Active Ingredients: Per gram: Polymyxin B Sulfate (10,000 IU), Bacitracin Zinc (500 IU), and Pramoxine HCl 10 mg.

How Supplied: 1/2 oz. plastic tube with an applicator tip. Store at room temperature.
*Formulated with Aquaphor® — a registered trademark of Beiersdorf AG.
Copyright 1998, 2003, The Purdue Frederick Company.
Shown in Product Identification Guide, page 522

Continued on next page

BETADINE® OINTMENT
(povidone-iodine, 10%)
BETADINE® SOLUTION
(povidone-iodine, 10%)
BETADINE ® SKIN CLEANSER
(povidone-iodine, 7.5%)
Topical Antiseptic
Bactericide/Virucide

Action: Topical microbicides active against organisms commonly encountered in minor skin wounds and burns.

Uses: Ointment—For the prevention of infection in minor burns, cuts and abrasions. Kills microorganisms promptly. **Solution**—Kills microorganisms in minor burns, cuts and scrapes. **Skin Cleanser**—Kills germs promptly. Skin sanitizer. Use routinely for general hygiene.

Directions: Ointment—For the prevention of infection in minor burns, cuts and abrasions, apply directly to affected areas as needed. Nonocclusive: allows air to reach the wound. May be bandaged. **Solution**—For minor cuts, scrapes and burns, apply directly to affected area as needed. May be covered with gauze or adhesive bandage. If bandaged, let dry first. **Skin Cleanser**—For handwashing, cleansing or bathing, wet skin and apply a sufficient amount to work up a rich, golden lather. Wash for at least 15 seconds. Repeat 2–3 times a day or as directed by physician.

Warnings: For External Use Only. Do not use in the eyes. Do not use if you are sensitive to iodine or other product ingredients. Do not use longer than one week unless directed by a doctor. In case of deep or puncture wounds, animal bites, or serious burns, consult physician. If redness, irritation, swelling or pain persists or increases, or if infection occurs, discontinue use and consult physician. If swallowed, get medical help or contact a Poison Control Center right away. Keep out of reach of children.

How Supplied:
Ointment: 1/32 oz. and 1/8 oz. packettes and 1 oz. tubes
Solution: 1/2 oz., 4 oz., 8 oz., 16 oz. (1 pt.), 32 oz. (1 qt.), and 1 gal. plastic bottles.
Skin Cleanser: 4 fl. oz. plastic bottles
Avoid storing at excessive heat.
Copyright 1991, 2003, The Purdue Frederick Company
Shown in Product Identification Guide, page 522

GENTLAX®
[jent' lax]
brand of bisacodyl USP, 5 mg
Tablets
Laxative

Indications: For relief of occasional constipation (irregularity).

Actions: This product generally causes bowel movement in 6–12 hours.

Directions: Take as follows or as directed by doctor. Adults and children 12 years and older, take 1 to 3 tablets (usually 2) in a single daily dose. Children 6 to under 12, take 1 tablet in a single daily dose. Children under 6 years of age: ask a doctor.

Warnings: Do not give to children under 6 years of age unless told to do so by a doctor, or to persons who cannot swallow without chewing unless told to do so by a doctor. Do not take laxative products for longer than 1 week unless directed by a doctor. Ask a doctor before use if you have stomach pain, nausea, vomiting, or if you have noticed a sudden change in bowel movements that continues over a period of 2 weeks. Do not chew or crush these tablets, do not use within 1 hour after taking an antacid or milk. When using this product, you may have stomach discomfort, faintness and cramps. Stop use and ask a doctor if you have rectal bleeding or fail to have a bowel movement after use of a laxative; these may indicate a serious condition. If you are pregnant or breast-feeding, ask a health professional before use. **Keep out of the reach of children.** In case of overdose, get medical help or contact a Poison Control Center right away.
Other information: Sodium content is less than 0.2 mg/tablet. Store at temperatures not above 86°F (30°C). Avoid excessive humidity.

Inactive Ingredients: calcium sulfate, carnauba wax, confectioner's sugar, croscarmellose sodium, D&C yellow no. 10, dibasic calcium phosphate, FD&C yellow no. 6, gelatin, kaolin, magnesium stearate, methacrylic acid copolymer, polyethylene glycol, powdered cellulose, pregelatinized starch, silicon dioxide, sucrose, talc, titanium dioxide, white wax.

How Supplied: Packages of 20 tablets and bottles of 100 tablets
Copyright 2003, The Purdue Frederick Company.
Shown in Product Identification Guide, page 522

SENOKOT® Tablets
(standardized senna concentrate)

Natural Vegetable Laxative

Actions: Senna provides a colon-specific action which is gentle, effective, and predictable, generally producing bowel movement in 6 to 12 hours.

Uses: For the relief of occasional constipation. Senokot Products generally produce bowel movement in 6 to 12 hours.

Directions: Take according to product-package instructions or as directed by a doctor. Take preferably at bedtime. For use of Senokot Laxatives in children under 2 years of age, consult a doctor.

Warnings: Ask a doctor before use if you have stomach pain, nausea or vomiting. If you have noticed a sudden change in bowel movements that persists over a period of 2 weeks, consult a doctor before using a laxative. Do not use laxative products for longer than 1 week unless directed by a doctor. Rectal bleeding or failure to have a bowel movement after the use of a laxative may indicate a serious condition. Discontinue use and consult your doctor. As with any drug, if you are pregnant or nursing a baby, seek the advice of a health professional before using this product. In case of accidental overdose, seek professional assistance or contact a Poison Control Center right away. Keep out of children's reach.

How Supplied: Senokot Tablets: Boxes of 20; bottles of 50, 100, and 1000; Unit Strip Packs in boxes of 100 individually sealed tablets. Each Senokot Tablet contains 8.6 mg sennosides.
Copyright 1991, 2003, The Purdue Frederick Company.
Shown in Product Identification Guide, page 522

EDUCATIONAL MATERIAL

Samples Available:
1) Betadine® Brand First Aid <u>Antibiotics</u> + Moisturizer Ointment Samples– 1 display of 48 packettes
2) Betadine® Brand Plus First Aid <u>Antibiotics</u> + Pain Reliever– 1 display of 48 packettes
3) **Up-to-date Information:** **www.senokot.com** provides dosing information for the Senokot® Products family of laxatives, as well as patient education about constipation and its causes. A special section on toilet training, written by a pediatrician, describes the popular child-centered approach.

Purdue Products L.P.
ONE STAMFORD FORUM
STAMFORD CT 06901-3431

For Medical Information Contact:
(888) 726-7535
Adverse Drug Experiences:
(888) 726-7535
Customer Service:
(800) 877-5666
FAX: (800) 877-3210

COLACE® CAPSULES,
COLACE® LIQUID 1% SOLUTION
[kō' lās]
docusate sodium

Actions: Colace® (docusate sodium) is a stool softener laxative. It helps moisten and soften hard, dry stools and facilitates natural defecation, providing effective relief usually within 12 to 72 hours.

Uses: Relieves occasional constipation (irregularity). Generally produces a bowel movement in 12 to 72 hours.

Directions: Take according to product-package instructions or as directed by a doctor. For use of Colace Capsules or Colace Liquid in children under 2 years of age, ask a doctor.

Warnings: Do not use laxative products for longer than 1 week unless told to do so by a doctor; if you are presently taking mineral oil, unless to do so by a doctor. **Ask a doctor before use if you have** stomach pain, nausea, vomiting, noticed a sudden change in bowel habits that lasts over 2 weeks. **Stop use and ask a doctor if** you have rectal bleeding or fail to have a bowel movement after use of a laxative. These could be signs of a serious condition. **If pregnant or breast-feeding,** ask a health professional before use. **Keep out of reach of children.** In case of overdose, get medical help or contact a Poison Control Center right away.

Other Information: Sodium content: 3 mg/50 mg capsule; 5 mg/100 mg capsule. VERY LOW SODIUM. Store at 25°C (77°F). Excursions permitted between 15–30°C (59–86°F). Keep bottle tightly closed.

Colace® Liquid 1% Solution: Each milliliter contains 10 mg of docusate sodium. Doses must be given in a 6–8 oz. glass of milk or fruit juice, or in infant's formula to prevent throat irritation. Sodium content 1 mg/mL. VERY LOW SODIUM. Supplied in 30 mL bottle with calibrated medicine dropper.

How Supplied: Colace Capsules **50 mg:** In boxes of 10 capsules. Bottles of 30 and 60 capsules. Colace Capsules **100 mg:** In boxes of 10 capsules. Bottles of 30, 60 and 250 capsules.
Copyright 2003, Purdue Products L.P., Stamford, CT 06901-3431
Shown in Product Identification Guide, page 522

COLACE® SYRUP
[kō' lās]
docusate sodium

Actions: Colace® Syrup (docusate sodium) is a stool softener laxative. It helps moisten and soften hard, dry stools and facilitates natural defecation, providing effective relief usually within 12 to 72 hours.
Uses: Relieves occasional constipation (irregularity). Generally produces a bowel movement in 12 to 72 hours.

Directions: Take according to product-package instructions or as directed by a doctor. Doses must be given in a 6–8 oz. glass of milk or fruit juice to prevent throat irritation. For use of Colace® Syrup in children under 2 years of age, ask a doctor.

Warnings: Do not use laxative products for longer than 1 week unless told to

do so by a doctor; if you are presently taking mineral oil, unless told to do so by a doctor; if you are on a sodium-restricted diet unless told to do so by a doctor. **Ask a doctor before use if you have** stomach pain, nausea, vomiting, noticed a sudden change in bowel habits that lasts over 2 weeks. **Stop use and ask a doctor if** you have rectal bleeding or fail to have a bowel movement after use of a laxative. These could be signs of a serious condition. **If pregnant or breast-feeding,** ask a health professional before use. **Keep out of reach of children.** In case of overdose, get medical help or contact a Poison Control Center right away.

Other Information: Each tablespoon (15 mL) contains 60 mg of docusate sodium. Sodium content: 36 mg/15 mL. Store at 20°–25°C (68°–77°F). Contains no sugar or alcohol.

How Supplied: Bottles of one pint (473 mL).
Copyright 2003, Purdue Products L.P., Stamford, CT 06901-3431

COLACE® GLYCERIN SUPPOSITORIES USP 1.2 GRAMS
[kō' lās]
glycerin
(Laxative for infants & children)
COLACE® GLYCERIN SUPPOSITORIES USP 2.1 GRAMS
glycerin
(Laxative for adults & children)

Action & Uses: Colace® suppositories are a laxative that relieves occasional constipation (irregularity). Generally produces a bowel movement in 1/4 to 1 hour.

Directions: Take according to product-package instructions or as directed by a doctor. For use of Colace Glycerin Suppositories in children under 2 years of age, ask a doctor.

Warnings: For rectal use only. Do not use laxative products for longer than 1 week unless told to do so by a doctor. **Ask a doctor before use if there is** stomach pain, nausea, vomiting, or a sudden change in bowel habits that lasts over 2 weeks. **When using this** product, there may be rectal discomfort or a burning sensation. **Stop use and ask a doctor if** there is rectal bleeding or a failure to have a bowel movement after use of a laxative. These could be signs of a serious condition. **If pregnant or breast-feeding,** ask a health professional before use. **Keep out of reach of children.** If swallowed, get medical help or contact a Poison Control Center right away.
Other Information: Avoid excessive heat. Keep jar tightly closed.

How Supplied: Infants and children suppositories: Jars of 12 and 24. Adults and children suppositories: Jars of 12, 24, 48 and 100.

Copyright 2003, Purdue Products L.P., Stamford, CT 06901-3431
Shown in Product Identification Guide, page 522

MINERAL OIL

Description: Intestinal lubricant laxative. Odorless, tasteless, crystal clear liquid.

Action & Uses: Relieves occasional constipation (irregularity). Generally produces a bowel movement in 6 to 8 hours.

Directions: Take according to product-package instructions or as directed by a doctor. For use in adults and children 12 years of age or older.

Warnings: Take only at bedtime and do not take with meals. **Do not use** for longer than 1 week, if you are presently taking a stool-softener laxative, if you are pregnant, in children under 12 years of age, in bedridden patients, in persons with difficulty swallowing. **Ask a doctor before use if you have** stomach pain, nausea, vomiting, noticed a sudden change in bowel habits that lasts over 2 weeks. **Stop use and ask a doctor if** you have rectal bleeding or fail to have a bowel movement after use of a laxative. These could be signs of a serious condition. **If pregnant or breast-feeding,** ask a health professional before use. **Keep out of reach of children.** In case of overdose, get medical help or contact a Poison Control Center right away.
Other Information: Store between 20°–25°C (68°–77°F). Keep bottle tightly closed. Protect from sunlight.

How Supplied: Bottles of 6 oz. and 16 oz.
Copyright 2003, Purdue Products L.P., Stamford, CT 06901-3431

PERI-COLACE® TABLETS
docusate sodium and standardized senna concentrate

Actions: This combination natural stimulant laxative and stool softener helps moisten and soften hard, dry stools and stimulates defecation, providing effective relief usually in 6 to 12 hours.

Uses: Relieves occasional constipation (irregularity). Generally produces a bowel movement in 6 to 12 hours.

Directions: Take according to product-package instructions or as directed by a doctor. For use of Peri-Colace Tablets in children under 2 years of age, consult a doctor.

Warnings: Do not use laxative products for longer than 1 week unless told to do so by a doctor; if you are presently taking mineral oil, unless to do so by a

Continued on next page

Peri-Colace—Cont.

doctor. **Ask a doctor before use if you have** stomach pain, nausea, vomiting, noticed a sudden change in bowel habits that lasts over 2 weeks. **Stop use and ask a doctor if** you have rectal bleeding or fail to have a bowel movement after use of a laxative. These could be signs of a serious condition. **If pregnant or breast-feeding,** ask a health professional before use. **Keep out of reach of children.** In case of overdose, get medical help or contact a Poison Control Center right away.

Other Information: Sodium content: 4 mg/tablet. VERY LOW SODIUM. Store at 25°C (77°F). Keep bottle tightly closed.

How Supplied: In boxes of 10 tablets. Bottles of 30 and 60 tablets. Copyright 2003, Purdue Products L.P., Stamford, CT 06901-3431
Shown in Product Identification Guide, page 522

Reese Pharmaceutical Company

10617 FRANK AVENUE CLEVELAND, OH 44106

Direct Inquiries to:
Voice: (800) 321-7178

REESE'S PINWORM MEDICINES
[rēsĭs]

Directions for Use: Take according to directions and do not exceed recommended dosage unless directed by a doctor. Medication should be taken only one time as a single dose: do not repeat treatment unless directed by a doctor. When one individual in a household has pinworms, the entire household should be treated unless otherwise advised. These products can be taken any time of day, with or without food. If you are pregnant, nursing a baby, or have liver disease, do not take this product unless directed by a doctor.

DOSAGE GUIDE

under 25 lbs or 2 yrs of age, consult a doctor

WEIGHT LBS.	DOSAGE TSP.	CAPS
25–37	1/2	2
38–62	1	4
63–87	1-1/2	6
88–112	2	8
113–137	2-1/2	10
138–162	3	12
163–187	3-1/2	14
188 & over	4	16

Liquid Dosage
NDC: 10956-618-01
Each 1 mL contains: 50 mg
Pyrantel base as Pyrantel Pamoate.
Pre-Measured Caplet Dosage
NDC: 10956-658-24
Packaged in boxes of 24 caplets.
Each caplet contains 62.5 mg
Pyrantel base as Pyrantel Pamoate.
Shown in Product Identification Guide, page 522

Schering-Plough HealthCare Products

3 CONNELL DRIVE BERKELEY HEIGHTS, NJ 07922

Direct Product Requests to:
Schering-Plough HealthCare Products
3 Connell Drive
Berkeley Heights, NJ 07922

For Medical Emergencies Contact:
Consumer Relations Department
P.O. Box 377
Memphis, TN 38151
(901) 320-2998 (Business Hours)
(901) 320-2364 (After Hours)

CLARITIN® NON-DROWSY 24 HOUR TABLETS
Brand of Loratadine

Drug Facts:

Active Ingredient (in each tablet): **Purpose:**
Loratadine 10 mg .... Antihistamine

Uses: temporarily relieves these symptoms due to hay fever or other upper respiratory allergies:
• runny nose • itchy, watery eyes
• sneezing • itching of the nose or throat

Warnings:
Do not use if you have ever had an allergic reaction to this product or any of its ingredients.
Ask a doctor before use if you have liver or kidney disease. Your doctor should determine if you need a different dose.
When using this product do not take more than directed. Taking more than directed may cause drowsiness.
Stop use and ask a doctor if an allergic reaction to this product occurs. Seek medical help right away.
If pregnant or breast-feeding, ask a health professional before use.
Keep out of reach of children. In case of overdose, get medical help or contact a Poison Control Center right away.

Directions:

adults and children 6 years and over	1 tablet daily; not more than 1 tablet in 24 hours
children under 6 years of age	ask a doctor
consumers with liver or kidney disease	ask a doctor

Other Information:
• safety sealed: do not use if the individual blister unit imprinted with Claritin® is open or torn
• store between 20°C to 25°C (68°F to 77°F)
• protect from excessive moisture

Inactive Ingredients: corn starch, lactose monohydrate, magnesium stearate

How Supplied: Boxes of 5, 10, 20, and 30 tablets
Questions or comments?
1-800-CLARITIN (1-800-252-7484) or **www.claritin.com**
Shown in Product Identification Guide, page 522

CLARITIN-D® NON-DROWSY 12 HOUR TABLETS

Drug Facts:

Active Ingredients (in each tablet): **Purpose:**
Loratadine 5 mg .... Antihistamine
Pseudoephedrine sulfate 120 mg .... Nasal decongestant

Uses:
• temporarily relieves these symptoms due to hay fever or other upper respiratory allergies:
  • nasal congestion • runny nose
  • sneezing • itchy, watery eyes
  • itching of the nose or throat
• reduces swelling of nasal passages
• temporarily relieves sinus congestion and pressure
• temporarily restores freer breathing through the nose

Warnings:
Do not use
• if you have ever had an allergic reaction to this product or any of its ingredients
• if you are now taking a prescription monoamine oxidase inhibitor (MAOI) (certain drugs for depression, psychiatric, or emotional conditions, or Parkinson's disease), or for 2 weeks after stopping the MAOI drug. If you do not know if your prescription drug contains an MAOI, ask a doctor or pharmacist before taking this product.
Ask a doctor before use if you have
• heart disease • thyroid disease
• high blood pressure • diabetes
• trouble urinating due to an enlarged prostate gland
• liver or kidney disease. Your doctor should determine if you need a different dose.

When using this product do not take more than directed. Taking more than directed may cause drowsiness.

Stop use and ask a doctor if
- an allergic reaction to this product occurs. Seek medical help right away.
- symptoms do not improve within 7 days or are accompanied by a fever
- nervousness, dizziness or sleeplessness occurs

If pregnant or breast-feeding, ask a health professional before use.

Keep out of reach of children. In case of overdose, get medical help or contact a Poison Control Center right away.

Directions:
- do not divide, crush, chew or dissolve the tablet

adults and children 12 years and over	1 tablet every 12 hours; not more than 2 tablets in 24 hours
children under 12 years of age	ask a doctor
consumers with liver or kidney disease	ask a doctor

Other Information:
- safety sealed: do not use if the individual blister unit imprinted with Claritin-D® 12 Hr. is open or torn
- store between 15°C to 25°C (59°F to 77°F)
- keep in a dry place

Inactive Ingredients: croscarmellose sodium, dibasic calcium phosphate, hypromellose, lactose monohydrate, magnesium stearate, pharmaceutical ink, povidone, titanium dioxide

How Supplied: Boxes of 10 and 30 tablets

Questions or comments?
1-800-CLARITIN (1-800-252-7484) or www.claritin.com
Shown in Product Identification Guide, page 522

CLARITIN-D® NON–DROWSY 24 HOUR TABLETS

Drug Facts:

Active Ingredients
(in each tablet): 　　　　　　**Purpose:**
Loratadine 10 mg .... Antihistamine
Pseudoephedrine
　sulfate 240 mg .... Nasal decongestant

Uses:
- temporarily relieves these symptoms due to hay fever or other upper respiratory allergies:
  - nasal congestion • runny nose
  - sneezing • itchy, watery eyes
  - itching of the nose or throat
- reduces swelling of nasal passages
- temporarily relieves sinus congestion and pressure
- temporarily restores freer breathing through the nose

Warnings:
Do not use
- if you have ever had an allergic reaction to this product or any of its ingredients
- if you are now taking a prescription monoamine oxidase inhibitor (MAOI) (certain drugs for depression, psychiatric, or emotional conditions, or Parkinson's disease), or for 2 weeks after stopping the MAOI drug. If you do not know if your prescription drug contains an MAOI, ask a doctor or pharmacist before taking this product.

Ask a doctor before use if you have
- heart disease
- thyroid disease
- high blood pressure
- diabetes
- trouble urinating due to an enlarged prostate gland
- liver or kidney disease. Your doctor should determine if you need a different dose.

When using this product do not take more than directed. Taking more than directed may cause drowsiness.

Stop use and ask a doctor if
- an allergic reaction to this product occurs. Seek medical help right away.
- symptoms do not improve within 7 days or are accompanied by a fever
- nervousness, dizziness or sleeplessness occurs

If pregnant or breast-feeding, ask a health professional before use.

Keep out of reach of children. In case of overdose, get medical help or contact a Poison Control Center right away.

Directions:
- do not divide, crush, chew or dissolve the tablet

adults and children 12 years and over	1 tablet daily with a full glass of water; not more than 1 tablet in 24 hours
children under 12 years of age	ask a doctor
consumers with liver or kidney disease	ask a doctor

Other Information:
- safety sealed: do not use if the individual blister unit imprinted with Claritin-D® 24 hour is open or torn
- store between 20° C to 25° C (68° F to 77° F)
- protect from light and store in a dry place

Inactive Ingredients: carnauba wax, dibasic calcium phosphate, ethylcellulose, hydroxypropyl cellulose, hypromellose, magnesium stearate, pharmaceutical ink, polyethylene glycol, povidone, silicon dioxide, sugar, titanium dioxide, white wax

How Supplied: Boxes of 5, 10, and 15 Tablets

Questions or comments?
1-800-CLARITIN (1-800-252-7484) or www.claritin.com
Shown in Product Identification Guide, page 522

CLARITIN® CHILDREN'S 24 HOUR NON-DROWSY ALLERGY SYRUP

Drug Facts:

Active Ingredient
(in each 5 mL): 　　　　　　**Purpose:**
Loratadine 5 mg .... Antihistamine

Uses: temporarily relieves these symptoms due to hay fever or other upper respiratory allergies:
- runny nose • itchy, watery eyes
- sneezing • itching of the nose or throat

Warnings:
Do not use if you have ever had an allergic reaction to this product or any of its ingredients.

Ask a doctor before use if you have liver or kidney disease. Your doctor should determine if you need a different dose.

When using this product do not take more than directed. Taking more than directed may cause drowsiness.

Stop use and ask a doctor if an allergic reaction to this product occurs. Seek medical help right away.

If pregnant or breast-feeding, ask a health professional before use.

Keep out of reach of children. In case of overdose, get medical help or contact a Poison Control Center right away.

Directions:

adults and children 6 years and over	2 teaspoonfuls daily; do not take more than 2 teaspoonfuls in 24 hours
children 2 to under 6 years of age	1 teaspoonful daily; do not take more than 1 teaspoonful in 24 hours
consumers with liver or kidney disease	ask a doctor

Other Information:
- safety sealed; do not use if Schering-Plough HealthCare imprinted bottle wrap is torn or missing
- store between 20°C to 25°C (68°F to 77°F)

Inactive Ingredients: citric acid, edetate disodium, flavor, glycerin, propylene glycol, sodium benzoate, sugar, water

How Supplied: 2 fl oz and 4 fl oz bottle
Questions or comments?
1-800-CLARITIN (1-800-252-7484) or www.claritin.com
Shown in Product Identification Guide, page 522

Continued on next page

Information on Schering-Plough HealthCare Products appearing on these pages is effective as of November 2003.

CLARITIN® REDITABS® 24 HOUR NON-DROWSY ORALLY DISINTEGRATING TABLETS
Brand of Loratadine

Drug Facts:

Active Ingredient

(in each tablet):   **Purpose:**
Loratadine 10 mg .... Antihistamine

Uses: temporarily relieves these symptoms due to hay fever or other upper respiratory allergies:
• runny nose • itchy, watery eyes
• sneezing • itching of the nose or throat

Warnings: **Do not use** if you have ever had an allergic reaction to this product or any of its ingredients.

Ask a doctor before use if you have liver or kidney disease. Your doctor should determine if you need a different dose.

When using this product do not take more than directed. Taking more than directed may cause drowsiness.

Stop use and ask a doctor if an allergic reaction to this product occurs. Seek medical help right away.

If pregnant or breast-feeding, ask a health professional before use.

Keep out of reach of children. In case of overdose, get medical help or contact a Poison Control Center right away.

Directions:
• place 1 tablet on tongue; tablet disintegrates, with or without water

adults and children 6 years and over	1 tablet daily; not more than 1 tablet in 24 hours
children under 6 years of age	ask a doctor
consumers with liver or kidney disease	ask a doctor

Other Information:
• safety sealed: do not use if interior foil pouch or individual blister unit imprinted with Claritin® RediTabs® inside the foil pouch is open or torn
• store between 20°C to 25°C (68°F to 77°F)
• keep in a dry place
• use within 6 months of opening foil pouch
• use tablet immediately after opening individual blister

Inactive Ingredients: citric acid, gelatin, mannitol, mint flavor

How Supplied: Boxes of 4, 10, and 20 tablets

Questions or comments?

1-800-CLARITIN **(1-800-252-7484)** or **www.claritin.com**

Shown in Product Identification Guide, page 523

LOTRIMIN® ULTRA™
[*lo-tre-min*]
Butenafine Hydrochloride Cream 1%
Antifungal
Athlete's Foot Cream
Jock Itch Cream

Drug Facts:

Active Ingredient: **Purpose:**
Butenafine
hydrochloride 1% .... Antifungal

Uses:
Athlete's Foot Cream:
• cures most athlete's foot between the toes. Effectiveness on the bottom or sides of foot is unknown.
• cures most jock itch and ringworm
• relieves itching, burning, cracking, and scaling which accompany these conditions
Jock Itch Cream:
• cures most jock itch
• relieves itching, burning, cracking, and scaling which accompany this condition

Warnings:
For external use only
Do not use
• on nails or scalp
• in or near the mouth or the eyes
• for vaginal yeast infections
When using this product do not get into the eyes. If eye contact occurs, rinse thoroughly with water.
Stop use and ask a doctor if too much irritation occurs or gets worse
Keep out of reach of children. If swallowed, get medical help or contact a Poison Control Center right away.

Directions:
Athlete's Foot Cream:
• adults and children 12 years and older
  • use the tip of the cap to break the seal and open the tube
  • wash the affected skin with soap and water and dry completely before applying

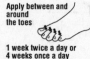
Apply between and around the toes

1 week twice a day or 4 weeks once a day

• **for athlete's foot between the toes:** apply to affected skin between and around the toes twice a day for 1 week (morning and night), or once a day for 4 weeks, or as directed by a doctor. Wear well-fitting, ventilated shoes. Change shoes and socks at least once daily.
• **for jock itch and ringworm** apply once a day to affected skin for 2 weeks or as directed by a doctor
  • wash hands after each use
• children under 12 years: ask a doctor
Jock Itch Cream:
• adults and children 12 years and over
  • use the tip of the cap to break the seal and open the tube
  • wash the affected skin with soap and water and dry completely before applying
  • apply once a day to affected skin for 2 weeks or as directed by a doctor
  • wash hands after each use
• children under 12 years: ask a doctor

Other Information:
• do not use if seal on tube is broken or is not visible
• store at 5°–30°C (41°–86°F)

Inactive Ingredients: Benzyl alcohol, cetyl alcohol, diethanolamine, glycerin, glyceryl monostearate SE, polyoxyethylene (23) cetyl ether, propylene glycol dicaprylate, purified water, sodium benzoate, stearic acid, white petrolatum

How Supplied: Available in 0.42 oz (12 gram) tubes for both athlete's foot and jock itch. Also available in a 0.85 oz (24 gram) tube for athlete's foot.
Shown in Product Identification Guide, page 522

SinoFresh HealthCare, Inc.
516 PAUL MORRIS DRIVE
ENGLEWOOD, FL 34223

Direct Inquiries to:
877-724-0587

SINOFRESH® Antiseptic Nasal Spray
Topical nasal, sinus, and pharyngeal antiseptic

Product Overview: SinoFresh Nasal Spray is a formulation of Cetylpyridinium Chloride blended with moisturizers and mint aromatics. SinoFresh has been shown, in vitro, to kill the most common pathogens found in the nose, sinuses, and nasopharynx. The organisms can trigger various allergic and non-allergic inflammatory reactions, cause post nasal drainage, and bad breath. SinoFresh cleanses and refreshes the nasal and pharyngeal tissues.
Drug Facts
Active Ingredient: **Purpose:**
Cetylpyridinium chloride
0.05% .... Antiseptic

Uses:
• Kills germs and bacteria
• Reduces germs and bacteria in the nasal passages

Warnings:
Ask a doctor before use if you have
• had any medical procedures for your nose or sinuses
• a bleeding or irritated nose
When using this product
• do not spray in eyes. If contact occurs, rinse eyes with water
• do not share dispenser with others
Stop use and ask a doctor if
• condition persists for more than 7 days or worsens
• a rash or irritation occurs
Keep out of reach of children.
In case of accidental overdose, get medical help or contact a Poison Control Center right away.

Directions:
• Adults and children 12 years and older, 1 to 3 sprays in each nostril morning and night
• Children under 12 years ask a doctor

Other Information: Store at room temperature and away from direct sunlight.

How Supplied: 1 fluid oz bottle with nasal sprayer

Inactive Ingredients: Benzalkonium chloride, dibasic sodium phosphate, eucalyptus oil, monobasic sodium phosphate, peppermint oil, polysorbate 80, propylene glycol, purified water, sodium chloride, sorbitol solution, spearmint oil, and wintergreen oil.

Questions? 877-724-0587

Tamper Evident Warning: Do not use this product if foil seal under cap is torn or missing.

DISTRIBUTED BY
SinoFresh HealthCare, Inc.
516 Paul Morris Drive
Englewood, Florida 34223
Toll Free: (877) 724-0587

SINOFRESH® is a registered trademark of SinoFresh HealthCare, Inc.
Patent Numbers: 5,785,988; 6,083,525; 6,344,210B2 Other patents pending.

Shown in Product Identification Guide, page 523

Standard Homeopathic Company

**210 WEST 131st STREET
BOX 61067
LOS ANGELES, CA 90061**

Direct Inquiries to:
Jay Borneman
(800) 624-9659 x20

HYLAND'S BACKACHE WITH ARNICA

Active Ingredients: BENZOICUM ACIDUM 3X HPUS, COLCHICUM AUTUMNALE 3X HPUS, SULPHUR 3X HPUS, ARNICA MONTANA 6X HPUS, RHUS TOXICODENDRON 6X HPUS.

Inactive Ingredients: Lactose, N.F.

Indications: A homeopathic medicine for the temporary relief of symptoms of low back pain due to strain or overexertion.

Directions: Adults and children over 12 years of age: Take 1–2 caplets with water every 4 hours or as needed.

Warnings: Do not use if imprinted cap band is broken or missing. If symptoms persist for more than seven days or worsen, contact a licensed health care professional. As with any drug, if you are pregnant or nursing a baby, seek the advice of a licensed health care professional before using this product. Keep this and

all medications out of the reach of children. In case of accidental overdose, contact a poison control center immediately. In case of emergency, the manufacturer may be reached 24 hours a day, 7 days a week at 800/624-9659.

How Supplied: Bottles of 40 5.5 grain caplets (NDC 54973-2965-2). Store at room temperature.

HYLAND'S BUMPS 'N BRUISES™ TABLETS

Active Ingredients: Arnica Montana 6X HPUS, Hypericum Perforatum 6X HPUS, Bellis Perennis 6X HPUS, Ruta Graveolens 6X HPUS.

Inactive Ingredients: Lactose, N.F.

Indications: A homeopathic medicine for the temporary relief of symptoms of bruising and swelling from falls, trauma or overexertion. Easy to take soft tablets dissolve instantly in the mouth.

Directions: For over 1 year of age: Dissolve 3–4 tablets in a teaspoon of water or on the tongue at the time of injury. May be repeated as needed every 15 minutes until relieved.

Warnings: Do not use if imprinted cap band is broken or missing. If symptoms persist for more than 7 days or worsen, consult a licensed health care professional. As with any drug, if you are pregnant or nursing a baby, consult a health care professional before using this product. Keep this and all medications out of the reach of children. In case of accidental overdose, contact a poison control center immediately. In case of emergency, the manufacturer may be reached 24 hours a day, 7 days a week at 800/624-9659.

How Supplied: Bottles of 125 1-grain sublingual tablets (NDC 54973-7508-1). Store at room temperature.

HYLAND'S CALMS FORTÉ™

Active Ingredients: *Passiflora* (Passion Flower) 1X triple strength HPUS, *Avena Sativa* (Oat) 1X double strength HPUS, *Humulus Lupulus* (Hops) 1X double strength HPUS, *Chamomilla* (Chamomile) 2X HPUS, *Calcarea Phosphorica* (Calcium Phosphate) 3X HPUS, *Ferrum Phosphorica* (Iron Phosphate) 3X HPUS, *Kali Phosphoricum* (Potassium Phosphate) 3X HPUS, *Natrum Phosphoricum* (Sodium Phosphate) 3X HPUS, *Magnesia Phosphoricum* (Magnesium Phosphate) 3X HPUS.

Inactive Ingredients: Lactose, N.F., Calcium Sulfate, Starch (Corn and Tapiocal), Magnesium Stearate.

Indications: Temporary symptomatic relief of simple nervous tension and sleeplessness.

Directions: Adults: As a relaxant: Swallow 1–2 tablets with water as needed, three times daily, preferably before meals. For insomnia: 1 to 3 tablets ½ to 1 hour before retiring. Repeat as needed without danger of side effects. Children: As a relaxant: Swallow 1 tablet with water as needed, three times daily, preferably before meals. For insomnia: 1 to 2 tablets ½ to 1 hour before retiring. Repeat as needed without danger of side effects.

Warning: Do not use if imprinted cap band is broken or missing. If symptoms persist for more than seven days or worsen, consult a licensed health care professional. As with any drug, if you are pregnant or nursing a baby, seek the advice of a licensed health care professional before using this product. Keep this and all medications out of the reach of children. In case of accidental overdose, contact a Poison Control Center immediately. In case of emergency, the manufacturer may be reached 24 hours a day, 7 days a week by calling 800/624-9659.

How Supplied: Bottles of 100 4-grain tablets (NDC 54973-1121-02), 50 4-grain tablets (NDC 54973-1121-01) and 32 5.5-grain caplets (NDC 54973-1121-48). Store at room temperature.

HYLAND'S COLIC TABLETS

Active Ingredients: *Disocorea* (Wild Yam) 3X HPUS, *Chamomilla* (Chamomile) 3X HPUS, *Colocynthinum* (Bitter Apple) 3X HPUS.

Inactive Ingredients: Lactose N.F.

Indications: A homeopathic combination for the temporary relief of symptoms of colic and gas pains caused by irritating food, feeding too quickly, swallowing air and similar conditions during teething, colds and other minor upset periods in children.

Directions: For children up to 2 years of age: Dissolve 2 tablets under the tongue every 15 minutes for up to 8 doses until relieved; then every 2 hours as required. If you prefer, tablets may first be dissolved in a teaspoon of water and then given to the child. Children over 2 years: Dissolve 3 tablets under the tongue as above; or as recommended by a licensed health care professional. Colic Tablets are very soft and dissolve almost instantly under the tongue. If your baby has been crying or has been very upset, your baby may fall asleep after using this product. This is because pain has been relieved and your child can rest.

Warnings: Do not use if imprinted cap band is broken or missing. If symptoms persist for more than seven days or worsen, consult a licensed health care professional. As with any drug, if you are

Continued on next page

Hyland's Colic—Cont.

pregnant or nursing a baby, seek the advice of a licensed health care professional before using this product. Keep this and all medications out of the reach of children. In case of accidental overdose, contact a poison control center immediately. In cases of emergency, the manufacturer may be contacted 24 hours a day, 7 days a week at 800/624-9659

How Supplied: Bottles of 125—one grain sublingual tablets (NDC 54973-7502-1). Store at room temperature.

HYLAND'S EARACHE TABLETS

Active Ingredients: Pulsatilla (Wind Flower) 30C, HPUS; Chamomilla (Chamomile) 30C, HPUS; Sulphur 30C, HPUS; Calcarea Carbonica (Carbonate of Lime) 30C, HPUS; Belladonna 30C, HPUS; (3×10^{-60} % Alkaloids) and Lycopodium (Club Moss) 30C, HPUS.

Inactive Ingredients: Lactose NF

Indications: For the relief of symptoms of fever, pain, irritability and sleeplessness associated with earaches in children after diagnosis by a physician. If symptoms persist for more than 48 hours or if there is a discharge from the ear, discontinue use and contact your health care professional.

Directions: Dissolve 4 tablets under the tongue 3 times per day for 48 hours or until symptoms subside. If you prefer, tablets may be dissolved in a teaspoon of water and then given to the child. Earache Tablets are very soft and dissolve almost instantly under the tongue.

Warnings: Do not use if imprinted blisters are broken or damaged. If symptoms persist for more than 48 hours, or if there is a discharge from the ear, discontinue use and consult a licensed health care professional. As with any drug, if you are pregnant or nursing a baby, seek the advice of a licensed health care professional before using this product. Keep this and all medications out of the reach of children. In case of accidental overdose, contact a poison control center immediately. In cases of emergency, the manufacturer may be contacted 24 hours a day, 7 days a week at 800/624-9659.

How Supplied: Blister pack of 40 tablets (NDC 54973-7507-1). Store at room temperature.

HYLAND'S LEG CRAMPS OINTMENT

Formula: Aconitum Nap. 3X HPUS, Arnica Montana 3X HPUS, Ledum Pal. 3X HPUS, Mag. Phos. 10X HPUS, Rhus Tox. 6X HPUS, Viscum Alb. 3X HPUS.

Indications: Temporarily relieves the symptoms of cramps and pains in legs and calves.

Directions: Apply liberally to affected area. Hyland's Leg Cramps Ointment will warm the area while easing the symptoms.

Warnings: For external use only. Do not use if tube seal is broken or missing. If symptoms persist for more than seven days or worsen, contact a licensed health care provider. Keep this and all medications out of reach of children.

How Supplied: Tube of 2.5 ounces (NDC 54973-75143-3).

HYLAND'S LEG CRAMPS WITH QUININE

Active Ingredients: Cinchona Officinalis 3X, HPUS (Quinine), Viscum Album 3X, HPUS; Gnaphalium Polycephalum 3X, HPUS; Rhus Toxicodendron 6X, HPUS; Aconitum Napellus 6X, HPUS; Ledum Palustre 6X, HPUS; Magnesia Phosphorica 6X, HPUS.

Inactive Ingredients: Lactose, N.F.

Indications: Hyland's Leg Cramps is a traditional homeopathic formula for the relief of symptoms of cramps and pains in lower back and legs often made worse by damp weather. Working without contraindications or side effects, Hyland's Leg Cramps stimulates your body's natural healing response to relieve symptoms. Hyland's Leg Cramps is safe for adults and can be used in conjuction with other medications.

Directions: Adults: Dissolve 2–3 tablets under tongue every 4 hours as needed.

Warnings: Do not use if imprinted cap band is missing or broken. If symptoms persist for more than seven days or worsen, contact a licensed health care professional. As with any drug, if you are pregnant or nursing a baby, seek the advice of a licensed health care professional before using this product. Do not use if pregnant, sensitive to quinine or under 12 years of age. Keep this and all medications out of the reach of children. In case of accidental overdose, contact a poison control center immediately. In case of emergency, the manufacturer may be reached 24 hours a day, 7 days a week at 800-624-9659.

How Supplied: Bottles of 100 three-grain sublingual tablets (NDC 54973-2956-02), Bottles of 50 three-grain sublingual tablets (NDC 54973-2956-01), Bottles of 40 5.5 grain caplets (NDC 54973-2956-68). Store at room temperature.

HYLAND'S MIGRAINE HEADACHE RELIEF TABLETS

Active Ingredients:
Glononium 12X HPUS, Belladonna 6X HPUS, Gelsemium 6X HPUS, Nux Vomica 6X HPUS, Iris Versicolor 6X HPUS, Sanguinaria Canadensis 6X HPUS.

Inactive Ingredients: Lactose NF.

Indications: Temporarily relieves the symptoms of migraine pain.

Directions: Adults and Children over 12 years of age: Dissolve 1 to 2 tablets on tongue every 4 hours or as needed.

Warnings: Ask a doctor before use if pregnant or nursing. Consult a physician if symptoms persist for more than 7 days or worsen. Keep out of the reach of children. Do not use if imprinted tamper band is broken or missing. In case of accidental overdose, contact a poison control center immediately. In case of emergency, the manufacturer may be contacted 24 hours a day, 7 days a week at 800/624-9659.

How Supplied: Bottles of 60 3-grain tablets. (NDC 54973-3013-01). Store at room temperature.
Hyland's, Inc.
Los Angeles, CA 90061
800/624-9659
www.hylands.com

HYLAND'S NERVE TONIC

Active Ingredients: Calcarea Phosphorica (Calcium Phosphate) 3X HPUS; Ferrum Phosphorica (Iron Phosphate) 3X HPUS; Kali Phosphoricum (Potassium Phosphate) 3X HPUS; Natrum Phosphoricum (Sodium Phosphate) 3X HPUS; Magnesia Phosphoricum (Magnesium Phosphate) 3X HPUS.

Inactive Ingredients: Lactose, N.F.

Indications: Temporary symptomatic relief of simple nervous tension and stress.

Directions: Adults take 2–6 tablets before each meal and at bedtime. Children: 2 tablets. In severe cases take 3 tablets every 2 hours.

Warnings: Do not use if imprinted cap band is broken or missing. If symptoms persist for more than seven days or worsen, contact a licensed health care professional. As with any drug, if you are pregnant or nursing a baby, seek the advice of a licensed health care professional before using this product. Keep this and all medications out of the reach of children. In case of accidental overdose, contact a poison control center immediately. In cases of emergency, the manufacturer may be contacted 24 hours a day, 7 days a week at 800/624-9659.

How Supplied: Bottles of 32 caplets (NDC 54973-1129-68), Bottles of 500 tablets (NDC 54973-1129-1), Bottles of 1000 tablets (NDC 54973-1129-2), Bottles of 100 tablets (NDC 54973-3014-02)

HYLAND'S SEASONAL ALLERGY TABLETS

Formula: Allium Cepa 6X HPUS, Natrum Muriaticum 6X HPUS Histaminum

Hydrochloricum 12X HPUS, Luffa Operculata 12X HPUS, Galphimia Glauca 12X HPUS, Nux Vomica 6X HPUS.

Indications: Temporarily relieves the runny eyes and nose symptoms of allergy from pollen, ragweed, grasses, mold and animal dander.

Directions: Adults and Children over 12 years of age: Dissolve 1 to 2 tablets on tongue every 4 hours as needed.

Warnings: Ask a doctor before use if pregnant or nursing. If symptoms persist for more than seven days or worsen, contact a licensed health care provider. Keep this and all medications out of reach of children. Do not use if imprinted tamper band is broken or missing. In case of accidental overdose, contact a poison control center immediately. In case of emergency, the manufacturer may be contacted 24 hours a day, 7 days a week at 800/624-9659.

How Supplied: Bottles of 60 tablets. (NDC 54973-3012-01).

SMILE'S PRID®

Contains: Acidum Carbolicum 2X HPUS, Ichthammol 2X HPUS, Arnica Montana 3X HPUS, Calendula Off 3X HPUS, Echinacea Ang 3X HPUS, Sulphur 12X HPUS, Hepar Sulph 12X HPUS, Silicea 12X HPUS, Rosin, Beeswax, Petrolatum, Stearyl Alcohol, Methyl & Propyl Paraben.

Indications: Temporary topical relief of pain symptoms associated with boils, minor skin eruptions, redness and irritation. Also aids in relieving the discomfort of superficial cuts, scratches and wounds.

Directions: Wash affected parts with hot water, dry and apply PRID® twice daily on clean bandage or gauze. Do not squeeze or pressure irritated skin area. After irritation subsides, repeat application once a day for several days. Children under two years: consult a physician. CAUTION: If symptoms persist for more than seven days or worsen, or if fever occurs, contact a licensed health care professional. Do not use on broken skin. Keep out of reach of children. In case of accidental ingestion, seek professional assistance or contact a poison control center. For external use only. Avoid contact with eyes.

How Supplied: 18GM tin (NDC 0619-4202-54). Keep in a cool dry place.

HYLAND'S TEETHING GEL

Active Ingredients: Calcarea Phosphorica (Calcium Phosphate) 12X, HPUS; Chamomilla (Chamomile) 6X, HPUS; Coffea Cruda (Coffee) 6X, HPUS; and Belladonna 6X, HPUS (Alkaloids 0.0000003%)

Inactive Ingredients: Deionized water, Vegetable Glycerin, Hydroxyethyl Cellulose, Methyl Paraben and Propyl Paraben.

Indications: A homeopathic combination for the temporary relief of symptoms of simple restlessness and wakeful irritability due to cutting teeth.

Directions: Apply to gums as necessary. If symptoms persist for more than seven days or worsen, discontinue use and contact your health care professional. Please note, if your baby has been crying or has been very upset, your baby may fall asleep after using this product because the pain has been relieved and your child can rest.

Warnings: Do not use if tube tip is broken or missing. If symptoms persist for more than seven days or if irritation persists, inflammation develops or fever or infection develop, discontinue use and consult a licensed health care professional. As with any drug, if you are pregnant or nursing a baby, seek the advice of a licensed health care professional before using this product. Keep this and all medications out of the reach of children. In case of accidental overdose, contact a poison control center immediately. In case of emergency, the manufacturer may be contacted 24 hours a day, 7 days a week at 800/624-9659.

How Supplied: Tubes of 1/3 OZ. (NDC 54973-7504-3). Store at room temperature.

HYLAND'S TEETHING TABLETS

Active Ingredients: *Calcarea Phosphorica* (Calcium Phosphate) 3X HPUS, *Chamomilla* (Chamomile) 3X HPUS, *Coffea Cruda* (Coffee) 3X HPUS, *Belladonna* 3X HPUS (Alkaloids 0.0003%).

Inactive Ingredients: Lactose N.F.

Indications: A homeopathic combination for the temporary relief of symptoms of simple restlessness and wakeful irritability due to cutting teeth.

Directions: Dissolve 2 to 3 tablets under the tongue 4 times per day. If you prefer, tablets may first be dissolved in a teaspoon of water and then given to the child. If the child is restless or wakeful, 2 tablets every hour for 6 doses or as recommended by a licensed health care professional. Teething Tablets are very soft and dissolve almost instantly under the tongue. Please note, if your baby has been crying or has been very upset, your baby may fall asleep after using this product because the pain has been relieved and your child can rest.

Warning: Do Not use if imprinted cap band is broken or missing. If symptoms persist for more than seven days, or if irritation persist, inflammation develops or fever or infection develop, discontinue use and consult a licensed health care professional. As with any drug, if you are pregnant or nursing a baby, seek the advice of a health care professional before using this product. Keep this and all medications out of the reach of children. In case of accidental overdose, contact a poison control center immediately. In case of emergency, the manufacturer may be contacted 24 hours a day, 7 days a week at 800/624-9659.

How Supplied: Bottles of 125—one grain sublingual tablets (NDC 54973-7504-01). Store at room temperature.

UAS Laboratories
9953 VALLEY VIEW RD
EDEN PRAIRIE, MN 55344

Direct Inquiries To:
Dr. S.K. Dash: (952) 935-1707
(952) 935-1650

Medical Emergency Contact:
Dr. S.K. Dash: (952) 935-1707
Fax: (952) 935-1650

DDS®-ACIDOPHILUS
Capsule, Tablet & Powder free of dairy products, corn, soy, and preservatives

Description: DDS®-Acidophilus is the source of a special strain of Lactobacillus acidophilus free of dairy products, corn, soy and preservatives. Each capsule or tablet contains one billion viable DDS®-1 L.acidophilus at the time of manufacturing. One gram of powder contains two billion viable DDS®-1 L.acidophilus.

Indications and Usages: An aid in implanting the gut with beneficial Lactobacillus acidophilus under conditions of digestive disorders, acne, yeast infections, and following antibiotic therapy.

Administration: One to two capsules or tablets twice daily before meals. One-fourth teaspoon powder can be substituted for two capsules or tablets.

How Supplied: Bottles of 100 capsules or tablets. 12 bottles per case. Powder is available in 2 oz. bottle; 12 bottles per case.

Storage: Keep refrigerated under 40°F.

EDUCATIONAL MATERIAL

DDS®-Acidophilus
Booklet describing superior-strain Acidophilus without dairy products, corn, soy, or preservatives. Two billion viable DDS®-1. L.acidopohilus per gram.

Upsher-Smith Laboratories, Inc.

6701 EVENSTAD DRIVE
MAPLE GROVE, MN 55369

Direct Inquiries to:
Professional Services
(800) 654-2299
(763) 315-2001

AMLACTIN® 12% Moisturizing Lotion and Cream
[ăm-lăk-tĭn]
Cosmetic Lotion and Cream

Description: AMLACTIN® Moisturizing Lotion and Cream are special formulations of 12% lactic acid neutralized with ammonium hydroxide to provide a lotion or cream pH of 4.5–5.5. Lactic acid, an alpha-hydroxy acid, is a naturally occurring humectant for the skin. AMLACTIN® moisturizes and softens rough, dry skin.

How Supplied: 225g (8oz) plastic bottle: List No. 0245-0023-22
400g (14oz) plastic bottle: List No. 0245-0023-40
140g (4.9oz) tube: List No. 0245-0024-14

AMLACTIN AP® Anti-Itch Moisturizing Cream
[ăm-lăk'-tĭn]
1% Pramoxine HCl

Description: AMLACTIN AP® Anti-Itch Moisturizing Cream is a special formulation containing 12% lactic acid neutralized with ammonium hydroxide to provide a cream pH of 4.5–5.5 with pramoxine HCl. Lactic acid, an alpha-hydroxy acid, is a naturally occurring humectant which moisturizes and softens rough, dry skin. Pramoxine HCl, USP, 1% is an effective antipruritic ingredient used to relieve itching associated with dry skin.

How Supplied: 140g (4.9oz) tube: NDC No. 0245-0025-14

UNKNOWN DRUG?
Consult the
Product Identification Guide
(Gray Pages)
for full-color photos of
leading over-the-counter
medications

Wellness International Network, Ltd.

5800 DEMOCRACY DRIVE
PLANO, TX 75024

Direct Inquiries to:
Product Coordinator
(972) 312-1100
FAX: (972) 943-5250

BIO-COMPLEX 5000™
Gentle Foaming Cleanser

Uses: BIO-COMPLEX 5000™ Gentle Foaming Cleanser, with alpha-hydroxy acids, aloe vera and botanical infusions, is an advanced cleansing gel designed for all skin types. BIO-COMPLEX 5000 Gentle Foaming Cleanser protects the skin and works to restore elasticity while gently removing surface impurities, make-up and pollution.

Ingredients: Water (Aqua), Ammonium Lauryl Sulfate, Lauramidopropyl Betaine, Salvia Officinalis (Sage) Leaf Extract, Anthemis Nobilis Flower Extract, Glycerin, Lauramide DEA, Cetyl Betaine, Tocopherol (Vitamin E), Ascorbic Acid (Vitamin C), Citric Acid, Methylchloroisothiazolinone, Methylisothiazolinone, Aloe Barbadensis Leaf Juice, Propylparaben, Methylparaben.

Directions: Splash warm water onto face. Place a small amount of gel on fingertips. Apply evenly to face and neck in circular motions, massaging skin gently but thoroughly. Rinse completely and pat dry with a soft towel.

How Supplied: 8 fluid ounce/236 ml. bottle.

BIO-COMPLEX 5000™
Revitalizing Conditioner

Uses: BIO-COMPLEX 5000™ Revitalizing Conditioner, with vitamins and anti-oxidants, helps restore moisture to dried-out, heat-styled hair. This advanced conditioner contains silkening agents which enhance the hair as well as detangle it after shampooing. Hair is left clean, soft, manageable, and protected against styling aids and environmental elements. BIO-COMPLEX 5000™ Revitalizing Conditioner is excellent for all hair types, especially damaged or over-processed hair.

Ingredients: Water, Stearyl Alcohol, Propylene Glycol, Stearamidopropyl Dimethylamine, Cyclomethicone, Polyquaternium - 11, Stearalkonium Chloride, Cetearyl Alcohol, PEG - 40 Hydrogenated Castor Oil, Citric Acid,

Tocopherol (Vitamin E), Ascorbic Acid (Vitamin C), Retinyl Palmitate (Vitamin A), Ethylhexyl Methoxycinnamate, Fragrance (Parfum), Ceteth - 20, Hydrolyzed Keratin, Sodium Chloride, Imidazolidinyl Urea, Methylparaben, Propylparaben.

Directions: After shampooing with BIO-COMPLEX 5000™ Revitalizing Shampoo, apply to wet hair. Massage through hair, paying special attention to the ends. Leave on 2–3 minutes. Rinse thoroughly. Towel dry and style as usual.

How Supplied: 12 fluid ounce bottle.

BIO-COMPLEX 5000™
Revitalizing Shampoo

Uses: BIO-COMPLEX 5000™ Revitalizing Shampoo, with vitamins and anti-oxidants, cleanses and moisturizes hair for excellent manageability. Specially formulated with the essence of awapuhi, a Hawaiian ginger plant extract known for its healing qualities, this formula contains the mildest blend of surfactants and a wealth of natural conditioning ingredients to provide body, luster and healthier-looking hair.

Ingredients: Water, Ammonium Lauryl Sulfate, Tea Lauryl Sulfate, Cocamidopropyl Betaine, Lauramide DEA, Cetyl Betaine, Glycerin, Ascorbic Acid (Vitamin C), Tocopherol (Vitamin E), Retinyl Palmitate (Vitamin A), Citric Acid, Hydrolyzed Wheat Protein, Fragrance (Parfum), Ethylhexyl Methoxycinnamate, PEG - 7 Glyceryl Cocoate, Methylchloroisothiazolinone, Methylisothiazolinone, Caramel.

Directions: Apply a small amount to wet hair and massage gently into scalp, creating a generous lather. Rinse and repeat if necessary. To further intensify this reconstructive process, follow with BIO-COMPLEX 5000™ Revitalizing Conditioner.

How Supplied: 12 fluid ounce bottle.

STEPHAN™ BIO-NUTRITIONAL
Daytime Hydrating Creme

Uses: Hypo-allergenic STEPHAN™ BIO-NUTRITIONAL Daytime Hydrating Creme hydrates the skin and preserves the moisture level of the upper layers of the epidermis. It is an excellent day cream for both men and women who wish to combat the visible signs of aging skin, the appearance of wrinkles or lines, and the inelastic look of facial features and contours. These light emulsions are absorbed rapidly, leaving an invisible protective film which hydrates the epidermis, regulates moisture levels and leaves skin feeling supple and soft.

Ingredients: Water (Aqua), Stearic Acid, Isodecyl Neopentanoate, Isostearyl Stearoyl Stearate, DEA-Cetyl Phosphate, C12-15 Alkyl Benzoate, Tocopherol (Vitamin E), Aloe Barbadensis Leaf Juice, Squalane, Cetyl Esters, Benzophenone-3, Dimethicone, Fragrance (Parfum), Carbomer, Triethanolamine, Imidazolidinyl Urea, Methylparaben, Propylparaben, Annatto.

Directions: Apply in the morning and during the day to clean skin. May be used around the eye area, avoiding direct contact with the eyes. Suitable for all skin types. For best results, use in conjunction with the complete STEPHAN BIO-NUTRITIONAL Skin Care line.

Warnings: For external use only. Avoid contact with eyes.

How Supplied: Net Wt. 1.75 oz.

STEPHAN™ BIO-NUTRITIONAL
Eye-Firming Concentrate

Uses: Hypo-allergenic STEPHAN™ BIO-NUTRITIONAL Eye-Firming Concentrate is specially formulated to revitalize the delicate area around the eyes. This non-oily fluid pampers sensitive eyes while reducing the look of puffiness and dark circles, and smoothing and softening the appearance of fine lines in the eye area.

Ingredients: Purified water, Cornflower extract, Methylsilanol hydroxyproline aspartate, Methyl Gluceth-20, Dimethicone copolyol, Peg-30, Glyceryl laurate, Horsetail extract, Panthenol, Propylene glycol, Carbomer, Disodium EDTA, Triethanolamine, Xanthan gum, Diazolidinyl urea, Methylparaben, Propylparaben.

Directions: Apply in the morning, or any time of the day, in small quantities to the skin around the eyes with light, tapping motions, avoiding direct contact with the eyes. In the evening, apply gently to the entire eye contour area. For best results, use in conjunction with the complete STEPHAN BIO-NUTRITIONAL Skin Care line.

Warnings: For external use only. Avoid direct contact with eyes.

How Supplied: 1 fl. oz.

STEPHAN™ BIO-NUTRITIONAL
Nighttime Moisture Creme

Uses: Hypo-allergenic STEPHAN™ BIO-NUTRITIONAL Nighttime Moisture Creme is a heavier, richer cream for mature, dry or sun-damaged skin. This advanced formula is excellent for dehydrated skin, promoting suppleness and moisture, while improving the appearance of fine lines and wrinkles.

Ingredients: Water (Aqua), Caprylic/ Capric Triglyceride, Propylene, Glycol/ Dicaprylate/Dicaprate, Stearic Acid, Polysorbate 60, Cetyl Alcohol, Ethylhexyl Palmitate, Cera Alba (Beeswax), Sorbitan Stearate, Canola Oil, Persea Gratissima (Avocado) Oil, Carthamus Tinctorius (safflower) Seed Oil, Squalane, Lecithin (Liposomes), Soluble Collagen, Dimethicone, Bisabolol, Aloe Barbadensis Leaf Juice, Fragrance (Parfum), C12–15 Alkyl Benzoate, Hydroxyethylcellulose, Alcohol, Ethylhexyl Methoxycinnamate, Disodium EDTA, Sodium Borate, Benzophenone-3, Allantoin, Potassium Sorbate, Phenoxyethanol, Methylparaben, Propylparaben, Butylparaben, Ethylparaben, Yellow 10, Caramel.

Directions: In the evening, apply by lightly massaging onto a thoroughly cleansed face and neck. Avoid direct contact with eyes. For drier skin, it may be used during the day as a moisturizer, under make-up or after sun bathing. For best results, use in conjunction with the complete STEPHAN BIO-NUTRITIONAL Skin Care line.

Warnings: For external use only. Avoid contact with eyes.

How Supplied: Net Wt. 1.75 oz.

STEPHAN™ BIO-NUTRITIONAL
Refreshing Moisture Gel

Uses: Hypo-allergenic STEPHAN™ BIO-NUTRITIONAL Refreshing Moisture Gel is specially formulated to refine pores and promote a clear, clean and smooth-looking complexion. It is designed to deeply cleanse and super-stimulate the skin. This gel is suitable for all skin types, especially problem areas. A quick "pick-me-up," STEPHAN BIO-NUTRITIONAL Refreshing Moisture Gel immediately restores the radiant, firm and youthful appearance of the face while acting as a cumulative, revitalizing beauty treatment.

Ingredients: Water (Aqua), Propylene Glycol, Glycerin, Hydroxyethylcellulose, Saccharum Officinarum (Sugar Cane) Extract, Citrus Unshiu Extract, Pyrus Malus (Apple) Extract, Camellia Oleifera Leaf Extract, Hydrolyzed Wheat Protein, Yeast Extract, Saccharomyces Lysate Extract, Panthenol, Aloe Barbadensis Leaf Juice, Phenethyl Alcohol, Laureth-4, Magnesium Aluminum Silicate, Tetrasodium EDTA, Benzophenone-3, Imidazolidinyl Urea, Methylchloroisothiazolinone, Methylisothiazolinone, Methylparaben, Propylparaben, Yellow 10, Red 40, Yellow 5.

Directions: Apply to clean skin at anytime. Remove after 20 minutes with warm water. Can be used around the eye area, avoiding direct contact with the eyes. Suitable for all skin types. For best results, use in conjunction with the complete STEPHAN BIO-NUTRITIONAL Skin Care line.

Warnings: For external use only. Avoid contact with eyes.

How Supplied: Net Wt. 1.75 oz.

STEPHAN™ BIO-NUTRITIONAL
Ultra Hydrating Fluid

Uses: Hypo-allergenic STEPHAN™ BIO-NUTRITIONAL Ultra Hydrating Fluid is a complete treatment formulated to soften fine lines and preserve youthful-looking, radiant skin. By utilizing ingredients focused on revitalization, STEPHAN BIO-NUTRITIONAL Ultra Hydrating Fluid possesses a progressive firming effect, helping to combat the aged look of skin due to external negative conditions.

Ingredients: Purified Water, Methyl Gluceth-20, Dimethicone Copolyol, Peg-30 Glyceryl Laurate, Panthenol Sugar Cane Extract, Citrus Extract, Apple Extract, Green Tea Extract, Live Yeast Cell Derivative, Laureth-4, Plant Pseudocollagen Methylsilanol Hydroxyproline Aspartate, Hydrolyzed Wheat Protein, Methylchloroisothiazolinone, Methylisothiazolinone, Phenethyl Alcohol, 2-Bromo-2-Nitropropane-1, 3-Diol, Xanthan Gum, Disodium EDTA, Methylparaben, Propylparaben.

Directions: Gently apply all over the face, neck and eye contour area, preferably in the morning. Make-up can be applied afterwards. Use as a part of a regular daily skin care routine or as an occasional preventive treatment. For best results, use in conjunction with the complete STEPHAN BIO-NUTRITIONAL Skin Care line.

Warnings: For external use only. Avoid direct contact with eyes.

How Supplied: 1 fl. oz.

Wyeth Consumer Healthcare
Wyeth

**FIVE GIRALDA FARMS
MADISON, NJ 07940**

Direct Inquiries to:
Wyeth Consumer Healthcare Product Information 800-322-3129

ADVIL®
**Ibuprofen Tablets, USP
Ibuprofen Caplets (Oval-Shaped Tablets)
Ibuprofen Gel Caplets (Oval-Shaped Gelatin Coated Tablets)
Ibuprofen Liqui-Gel Capsules
Fever reducer/Pain reliever**

Active Ingredient: Each tablet, caplet, gel caplet, or liquigel capsule contains Ibuprofen 200 mg

Uses: temporarily relieves minor aches and pains due to the common cold, headache, toothache, muscular aches, backache, minor pain of arthritis, menstrual cramps; and temporarily reduces fever.

Warnings
Allergy alert: ibuprofen may cause a severe allergic reaction which may include:
- hives
- facial swelling
- asthma (wheezing)
- shock

Stomach bleeding warning: Taking more than recommended may cause stomach bleeding.
Alcohol warning: if you consume 3 or more alcoholic drinks every day, ask your doctor whether you should take ibuprofen or other pain relievers/fever reducers. Ibuprofen may cause stomach bleeding.
Do not use if you have ever had an allergic reaction to any other pain reliever/fever reducer
Ask a doctor before use if you have
- problems or serious side effects from taking pain relievers or fever reducers
- stomach problems that last or come back, such as heartburn, upset stomach, or pain
- ulcers
- bleeding problems
- high blood pressure, heart or kidney disease, are taking a diuretic, or are over 65 years of age

Ask a doctor or pharmacist before use if you are
- under a doctor's care for any serious condition
- taking any other product containing ibuprofen, or any other pain reliever/fever reducer
- taking a prescription drug for anticoagulation (blood thinning)
- taking any other drug

When using this product take with food or milk if stomach upset occurs
Stop use and ask a doctor if
- an allergic reaction occurs. Seek medical help right away.
- pain gets worse or lasts more than 10 days

- fever gets worse or lasts more than 3 days
- stomach pain or upset gets worse or lasts
- redness or swelling is present in the painful area
- any new symptoms appear

If pregnant or breast-feeding, ask a health professional before use. It is especially important not to use ibuprofen during the last 3 months of pregnancy unless definitely directed to do so by a doctor because it may cause problems in the unborn child or complications during delivery.

Keep out of reach of children. In case of overdose, get medical help or contact a Poison Control Center right away.

Dosage and Administration:

Directions—**Do not take more than directed**
Adults and children 12 years and over:
- take 1 tablet, caplet, gelcap or liquigel capsule every 4 to 6 hours while symptoms persist
- if pain or fever does not respond to 1 tablet, caplet, gelcap, or liquigel capsule, 2 tablets, caplets, gelcaps or liquigel capsules may be used • do not exceed 6 tablets, caplets, gelcaps or liquigel capsules in 24 hours, unless directed by a doctor
- the smallest effective dose should be used

Children under 12 years: ask a doctor

Inactive Ingredients:

Tablets and Caplets: acetylated monoglyceride, beeswax and/or carnauba wax, croscarmellose sodium, iron oxides, lecithin, methylparaben, microcrystalline cellulose, pharmaceutical glaze, povidone, propylparaben, silicon dioxide, simethicone, sodium benzoate, sodium lauryl sulfate, starch, stearic acid, sucrose, titanium dioxide.

Gel Caplets: croscarmellose sodium, FD&C red no. 40, FD&C yellow no. 6, gelatin, glycerin, hypromellose, iron oxides, medium chain triglycerides, pharmaceutical ink, propyl gallate, silicon dioxide, sodium lauryl sulfate, starch, stearic acid, titanium dioxide, triacetin

Liqui-Gels: FD&C green no. 3, gelatin, light mineral oil, pharmaceutical ink, polyethylene glycol, potassium hydroxide, purified water, sorbitan, sorbitol.

Storage: Store at 20–25°C (68–77°F)
Avoid excessive heat 40°C (above 104°F)

How Supplied:
Coated tablets in a 10 ct. vial and bottles of 8, 24, 50, 100, 165 (non-child resistant), and 225. Coated caplets in bottles of 24, 50, 100, 165 (non-child resistant), and 225.

Gel caplets in bottles of 24, 50, 100, 165 (non-child resistant) and 225.

Liqui-Gels in bottles of 20, 40, 80, 135 (non-child resistant) and 180.

ADVIL® ALLERGY SINUS CAPLETS
**Pain Reliever/Fever Reducer
Nasal Decongestant
Antihistamine**

Active Ingredients (in each caplet):
Chlorpheniramine maleate 2 mg
Ibuprofen 200 mg
Pseudoephedrine HCl 30 mg

Uses:
- temporarily relieves these symptoms associated with hay fever or other upper respiratory allergies, and the common cold:
  - runny nose • sneezing • headache
  - itchy, watery eyes
  - nasal congestion • minor aches and pains • itching of the nose or throat
  - sinus pressure • fever

Warnings:
Allergy alert: Ibuprofen may cause a severe allergic reaction which may include:
- hives • facial swelling • asthma (wheezing) • shock

Stomach bleeding warning: Taking more than recommended may cause stomach bleeding.
Alcohol warning: If you consume 3 or more alcoholic drinks every day, ask your doctor whether you should take ibuprofen or other pain relievers/fever reducers. Ibuprofen may cause stomach bleeding.
Do not use
- if you have ever had an allergic reaction to any other pain reliever/fever reducer
- if you are now taking a prescription monoamine oxidase inhibitor (MAOI) (certain drugs for depression, psychiatric, or emotional conditions, or Parkinson's disease), or for 2 weeks after stopping the MAOI drug. If you do not know if your prescription drug contains an MAOI, ask a doctor or pharmacist before taking this product.

Ask a doctor before use is you have
- a breathing problem such as emphysema or chronic bronchitis
- heart disease • high blood pressure • thyroid disease • diabetes • kidney disease • ulcers • bleeding problems • glaucoma
- problems or serious side effects from taking pain relievers or fever reducers
- stomach problems that last or come back, such as heartburn, upset stomach, or pain
- trouble urinating due to an enlarged prostate gland

Ask a doctor or pharmacist before use if you are
- under a doctor's care for any serious condition
- taking sedatives or tranquilizers
- over 65 years of age
- taking any other product that contains ibuprofen, or any other pain reliever/fever reducer
- taking any other product that contains pseudoephedrine, chlorpheniramine or any other nasal decongestant or antihistamine
- taking a prescription drug for anticoagulation (blood thinning), or a diuretic
- taking any other drug

When using this product
- **do not use more than directed**
- avoid alcoholic drinks
- be careful when driving a motor vehicle or operating machinery
- drowsiness may occur
- take with food or milk if stomach upset occurs
- alcohol, sedatives, and tranquilizers may increase drowsiness

Stop use and ask a doctor if
- an allergic reaction occurs. Seek medical help right away.
- nasal congestion lasts for more than 7 days
- fever lasts for more than 3 days
- you get nervous, dizzy, or sleepless
- symptoms continue or get worse
- stomach pain occurs with the use of this product even if mild pain persists
- any new symptoms appear

If pregnant or breast-feeding, ask a health professional before use. It is especially important not to use this product during the last 3 months of pregnancy unless definitely directed to do so by a doctor because it may cause problems in the unborn child or complications during delivery.

Keep out of reach of children. In case of overdose, get medical help or contact a Poison Control Center right away.

Directions:
- adults: take 1 caplet every 4–6 hours while symptoms persist.
- do not take more than 6 caplets in any 24-hour period, unless directed by a doctor
- children under 12 years of age: consult a doctor

Other Information:
- read all warnings and directions before use. Keep carton.
- store in a dry place 20–25°C (68–77°F)
- avoid excessive heat above 40°C (104°F)

Inactive Ingredients: carnauba wax, croscarmellose sodium, FD&C red no. 40 aluminum lake, FD&C yellow no. 6 aluminum lake, glyceryl behenate, hypromellose, iron oxide black, microcrystalline cellulose, polydextrose, polyethylene glycol, pregelatinized starch, propylene glycol, silicon dioxide, starch, titanium dioxide

How Supplied: Packages of 10 and 20 caplets

ADVIL® COLD & SINUS
Caplets, Tablets and Liqui-Gels
Pain Reliever/Fever Reducer/Nasal Decongestant

Active Ingredients (in each tablet or caplet):
Ibuprofen 200 mg
Pseudoephedrine HCl 30 mg

Active Ingredients (in each Liqui-Gel):
Solubilized Ibuprofen equal to 200 mg ibuprofen (present as the free acid and potassium salt)
Pseudoephedrine HCl 30 mg

Uses: Temporarily relieves these symptoms associated with the common cold, sinusitis or flu:

- headache • fever • nasal congestion
- minor body aches and pains

Warnings:
Allergy Alert: Ibuprofen may cause a severe allergic reaction which may include: • hives • facial swelling • asthma (wheezing) • shock
Stomach bleeding warning: Taking more than recommended may cause stomach bleeding

Alcohol warning: If you consume 3 or more alcoholic drinks every day, ask your doctor whether you should take ibuprofen or other pain relievers/fever reducers. Ibuprofen may cause stomach bleeding.
Do not use
- if you have ever had an allergic reaction to any other pain reliever/fever reducer
- if you are now taking a prescription monoamine oxidase inhibitor (MAOI) (certain drugs for depression, psychiatric, or emotional conditions, or Parkinson's disease), or for 2 weeks after stopping the MAOI drug. If you do not know if your prescription drug contains an MAOI, ask a doctor or pharmacist before taking this product

Ask a doctor before use if you have
- heart disease • high blood pressure
- thyroid disease • diabetes
- trouble urinating due to an enlarged prostate gland
- had serious side effects from any pain reliever/fever reducer
- ulcers
- bleeding problems
- stomach problems that last or come back, such as heartburn, upset stomach or pain

Ask a doctor or pharmacist before use if you are
- taking any other product that contains ibuprofen or pseudoephedrine
- taking any other pain reliever/fever reducer or nasal decongestant
- under a doctor's care for any continuing medical condition
- taking a prescription product for anticoagulation (blood thinning) or a diuretic
- taking other drugs on a regular basis

When using this product
- **do not use more than directed**
- take with food or milk if stomach upset occurs

Stop use and ask a doctor if
- an allergic reaction occurs. Seek medical help right away.
- you get nervous, dizzy, or sleepless
- nasal congestion lasts for more than 7 days
- fever lasts for more than 3 days
- symptoms continue or get worse
- new or unexpected symptoms occur
- stomach pain occurs with use of this product or if even mild symptoms persist

If pregnant or breast-feeding, ask a health professional before use. It is especially important not to use this product during the last 3 months of pregnancy unless definitely directed to do so by a doctor because it may cause problems in the unborn child or complications during delivery.

Keep out of reach of children. In case of overdose, get medical help or contact a Poison Control Center right away.

Directions:
- adults and children 12 years of age and over:
  - take 1 tablet, caplet or liqui-gel every 4 to 6 hours while symptoms persist. If symptoms do not respond to 1 tablet, caplet or liqui-gel, 2 tablets, caplets or liqui-gels may be used.
  - do not use more than 6 tablets, caplets or liqui-gels in any 24-hour period unless directed by a doctor
  - the smallest effective dose should be used
- children under 12 years of age: consult a doctor

Other Information:
- store at 20–25°C (68–77°F). Avoid excessive heat above 40°C (104°F).
- read all warnings and directions before use. Keep carton.

Inactive Ingredients (tablets and caplets): carnauba or equivalent wax, croscarmellose sodium, iron oxides, methylparaben, microcrystalline cellulose, propylparaben, silicon dioxide, sodium benzoate, sodium lauryl sulfate, starch, stearic acid, sucrose, titanium dioxide

Inactive Ingredients (liqui-gels): D&C yellow no. 10, FD&C red no. 40, fractionated coconut oil, gelatin, pharmaceutical ink, polyethylene glycol, potassium hydroxide, purified water, sorbitan, sorbitol

How Supplied: Advil® Cold and Sinus is an oval-shaped, tan-colored caplet, a tan-colored tablet or a liqui-gel. The caplet is supplied in blister packs of 20 and 40. The tablet is available in blister packs of 20. The liqui-gel is available in blister packs of 16 and 32.

ADVIL®
FLU & BODY ACHE Caplets
Pain Reliever/Fever Reducer/Nasal Decongestant

Active Ingredients (in each caplet)
Ibuprofen 200 mg
Pseudoephedrine HCl 30 mg

Uses:
- temporarily relieves these symptoms associated with the common cold, sinusitis, or flu
  - headache
  - fever
  - nasal congestion
  - minor body aches and pains

Warnings:
Allergy alert: Ibuprofen may cause a severe allergic reaction which may include: • hives • facial swelling • asthma (wheezing) • shock
Stomach bleeding warning: Taking more than recommended may cause stomach bleeding
Alcohol warning: If you consume 3 or more alcoholic drinks every day, ask your doctor whether you should take ibuprofen or other pain relievers/fever reducers. Ibuprofen may cause stomach bleeding.

Continued on next page

Advil Flu/Body Ache—Cont.

Do not use
- if you have ever had an allergic reaction to any other pain reliever/fever reducer
- if you are now taking a prescription monoamine oxidase inhibitor (MAOI) (certain drugs for depression, psychiatric, or emotional conditions, or Parkinson's disease), or for 2 weeks after stopping the MAOI drug. If you do not know if your prescription drug contains an MAOI, ask a doctor or pharmacist before taking this product

Ask a doctor before use if you have
- heart disease • high blood pressure
- thyroid disease • diabetes
- ulcers
- bleeding problems
- stomach problems that last or come back, such as heartburn, upset stomach or pain
- trouble urinating due to an enlarged prostate gland
- had serious side effects from any pain reliever/fever reducer

Ask a doctor or pharmacist before use if you are
- taking any other product that contains ibuprofen or pseudoephedrine
- taking any other pain reliever/fever reducer or nasal decongestant
- under a doctor's care for any continuing medical condition
- taking other drugs on a regular basis
- taking a prescription product for anticoagulation (blood thinning) or a diuretic

When using this product
- **do not use more than directed**
- take with food or milk if stomach upset occurs

Stop use and ask a doctor if
- an allergic reaction occurs. Seek medical help right away.
- you get nervous, dizzy, or sleepless
- nasal congestion lasts for more than 7 days
- fever lasts for more than 3 days
- symptoms continue or get worse
- new or unexpected symptoms occur
- stomach pain occurs with use of this product or if even mild symptoms persist

If pregnant or breast-feeding, ask a health professional before use. It is especially important not to use this product during the last 3 months of pregnancy unless definitely directed to do so by a doctor because it may cause problems in the unborn child or complications during delivery.

Keep out of reach of children. In case of overdose, get medical help or contact a Poison Control Center right away.

Directions:
- adults and children 12 years of age and over: Take 1 caplet every 4 to 6 hours while symptoms persist. If symptoms do not respond to 1 caplet, 2 caplets may be used.
- do not use more than 6 caplets in any 24-hour period unless directed by a doctor
- the smallest effective dose should be used
- children under 12 years of age: consult a doctor

Other Information:
- store at 20–25°C (68–77°F). Avoid excessive heat above 40°C (104°F).

- read all warnings and directions before use. Keep carton.

Inactive Ingredients: carnauba or equivalent wax, croscarmellose sodium, iron oxide, methylparaben, microcrystalline cellulose, propylparaben, silicon dioxide, sodium benzoate, sodium lauryl sulfate, starch, stearic acid, sucrose, titanium dioxide

How Supplied:
Blister packs of 20 caplets.

ADVIL®
MIGRAINE Liquigels

Use: Treats migraine

Active Ingredient:
Each brown, oval capsule contains solubilized ibuprofen, a pain reliever, equal to 200 mg ibuprofen (present as the free acid and potassium salt)

Warnings:
Allergy alert: Ibuprofen may cause a severe allergic reaction which may include:
- hives
- facial swelling
- asthma (wheezing)
- shock

Stomach bleeding warning: Taking more than recommended may cause stomach bleeding.

Alcohol warning: If you consume 3 or more alcoholic drinks every day, ask your doctor whether you should take ibuprofen or other pain relievers/fever reducers. Ibuprofen may cause stomach bleeding.

Do not use if you have ever had an allergic reaction to any other pain reliever/fever reducer

Ask a doctor before use if you have
- never had migraines diagnosed by a health professional
- a headache that is different from your usual migraines
- the worse headache of your life
- fever and stiff neck
- headaches beginning after, or caused by head injury, exertion, coughing or bending
- experienced your first headache after the age of 50
- daily headaches
- a migraine so severe as to require bed rest
- problems or serious side effects from taking pain relievers or fever reducers
- stomach problems that last or come back, such as heartburn, upset stomach, or pain
- ulcers
- bleeding problems
- high blood pressure, heart or kidney disease, are taking a diuretic, or are over 65 years of age

Ask a doctor or pharmacist before use if you are
- under a doctor's care for any serious condition
- taking another product containing ibuprofen, or any other pain reliever/fever reducer
- taking a prescription drug for anticoagulation (blood thinning)

- taking any other drug

When using this product take with food or milk of stomach upset occurs.

Stop use and ask a doctor if
- an allergic reaction occurs. Seek medical help right away.
- migraine headache pain is not relieved or gets worse after first dose
- stomach pain occurs with the use of this product
- any new symptoms appear

If pregnant or breast-feeding, ask a health professional before use. It is especially important not to use ibuprofen during the last 3 months of pregnancy unless definitely directed to do so by a doctor because it may cause problems in the unborn child or complications during delivery.

Keep out of reach of children. In case of overdose, get medical help or contact a Poison Control Center right away.

Directions:

Adults:	• take 2 capsules with a glass of water • if symptoms persist or worsen, ask your doctor • do not take more than 2 capsules in 24 hours, unless directed by a doctor
Under 18 years of age:	• ask a doctor

Other Information:
- read all directions and warnings before use. Keep carton.
- store at 20–25°C (68–77°F)
- avoid excessive heat 40°C (above 104°F)

Inactive Ingredients:
D&C yellow no. 10, FD&C green no. 3, FD&C red no. 40, gelatin, light mineral oil, pharmaceutical ink, polyethylene glycol, potassium hydroxide, purified water, sorbitan, sorbitol

How Supplied: Bottles of 20, 40, & 80 liquigels.

JUNIOR STRENGTH ADVIL
Chewable Tablets
Fever Reducer/Pain Reliever

Active Ingredient:
(in each tablet)
Ibuprofen 100 mg

Uses: temporarily:
- reduces fever
- relieves minor aches and pains due to the common cold, flu, sore throat, headaches and toothaches

Warnings:
Allergy alert: Ibuprofen may cause a severe allergic reaction which may include:
- hives • asthma (wheezing)
- facial swelling • shock

Dosing Chart

Weight (lb)	Age (yr)	Dose (tablets)
under 48 lb	under 6 yr	ask a doctor
48–59 lb	6–8 yr	2 tablets
60–71 lb	9–10 yr	2 ½ tablets
72–95 lb	11 yr	3 tablets

Stomach bleeding warning: Taking more than recommended may cause stomach bleeding

Sore throat warning: Severe or persistent sore throat or sore throat accompanied by high fever, headache, nausea, and vomiting may be serious. Consult doctor promptly. Do not use more than 2 days or administer to children under 3 years of age unless directed by doctor.

Do not use if the child has ever had an allergic reaction to any other fever reducer/pain reliever

Ask a doctor before use if the child has
• ulcers
• bleeding problems
• stomach problems that last or come back, such as heartburn, upset stomach or pain
• high blood pressure, heart or kidney disease or is taking a diuretic
• not been drinking fluids
• lost a lot of fluid due to continued vomiting or diarrhea
• problems or serious side effects from taking fever reducers or pain relievers

Ask a doctor or pharmacist before use if the child is
• under a doctor's care for any serious condition
• taking any other drug
• taking a prescription product for anticoagulation (blood thinning)
• taking any other product that contains ibuprofen, or any other pain reliever/fever reducer

When using this product give with food or milk if stomach upset occurs

Stop use and ask a doctor if
• an allergic reaction occurs. Seek medical help right away.
• fever or pain gets worse or lasts more than 3 days
• the child does not get any relief within first day (24 hours) of treatment
• stomach pain or upset gets worse or lasts
• redness or swelling is present in the painful area
• any new symptoms appear

Keep out of reach of children. In case of overdose, get medical help or contact a Poison Control Center right away.

Directions:
• **do not give more than directed**
• find right dose on chart below. If possible, use weight to dose; otherwise use age.
• repeat dose every 6–8 hours, if needed
• do not use more than 4 times a day [See table above]

Other Information:
• **Phenylketonurics:** contains phenylalanine 4.2 mg per tablet
• one dose lasts 6–8 hours
• store at 20–25°C (68–77°F)

Inactive Ingredients: (GRAPE FLAVOR) artificial flavor, aspartame, cellulose acetate phthalate, D&C red no. 30 lake, FD&C blue no. 2 lake, gelatin, magnasweet, magnesium stearate, mannitol, microcrystalline cellulose, silicon dioxide, sodium starch glycolate

Inactive Ingredients: (FRUIT FLAVOR) aspartame, cellulose acetate phthalate, D&C red no. 27 lake, FD&C red no. 40 lake, gelatin, magnasweet, magnesium stearate, mannitol, microcrystalline cellulose, natural and artificial flavors, silicon dioxide, sodium starch glycolate

How Supplied:
Chewable Tablets: bottles of 24 (fruit and grape flavors).

JUNIOR STRENGTH ADVIL SWALLOW TABLETS
Fever Reducer/Pain Reliever

Active Ingredient:
(in each tablet)
Ibuprofen 100 mg

Uses: temporarily:
• reduces fever
• relieves minor aches and pains due to the common cold, flu, sore throat, headaches and toothaches

Warnings:
Allergy alert: Ibuprofen may cause a severe allergic reaction which may include:
• hives • asthma (wheezing)
• facial swelling • shock

Stomach bleeding warning: Taking more than recommended may cause stomach bleeding

Sore throat warning: Severe or persistent sore throat or sore throat accompanied by high fever, headache, nausea, and vomiting may be serious. Consult doctor promptly. Do not use more than 2 days or administer to children under 3 years of age unless directed by doctor.

Do not use if the child has ever had an allergic reaction to any other fever reducer/pain reliever

Ask a doctor before use if the child has
• not been drinking fluids • ulcers
• bleeding problems
• stomach problems that last or come back, such as heartburn, upset stomach or pain
• high blood pressure, heart or kidney disease or is taking a diuretic
• lost a lot of fluid due to continued vomiting or diarrhea
• problems or serious side effects from taking fever reducers or pain relievers

Ask a doctor or pharmacist before use if the child is
• under a doctor's care for any serious condition
• taking any other drug
• taking any other product that contains ibuprofen, or any other pain reliever/fever reducer
• taking a prescription product for anticoagulation (blood thinning)

When using this product give with food or milk if stomach upset occurs

Stop use and ask a doctor if
• an allergic reaction occurs. Seek medical help right away.
• fever or pain gets worse or lasts more than 3 days
• the child does not get any relief within first day (24 hours) of treatment
• stomach pain or upset gets worse or lasts
• redness or swelling is present in the painful area
• any new symptoms appear

Keep out of reach of children. In case of overdose, get medical help or contact a Poison Control Center right away.

Directions:
• **do not give more than directed**
• find right dose on chart below. If possible, use weight to dose; otherwise use age.
• repeat dose every 6–8 hours, if needed
• do not use more than 4 times a day

Dosing Chart

Weight (lb)	Age (yr)	Dose (tablets)
under 48 lb	under 6 yr	ask a doctor
48–71 lb	6–10 yr	2 tablets
72–95 lb	11 yr	3 tablets

Other Information:
• one dose lasts 6–8 hours
• store at 20–25°C (68–77°F)

Inactive Ingredients: acetylated monoglycerides, carnauba wax, colloidal silicon dioxide, croscarmellose sodium, iron oxides, methylparaben, microcrystalline cellulose, povidone, pregelatinized starch, propylene glycol, propylparaben, shellac, sodium benzoate, starch, stearic acid, sucrose, titanium dioxide

How Supplied: Coated Tablets in bottles of 24.

CHILDREN'S ADVIL CHEWABLE TABLETS
Fever Reducer/Pain Reliever

Active Ingredient:
(in each tablet)
Ibuprofen 50 mg

Uses: temporarily:
• reduces fever
• relieves minor aches and pains due to the common cold, flu, sore throat, headaches and toothaches

Continued on next page

Children's Advil Chew.—Cont.

Warnings:

Allergy alert: Ibuprofen may cause a severe allergic reaction which may include:
- hives • asthma (wheezing)
- facial swelling • shock

Stomach bleeding warning: Taking more than recommended may cause stomach bleeding

Sore throat warning: Severe or persistent sore throat or sore throat accompanied by high fever, headache, nausea, and vomiting may be serious. Consult doctor promptly. Do not use more than 2 days or administer to children under 3 years of age unless directed by doctor.

Do not use if the child has ever had an allergic reaction to any other fever reducer/pain reliever

Ask a doctor before use if the child has
- not been drinking fluids
- lost a lot of fluid due to continued vomiting or diarrhea
- ulcers
- bleeding problems
- stomach problems that last or come back, such as heartburn, upset stomach or pain
- high blood pressure, heart or kidney disease or is taking a diuretic
- problems or serious side effects from taking fever reducers or pain relievers

Ask a doctor or pharmacist before use if the child is
- under a doctor's care for any serious condition
- taking any other drug
- taking a prescription product for anticoagulation (blood thinning)
- taking any other product that contains ibuprofen, or any other pain reliever/fever reducer

When using this product give with food or milk if stomach upset occurs

Stop use and ask a doctor if
- an allergic reaction occurs. Seek medical help right away.
- fever or pain gets worse or lasts more than 3 days
- the child does not get any relief within first day (24 hours) of treatment
- stomach pain or upset gets worse or lasts
- redness or swelling is present in the painful area
- any new symptoms appear

Keep out of reach of children. In case of overdose, get medical help or contact a Poison Control Center right away.

Directions:
- **do not give more than directed**
- find right dose on chart below. If possible, use weight to dose; otherwise use age.
- repeat dose every 6–8 hours, if needed
- do not use more than 4 times a day

[See table below]

Other Information:
- **Phenylketonurics:** contains phenylalanine 2.1 mg per tablet
- one dose lasts 6–8 hours
- store in a dry place at 20–25°C (68–77°F)

Inactive Ingredients: (GRAPE FLAVOR) artificial flavor, aspartame, cellulose acetate phthalate, D&C red no. 30 lake, FD&C blue no. 2 lake, gelatin, magnasweet, magnesium stearate, mannitol, microcrystalline cellulose, silicon dioxide, sodium starch glycolate

Inactive Ingredients: (FRUIT FLAVOR) aspartame, cellulose acetate phthalate, D&C red no. 27 lake, FD&C red no. 40 lake, gelatin, magnasweet, magnesium stearate, mannitol, microcrystalline cellulose, natural and artifical flavors, silicon dioxide, sodium starch glycolate

How Supplied: Blister of 24 (fruit and grape flavors).

CHILDREN'S ADVIL COLD SUSPENSION

Pain Reliever/Fever Reducer/Nasal Decongestant

Active Ingredients:
(in each 5mL teaspoon)
Ibuprofen 100 mg
Pseudoephedrine HCl 15mg

Uses: temporarily relieves these cold, sinus and flu symptoms:
- nasal and sinus congestion • headache
- stuffy nose • sore throat
- minor aches and pains • fever

Warnings:

Allergy alert: Ibuprofen may cause a severe allergic reaction which may include: • hives • facial swelling • asthma (wheezing) • shock

Stomach bleeding warning: Taking more than recommended may cause stomach bleeding

Sore throat warning: Severe or persistent sore throat or sore throat accompanied by high fever, headache, nausea, and vomiting may be serious. Consult a doctor right away. Do not use more than 2 days or give to children under 3 years of age unless directed by a doctor.

Do not use:
- if the child has ever had an allergic reaction to any pain reliever, fever reducer or nasal decongestant
- in a child who is taking a prescription monoamine oxidase inhibitor (MAOI) (certain drugs for depression, psychiatric, or emotional conditions, or Parkinson's disease), or for 2 weeks after stopping the MAOI drug. If you do not know if your child's prescription drug contains an MAOI, ask a doctor or pharmacist before giving this product.

Ask a doctor before use if the child has
- not been drinking fluids
- lost a lot of fluid due to continued vomiting or diarrhea
- problems or serious side effects from taking any pain reliever, fever reducer or nasal decongestant
- stomach problems that last or come back, such as heartburn, upset stomach or pain • diabetes
- high blood pressure, heart or kidney disease or is taking a diuretic
- thyroid disease • ulcers • bleeding problems

Ask a doctor or pharmacist before use if the child is
- under a doctor's care for any continuing medical condition
- taking any other drug
- taking any other product that contains ibuprofen or any other pain reliever/fever reducer
- taking any other product that contains pseudoephedrine or any other nasal decongestant
- taking a prescription product for anticoagulation (blood thinning)

When using this product
- **do not use more than directed**
- give with food or milk if stomach upset occurs

Stop use and ask a doctor if
- an allergic reaction occurs. Seek medical help right away.
- the child does not get any relief within first day (24 hours) of treatment
- fever or pain or nasal congestion gets worse or lasts for more than 3 days
- stomach pain or upset gets worse or lasts
- symptoms continue or get worse
- redness or swelling is present in the painful area
- the child gets nervous, dizzy, sleepless or sleepy
- any new symptoms appear

Keep out of reach of children. In case of overdose, get medical help or contact a Poison Control Center right away.

Directions:
- **do not give more than directed**
- **shake well before using**
- find right dose on chart below. If possible, use weight to dose; otherwise use age.
- if needed, repeat dose every **6 hours**

Dosing Chart

Weight (lb)	Age (yr)	Dose (tablets)
under 24 lb	under 2 yr	ask a doctor
24–35 lb	2–3 yr	2 tablets
36–47 lb	4–5 yr	3 tablets
48–59 lb	6–8 yr	4 tablets
60–71 lb	9–10 yr	5 tablets
72–95 lb	11 yr	6 tablets

- do not use more than **4 times a day**
- replace original bottle cap to maintain child resistance
- measure only with dosing cup provided. Dosing cup to be used with Children's Advil Cold Suspension only. Do not use with other products. Dose lines account for product remaining in cup due to thickness of suspension.

Dosing Chart

Weight (lb)	Age (yr)	Dose (teaspoons)
under 24	under 2 yr	ask a doctor
24–47	2–5 yr	1 teaspoon
48–95	6–11 yr	2 teaspoons

Other Information:
- store a room temperature 20–25°C (68–77°F)
- alcohol free

Inactive Ingredients: carboxymethylcellulose sodium, citric acid, edetate disodium, FD&C blue no. 1, FD&C red no. 40, flavor, glycerin, microcrystalline cellulose, polysorbate 80, purified water, sodium benzoate, sorbitol solution, sucrose, xanthan gum

How Supplied: Bottles of 4 fl. oz. in grape flavor.

CHILDREN'S ADVIL SUSPENSION
Fever Reducer/Pain Reliever

Active Ingredient:
(in each 5 mL)
Ibuprofen 100 mg

Uses: temporarily:
- reduces fever
- relieves minor aches and pains due to the common cold, flu, sore throat, headaches and toothaches

Warnings:
Allergy alert: Ibuprofen may cause a severe allergic reaction which may include:
- hives • asthma (wheezing)
- facial swelling • shock

Stomach bleeding warning: Taking more than recommended may cause stomach bleeding.
Sore throat warning: Severe or persistent sore throat or sore throat accompanied by high fever, headache, nausea, and vomiting may be serious. Consult doctor promptly. Do not use more than 2 days or administer to children under 3 years of age unless directed by doctor.

Do not use if the child has ever had an allergic reaction to any other fever reducer/pain reliever

Ask a doctor before use if the child has
- ulcers
- bleeding problems
- stomach problems that last or come back, such as heartburn, upset stomach or pain
- high blood pressure, heart or kidney disease or is taking a diuretic
- not been drinking fluids
- lost a lot of fluid due to continued vomiting or diarrhea
- problems or serious side effects from taking fever reducers or pain relievers

Ask a doctor or pharmacist before use if the child is
- under a doctor's care for any serious condition
- taking a prescription product for anticoagulation (blood thinning)
- taking any other drug
- taking any other product that contains ibuprofen, or any other pain reliever/fever reducer

When using this product give with food or milk if stomach upset occurs

Stop use and ask a doctor if
- an allergic reaction occurs. Seek medical help right away.
- fever or pain gets worse or lasts more than 3 days
- the child does not get any relief within first day (24 hours) of treatment
- stomach pain or upset gets worse or lasts
- redness or swelling is present in the painful area
- any new symptoms appear

Keep out of reach of children. In case of overdose, get medical help or contact a Poison Control Center right away.

Directions:
- **do not give more than directed**
- **shake well before using**
- find right dose on chart below. If possible, use weight to dose; otherwise use age.
- repeat dose every 6–8 hours, if needed
- do not use more than 4 times a day
- measure only with the blue dosing cup provided. Blue dosing cup to be used with Children's Advil Suspension only. Do not use with other products. Dose lines account for product remaining in cup due to thickness of suspension.
[See table below]

Other Information:
- one dose lasts 6–8 hours
- store at 20–25°C (68–77°F)

Inactive Ingredients: (FRUIT FLAVOR) artifical flavors, carboxymethylcellulose sodium, citric acid, edetate disodium, FD&C red no. 40, glycerin, microcrystalline cellulose, polysorbate 80, purified water, sodium benzoate, sorbitol solution, sucrose, xanthan gum

Inactive Ingredients: (GRAPE FLAVOR) artifical flavor, carboxymethylcellulose sodium, citric acid, edetate disodium, FD&C blue no. 1, FD&C red no. 40, glycerin, microcrystalline cellulose, polysorbate 80, purified water, sodium benzoate, sorbitol solution, sucrose, xanthan gum

Inactive Ingredients: (BLUE RASPBERRY FLAVOR) carboxymethylcellulose sodium, citric acid, edetate disodium, FD&C blue no. 1, flavors, glycerin, microcrystalline cellulose, polysorbate 80, purified water, sodium benzoate, sodium citrate, sorbitol solution, sucrose, xanthan gum

How Supplied: Bottles of 2 fl. oz. and 4 fl. oz. in grape, fruit, and blue raspberry flavors.

INFANTS' ADVIL CONCENTRATED DROPS
Fever Reducer/Pain Reliever

Active Ingredient:
(in each 1.25 mL)
Ibuprofen 50 mg

Uses: temporarily:
- reduces fever
- relieves minor aches and pains due to the common cold, flu, headaches and toothaches

Warnings:

Allergy Alert: Ibuprofen may cause a severe allergic reaction which may include:
- hives • asthma (wheezing)
- facial swelling • shock

Stomach bleeding warning: Taking more than recommended may cause stomach bleeding.

Do not use if the child has ever had an allergic reaction to any other fever reducer/pain reliever

Ask a doctor before use if the child has
- not been drinking fluids
- lost a lot of fluid due to continued vomiting or diarrhea
- problems or serious side effects from taking fever reducers or pain relievers
- ulcers

Continued on next page

Dosing Chart

Weight (lb)	Age (yr)	Dose (tsp)
under 24 lb	under 2 yr	ask a doctor
24–35 lb	2–3 yr	1 tsp
36–47 lb	4–5 yr	1½ tsp
48–59 lb	6–8 yr	2 tsp
60–71 lb	9–10 yr	2½ tsp
72–95 lb	11 yr	3 tsp

Infant's Advil Drops—Cont.

- bleeding problems
- stomach problems that last or come back, such as heartburn, upset stomach or pain
- high blood pressure, heart or kidney disease or is taking a diuretic

Ask a doctor or pharmacist before use if the child is

- under a doctor's care for any serious condition
- taking any other drug
- taking any other product that contains ibuprofen, or any other pain reliever/fever reducer
- taking a prescription product for anticoagulation (blood thinning)

When using this product give with food or milk if upset stomach occurs

Stop use and ask a doctor if

- an allergic reaction occurs. Seek medical help right away.
- fever or pain gets worse or lasts more than 3 days
- the child does not get any relief within first day (24 hours) of treatment
- stomach pain or upset gets worse or lasts
- redness or swelling is present in the painful area
- any new symptoms appear

Keep out of reach of children. In case of overdose, get medical help or contact a Poison Control Center right away.

Directions:

- **do not give more than directed**
- **shake well before using**
- find right dose on chart below. If possible, use weight to dose; otherwise use age.
- repeat dose every 6–8 hours, if needed
- do not use more than 4 times a day
- measure with the dosing device provided. Do not use with any other device.

[See table below]

Other Information:

- one dose lasts 6–8 hours
- store at 20–25°C (68–77°F)

Inactive Ingredients: (FRUIT FLAVOR) artificial flavors, carboxymethylcellulose sodium, citric acid, edetate disodium, FD&C red no. 40, glycerin, microcrystalline cellulose, polysorbate 80, purified water, sodium benzoate, sorbitol solution, sucrose, xanthan gum

Inactive Ingredients: (GRAPE FLAVOR) artificial flavor, carboxymethylcellulose sodium, citric acid, edetate disodium, FD&C blue no. 1, FD&C red no. 40, glycerin, microcrystalline cellulose, polysorbate 80, purified water, sodium benzoate, sorbitol solution, sucrose, xanthan gum

How Supplied: Bottles of ½ fl. oz. in grape and fruit flavors.

ALAVERT
Loratadine orally disintegrating tablets
Loratadine swallow tablets
Antihistamine

Active Ingredient (in each tablet):
Loratadine 10 mg

Uses:

- temporarily relieves these symptoms due to hay fever or other upper respiratory allergies:
  - runny nose • sneezing • itchy, watery eyes
  - itching of the nose or throat

Warnings:

Do not use if you have ever had an allergic reaction to this product or any of its ingredients

Ask a doctor before use if you have liver or kidney disease. Your doctor should determine if you need a different dose.

When using this product do not use more than directed. Taking more than recommended may cause drowsiness.

Stop use and ask a doctor if an allergic reaction to this product occurs. Seek medical help right away.

If pregnant or breast-feeding, ask a health professional before use.

Keep out of reach of children. In case of overdose, get medical help or contact a Poison Control Center right away.

Directions:

- tablet melts in mouth. Can be taken with or without water.

Age	Dose
adults and children 6 years and over	1 tablet daily; do not use more than 1 tablet daily
children under 6	ask a doctor
consumers who have liver or kidney disease	ask a doctor

Other Information:

- Phenylketonurics: Contains Phenylalanine 8.4 mg per tablet
- store at 20–25°C (68–77°F)
- keep in a dry place

Inactive Ingredients (Loratadine orally disintegrating tablets): artificial & natural flavor, aspartame, citric acid, colloidal silicon dioxide, corn syrup solids, crospovidone, magnesium stearate, mannitol, microcrystalline cellulose, modified food starch, sodium bicarbonate

Inactive Ingredients (Loratadine swallow tablets): lactose monohydrate, magnesium stearate, microcrystalline cellulose, sodium starch glycolate

How Supplied: Loratadine orally disintegrating tablets in packages of 6, 12, 24 & 48

How Supplied: Loratadine swallow tablets in packages of 15 and 30 tablets

---

ALAVERT ALLERGY & SINUS D-12 HOUR TABLETS
Loratadine/Pseudoephedrine Sulfate Extended Release Tablets
Antihistamine/Nasal Decongestant

Active Ingredients (in each tablet):
Loratadine 5 mg
Pseudoephedrine sulfate 120 mg

Uses:

- temporarily relieves these symptoms due to hay fever or other upper respiratory allergies:
  - nasal congestion • runny nose
  - sneezing • itchy, watery eyes
  - itching of the nose or throat
- reduces swelling of nasal passages
- temporarily relieves sinus congestion and pressure
- temporarily restores freer breathing through the nose

Warnings:

Do not use

- if you have ever had an allergic reaction to this product or any of its ingredients
- if you are now taking a prescription monoamine oxidase inhibitor (MAOI) (certain drugs for depression, psychiatric, or emotional conditions, or Parkinson's disease), or for 2 weeks after stopping the MAOI drug. If you do not know if your prescription drug contains an MAOI, ask a doctor or pharmacist before taking this product.

Ask a doctor before use if you have

- heart disease • high blood pressure
- thyroid disease • diabetes
- trouble urinating due to an enlarged prostate gland
- liver or kidney disease. Your doctor should determine if you need a different dose.

When using this product do not take more than directed. Taking more than directed may cause drowsiness.

Stop use and ask a doctor if

- an allergic reaction to this product occurs. Seek medical help right away.
- symptoms do not improve within 7 days or are accompanied by a fever
- nervousness, dizziness or sleeplessness occurs

If pregnant or breast-feeding, ask a health professional before use.

Keep out of reach of children. In case of overdose, get medical help or contact a Poison Control Center right away.

Directions:

- do not divide, crush, chew or dissolve the tablet

Dosing Chart		
Weight (lb)	Age (mos)	Dose (mL)
under 6 mos		ask a doctor
12–17 lb	6–11 mos	1.25 mL
18–23 lb	12–23 mos	1.875 mL

Age	Dose
adults and children 12 years and over	1 tablet every 12 hours; not more than 2 tablets in 24 hours
children under 12 years of age	ask a doctor
consumers with liver or kidney disease	ask a doctor

Other Information:
• store between 15° and 25°C (59° and 77°F)
• keep in a dry place

Inactive Ingredients: croscarmellose sodium, dibasic calcium phosphate, hypromellose, lactose monohydrate, magnesium stearate, pharmaceutical ink, povidone, titanium dioxide

How Supplied: Blister packs of 12 and 24 tablets.

MAXIMUM STRENGTH
ANBESOL® Gel and Liquid
Oral Anesthetic

ANBESOL JUNIOR® Gel
Oral Anesthetic

BABY ANBESOL®
Grape Flavor
Oral Anesthetic

Active Ingredients: Anbesol is an oral anesthetic which is available in a Maximum Strength gel and liquid. Anbesol Junior, available in a gel, is an oral anesthetic. Baby Anbesol, available in a grape-flavored gel, is an oral anesthetic and is alcohol-free.
Maximum Strength Anbesol Gel and Liquid contain Benzocaine 20%.
Anbesol Junior Gel contains Benzocaine 10%.
Baby Anbesol Gel contains Benzocaine 7.5%.

Uses: Maximum Strength Anbesol temporarily relieves pain associated with toothache, canker sores, minor dental procedures, sore gums, braces, and dentures. Anbesol Junior temporarily relieves pain associated with braces, sore gums, canker sores, toothaches, and minor dental procedures. Baby Anbesol Gel temporarily relieves sore gums due to teething in infants and children 4 months of age and older.

Warnings: **Allergy alert:** Do not use these products if you have a history of allergy to local anesthetics such as procaine, butacaine, benzocaine, or other "caine" anesthetics.
Baby Anbesol: **Do not use** to treat fever and nasal congestion. These are not symptoms of teething and may indicate the presence of infection. If these symptoms persist, consult your doctor.

Maximum Strength Anbesol, Anbesol Junior and Baby Anbesol:
When using this product
• avoid contact with the eyes
• do not exceed recommended dosage
• do not use for more than 7 days unless directed by a doctor/dentist
Stop use and ask a doctor if
• sore mouth symptoms do not improve in 7 days
• irritation, pain, or redness persists or worsens
• swelling, rash, or fever develops
Keep out of reach of children. If more than used for pain is accidentally swallowed, get medical help or contact a Poison Control Center right away.

Directions: Maximum Strength Anbesol: Gel—
• to open tube, cut tip of the tube on score mark with scissors
• adults and children 2 years of age and older: apply to the affected area up to 4 times daily or as directed by a doctor/dentist
• children under 12 years of age: adult supervision should be given in the use of this product
• children under 2 years of age: consult a doctor/dentist
• for denture irritation:
  • apply thin layer to the affected area
  • do not reinsert dental work until irritation/pain is relieved
  • rinse mouth well before reinserting
Do not refrigerate.
Tamper-Evident: Safety Sealed Tube. Do Not Use if tube tip is cut prior to opening.
Liquid—
• adults and children 2 years of age and older:
  • wipe liquid on with cotton, or cotton swab, or fingertip
  • apply to the affected area up to 4 times daily or as directed by a doctor/dentist
• children under 12 years of age: adult supervision should be given in the use of this product
• children under 2 years of age; consult a doctor/dentist
Tamper-Evident: Do Not Use if plastic blister or backing material is broken or if backing material is separated from the plastic.

Anbesol Junior Gel:
• to open tube, cut tip of the tube on score mark with scissors
• adults and children 2 years of age and older: apply to the affected area up to 4 times daily or as directed by a doctor/dentist
• children under 12 years of age: adult supervision should be given in the use of this product
• children under 2 years of age: consult a doctor/dentist
Tamper-Evident: Safety Sealed Tube. Do Not Use if tube tip is cut prior to opening.

Grape Baby Anbesol Gel:
• to open tube, cut tip of the tube on score mark with scissors
• children 4 months of age and older: apply to the affected area not more than 4 times daily or as directed by a doctor/dentist

• infants under 4 months of age: no recommended dosage or treatment except under the advice and supervision of a doctor/dentist
Tamper-Evident: Safety Sealed Tube. Do Not Use if tube tip is cut prior to opening.

Inactive Ingredients:
Maximum Strength Gel: benzyl alcohol, carbomer 934P, D&C yellow no. 10, FD&C blue no. 1, FD&C red no. 40, flavor, glycerin, methylparaben, polyethylene glycol, propylene glycol, saccharin.
Maximum Strength Liquid: benzyl alcohol, D&C yellow no. 10, FD&C blue no. 1, FD&C red no. 40, flavor, methylparaben, polyethylene glycol, propylene glycol, saccharin.
Junior Gel: artificial flavor, benzyl alcohol, carbomer 934P, D&C red no. 33, glycerin, methylparaben, polyethylene glycol, potassium acesulfame
Grape Baby Gel: benzoic acid, carbomer 934P, D&C red no. 33, edetate disodium, FD&C blue no. 1, flavor, glycerin, methylparaben, polyethylene glycol, propylparaben, saccharin, water

Storage: Store at 20–25°C (68–77°F)

How Supplied: All Gels in .25 oz (7.1 g) tubes, Maximum Strength Liquid in .31 fl oz (9 mL) bottle.

ANBESOL COLD SORE THERAPY
Fever blister/Cold sore treatment

Active Ingredients:
Allantoin 1%,
Benzocaine 20%,
Camphor 3%,
White petrolatum 64.9%

Uses:
• temporarily relieves pain associated with fever blisters and cold sores
• relieves dryness and softens fever blisters and cold sores

Warnings: **For external use only**
Allergy alert: Do not use this product if you have a history of allergy to local anesthetics such as procaine, butacaine, benzocaine, or other "caine" anesthetics.
Do not use over deep or puncture wounds, infections, or lacerations. Consult a doctor.
When using this product • avoid contact with the eyes
• do not exceed recommended dosage
Stop use and ask a doctor if
• condition worsens
• symptoms persist for more than 7 days
• symptoms clear up and occur again within a few days
Keep out of reach of children. If swallowed, get medical help or contact a Poison Control Center right away.

Directions:
• to open tube, cut tip of the tube on score mark with scissors
• adults and children 2 years of age and older: apply to the affected area not more than 3 to 4 times daily

Continued on next page

Anbesol Cold Sore—Cont.

- children under 12 years of age: adult supervision should be given in the use of this product
- children under 2 years of age: consult a doctor

Tamper-Evident:
Safety Sealed Tube.
Do Not Use if tube tip is cut prior to opening.

Inactive Ingredients: aloe extract, benzyl alcohol, butylparaben, glyceryl stearate, isocetyl stearate, menthol, methylparaben, propylparaben, sodium lauryl sulfate, vitamin E, white wax

Other Information:
- store at 20–25°C (68–77°F)

How Supplied: 0.25 oz Tube

CHILDREN'S DIMETAPP® Cold & Allergy Elixir
Nasal Decongestant, Antihistamine

Active Ingredients:
Each 5 mL (1 teaspoonful) contains:
Brompheniramine Maleate, USP 1 mg
Pseudoephedrine Hydrochloride, USP 15 mg

Uses:
- temporarily relieves nasal congestion due to the common cold, hay fever or other upper respiratory allergies, or associated with sinusitis
- temporarily relieves these symptoms due to hay fever (allergic rhinitis):
  - runny nose
  - sneezing
  - itchy, watery eyes
  - itching of the nose or throat
- temporarily restores freer breathing through the nose

Warnings:
Do not use if you are now taking a prescription monoamine oxidase inhibitor (MAOI) (certain drugs for depression, psychiatric, or emotional conditions, or Parkinson's disease), or for 2 weeks after stopping the MAOI drug. If you do not know if your prescription drug contains an MAOI, ask a doctor or pharmacist before taking this product.

Ask a doctor before use if you have
- heart disease
- high blood pressure
- thyroid disease
- diabetes
- trouble urinating due to an enlarged prostate gland
- glaucoma
- a breathing problem such as emphysema or chronic bronchitis

Ask a doctor or pharmacist before use if you are taking sedatives or tranquilizers.

When using this product
- **do not use more than directed**
- drowsiness may occur
- avoid alcoholic beverages
- alcohol, sedatives, and tranquilizers may increase drowsiness
- be careful when driving a motor vehicle or operating machinery
- excitability may occur, especially in children

Stop use and ask a doctor if
- you get nervous, dizzy, or sleepless
- symptoms do not get better within 7 days or are accompanied by fever

If pregnant or breast-feeding, ask a health professional before use.

Keep out of reach of children. In case of overdose, get medical help or contact a Poison Control Center right away.

Directions:
- do not take more than 4 doses in any 24-hour period

age	dose
adults and children 12 years and over	4 tsp every 4 hours
children 6 to under 12 years	2 tsp every 4 hours
children under 6 years	ask a doctor

Each teaspoon contains: sodium 3 mg.
Store at 20–25°C (68–77°F).
Dosage cup provided.

Inactive Ingredients: artificial flavor, citric acid, FD&C blue no. 1, FD&C red no. 40, glycerin, propylene glycol, purified water, sodium benzoate, sodium citrate, sorbitol solution, sucralose

How Supplied: Purple, grape-flavored liquid in bottles of 4 fl oz, 8 fl oz, and 12 fl oz. Not a USP elixir.

CHILDREN'S DIMETAPP® DM COLD & COUGH Elixir
Nasal Decongestant, Antihistamine, Cough Suppressant

Active Ingredients: Each 5 mL (1 teaspoonful) of DIMETAPP DM Elixir contains

Brompheniramine Maleate, USP 1 mg
Dextromethorphan Hydrobromide, USP 5 mg
Pseudoephedrine Hydrochloride, USP 15 mg

Uses:
- temporarily relieves cough due to minor throat and bronchial irritation occurring with a cold, and nasal congestion due to the common cold, hay fever or other upper respiratory allergies, or associated with sinusitis
- temporarily relieves these symptoms due to hay fever (allergic rhinitis):
  - runny nose
  - sneezing
  - itchy, watery eyes
  - itching of the nose or throat
- temporarily restores freer breathing through the nose

Warnings:
Do not use if you are now taking a prescription monoamine oxidase inhibitor (MAOI) (certain drugs for depression,

psychiatric, or emotional conditions, or Parkinson's disease), or for 2 weeks after stopping the MAOI drug. If you do not know if your prescription drug contains an MAOI, ask a doctor or pharmacist before taking this product.

Ask a doctor before use if you have
- heart disease
- high blood pressure
- thyroid disease
- diabetes
- trouble urinating due to an enlarged prostate gland
- glaucoma
- cough that occurs with too much phlegm (mucus)
- a breathing problem or persistent or chronic cough that lasts such as occurs with smoking, asthma, chronic bronchitis, or emphysema

Ask a doctor or pharmacist before use if you are taking sedatives or tranquilizers.

When using this product
- **do not use more than directed**
- may cause marked drowsiness
- avoid alcoholic beverages
- alcohol, sedatives, and tranquilizers may increase drowsiness
- be careful when driving a motor vehicle or operating machinery
- excitability may occur, especially in children

Stop use and ask a doctor if
- you get nervous, dizzy, or sleepless
- symptoms do not get better within 7 days or are accompanied by fever
- cough lasts more than 7 days, comes back, or is accompanied by fever, rash, or persistent headache. These could be signs of a serious condition

If pregnant or breast-feeding, ask a health professional before use.

Keep out of reach of children. In case of overdose, get medical help or contact a Poison Control Center right away.

Directions:
- do not take more than 4 doses in any 24-hour period

Age	Dose
adults and children 12 years and over	4 tsp every 4 hours
children 6 to under 12 years	2 tsp every 4 hours
children under 6 years	ask a doctor

Store at 20–25°C (68–77°F). Dosage cap provided.

Inactive Ingredients: artificial flavor, citric acid, FD&C blue no. 1, FD&C red no. 40, glycerin, high fructose corn syrup, propylene glycol, saccharin sodium, sodium benzoate, sorbitol, water

How Supplied: Red, grape-flavored liquid in bottles of 4 fl oz and 8 fl oz. Not a USP Elixir.

CHILDREN'S DIMETAPP® LONG ACTING COUGH PLUS COLD SYRUP
Cough suppressant/Nasal decongestant

Active Ingredients (in each 5 mL tsp):
Dextromethorphan HBr, USP 7.5 mg
Pseudoephedrine HCl, USP 15 mg

Uses:
- temporarily relieves these symptoms occurring with a cold:
  - nasal congestion
  - cough due to minor throat and bronchial irritation

Warnings:
Do not use if you are now taking a prescription monoamine oxidase inhibitor (MAOI) (certain drugs for depression, psychiatric, or emotional conditions, or Parkinson's disease), or for 2 weeks after stopping the MAOI drug. If you do not know if your prescription drug contains an MAOI, ask a doctor or pharmacist before taking this product.

Ask a doctor before use if you have
- heart disease • high blood pressure
- thyroid disease • diabetes
- trouble urinating due to an enlarged prostate gland
- cough that occurs with too much phlegm (mucus)
- cough that lasts or is chronic such as occurs with smoking, asthma, or emphysema

When using this product do not use more than directed.

Stop use and ask a doctor if
- you get nervous, dizzy, or sleepless
- symptoms do not get better within 7 days or are accompanied by fever
- cough lasts more than 7 days, comes back, or is accompanied by fever, rash, or persistent headache. These could be signs of a serious condition.

If pregnant or breast-feeding, ask a health professional before use.

Keep out of reach of children. In case of overdose, get medical help or contact a Poison Control Center right away.

Directions:
- do not take more than 4 doses in any 24-hour period
- repeat every 6 hours

age	dose
12 years and older	4 tsp every 6 hours
6 to under 12 years	2 tsp every 6 hours
2 to under 6 years	1 tsp every 6 hours
under 2 years	ask a doctor

Other Information: • store at 20–25°C (68–77°F)
• dosage cup provided

Inactive Ingredients: citric acid, FD&C red no. 40, flavor, glycerin, high fructose corn syrup, propylene glycol, purified water, saccharin sodium, sodium benzoate, sodium chloride, sodium citrate

How Supplied: Bottles of 4 fl. oz.

DIMETAPP® Infant Drops Decongestant
Nasal Decongestant

Alcohol-Free

Active Ingredient: Each 0.8 mL contains: 7.5 mg Pseudoephedrine Hydrochloride, USP.

Uses: temporarily relieves nasal congestion due to the common cold, hay fever, other upper respiratory allergies, or associated with sinusitis.

Warnings:
Do not use in a child who is taking a prescription monoamine oxidase inhibitor (MAOI) (certain drugs for depression, psychiatric, or emotional conditions, or Parkinson's disease), or for 2 weeks after stopping the MAOI drug. If you do not know if your child's prescription drug contains an MAOI, ask a doctor or pharmacist before giving this product.

Ask a doctor before use if your child has
- heart disease
- high blood pressure
- thyroid disease
- diabetes

When using this product
- do not use more than directed

Stop use and ask a doctor if
- your child gets nervous, dizzy, or sleepless
- symptoms do not get better within 7 days or are accompanied by fever

Keep out of reach of children. In case of overdose, get medical help or contact a Poison Control Center right away.

Directions:
- do not give more than 4 doses in any 24-hour period
- children 2 to 3 years: 1.6 mL every 4 to 6 hours or as directed by a physician
- children under 2 years: ask a doctor
- measure with the dosing device provided. Do not use with any other device.

Storage: Store at 20-25°C (68-77°F).

Inactive Ingredients: caramel, citric acid, D&C red no. 33, FD&C blue no. 1, flavors, glycerin, high fructose corn syrup, maltol, menthol, polyethylene glycol, propylene glycol, sodium benzoate, sorbitol, sucrose, water

How Supplied: ½ oz bottle with oral dosing device.

DIMETAPP®
Infant Drops Decongestant Plus Cough
Nasal decongestant/cough suppressant
Alcohol-Free/non-staining

Active Ingredients: Each 0.8 mL contains: 2.5 mg Dextromethorphan Hydrobromide, USP; 7.5 mg Pseudoephedrine Hydrochloride, USP.

Indications: Temporarily relieves cough occurring with the common cold and temporarily relieves nasal congestion due to the common cold, hay fever, or other upper respiratory allergies, or associated with sinusitis

Warnings:
Do not use in a child who is taking a prescription monoamine oxidase inhibitor (MAOI) (certain drugs for depression, psychiatric, or emotional conditions, or Parkinson's disease), or for 2 weeks after stopping the MAOI drug. If you do not know if your child's prescription drug contains an MAOI, ask a doctor or pharmacist before giving this product.

Ask a doctor before use if your child has
- heart disease
- high blood pressure
- thyroid disease
- diabetes
- cough that occurs with too much phlegm (mucus)
- cough that lasts or is chronic such as occurs with asthma

When using this product
- do not use more than directed

Stop use and ask a doctor if
- your child gets nervous, dizzy, or sleepless
- symptoms do not get better within 7 days or are accompanied by fever
- cough lasts more than 7 days, comes back, or is accompanied by fever, rash, or persistent headache. These could be signs of a serious condition.

Keep out of reach of children. In case of overdose, get medical help or contact a Poison Control Center right away.

Directions: do not give more than 4 doses in any 24-hour period
- children 2–3 years: 1.6 mL every 4–6 hours or as directed by a physician
- children under 2 years: ask a doctor
- measure with the dosing device provided. Do not use with any other device.

Storage: Store at 20–25°C (68–77°F).

Inactive Ingredients: citric acid, flavors, glycerin, high fructose corn syrup, maltol, menthol, polyethylene glycol, propylene glycol, sodium benzoate, sorbitol, sucrose, water.

How Supplied: ½ oz bottle with oral dosing device.

FIBERCON®
Calcium Polycarbophil
Bulk-Forming Laxative

Active Ingredient
(in each caplet):
Calcium polycarbophil 625 mg (equivalent to 500 mg polycarbophil)

Continued on next page

Fibercon—Cont.

Uses:
- relieves constipation to help restore and maintain regularity
- this product generally produces bowel movement in 12 to 72 hours

Warnings:
Choking: Taking this product without adequate fluid may cause it to swell and block your throat or esophagus and may cause choking. Do not take this product if you have difficulty in swallowing. If you experience chest pain, vomiting, or difficulty in swallowing or breathing after taking this product, seek immediate medical attention.

Ask a doctor before use if you have
- abdominal pain, nausea, or vomiting
- a sudden change in bowel habits that persists over a period of 2 weeks

Ask a doctor or pharmacist before use if you are taking any other drug. Take this product 2 or more hours before or after other drugs. All laxatives may affect how other drugs work.

When using this product
- do not use for more than 7 days unless directed by a doctor
- do not take caplets more than 4 times in a 24 hour period unless directed by a doctor

Stop use and ask a doctor if rectal bleeding occurs or if you fail to have a bowel movement after use of this or any other laxative These could be signs of a serious condition.

Keep out of reach of children. In case of overdose, get medical help or contact a Poison Control Center right away.

Directions:
- take each dose of this product with at least 8 ounces (a full glass) of water or other fluid. Taking this product without enough liquid may cause choking. See choking warning
- FiberCon works naturally so continued use for one to three days is normally required to provide full benefit. Dosage may vary according to diet, exercise, previous laxative use or severity of constipation.
[See first table above]

Inactive Ingredients: calcium carbonate, caramel, crospovidone, hypromellose, light mineral oil, magnesium stearate, microcrystalline cellulose, povidone, silicon dioxide, sodium lauryl sulfate
Each caplet contains: 122 mg calcium.
Storage Protect contents from moisture. Store at 20–25°C (68–77°F)

How Supplied: Film-coated scored caplets.
Package of 36 caplets, and
Bottles of 60, 90, 140 and 200 caplets.

FREELAX
Magnesium hydroxide
Saline laxative

Active Ingredient (in each caplet):
Magnesium hydroxide 1200 mg (equivalent to magnesium 500 mg)

Age	Recommended dose	Daily maximum
adults & children 12 years of age and over	2 caplets once a day	up to 4 times a day
children under 12 years	consult a physician	

age	recommended dose	daily maximum
adults and children 12 years of age and over	2 caplets	up to 4 caplets a day
children under 12 years	consult a physician	

Uses:
for relief of occasional constipation (irregularity)
this product generally produces bowel movement in ½ to 6 hours

Warnings:
Ask a doctor before us if you have
- kidney disease
- been told to follow a magnesium-restricted diet
- abdominal pain, nausea, or vomiting
- a sudden change in bowel habits that persists over a period of 2 weeks

Ask a doctor or pharmacist before use if you are taking any other drug. Take this product 2 or more hours before or after other drugs. All laxatives may affect how other drugs work.

When using this product do not use for more than 7 days unless directed by a doctor

Stop use and ask a doctor if rectal bleeding occurs or if you fail to have a bowel movement after use of this or any other laxative. These could be signs of a serious condition.

If pregnant or breast-feeding, ask a health professional before use.

Keep out of reach of children. In case of overdose, get medical help or contact a Poison Control Center right away.

Directions:
Take each dose of this product with at least 8 ounces (a full glass) of water or other fluid
[See table above]

Other Information:
- **each caplet contains:** 500 mg magnesium
- store at 20–25°C (68–77°F)

Inactive Ingredients: crospovidone, D&C yellow no. 10 aluminum lake, FD&C yellow no. 6 aluminum lake, glyceryl behenate, hydroxypropyl cellulose, hypromellose, microcrystalline cellulose, polydextrose, polyethylene glycol, silicon dioxide, titanium dioxide, triacetin

How Supplied:
packages of 30 caplets

PREPARATION H®
Hemorrhoidal Ointment and Cream
PREPARATION H®
Hemorrhoidal Suppositories
PREPARATION H®
Hemorrhoidal Cooling Gel

Active Ingredients: Preparation H is available in ointment, cream, gel, and suppository product forms. The **Ointment** contains Petrolatum 71.9%, Mineral Oil 14%, Shark Liver Oil 3% and Phenylephrine HCl 0.25%.
The **Cream** contains Petrolatum 18%, Glycerin 12%, Shark Liver Oil 3% and Phenylephrine HCl 0.25%.
The **Suppositories** contain Cocoa Butter 85.5%, Shark Liver Oil 3%, and Phenylephrine HCl 0.25%.
The **Cooling Gel** contains Phenylephrine HCl 0.25% and Witch Hazel 50%.

Uses: Preparation H Ointment, Cream, and Suppositories
- help relieve the local itching and discomfort associated with hemorrhoids
- temporarily shrink hemorrhoidal tissue and relieve burning
- temporarily provide a coating for relief of anorectal discomforts
- temporarily protect the inflamed, irritated anorectal surface to help make bowel movements less painful
Cooling Gel
- helps relieve the local itching and discomfort associated with hemorrhoids
- temporarily relieves irritation and burning
- temporarily shrinks hemorrhoidal tissue
- aids in protecting irritated anorectal areas

Warnings:
For all product forms:
Ask a doctor before use if you have
- heart disease
- high blood pressure
- thyroid disease
- diabetes
- difficulty in urination due to enlargement of the prostate gland

Ask a doctor or pharmacist before use if you are presently taking a prescription drug for high blood pressure or depression.

When using this product do not exceed the recommended daily dosage unless directed by a doctor.

Stop use and ask a doctor if
- bleeding occurs
- condition worsens or does not improve within 7 days

If pregnant or breast-feeding, ask a health professional before use.

Keep out of reach of children. If swallowed, get medical help or contact a Poison Control Center right away.

Ointment: Stop use and ask a doctor if introduction of applicator into the rectum causes additional pain. For external and/or intrarectal use only.

Cream/Cooling Gel: For external use only. Do not put into the rectum by using fingers or any mechanical device or applicator.

Suppositories: For rectal use only.

Directions:

Ointment—
- adults: when practical, cleanse the affected area by patting or blotting with an appropriate cleansing wipe. Gently dry by patting or blotting with a tissue or a soft cloth before applying ointment.
- when first opening the tube, puncture foil seal with top end of cap
- apply to the affected area up to 4 times daily, especially at night, in the morning or after each bowel movement
- intrarectal use:
  - remove cover from applicator, attach applicator to tube, lubricate applicator well and gently insert applicator into the rectum
  - thoroughly cleanse applicator after each use and replace cover
- also apply ointment to external area
- regular use provides continual therapy for relief of symptoms
- children under 12 years of age: ask a doctor

Tamper-Evident: Do Not Use if tube seal under cap embossed with "H" is broken or missing.

Cream—
- adults: when practical, cleanse the affected area by patting or blotting with an appropriate cleansing wipe. Gently dry by patting or blotting with a tissue or a soft cloth before applying cream.
- when first opening the tube, puncture foil seal with top end of cap
- apply externally or in the lower portion of the anal canal only
- apply externally to the affected area up to 4 times daily, especially at night, in the morning or after each bowel movement
- for application in the lower anal canal: remove cover from dispensing cap. Attach dispensing cap to tube. Lubricate dispensing cap well, then gently insert dispensing cap partway into the anus.
- thoroughly cleanse dispensing cap after each use and replace cover
- children under 12 years of age: ask a doctor

Tamper-Evident: Do Not Use if tube seal under cap embossed with "H" is broken or missing.

Suppositories—
- adults: when practical, cleanse the affected area by patting or blotting with an appropriate cleansing wipe. Gently dry by patting or blotting with a tissue or a soft cloth before insertion of this product.
- detach one suppository from the strip; remove the foil wrapper before inserting into the rectum as follows:
  - hold suppository with rounded end up
  - carefully separate foil tabs by inserting tip of fingernail at end marked "peel down"
  - slowly and evenly peel apart (do not tear) foil by pulling tabs down both sides, to expose the suppository
  - remove exposed suppository from wrapper

- insert one suppository into the rectum up to 4 times daily, especially at night, in the morning or after each bowel movement
- children under 12 years of age: ask a doctor

Tamper-Evident: Individually quality sealed for your protection. Do Not Use if foil imprinted "PREPARATION H" is torn or damaged.

Cooling Gel—
- adults: when practical, cleanse the affected area by patting or blotting with an appropriate cleansing wipe. Gently dry by patting or blotting with a tissue or a soft cloth before applying gel.
- when first opening the tube, puncture foil seal with top end of cap
- apply externally to the affected area up to 4 times daily, especially at night, in the morning or after each bowel movement
- children under 12 years of age: ask a doctor

Tamper-Evident: Do Not Use if tube seal under cap embossed with "H" is broken or missing.

Inactive Ingredients: Ointment— benzoic acid, BHA, BHT, corn oil, glycerin, lanolin, lanolin alcohol, methylparaben, paraffin, propylparaben, thyme oil, tocopherol, water, wax

Cream— BHA, carboxymethylcellulose sodium, cetyl alcohol, citric acid, edetate disodium, glyceryl oleate, glyceryl stearate, lanolin, methylparaben, propyl gallate, propylene glycol, propylparaben, simethicone, sodium benzoate, sodium lauryl sulfate, stearyl alcohol, tocopherol, water, xanthan gum.

Suppositories— methylparaben, propylparaben, starch

Cooling Gel— aloe barbadensis gel, benzophenone-4, edetate disodium, hydroxyethylcellulose, methylparaben, polysorbate 80, propylene glycol, propylparaben, sodium citrate, vitamin E, water

Storage: Store at 20–25°C (68–77°F).

How Supplied: Ointment: Net Wt. 1 oz and 2 oz **Cream:** Net Wt. 0.9 oz and 1.8 oz **Suppositories:** 12's, 24's and 48's. **Cooling Gel:** Net Wt. 0.9 oz and 1.8 oz

---

PREPARATION H HYDROCORTISONE CREAM
Anti-itch cream

Active Ingredient:
Hydrocortisone 1%

Uses:
- temporary relief of external anal itching
- temporary relief of itching associated with minor skin irritations and rashes
- other uses of this product should be only under the advice and supervision of a doctor

Warnings:
For external use only
Do not use for the treatment of diaper rash. Consult a doctor.

When using this product
- avoid contact with the eyes
- do not exceed the recommended daily dosage unless directed by a doctor
- do not put into the rectum by using fingers or any mechanical device or applicator

Stop use and ask a doctor if
- bleeding occurs
- condition worsens
- symptoms persist for more than 7 days or clear up and occur again within a few days. Do not begin use of any other hydrocortisone product unless you have consulted a doctor.

Keep out of reach of children. If swallowed, get medical help or contact a Poison Control Center right away.

Directions:
- adults: when practical, cleanse the affected area by patting or blotting with an appropriate cleansing wipe. Gently dry by patting or blotting with a tissue or soft cloth before application of this product.
- when first opening the tube, puncture foil seal with top end of cap
- adults and children 12 years of age and older: apply to the affected area not more than 3 to 4 times daily
- children under 12 years of age: do not use, consult a doctor

Tamper-Evident: Do Not Use if tube seal under cap embossed with "H" is broken or missing.

Inactive Ingredients: BHA, carboxymethylcellulose sodium, cetyl alcohol, citric acid, edetate disodium, glycerin, glyceryl oleate, glyceryl stearate, lanolin, methylparaben, petrolatum, propyl gallate, propylene glycol, propylparaben, simethicone, sodium benzoate, sodium lauryl sulfate, stearyl alcohol, water, xanthan gum.

Storage: Store at 20–25 °C (68–77 °F)

How Supplied: 0.9 oz. tubes

PREPARATION H®
MEDICATED WIPES

Active Ingredient: Witch Hazel 50%.

Uses:
- helps relieve the local itching and discomfort associated with hemorrhoids
- temporary relief of irritation and burning
- aids in protecting irritated anorectal areas
- **for vaginal care**—cleanse the area by gently wiping, patting or blotting. Repeat as needed.
- **for use as a moist compress**—if necessary, first cleanse the area as described below. Fold wipe to desired size and place in contact with tissue for a soothing and cooling effect. Leave in place for up to 15 minutes and repeat as needed.

Warnings:
For external use only
When using this product
- do not exceed the recommended daily dosage unless directed by a doctor
- do not put this product into the rectum by using fingers or any mechanical device or applicator

Continued on next page

Preparation H Wipes—Cont.

Stop use and ask a doctor if
• bleeding occurs
• condition worsens or does not improve within 7 days

If pregnant or breast-feeding, ask a health professional before use. **Keep out of reach of children.** If swallowed, get medical help or contact a Poison Control Center right away.

Directions:
• remove tab on right side of wipes pouch label and peel back to open
• grab the top wipe at the edge of the center fold and pull out of pouch
• carefully reseal label on pouch after each use to retain moistness
• adults: unfold wipe and cleanse the area by gently wiping, patting or blotting. If necessary, repeat until all matter is removed from the area.
• use up to 6 times daily or after each bowel movement and before applying topical hemorrhoidal treatments
• children under 12 years of age: consult a doctor
• store at 20–25°C (68–77°F)
• for best results, flush only one or two wipes at a time
Tamper-Evident: Pouch quality sealed for your protection. Do Not Use if tear strip imprinted "Safety Sealed" is torn or missing

Inactive Ingredients: aloe barbadensis gel, capryl/capramidopropyl betaine, citric acid, diazolidinyl urea, glycerin, methylparaben, propylene glycol, propylparaben, sodium citrate, water.

How Supplied: Containers of 48 wipes. Refills of 48 wipes. 8 count travel pack.

PRIMATENE® Mist
Epinephrine Inhalation Aerosol
Bronchodilator

Active Ingredient: (in each inhalation)
Epinephrine 0.22 mg

Uses:
• temporarily relieves shortness of breath, tightness of chest, and wheezing due to bronchial asthma
• eases breathing for asthma patients by reducing spasms of bronchial muscles

Warnings:
For inhalation only
Do not use
• unless a doctor has said you have asthma
• if you are now taking a prescription monoamine oxidase inhibitor (MAOI) (certain drugs for depression, psychiatric, or emotional conditions, or Parkinson's disease), or for 2 weeks after stopping the MAOI drug If you do not know if your prescription drug contains an MAOI, ask a doctor or pharmacist before taking this product
Ask a doctor before use if you have
• heart disease • thyroid disease
• diabetes • high blood pressure
• ever been hospitalized for asthma
• trouble urinating due to an enlarged prostate gland

Ask a doctor or pharmacist before use if you are taking any prescription drug for asthma
When using this product
• overuse may cause nervousness, rapid heart beat, and heart problems
• do not continue to use, but seek medical assistance immediately if symptoms are not relieved within 20 minutes or become worse
• do not puncture or throw into incinerator. Contents under pressure.
• do not use or store near open flame or heat above 120°F (49°C). May cause bursting.
Contains CFC 12, 114, substances which harm public health and environment by destroying ozone in the upper atmosphere
If pregnant or breast-feeding, ask a health professional before use.
Keep out of reach of children. In case of overdose, get medical help or contact a Poison Control Center right away.

Directions:
• do not use more often or at higher doses unless directed by a doctor
• supervise children using this product
• adults and children 4 years and over: start with one inhalation, then wait at least 1 minute. If not relieved, use once more. Do not use again for at least 3 hours.
• children under 4 years of age: ask a doctor

Directions For Use of Mouthpiece:
The Primatene Mist mouthpiece, which is enclosed in the Primatene Mist 15 mL size (not the refill size), should be used for inhalation only with Primatene Mist.
1. Take plastic cap off mouthpiece. (For refills, use mouthpiece from previous purchase.)
2. Take plastic mouthpiece off bottle.
3. Place other end of mouthpiece on bottle.
4. Turn bottle upside down. Place thumb on bottom of mouthpiece over circular button and forefinger on top of vial. Empty the lungs as completely as possible by exhaling.
5. Place mouthpiece in mouth with lips closed around opening. Inhale deeply while squeezing mouthpiece and bottle together. Release immediately and remove unit from mouth. Complete taking the deep breath, drawing the medication into your lungs and holding breath as long as comfortable.
6. Exhale slowly keeping lips nearly closed. This helps distribute the medication in the lungs.
7. Replace plastic cap on mouthpiece.

Care of the Mouthpiece:
The Primatene Mist mouthpiece should be washed once daily with soap and hot water, and rinsed thoroughly. Then it should be dried with a clean, lint-free cloth.

Other Information:
• store at room temperature, between 20–25°C (68–77°F) • contains no sulfites

Inactive Ingredients: ascorbic acid, dehydrated alcohol (34%), dichlorodifluoromethane (CFC 12), dichlorotetrafluoroethane (CFC 114), hydrochloric acid, nitric acid, purified water

How Supplied:
$1/2$ Fl oz (15 mL) With Mouthpiece.
$1/2$ Fl oz (15 mL) Refill
$3/4$ Fl oz (22.5 mL) Refill

PRIMATENE® Tablets
Bronchodilator, Expectorant

Active Ingredients (in each tablet):
Ephedrine HCl, USP   12.5 mg
Guaifenesin, USP   200 mg

Uses:
• temporarily relieves shortness of breath, tightness of chest, and wheezing due to bronchial asthma
• eases breathing for asthma patients by reducing spasms of bronchial muscles
• helps loosen phlegm (mucus) and thin bronchial secretions to rid bronchial passageways of bothersome mucus, and to make coughs more productive

Warnings:
Do not use
• unless a diagnosis of asthma has been made by a doctor
• if you are now taking a prescription monoamine oxidase inhibitor (MAOI) (certain drugs for depression, psychiatric, or emotional conditions, or Parkinson's disease), or for 2 weeks after stopping the MAOI drug If you do not know if your prescription drug contains an MAOI, ask a doctor or pharmacist before taking this product
Ask a doctor before use if you have
• heart disease • high blood pressure
• thyroid disease • diabetes
• trouble urinating due to an enlarged prostate gland
• ever been hospitalized for asthma
• cough that occurs with too much phlegm (mucus)
• cough that lasts or is chronic such as occurs with smoking, asthma, chronic bronchitis, or emphysema
Ask a doctor or pharmacist before use if you are taking any prescription drug for asthma

When using this product some users may experience nervousness, tremor, sleeplessness, nausea, and loss of appetite

Stop use and ask a doctor if
• symptoms are not relieved within 1 hour or become worse
• nervousness, tremor, sleeplessness, nausea, and loss of appetite persist or become worse
• cough lasts more than 7 days, comes back, or occurs with fever, rash, or persistent headache These could be signs of a serious condition
If pregnant or breast-feeding, ask a health professional before use.
Keep out of reach of children. In case of overdose, get medical help or contact a Poison Control Center right away.

Directions:
• do not use more than dosage below unless directed by a doctor
• adults and children 12 years and over: take 2 tablets initially, then 2 tablets

every 4 hours, as needed, not to exceed 12 tablets in 24 hours
- children under 12 years: ask a doctor

Other Information:
- store at 20–25°C (68–77°F)

Inactive Ingredients: crospovidone, D&C yellow no. 10 aluminum lake, FD&C yellow no. 6 aluminum lake, magnesium stearate, microcrystalline cellulose, povidone, silicon dioxide (colloidal)

How Supplied: Available in 24 and 60 tablet thermoform blister cartons.

ROBITUSSIN® Expectorant

Active Ingredient: (in each 5 mL tsp) Guaifenesin, USP 100 mg

Use: helps loosen phlegm (mucus) and thin bronchial secretions to make coughs more productive

Warnings:
Ask a doctor before use if you have
- cough that occurs with too much phlegm (mucus)
- cough that lasts or is chronic such as occurs with smoking, asthma, chronic bronchitis, or emphysema

Stop use and ask a doctor if cough lasts more than 7 days, comes back, or is accompanied by fever, rash, or persistent headache. These could be signs of a serious condition.

If pregnant or breast-feeding, ask a health professional before use.

Keep out of reach of children. In case of overdose, get medical help or contact a Poison Control Center right away.

Directions:
- do not take more than 6 doses in any 24-hour period
- adults and children 12 yrs and over: 2–4 tsp every 4 hours
- children 6 to under 12 yrs: 1–2 tsp every 4 hours
- children 2 to under 6 yrs: ½–1 tsp every 4 hours
- children under 2 yrs: ask a doctor

Other Information:
- store at 20–25°C (68–77°F)
- alcohol-free
- dosage cup provided

Inactive Ingredients: caramel, citric acid, FD&C red no. 40, flavors, glucose, glycerin, high fructose corn syrup, menthol, saccharin sodium, sodium benzoate, water.

How Supplied: Bottles of 4 fl oz, 8 fl oz.

ROBITUSSIN® ALLERGY & COUGH SYRUP
Nasal Decongestant, Cough Suppressant, Antihistamine

Active Ingredients: (in each 5 mL tsp)
Brompheniramine maleate, USP 2 mg
Dextromethorphan HBr, USP 10 mg
Pseudoephedrine HCl, USP 30 mg

Uses:
- temporarily relieves these symptoms due to hay fever (allergic rhinitis):
  - runny nose • sneezing • itchy, watery eyes • itching of the nose or throat
  - nasal congestion
- temporarily controls cough due to minor throat and bronchial irritation associated with inhaled irritants
- temporarily restores freer breathing through the nose

Warnings:
Do not use if you are now taking a prescription monoamine oxidase inhibitor (MAOI) (certain drugs for depression, psychiatric, or emotional conditions, or Parkinson's disease), or for 2 weeks after stopping the MAOI drug. If you do not know if your prescription drug contains an MAOI, ask a doctor or pharmacist before taking this product.

Ask a doctor before use if you have
- heart disease • high blood pressure
- thyroid disease • diabetes
- trouble urinating due to an enlarged prostate gland • glaucoma
- cough that occurs with too much phlegm (mucus)
- cough that lasts or is chronic such as occurs with smoking, asthma, chronic bronchitis or emphysema

Ask a doctor or pharmacist before use if you are taking sedatives or tranquilizers

When using this product
- **do not use more than directed**
- marked drowsiness may occur
- avoid alcoholic beverages
- alcohol, sedatives, and tranquilizers may increase drowsiness
- be careful when driving a motor vehicle or operating machinery
- excitability may occur, especially in children

Stop use and ask a doctor if
- you get nervous, dizzy, or sleepless
- symptoms do not get better within 7 days or are accompanied by fever
- cough lasts more than 7 days, comes back, or is accompanied by fever, rash, or persistent headache. These could be signs of a serious condition.

If pregnant or breast-feeding, ask a health professional before use.

Keep out of reach of children. In case of overdose, get medical help or contact a Poison Control Center right away.

Directions:
- do not take more than 4 doses in any 24-hour period
- adults and children 12 yrs and over: 2 tsp every 4 hours
- children 6 to under 12 yrs: 1 tsp every 4 hours
- children under 6 yrs: ask a doctor

Other Information:
- store at 20–25°C (68–77°F)
- alcohol free
- dosage cup provided

Inactive Ingredients: artificial flavor, citric acid, glycerin, propylene glycol, saccharin sodium, sodium benzoate, sorbitol, water

How Supplied: Bottles of 4 fl. oz.

ROBITUSSIN® COLD
COUGH & COLD
Liquid-filled Capsules
Nasal Decongestant, Expectorant, Cough Suppressant

Active Ingredients
(in each capsule):
Dextromethorphan HBr, USP 10 mg
Guaifenesin, USP 200 mg
Pseudoephedrine HCl, USP 30 mg

Uses:
- temporarily relieves nasal congestion, and cough due to minor throat and bronchial irritation occurring with the common cold
- helps loosen phlegm (mucus) and thin bronchial secretions to make coughs more productive
- temporarily relieves nasal congestion associated with hay fever or other upper respiratory allergies, or associated with sinusitis

Warnings:
Do not use if you are now taking a prescription monoamine oxidase inhibitor (MAOI) (certain drugs for depression, psychiatric, or emotional conditions, or Parkinson's disease), or for 2 weeks after stopping the MAOI drug. If you do not know if your prescription drug contains an MAOI, ask a doctor or pharmacist before taking this product.

Ask a doctor before use if you have
- heart disease • high blood pressure
- thyroid disease • diabetes
- trouble urinating due to an enlarged prostate gland
- cough that occurs with too much phlegm (mucus)
- cough that lasts or is chronic such as occurs with smoking, asthma, chronic bronchitis, or emphysema

When using this product do not use more than directed.

Stop use and ask a doctor if
- you get nervous, dizzy, or sleepless
- symptoms do not get better within 7 days or are accompanied by fever
- cough lasts more than 7 days, comes back, or is accompanied by fever, rash, or persistent headache. These could be signs of a serious condition.

If pregnant or breast-feeding, ask a health professional before use.

Keep out of reach of children. In case of overdose, get medical help or contact a Poison Control Center right away.

Directions:
- do not use more than 4 doses in any 24-hr period
- adults and children 12 yrs and over: 2 capsules every 4 hours
- children 6 to under 12 yrs: 1 capsule every 4 hours
- children under 6 years: ask a doctor

Other Information:
- store at 20–25°C (68–77°F)

Inactive Ingredients (Capsules): FD&C blue no. 1, FD&C red no. 40, gelatin, glycerin, mannitol, pharmaceutical glaze, polyethylene glycol, povidone,

Continued on next page

Robitussin—Cont.

propylene glycol, sorbitan, sorbitol, titanium dioxide, water

How Supplied: Capsules in packages of 12 (individually packaged).

ROBITUSSIN® COUGH, COLD & FLU Liquid-filled Capsules
Pain Reliever/Fever Reducer, Cough Suppressant, Nasal Decongestant, Expectorant

Active Ingredients (in each capsule):
Acetaminophen, USP 250 mg
Dextromethorphan HBr, USP 10 mg
Guaifenesin, USP 100 mg
Pseudoephedrine HCl, USP 30 mg

Uses:
- temporarily relieves these symptoms associated with a cold, or flu:
  - headache • sore throat • fever
  - muscular aches • minor aches and pains
- temporarily relieves nasal congestion, and cough due to minor throat and bronchial irritation occurring with a cold
- helps loosen phlegm (mucus) and thin bronchial secretions to make coughs more productive

Warnings:
Alcohol warning: If you consume 3 or more alcoholic drinks every day, ask your doctor whether you should take acetaminophen or other pain relievers/fever reducers. Acetaminophen may cause liver damage.
Taking more than the recommended dose (overdose) may cause serious liver damage.
Sore throat warning: If sore throat is severe, persists for more than two days, is accompanied or followed by fever, headache, rash, nausea, or vomiting, consult a doctor promptly
Do not use
- if you are now taking a prescription monoamine oxidase inhibitor (MAOI) (certain drugs for depression, psychiatric, or emotional conditions, or Parkinson's disease), or for 2 weeks after stopping the MAOI drug. If you do not know if your prescription drug contains an MAOI, ask a doctor or pharmacist before taking this product.
- with any other product containing acetaminophen as this may lead to an overdose. Overdose requires prompt medical attention even if you do not notice any signs or symptoms.
Ask a doctor before use if you have
- heart disease • high blood pressure
- thyroid disease • diabetes
- trouble urinating due to an enlarged prostate gland
- cough that occurs with too much phlegm (mucus)
- cough that lasts or is chronic such as occurs with smoking, asthma, chronic bronchitis, or emphysema
Ask a doctor or pharmacist before use if you are taking any other product containing acetaminophen, or any other pain reliever/fever reducer.
When using this product do not use more than directed.

Stop use and ask a doctor if
- you get nervous, dizzy, or sleepless
- pain, cough, or nasal congestion gets worse or lasts more than 5 days (children) or 7 days (adults)
- fever gets worse or lasts more than 3 days
- redness or swelling is present
- new symptoms occur
- cough comes back or occurs with rash or headache that lasts. These could be signs of a serious condition.
If pregnant or breast-feeding, ask a health professional before use.
Keep out of reach of children. In case of overdose, get medical help or contact a Poison Control Center right away. Prompt medical attention is critical for adults as well as for children, even if you do not notice any signs or symptoms.

Directions:
- do not use more than 4 doses in any 24-hour period
- do not exceed recommended dosage. Taking more than the recommended dose (overdose) may cause serious liver damage.
- adults and children 12 yrs and over: 2 capsules every 4 hours
- children under 12 years: ask a doctor

Other Information:
store at 20–25°C (68–77°F)

Inactive Ingredients: D&C yellow no. 10, FD&C red no. 40, gelatin, glycerin, iron oxides, lecithin, mannitol, pharmaceutical glaze, polyethylene glycol, povidone, propylene glycol, simethicone, sorbitan, sorbitol, water

How Supplied: In blister packs of 12 liquid-filled capsules.

ROBITUSSIN® COLD SEVERE CONGESTION Liquid-filled Capsules
Nasal Decongestant, Expectorant

Active Ingredients:
(in each capsule)
Guaifenesin, USP 200 mg
Pseudoephedrine HCl USP 30 mg

Uses:
- temporarily relieves nasal congestion associated with
  - the common cold
  - hay fever
  - upper respiratory allergies
  - sinusitis
- helps loosen phlegm (mucus) and thin bronchial secretions to make coughs more productive

Warnings:
Do not use if you are now taking a prescription monoamine oxidase inhibitor (MAOI) (certain drugs for depression, psychiatric, or emotional conditions, or Parkinson's disease), or for 2 weeks after stopping the MAOI drug. If you do not know if your prescription drug contains an MAOI, ask a doctor or pharmacist before taking this product.
Ask a doctor before use if you have
- heart disease • high blood pressure
- thyroid disease • diabetes
- trouble urinating due to an enlarged prostate gland

- cough that occurs with too much phlegm (mucus)
- cough that lasts or is chronic such as occurs with smoking, asthma, chronic bronchitis, or emphysema
When using this product do not use more than directed.
Stop use and ask a doctor if
- you get nervous, dizzy, or sleepless
- symptoms do not get better within 7 days or are accompanied by fever
- cough lasts more than 7 days, comes back, or is accompanied by fever, rash, or persistent headache. These could be signs of a serious condition.
If pregnant or breast-feeding, ask a health professional before use.
Keep out of reach of children. In case of overdose, get medical help or contact a Poison Control Center right away.

Directions:
- do not use more than 4 doses in any 24-hr period
- adults and children 12 yrs and over: 2 capsules every 4 hours
- children 6 to under 12 yrs: 1 capsule every 4 hours
- children under 6 yrs: ask a doctor

Other Information: store at 20–25°C (68–77°F).

Inactive Ingredients: FD&C green no. 3, gelatin, glycerin, mannitol, pharmaceutical glaze, polyethylene glycol, povidone, propylene glycol, sorbitan, sorbitol, titanium dioxide, water

How Supplied: Blister Packs of 12's.

ROBITUSSIN® COUGH DROPS
Menthol Eucalyptus, Cherry, and Honey-Lemon Flavors

Active Ingredient: (in each drop)
Menthol Eucalyptus:
Menthol, USP 10 mg
Cherry and Honey-Lemon:
Menthol, USP 5 mg

Uses:
- temporarily relieves
  - occasional minor irritation, pain, sore mouth, and sore throat
  - cough associated with a cold or inhaled irritants

Warnings:
Sore throat warning: Severe or persistent sore throat or sore throat accompanied by high fever, headache, nausea, and vomiting may be serious. Consult a doctor right away. Do not use more than 2 days or give to children under 3 years of age unless directed by a doctor
Ask a doctor before use if you have
- cough that occurs with too much phlegm (mucus)
- cough that lasts or is chronic such as occurs with smoking, asthma, or emphysema
Stop use and ask a doctor if cough lasts more than 7 days, comes back, or is accompanied by fever, rash, or persistent headache. These could be signs of a serious condition.
If pregnant or breast-feeding, ask a health professional before use.

Keep out of reach of children.

Directions:
- adults and children 4 years and over: allow 1 drop to dissolve slowly in the mouth
  - for sore throat: may be repeated every 2 hours, as needed, or as directed by a doctor
  - for cough: may be repeated every hour, as needed, or as directed by a doctor
- children under 4 years of age: ask a doctor

Other Information: store at 20–25°C (68–77°F).

Inactive Ingredients:
Menthol Eucalyptus: corn syrup, eucalyptus oil, flavor, sucrose
Cherry: corn syrup, FD&C red no. 40, flavor, methylparaben, propylparaben, sodium benzoate, sucrose
Honey-Lemon: citric acid, corn syrup, D&C yellow no. 10, FD&C yellow no. 6, honey, lemon oil, methylparaben, povidone, propylparaben, sodium benzoate, sucrose

How Supplied: All 3 flavors of Robitussin Cough Drops are available in bags of 25 drops.

ROBITUSSIN® FLU
Pain Reliever/Fever Reducer, Nasal Decongestant, Cough Suppressant, Antihistamine

Active Ingredients: (in each 5 mL tsp)
Acetaminophen, USP 160 mg
Chlorpheniramine maleate, USP 1 mg
Dextromethorphan HBr, USP 5 mg
Pseudoephedrine HCl, USP 15 mg

Uses:
- temporarily relieves these symptoms occurring with a cold or flu, hay fever, or other upper respiratory allergies:
- headache • cough • runny nose • itching of the nose or throat • nasal congestion • muscular aches • sneezing • sore throat • minor aches and pains • itchy, watery eyes • fever

Warnings:
Alcohol warning: If you consume 3 or more alcoholic drinks every day, ask your doctor whether you should take acetaminophen or other pain relievers/fever reducers. Acetaminophen may cause liver damage.
Taking more than the recommended dose (overdose) may cause serious liver damage.
Sore throat warning: If sore throat is severe, persists for more than 2 days, is accompanied or followed by fever, headache, rash, nausea, or vomiting, consult a doctor promptly
Do not use:
- if you are now taking a prescription monoamine oxidase inhibitor (MAOI) (certain drugs for depression, psychiatric, or emotional conditions, or Parkinson's disease), or for 2 weeks after stopping the MAOI drug. If you do not know if your prescription drug contains an MAOI, ask a doctor or pharmacist before taking this product.

- with any other product containing acetaminophen as this may lead to an overdose. Overdose requires prompt medical attention even if you do not notice any signs or symptoms.

Ask a doctor before use if you have
- heart disease • thyroid disease
- trouble urinating due to an enlarged prostate gland • diabetes
- cough that occurs with too much phlegm (mucus) • glaucoma
- a breathing problem or chronic cough that lasts or as occurs with smoking, asthma, chronic bronchitis, or emphysema • high blood pressure

Ask a doctor or pharmacist before use if you are • taking any other product containing acetaminophen, or any other pain reliever/fever reducer
- taking sedatives or tranquilizers

When using this product
- **do not use more than directed**
- marked drowsiness may occur
- alcohol, sedatives, and tranquilizers may increase drowsiness
- be careful when driving a motor vehicle or operating machinery
- excitability may occur, especially in children • avoid alcoholic drinks

Stop use and ask a doctor if
- you get nervous, dizzy, or sleepless
- pain, cough, or nasal congestion gets worse or lasts more than 5 days (children) or 7 days (adults)
- fever gets worse or lasts more than 3 days
- redness or swelling is present
- cough comes back or occurs with rash or headache that lasts. These could be signs of a serious condition.
- new symptoms occur

If pregnant or breast-feeding, ask a health professional before use.

Keep out of reach of children. In case of overdose, get medical help or contact a Poison Control Center right away. Prompt medical attention is critical for adults as well as for children, even if you do not notice any signs or symptoms.

Directions:
- do not take more than 4 doses in any 24-hour period
- do not exceed recommended dosage. Taking more than the recommended dose (overdose) may cause serious liver damage.
- adults and children 12 yrs and over: 4 tsp every 4 hours
- children 6 to under 12 yrs: 2 tsp every 4 hours
- children under 6 yrs: ask a doctor

Other Information:
- **each teaspoon contains:** sodium 4 mg
- store at 20–25°C (68–77°F)
- alcohol free

Inactive Ingredients: citric acid, D&C red no. 33, FD&C yellow no. 6, flavor, glycerin, high fructose corn syrup, polyethylene glycol, purified water, sodium benzoate, sodium citrate, sorbitol solution, sucralose

How Supplied: Bottles of 4 fl. oz.

ROBITUSSIN®
HONEY CALMERS THROAT DROPS (BERRY)
Oral Pain Reliever

Active Ingredient
(in each drop):
Menthol, USP 1 mg

Use: Temporarily relieves occasional minor irritation, pain, sore mouth, and sore throat.

Warnings
Sore throat warning: Severe or persistent sore throat or sore throat accompanied by high fever, headache, nausea, and vomiting may be serious. Consult a doctor right away. Do not use more than 2 days or give to children under 3 years of age unless directed by a doctor.
If pregnant or breast-feeding, ask a health professional before use.
Keep out of reach of children.

Directions:
- adults and children 4 years and over: allow 2 drops to dissolve slowly in the mouth. May be repeated every 2 hours, as needed, or as directed by a doctor.
- children under 4 years of age: ask a doctor

Other Information: store at 20–25°C (68–77°F)

Inactive Ingredients carmine, citric acid, cochineal extract, corn syrup, glycerin, natural flavor blend, natural grade A wildflower honey, sucrose

How Supplied: Packages of 25 drops.

ROBITUSSIN®
HONEY COUGH™ LIQUID
Cough Suppressant

Active Ingredient: (in each 5 mL tsp)
Dextromethorphan HBr, USP 10 mg

Use: temporarily relieves cough due to minor throat and bronchial irritation as may occur with a cold

Warnings:
Do not use if you are now taking a prescription monoamine oxidase inhibitor (MAOI) (certain drugs for depression, psychiatric, or emotional conditions, or Parkinson's disease), or for 2 weeks after stopping the MAOI drug. If you do not know if your prescription drug contains an MAOI, ask a doctor or pharmacist before taking this product.
Ask a doctor before use if you have
- cough that occurs with too much phlegm (mucus)
- cough that lasts or is chronic such as occurs with smoking, asthma, or emphysema

Stop use and ask a doctor if cough lasts more than 7 days, comes back, or is accompanied by fever, rash, or persistent headache. These could be signs of a serious condition.

If pregnant or breast-feeding, ask a health professional before use.

Continued on next page

Robitussin Honey Cough—Cont.

Keep out of reach of children. In case of overdose, get medical help or contact a Poison Control Center right away.

Directions:
- do not take more than 4 doses in any 24-hr period
- adults and children 12 yrs and over: 3 tsp every 6 to 8 hours
- children 6 to under 12 yrs: 1.5 tsp every 6 to 8 hours
- children under 6 yrs: not recommended

Other Information: • store at 20–25°C (68°–77°F)
- alcohol-free
- dosage cup provided

Inactive Ingredients: flavors, glucose, glycerin, honey, maltol, methylparaben, propylene glycol, sodium benzoate, water

How Supplied: Bottles of 4 fl. oz. and 8 fl. oz.

ROBITUSSIN®
HONEY COUGH Drops
Honey-Lemon Tea, Herbal Honey Citrus, Herbal and Herbal Almond with Natural Honey Center

Active Ingredient (in each drop):
Herbal with Natural Honey Center and *Honey Lemon Tea:*
Menthol, USP 5 mg
Herbal Honey Citrus and Herbal Almond with Natural Honey Center:
Menthol, USP 2.5 mg

Uses:
- temporarily relieves
  - occasional minor irritation, pain, sore mouth, and sore throat
  - cough associated with a cold or inhaled irritants

Warnings:
Sore throat warning: Severe or persistent sore throat or sore throat accompanied by high fever, headache, nausea, and vomiting may be serious. Consult a doctor right away. Do not use more than 2 days or give to children under 3 years of age unless directed by a doctor.
Ask a doctor before use if you have
- cough that occurs with too much phlegm (mucus)
- cough that lasts or is chronic such as occurs with smoking, asthma, or emphysema
Stop use and ask a doctor if cough lasts more than 7 days, comes back, or is accompanied by fever, rash, or persistent headache. These could be signs of a serious condition.
If pregnant or breast-feeding, ask a health professional before use.
Keep out of reach of children.

Directions:
- adults and children 4 years and over:
  - for sore throat: allow 1 drop to dissolve slowly in the mouth. May be repeated every 2 hours, as needed, or as directed by a doctor.

- for cough: *Honey Lemon Tea and Herbal with Natural Honey Center*—allow 1 drop to dissolve slowly in mouth.
  Herbal Honey Citrus and Herbal Almond with Natural Honey Center—allow 2 drops to dissolve slowly in mouth.
  May be repeated every hour, as needed, or as directed by a doctor.
- children under 4 years: ask a doctor

Other Information: store at 20–25°C (68–77°F).

Inactive Ingredients:
Herbal with Natural Honey Center: caramel, corn syrup, glycerin, high fructose corn syrup, honey, natural herbal flavor, sorbitol, sucrose
Honey Lemon Tea: caramel, citric acid, corn syrup, honey, natural flavor, sucrose, tea extract
Herbal Honey Citrus: citric acid, corn syrup, flavors, honey, sucrose
Herbal Almond with Natural Honey Center: caramel, corn syrup, glycerin, honey, natural almond flavor, natural anise flavor, natural coriander flavor, natural fennel flavor, natural honey flavor and other natural flavors, sorbitol, sucrose

How Supplied: Honey Lemon Tea and Herbal Honey Citrus in bags of 25 drops. Herbal and Herbal Almond with Natural Honey center in bags of 20 drops.

ROBITUSSIN® PM Cough & Cold
Nasal Decongestant, Cough Suppressant, Antihistamine

Active Ingredients: (in each 5 mL tsp):
Chlorpheniramine maleate, USP 1 mg
Dextromethorphan HBr, USP 7.5 mg
Pseudoephedrine HCl, USP 15 mg

Uses:
- temporarily relieves these symptoms occurring with a cold:
  - cough due to minor throat and bronchial irritation
  - nasal congestion
- temporarily relieves these symptoms due to hay fever or other upper respiratory allergies: • runny nose • sneezing • itchy, watery eyes • itching of the nose or throat

Warnings:
Do not use if you are now taking a prescription monoamine oxidase inhibitor (MAOI) (certain drugs for depression, psychiatric, or emotional conditions, or Parkinson's disease), or for 2 weeks after stopping the MAOI drug. If you do not know if your prescription drug contains an MAOI, ask a doctor or pharmacist before taking this product.
Ask a doctor before use if you have
• heart disease • high blood pressure • thyroid disease • diabetes • trouble urinating due to an enlarged prostate gland • glaucoma • cough that occurs with too much phlegm (mucus) • a breathing problem or chronic cough that lasts or as occurs with smoking, asthma, chronic bronchitis, or emphysema

Ask a doctor or pharmacist before use if you are taking sedatives or tranquilizers.
When using this product
- do not use more than directed
- marked drowsiness may occur
- avoid alcoholic drinks
- alcohol, sedatives, and tranquilizers may increase drowsiness
- be careful when driving a motor vehicle or operating machinery
- excitability may occur, especially in children
Stop use and ask a doctor if
- you get nervous, dizzy, or sleepless
- symptoms do not get better within 7 days or are accompanied by fever
- cough lasts more than 7 days, comes back, or is accompanied by fever, rash, or persistent headache. These could be signs of a serious condition.
If pregnant or breast-feeding, ask a health professional before use.
Keep out of reach of children. In case of overdose, get medical help or contact a Poison Control Center right away.

Directions:
- do not take more than 4 doses in any 24-hour period
- adults and children 12 years and older: 4 tsp every 6 hours
- children 6 to under 12 years: 2 tsp every 6 hours
- children under 6 years: ask a doctor
Other Information:
- store at 20–25°C (68–77°F)
- not USP. Meets specifications when tested with a validated non-USP assay method
- dosage cup provided

Inactive Ingredients: citric acid, FD&C red no. 40, glycerin, high fructose corn syrup, natural and artificial flavors, propylene glycol, purified water, saccharin sodium, sodium benzoate, sodium chloride, sodium citrate

How Supplied:
Bottles of 4 fl. oz.

ROBITUSSIN® PE Syrup
Nasal Decongestant, Expectorant

Active Ingredients:
(in each 5 mL tsp):

Guaifenesin, USP 100 mg
Pseudoephedrine HCl, USP 30 mg

Uses: • temporarily relieves nasal congestion due to a cold • helps loosen phlegm (mucus) and thin bronchial secretions to make coughs more productive.

Warnings:
Do not use if you are now taking a prescription monoamine oxidase inhibitor (MAOI) (certain drugs for depression, psychiatric, or emotional conditions, or Parkinson's disease), or for 2 weeks after stopping the MAOI drug. If you do not know if your prescription drug contains an MAOI, ask a doctor or pharmacist before taking this product.
Ask a doctor before use if you have
• heart disease • high blood pressure
• thyroid disease • diabetes
• trouble urinating due to an enlarged prostate gland

- cough that occurs with too much phlegm (mucus)
- cough that lasts or is chronic such as occurs with smoking, asthma, chronic bronchitis, or emphysema

When using this product do not use more than directed.

Stop use and ask a doctor if
- you get nervous, dizzy, or sleepless
- symptoms do not get better within 7 days or are accompanied by fever
- cough lasts more than 7 days, comes back, or is accompanied by fever, rash, or persistent headache. These could be signs of a serious condition.

If pregnant or breast-feeding, ask a health professional before use.

Keep out of reach of children. In case of overdose, get medical help or contact a Poison Control Center right away.

Directions:
- do not take more than 4 doses in any 24-hr period
- adults and children 12 yrs and over: 2 tsp every 4 hours
- children 6 to under 12 yrs: 1 tsp every 4 hours
- children 2 to under 6 yrs: ½ tsp every 4 hours
- children under 2 yrs: ask a doctor

Other Information:
- store at 20–25°C (68–77°F)
- alcohol-free
- dosage cup provided

Inactive Ingredients:
citric acid, FD&C red no. 40, flavors, glucose, glycerin, high fructose corn syrup, maltol, menthol, propylene glycol, saccharin sodium, sodium benzoate, water

How Supplied: Bottles of 4 fl oz, and 8 fl oz.

ROBITUSSIN® DM SYRUP
ROBITUSSIN® SUGAR FREE COUGH

ROBITUSSIN® DM INFANT DROPS
Cough Suppressant, Expectorant

Active Ingredients: (in each 5 mL tsp: Robitussin DM, Robitussin Sugar Free Cough)
Dextromethorphan HBr, USP 10 mg
Guaifenesin, USP 100 mg

Active Ingredients: (in each 2.5 mL Robitussin DM Infant Drops)
Dextromethorphan HBr, USP 5 mg
Guaifenesin, USP 100 mg

Uses:
- temporarily relieves cough due to minor throat and bronchial irritation as may occur with a cold
- helps loosen phlegm (mucus) and thin bronchial secretions to make coughs more productive

Warnings:
Do not use if you or your child are now taking a prescription monoamine oxidase inhibitor (MAOI) (certain drugs for depression, psychiatric, or emotional conditions, or Parkinson's disease), or for 2 weeks after stopping the MAOI drug. If you do not know if your child's or your

prescription drug contains an MAOI, ask a doctor or pharmacist before taking this product or giving it to your child.

Ask a doctor before use if you or your child has
- cough that occurs with too much phlegm (mucus)
- cough that lasts or is chronic such as occurs with smoking, asthma, chronic bronchitis, or emphysema

Stop use and ask a doctor if cough lasts more than 7 days, comes back, or is accompanied by fever, rash, or persistent headache. These could be signs of a serious condition.

If pregnant or breast-feeding, ask a health professional before use.

Keep out of reach of children. In case of overdose, get medical help or contact a Poison Control Center right away.

Directions: (Robitussin DM, Robitussin Sugar Free Cough):
- do not take more than 6 doses in any 24-hour period
- adults and children 12 yrs and over: 2 tsp every 4 hours
- children 6 to under 12 yrs: 1 tsp every 4 hours
- children 2 to under 6 yrs: ½ tsp every 4 hours
- children under 2 yrs: ask a doctor

Directions: (Robitussin DM Infant Drops):
- repeat dose every 4 hrs, as needed
- do not use more than 6 doses in any 24-hr period
- choose by weight (if weight not known, choose by age)
- measure with the dosing device provided. Do not use with any other device.
- 24–47 lbs (2 to under 6 yrs): 2.5 mL
- under 24 lbs (under 2 yrs): ask a doctor

Inactive Ingredients: (Robitussin DM): citric acid, FD&C red no. 40, flavors, glucose, glycerin, high fructose corn syrup, menthol, saccharin sodium, sodium benzoate, water

Inactive Ingredients: (Robitussin Sugar Free Cough): acesulfame potassium, citric acid, flavors, glycerin, methylparaben, polyethylene glycol, povidone, propylene glycol, saccharin sodium, sodium benzoate, water

Inactive Ingredients: (Robitussin DM Infant Drops): citric acid, FD&C red no. 40, flavors, glycerin, high fructose corn syrup, maltitol, maltol, polyethylene glycol, povidone, propylene glycol, saccharin sodium, sodium benzoate, sodium chloride, sodium citrate, water

Other Information:
- store at 20–25°C (68–77°F)
- alcohol-free
- dosage cup or oral dosing device provided

How Supplied: Robitussin DM (cherry-colored) in bottles of 4, 8 and 12 fl oz, and single doses (premeasured doses 1/3 fl oz each)
Robitussin Sugar Free Cough in bottles of 4 fl oz
Robitussin DM Infant Drops (berry flavor) in 1 fl oz bottles

ROBITUSSIN®
SUGAR FREE Throat Drops
(Natural Citrus and Tropical Fruit Flavors)

Active Ingredient (in each drop):
Menthol, USP 2.5 mg

Uses:
- temporarily relieves
  - occasional minor irritation, pain, sore mouth, and sore throat
  - cough associated with a cold or inhaled irritants

Warnings:
Sore throat warning: Severe or persistent sore throat or sore throat accompanied by high fever, headache, nausea, and vomiting may be serious. Consult a doctor right away. Do not use more than 2 days or give to children under 3 years of age unless directed by a doctor.

Ask a doctor before use if you have
- cough that occurs with too much phlegm (mucus)
- cough that lasts or is chronic such as occurs with smoking, asthma, or emphysema

When using this product excessive use may have a laxative effect

Stop use and ask a doctor if cough lasts more than 7 days, comes back, or is accompanied by fever, rash, or persistent headache. These could be signs of a serious condition.

If pregnant or breast-feeding, ask a health professional before use.

Keep out of reach of children.

Directions:
- adults and children 4 years and over: allow 2 drops to dissolve slowly in the mouth
  - for sore throat: may be repeated every 2 hours, as needed, up to 9 drops per day, or as directed by a doctor
  - for cough: may be repeated every hour, as needed, up to 9 drops per day, as or as directed by a doctor
- children under 4 years: ask a doctor

Other Information:
- each drop contains: **phenylalanine 3.37 mg**
- store at 20–25°C (68–77°F)
- does not promote tooth decay
- product may be useful in a diabetic's diet on the advice of a doctor.
Exchange information*:

    3 Drops = FREE Exchange
    9 Drops = 1 Fruit

*The dietary exchanges are based on Exchange Lists for Meal Planning. Copyright 1995 by the American Diabetes Association Inc. and the American Dietetic Association.

Inactive Ingredients: aspartame, canola oil, citric acid, D&C yellow no. 10 aluminum lake (natural citrus only), FD&C blue no. 1 (natural citrus only), FD&C yellow no. 6 (tropical fruit only), isomalt, maltitol, natural flavor

How Supplied: Packages of 18 drops.

Continued on next page

ROBITUSSIN SUNNY ORANGE and RASPBERRY VITAMIN C SUPPLEMENT DROPS

Each soothing, refreshing drop provides a great tasting and convenient way to get 100% of the Daily Value of Vitamin C.
Made with 5% real orange juice.

Supplement Facts:
Serving Size: 1 drop

Amount Per Drop		% Daily Value
Calories		
Sunny Orange	15	
Sunny Raspberry	10	
Total Carbohydrate	3 g	1%†
Sugars	3 g	*
Vitamin C	60 mg	100%
(as sodium ascorbate and ascorbic acid)		
Sodium		
Sunny Orange	10 mg	<1%†
Sunny Raspberry	8 mg	

*Daily Value (%DV) not established.
†Percent Daily Values are based on a 2,000 calorie diet.

Other Ingredients: Corn syrup, sucrose.
Contains less than 2 % of the following (Sunny Orange): ascorbyl palmitate, beta carotene, citric acid, citrus aurantium dulcis (orange) juice (concentrate), corn oil, gelatin, menthol, methylparaben, natural flavor, phosphoric acid, potassium sorbate, propylparaben, sodium benzoate, sorbitol, tocopherols.
(Sunny Raspberry): citric acid, citrus aurantium dulcis (orange) juice (concentrate), FD&C blue no. 1, FD&C red no. 40, menthol, methylparaben, natural and artificial raspberry flavor, potassium sorbate, povidone, propylparaben, sodium benzoate

Directions: Take a minimum of 3 to 4 drops a day, not to exceed 15 drops per day. Allow drop to dissolve fully in mouth and swallow. Not formulated for use in children.

Warnings: Keep out of reach of children.
If you are pregnant or nursing a baby, contact your physician before taking this product.
Storage: Store at 20–25°C (68–77°F)

How Supplied: 25 Drops

ROBITUSSIN® MAXIMUM STRENGTH COUGH ROBITUSSIN® PEDIATRIC COUGH Formula
Cough Suppressant

Active Ingredients (in each 5 mL tsp Robitussin Maximum Strength Cough):
Dextromethorphan HBr, USP 15 mg
(in each 5 mL tsp Robitussin Pediatric Cough Formula):
Dextromethorphan HBr, USP 7.5 mg

Uses: temporarily relieves cough due to minor throat and bronchial irritation as may occur with a cold

Warnings:
Do not use if you are now taking a prescription monoamine oxidase inhibitor (MAOI) (certain drugs for depression, psychiatric, or emotional conditions, or Parkinson's disease), or for 2 weeks after stopping the MAOI drug. If you do not know if your prescription drug contains an MAOI, ask a doctor or pharmacist before taking this product.
Ask a doctor before use if you have
• cough that occurs with too much phlegm (mucus)
• cough that lasts or is chronic such as occurs with smoking, asthma, or emphysema
Stop use and ask a doctor if cough lasts more than 7 days, comes back, or is accompanied by fever, rash, or persistent headache. These could be signs of a serious condition.
If pregnant or breast-feeding, ask a health professional before use.
Keep out of reach of children. In case of overdose, get medical help or contact a Poison Control Center right away.

Directions:
• do not take more than 4 doses in any 24-hr period
Robitussin Maximum Strength Cough Suppressant
• adults and children 12 yrs and over: 2 tsp every 6 to 8 hours, as needed
• children under 12 yrs: ask a doctor
Robitussin Pediatric Cough Suppressant
• choose dosage by weight (if weight is not known, choose by age)
• under 24 lbs (under 2 yrs): ask a doctor
• 24–47 lbs (2 to under 6 yrs): 1 tsp every 6 to 8 hours
• 48–95 lbs (6–under 12 yrs): 2 tsp every 6 to 8 hours
• 96 lbs and over (12 yrs and older): 4 tsp every 6 to 8 hours

Other Information:
• store at 20–25°C (68–77°F)
• dosage cup provided

Inactive Ingredients (Robitussin Maximum Strength Cough): alcohol, citric acid, FD&C red no. 40, flavors, glucose, glycerin, high fructose corn syrup, menthol, saccharin sodium, sodium benzoate, water

(Robitussin Pediatric Cough Formula): citric acid, FD&C red no. 40, flavor, glycerin, high fructose corn syrup, saccharin sodium, sodium benzoate, sodium chloride, sodium citrate, water

How Supplied: Robitussin Maximum Strength (dark red-colored) in bottles of 4 and 8 fl oz.
Robitussin Pediatric (cherry-colored) in bottles of 4 fl oz.

ROBITUSSIN® MAXIMUM STRENGTH COUGH& COLD ROBITUSSIN® PEDIATRIC COUGH & COLD Formula
Cough Suppressant, Nasal Decongestant

Active Ingredients: (in each 5 mL tsp Robitussin Maximum Strength Cough & Cold)
Dextromethorphan HBr, USP 15 mg
Pseudoephedrine HCl, USP 30 mg
(in each 5 mL tsp Robitussin Pediatric Cough & Cold Formula)
Dextromethorphan HBr, USP 7.5 mg
Pseudoephedrine HCl, USP 15 mg

Active Ingredients:

Uses:
• temporarily relieves these symptoms occurring with a cold:
  • nasal congestion • cough due to minor throat and bronchial irritation

Warnings:
Do not use if you are now taking a prescription monoamine oxidase inhibitor (MAOI) (certain drugs for depression, psychiatric, or emotional conditions, or Parkinson's disease), or for 2 weeks after stopping the MAOI drug. If you do not know if your prescription drug contains an MAOI, ask a doctor or pharmacist before taking this product.
Ask a doctor before use if you have
• heart disease • high blood pressure
• thyroid disease • diabetes
• trouble urinating due to an enlarged prostate gland
• cough that occurs with too much phlegm (mucus)
• cough that lasts or is chronic such as occurs with smoking, asthma, or emphysema
When using this product do not use more than directed.
Stop use and ask a doctor if
• you get nervous, dizzy, or sleepless
• symptoms do not get better within 7 days or are accompanied by fever
• cough lasts more than 7 days, comes back, or is accompanied by fever, rash, or persistent headache. These could be signs of a serious condition.
If pregnant or breast-feeding, ask a health professional before use.
Keep out of reach of children. In case of overdose, get medical help or contact a Poison Control Center right away.

Directions:
• repeat dose every 6 hrs, as needed
• do not take more than 4 doses in any 24-hr period
Robitussin Maximum Strength Cough & Cold. • adults and children 12 yrs and over: 2 tsp • children under 12 yrs: ask a doctor
Robitussin Pediatric Cough & Cold Formula • choose dosage by weight (if weight is not known, choose by age)
• under 24 lbs (under 2 yrs): ask a doctor
• 24–47 lbs (2 to under 6 yrs): 1 tsp
• 48–95 lbs (6 to under 12 yrs): 2 tsp
• 96 lbs and over (12 yrs and older): 4 tsp

Other Information: • store at 20–25°C (68–77°F)
• dosage cup provided

Inactive Ingredients (Robitussin Maximum Strength Cough & Cold): alcohol, citric acid, FD&C red no. 40, flavors, glucose, glycerin, high fructose corn syrup, menthol, saccharin sodium, sodium benzoate, water
(Robitussin Pediatric Cough & Cold Formula): citric acid, FD&C red no. 40, flavor, glycerin, high fructose corn syrup, saccharin sodium, sodium benzoate, sodium chloride, sodium citrate, water

How Supplied:
Robitussin Maximum Strength Cough & Cold: Red syrup in bottles of 4 fl oz and 8 fl oz.
Robitussin Pediatric Cough & Cold Formula: (bright red) in bottles of 4 fl oz.

ROBITUSSIN®-CF Syrup
ROBITUSSIN® COUGH & COLD INFANT DROPS
Nasal Decongestant, Cough Suppressant, Expectorant

Active Ingredients: (in each 5 mL tsp Robitussin CF)
Dextromethorphan HBr, USP 10 mg
Guaifenesin, USP 100 mg
Pseudoephedrine HCl, USP 30 mg
(in each 2.5 mL Robitussin Cough & Cold Infant Drops)
Dextromethorphan HBr, USP 5 mg
Guaifenesin, USP 100 mg
Pseudoephedrine HCl, USP 15 mg

Uses:
• temporarily relieves these symptoms occurring with a cold:
  • nasal congestion
  • cough due to minor throat and bronchial irritation
• helps loosen phlegm (mucus) and thin bronchial secretions to make coughs more productive

Warnings:
Do not use if you or your child are taking a prescription monoamine oxidase inhibitor (MAOI) (certain drugs for depression, psychiatric, or emotional conditions, or Parkinson's disease), or for 2 weeks after stopping the MAOI drug. If you do not know if your child's or your prescription drug contains an MAOI, ask a doctor or pharmacist before taking this product or giving it to your child.
Ask a doctor before use if you or your child has
• heart disease • high blood pressure
• thyroid disease • diabetes
• trouble urinating due to an enlarged prostate gland

• cough that occurs with too much phlegm (mucus)
• cough that lasts or is chronic such as occurs with asthma
When using this product do not use more than directed.
Stop use and ask a doctor if
• you or your child gets nervous, dizzy, or sleepless
• symptoms do not get better within 7 days or are accompanied by fever
• cough lasts more than 7 days, comes back, or is accompanied by fever, rash, or persistent headache. These could be signs of a serious condition.
If pregnant or breast-feeding, ask a health professional before use.
Keep out of reach of children. In case of overdose, get medical help or contact a Poison Control Center right away.

Directions: (Robitussin CF Syrup):
• do not take more than 4 doses in any 24-hr period
• adults and children 12 yrs and over: 2 tsp every 4 hours
• children 6 to under 12 yrs: 1 tsp every 4 hours
• children 2 to under 6 yrs: ½ tsp or 2.5 mL
• children under 2 yrs: ask a doctor

Directions: (Robitussin Cough & Cold Infant Drops):
• do not use more than 4 doses in any 24-hour period
• repeat every 4 hours, as needed
• choose dosage by weight (if weight is not known, choose by age)
• measure with the dosing device provided. Do not use with any other device.
• 27–47 lbs (2 to under 6 yrs): 2.5 mL
• under 24 lbs (under 2 yrs): ask a doctor

Other Information:
• store at 20–25°C (68–77°F)
• alcohol-free
• dosage cup or oral dosing device provided

Inactive Ingredients: (Robitussin CF) citric acid, FD&C red no. 40, flavors, glycerin, propylene glycol, saccharin sodium, sodium benzoate, sorbitol, water
(Robitussin Cough & Cold Infant Drops) citric acid, FD&C red no. 40, flavors, glycerin, high fructose corn syrup, maltitol, maltol, polyethylene glycol, povidone, propylene glycol, saccharin sodium, sodium benzoate, sodium citrate, water

How Supplied: Robitussin CF (red-colored) in bottles of 4, 8, and 12 fl oz. Robitussin Cough & Cold Infant Drops in 1 fl oz bottles

ROBITUSSIN COUGHGELS/ LIQUIGELS
Cough suppressant

Active Ingredient
(in each liquid-filled capsule):
Dextromethorphan HBr, USP 15 mg

Use: temporarily relieves cough due to minor throat and bronchial irritation as may occur with a cold.

Warnings:
Do not use if you are now taking a prescription monoamine oxidase inhibitor (MAOI) (certain drugs for depression, psychiatric, or emotional conditions, or Parkinson's disease), or for 2 weeks after stopping the MAOI drug. If you do not know if your prescription drug contains an MAOI, ask a doctor or pharmacist before taking this product.
Ask a doctor before use if you have
• a cough that occurs with too much phlegm (mucus)
• a cough that lasts or is chronic as occurs with smoking, asthma, or emphysema
Stop use and ask a doctor if cough lasts for more than 7 days, comes back, or is accompanied by fever, rash, or persistent headache. These could be signs of a serious condition.
If pregnant or breast-feeding, ask a health professional before use.
Keep out of reach of children. In case of overdose, get medical help or contact a Poison Control Center right away.

Directions:
• do not take more than 8 capsules in any 24-hour period
• adults and children 12 years and over: take 2 capsules every 6 to 8 hours, as needed
• children under 12 years: ask a doctor
Other Information:
• store at 20-25°C (68-77°F)
• avoid excessive heat above 40°C (104°F)
• protect from light

Inactive Ingredients: FD&C blue no. 1, FD&C red no. 40, fractionated coconut oil, gelatin, glycerin, mannitol, pharmaceutical ink, polyethylene glycol, povidone, propyl gallate, propylene glycol, purified water, sorbitol, sorbitol anhydrides

How Supplied: Blister packs of 20 capsules.

DIETARY SUPPLEMENT INFORMATION

This section presents information on natural remedies and nutritional supplements marketed under the Dietary Supplement Health and Education Act of 1994. It is made possible through the courtesy of the manufacturers whose products appear on the following pages. The information concerning each product has been prepared, edited, and approved by the manufacturer's professional staff.

Products found in this section include vitamins, minerals, herbs and other botanicals, amino acids, other substances intended to supplement the diet, and concentrates, metabolites, constituents, extracts, and combinations of these ingredients. The descriptions of these products are designed to provide all information necessary for informed use, including, when applicable, active ingredients, inactive ingredients, actions, warnings, cautions, interactions, symptoms and treatment of oral overdosage, dosage and directions for use, and how supplied. Descriptions in this section must be in full compliance with the Dietary Supplement Health and Education Act, which permits claims regarding a product's effect on the structure or functioning of the body, but forbids claims regarding a product's ability to treat, diagnose, cure, or prevent any specific disease. Descriptions of products marketed under the act do not receive formal evaluation or approval from the Food and Drug Administration.

In compiling this section, the publisher has emphasized the necessity of describing products comprehensively. The descriptions seen here include all information made available by the manufacturer. The publisher does not warrant or guarantee any product described here, and does not perform any independent analysis of the information provided. Inclusion of a product in this book does not represent an endorsement, and the publisher does not necessarily advocate the use of any product listed.

A & Z Pharmaceutical Inc.

180 OSER AVENUE, SUITE 300 HAUPPAUGE, NY 11788

Direct Inquiries to:
Customer Service
(631) 952-3800
Fax: (631) 952-3900

D-CAL™
Calcium Supplement with Vitamin D Chewable Caplets

Ingredients: Calcium Carbonate, Vitamin D, Sorbitol, Flavor, D&C Red #27 Lake, Magnesium Stearate. No sugar, No salt, No lactose, No preservative.

Supplement Facts

Serving Size One Caplet

Each Caplet Contains		% Daily Value
Calcium (as calcium carbonate)	300 mg	30%
Vitamin D	100 IU	25%

Recommended Intake: Take two caplets daily for adult and one caplet for child, or as directed by your physician.

Warnings: KEEP OUT OF REACH OF CHILDREN. Do not accept if safety seal under cap is broken or missing.

Actions: D-Cal™ provides a concentrated form of calcium to help build healthy bones. It contains Vitamin D to help the body absorb calcium. D-Cal™ can also help prevent osteoporosis. It is helpful to pregnant and nursing women, children's growth, and calcium deficiency at all ages.

How Supplied: Bottles of 30 and 60 caplets

Shown in Product Identification Guide, page 503

AkPharma Inc.

**P.O. BOX 111
PLEASANTVILLE, NJ
08232-0111**

Direct Inquiries To:
Elizabeth Klein: (609) 645-5100
FAX: (609) 645-0767

Medical Emergency Contact:
Alan E. Kligerman: (609) 645-5100

PRELIEF®

PRODUCT OVERVIEW
Key Facts: Prelief is AkPharma's brand name for calcium glycerophosphate. It is used to take acid out of acidic foods and beverages for more comfortable consumption. Prelief tablets are swallowed with the first bite or drink of acidic food or beverage. Prelief powder is added to each serving of acidic food or beverage. It is classified as a dietary supplement.

Major Uses: Takes acid out of acidic foods such as tomato sauce, citrus, fruit drinks, coffee, wine, beer and colas. Acid foods are now established as problematic for persons with interstitial cystitis, overactive bladder and are suspect in some situations of intestinal irritation. Those with interstitial cystitis or overactive bladder, whose symptoms may be exacerbated by acidic foods, may particularly benefit.

Safety Information: Prelief is made from an FDA Generally Recognized as Safe (GRAS)[1] dietary supplement ingredient and is also listed as a food ingredient in the US Government Food Chemicals Codex (FCC)[2]

PRODUCT INFORMATION
Prelief®

Description: Prelief Tablets: Each tablet contains 65 mg elemental calcium as calcium glycerophosphate. The tablets also contain 0.025% magnesium stearate as a processing aid. Two tablets should be swallowed with the average serving of food or beverage. (See chart)

Prelief Powder: Each packet contains 65 mg elemental calcium as calcium glycerophosphate. Add 2 packets of powder to each average serving of acidic food or beverage. The powder dissolves rapidly in acidic food or non-alcoholic beverages. Tablets are recommended for taking with alcoholic beverages. An additional 1–2 tablets or packets may be needed with foods that may be particularly high in acid. (See chart)

One tablet or packet of powder supplies 6% (65 mg) of the US Recommended Daily Intake (RDI) for calcium and 5% (50 mg) of the RDI for phosphorus. No sodium; no aluminum; no sugar.

[1]reference 21 CFR §184.1201
[2]reference Food Chemicals Codex, 3rd Edition, pp 51–52

Reasons for Use: Prelief is for use with acidic foods and beverages. It is a dietary intervention used to take acid out of these foods for persons who identify acid discomfort with the ingestion of acidic foods and beverages.

Action: Prelief neutralizes the acid found in a large number of foods which many people find cause them discomfort. **See Table.**

Usage: Take 2 tablets 3 times a day. Best with meals; also 2 tablets at bedtime if desired.

How Supplied: Prelief is supplied in both tablet form (30, 60, 120 and 300 tablet bottle sizes and 24 tablets in 12–2 tablet packets), and powder form (36 count packet boxes, 40-serving squeeze bottle and 150-serving shaker).

Kosher: Prelief is Kosher and Pareve.
Use Limitations: None, except as may apply below.

Adverse Reactions: None known
Toxicity: None known
Interactions with Drugs: Calcium may interfere with efficacy of some medications. Check with drug publications.

Precautions: None, except for people who have been advised by their physician not to take calcium, phosphorus or glycerin/glycerol.

Prelief is classified as a dietary supplement, not a drug.

Typical Food Acid Removal by Prelief			
Product	1 Packet or 1 Tablet	2 Packets or 2 Tablets	3 Packets or 3 Tablets
Pepsi Cola® – 8 oz.	98%	99.8%	–
Mott's® 100% Apple Juice – 4 oz.	49.8%	74.9%	90%
Tropicana® Orange Juice – 4 oz.	20.6%	36.9%	60%
Coors Light® Beer – 12 oz.	80.1%	95%	96.8%
Monty's Hill® Chardonnay – 4 oz.	37%	60.1%	80%
Ireland® Coffee – 6 oz.	93.7%	96.8%	98%
Tetley® Iced Tea – 8 oz.	99%	99.5%	–
Seven Seas® Red Wine & Vinegar Salad Dressing – 31 gm	90%	95%	98%
Old El Paso® Thick'n Chunky Salsa Medium – 2 Tbsp.	80.1%	95%	97.5%
Heinz® Tomato Ketchup – 1 Tbsp.	68.4%	87.4%	92.1%
Kraft® Original Barbeque Sauce 2 Tbsp.	60.2%	80%	90%
Ragu® Old World Style Traditional Sauce – 125 gm	20.6%	36.9%	60.2%
Dannon® Strawberry Lowfat Yogurt (fully mixed) – 116 gm	49.9%	68.4%	80.1%
Grapefruit Sections – 150 gm	36.9%	50%	68.3%
Sauerkraut – 2 Tbsp.	60.3%	80%	92.1%
Red Cabbage – 130 gm	49.7%	68.3%	74.8%

For more information and samples, please write or call toll-free 1-800-994-4711.
[See table at bottom of previous page]
Shown in Product Identification Guide, page 503

American Longevity
**2400 BOSWELL ROAD
CHULA VISTA, CA 91914**

Direct Inquiries to:
Customer Service
800-982-3189
Fax:
619-934-3205
www.americanlongevity.net

Plant Derived Minerals

Description: Minerals which are so important to our health are not so readily available. Minerals never occured in a uniform blanket on the crust of the Earth. Therefore, unless you supplement with minerals, you can't guarantee that you will get all you need through the 4 food groups. Our Plant Derived Mineral products are liquid concentrates containing a natural assortment of up to 77 minerals from prehistoric plants in their unaltered colloidal form. A mineral deficiency can lead to disease or even death. Plant Derived Minerals can help you in your fight against deficiencies. Now, it even comes in a great tasting cherry flavor.

Supplement Facts:
Calories <5
Majestic Earth Plant   600mg *
   Derived Minerals
*daily value not established

Directions:
1) Store in cool environment after opening
2) Suggested as a dietary supplement. For adults, mix 1 or 2 ounces in a small glass of fruit or vegetable juice of your choice. Drink during or after meals, 1 to 3 times a day or as desired. For children reduce amount by two-thirds

Other Ingredients: Calcium, Chlorine, Magnesium, Phosphorus, Potassium, Sodium, Sulfur, Antimony, Arsenic, Aluminum Hydroxide, Barium, Beryllium, Bismuth, Boron, Bromine, Cadmium, Carbon, Cerium Cesium, Chromium, Cobalt, Copper, Dysprosium, Erbium, Europium, Fluorine, Gadolinium, Gallium, Germanium, Gold, Hafnium, Holmium Hydrogen, Indium, Iodine, Iridium, Iron, Lanthanum, Lead, Lithium, Lutetium, Manganese, Mercury, Molybdenum, Neodymium, Nickel, Niobium, Nitrogen, Osmium, Oxygen, Palladium, Platinum, Praseodymium, Rhenium, Rhodium, Rubidium, Ruthenium, Samarium, Scandium, Selenium, Silicon,

Silver, Strontium, Tantalum, Tellurium, Terbium, Thallium, Thorium, Thulium, Tin, Titanium, Tungsten, Vanadium, Ytterbium, Yttrium, Zinc, Zirconium.

MAJESTIC EARTH
(Ultimate Osteo-FX)

Description: *Majestic Earth Ultimate Osteo-FX was formulated to support healthy bones and joints. With todays fast paced life styles it is becoming increasingly difficult to get enough nutrients in our diets. For many people Majestic Earth Osteo-FX fills the gap! American Longevity is proud to include Majestic Earth Ultimate Osteo-FX in our popular line of Majestic Earth products. Note Majestic Earth Ultimate Osteo-FX goes great with an Ultimate Natures Whey Chocolate or Vanilla shake also. Each quart of Majestic Earth Ultimate Osteo-FX contains Majestic Earth plant derived minerals. These minerals come from a unique source in Southern Utah. They are leached from humic shale with purified water only. The balance of Majestic Earth Ultimate Osteo-FX contains vitamins, major minerals and other beneficial nutrients.

Supplement Facts:

Calories	0
Calories from Fat	0
Total Fat	0
Saturated Fat	0g
Cholesterol	0g
Total Carbohydrates	0g
Dietary Fiber	0g
Sugars	0g
Sodium	0g
Protein	0g
Vitamin D3	100 IU
	25% of Daily Value
Calcium (as tricalcium phosphate, calcium citrate)	1200mg
	120% of Daily Value
Magnesium (as citrate)	200mg
	50% of Daily Value
Zinc (as gluconate)	5mg
	33% of Daily Value
Boron (as chelated amino acid complex)	1mg T
MSM (methyl sulffonyl methane)	250mg T
Glucosamine sulphate KCl	100mg T

*Percent Daily values are based on a 2,000 calorie diet.
T Daily value not established

Directions:
1) Shake well before using.
2) Store in cool environment after opening.
3) Suggested as a food for special dietary use.
4) As with any nutritional supplement program, seek the advice of your health care professional.

Other Ingredients: Water, Majestic Earth Plant Derived Minerals complex, citric acid, potassium benzoate, sodium benzoate, vanillain, natural flavors, sucralose.

Amerifit Nutrition, Inc.
**166 HIGHLAND PARK DRIVE
BLOOMFIELD, CT 06002**

Direct Inquiries to:
Consumer Resources
(800) 722-3476
FAX: (860) 243-9400
www.amerifit.com

ESTROVEN®
Dietary supplement for perimenopause, menopause and post-menopause

Uses: Estroven contains natural ingredients to help reduce physical and psychological effects of hormonal imbalance. Clinical studies of the specific ingredients in Estroven when used by women experiencing climacteric symptoms have shown significant reduction in vasomotor symptoms including night sweats and hot flashes; reduction of menopause-related irritability; support for a restful sleep; and protective effects on bones and the cardiovascular system.

Directions: Take one caplet or gelcap daily before bedtime with food.

Ingredients: Each caplet or gelcap contains: Vitamin E 30IU; Thiamin 2mg; Riboflavin 2mg; Niacin 20mg; Vitamin B-6 10mg; Folate 400mcg; Vitamin B-12 6mcg; Calcium 150mg; Selenium 70mcg; Boron 1.5mg; Isoflavones (from *Pueraria lobata* root extract and GMO-free soybeans) 55mg; Estroven Calming Herbal Blend (proprietary blend of Date seed extract [*Zizyphus spinosa*] and Magnolia bark extract) 150mg; Black cohosh root standardized extract 40mg.

Other Ingredients: cellulose, croscarmellose sodium, silica, vegetable magnesium stearate, titanium dioxide (natural mineral source), vanilla and caramel color.
Estroven contains no artificial dyes, colors, preservatives, flavors, yeast, wheat, gluten or lactose.

Precautions: Do not take if pregnant, lactating or trying to conceive. Keep out of reach of children.

How Supplied: Box of 30 Caplets
Box of 40 Easy-to-Swallow Gelcaps
Shown in Product Identification Guide, page 503

EXTRA STRENGTH ESTROVEN®
Dietary supplement for menopause

Uses: Extra Strength Estroven contains a high level of natural ingredients clinically shown to help relieve vasomotor symptoms of menopause such as hot flashes and night sweats. Extra Strength

Continued on next page

Estroven Extra Strength—Cont.

Estroven has also been shown to improve mental clarity, reduce irritability and the risk of osteoporosis, as well as support cardiovascular and urinary tract health.

Directions: Take two caplets daily. Best taken near mealtime.

Ingredients: Each caplet contains: Vitamin E 30IU; Thiamin 5mg; Riboflavin 5mg; Niacin 20mg; Vitamin B-6 25mg; Folate 400mcg; Vitamin B-12 25mcg; Calcium 200mg; Selenium 70mcg; Chromium 120mcg; Boron 1.5mg; Isoflavones (from GMO-free soybeans and *Pueraria lobata* root extract, optimized with Isolase™ enzymes) 80mg; Estroven Balancing Herbal Blend (Green tea extract, Date seed extract [*Zizyphus spinosa*] Cinnamon twig extract, Galangal root extract and Magnolia bark extract) 200mg; Black cohosh root standardized extract 40mg; Cranberry juice 300mg.

Other Ingredients: microcrystalline cellulose, croscarmellose sodium, vegetable stearic acid, Isolase™ enzymes, vegetable magnesium stearate, silica, cellulose, titanium dioxide, riboflavin and sodium citrate.

Extra Strength Estroven contains no artificial dyes, colors, preservatives, flavors, yeast, wheat, gluten, lactose or animal products.

Precautions: Do not take if pregnant, lactating or trying to conceive. Keep out of reach of children.

How Supplied: Box of 56 Caplets
Shown in Product Identification Guide, page 503

VITABALL® VITAMIN GUMBALLS
Multi-vitamin supplement

Uses: Vitaball is a fun and great tasting way to take vitamins. Each bubble gum gumball delivers 100% of the Daily Value of 11 essential vitamins. Offered in a variety of flavors.

Directions: For adults and children over five years of age, chew one gumball daily for 5–10 minutes to ensure release of vitamins. Discard gum after chewing, although not harmful if swallowed. Best taken near mealtime. Adults should supervise children's use.

Nutrition Facts
Serving Size 1 Gumball
Total Calories 15
Total Fat 0g
Total Carbohydrates 4g
   Sugars 4g

	Amount Per Serving	% Daily Value
Vitamin A	5000IU	100
Vitamin C	60mg	100
Vitamin D	400IU	100
Vitamin E	30IU	100
Thiamin	1.5mg	100
Riboflavin	1.7mg	100
Niacin	20mg	100
Vitamin B-6	2mg	100
Folic Acid	400mcg	100
Vitamin B-12	6mcg	100
Biotin	45mcg	15
Pantothenic Acid	10mg	100

*Percent Daily Values (DV) for adults and children 4 years of age and over, based on a 2000 calorie diet.
Not a significant source of dietary fiber, calcium or iron.

Other Ingredients: sucrose, gum base, corn syrup, natural and artificial flavors, sucralose, carnauba wax, artificial colors* and BHT (to maintain freshness).
May also contain one or more of the following: citric acid, tapioca dextrine or maltodextrine, confectioners or resinous glaze, corn starch, beeswax.

---

*Bubble gum – FD&C Red 3, Red 40; Watermelon – FD&C Blue 1, Yellow 5; Grape – FD&C Red 3, Blue 1; Cherry – FD&C Red 40; Blue raspberry – FD&C Blue 1.
Vitaball contains no yeast, wheat, gluten, nuts or dairy products.

Precautions: Keep out of reach of children. Store at room temperature. Secure lid tightly.
Shown in Product Identification Guide, page 503

Awareness Corporation/ dba AwarenessLife
25 SOUTH ARIZONA PLACE, SUITE 500 CHANDLER, ARIZONA 85225

Direct Inquiries to:
1-800-69AWARE
www.awarecorp.com
www.awarenesslife.com

AWARENESS CLEAR™

Description: May help with general digestion.*

Ingredients: Proprietary blend of Oregano Leaf, Clove Flowers, Black Walnut Seed Husk, Peppermint Leaf, Nigella, Grapefruit, Winter Melon Seed, Gentian, Hyssop Leaf, Crampbark, Thyme Leaf, Fennel.

Directions: Take 2 capsules each morning on an empty stomach, 1–2 hours before eating with 1 glass of water

Warnings: Do not use if Pregnant or Breastfeeding. Keep out of reach of children.

How Supplied: 90 Vegetarian Capsules per Bottle

---

*These statements have not been evaluated by the Food and Drug Administration. These products are not intended to diagnose, treat, cure, or prevent any disease.

AWARENESS FEMALE BALANCE™

Description: For relief of mild Menopausal & PMS symptoms*

Ingredients: Angelica Root, Black Cohosh Root, Chinese Peony Root, Oyster Shell, Damiana Leaf, Peppermint Leaf, Passionflower, Hemidesmus Indicus (East Indian Saraparilla)(root), Crampbark, Partridge Berry Fruit, Polygonatum (many-flower Solomon's Seal) (rhizome), Valerian Root, Dandelion Root, Chaste Tree Fruit, Rosemary Leaf, Caraway Seed, Nigella Black cumin seed, Joe Pye (Queen of the Meadow Leaf, Herba Epimedi Barronwort & Epimedium Leaf, Ligusticum Wallichii Chuan Xiong rhizome, Schisandra Berry, Raspberry Leaf.

Directions: Menopause: Use 1 to 2 capsules twice a day (morning & evening) with a glass of water. **Menstruation:** Use during cycle.

Warnings: Do not use this product if you are pregnant or breastfeeding. Consult your doctor prior to using this product if you are taking any prescription medication. Keep out of reach of children.

How Supplied: 60 Vegetarian Capsules per bottle, Clinically Test

---

*These statements have not been evaluated by the Food and Drug Administration. These products are not intended to diagnose, treat, cure, or prevent any disease.
Shown in Product Identification Guide, page 503

DAILY COMPLETE®

Description: Liquid Supplement. 100% vegetarian ingredients delivers 211 vitamins, minerals, antioxidants, enzymes, fruits and vegetables, amino acids and herbs, in one ounce liquid a day* (great orange taste) Helps to Provide Energy & Reduce Stress Levels

Ingredients: Rich in Vitamins & Minerals, Ionic Plant Minerals, Botanical Antioxidants with Phenalgrin™, 32 Fruit & Vegetable Whole Juice Complex, Whole Superfood Green complex, 34 Herbal Ingredients, Essential Fatty Acid Complex, Special Ocean Vegetable Blend

Directions: Take 1 ounce (30 ml) per day, during or immediately after a meal

Warnings: Do not use if pregnant or breast-feeding. Keep out of reach of children.

How Supplied: 30 ounces per Bottle, Clinically tested

———
*These statements have not been evaluated by the Food and Drug Administration. These products are not intended to diagnose, treat, cure, or prevent any disease.
Shown in Product Identification Guide, page 503

EXPERIENCE®

Description: Promotes Regularity & Cleanses the Colon

Ingredients: Proprietary Blend of Senna, Blonde Psyllium Seed Husk, Fennel Seed, Cornsilk, Solomon's seal, Rhubarb Root, Kelp

Directions: Take 1 to 2 Capsules before bedtime with a full glass of water.

Warnings: Do not use if pregnant or breast-feeding or if you have colitis. Keep out of reach of children.

How Supplied: 90 Capsules per bottle, Clinically tested

———
*These statements have not been evaluated by the Food and Drug Administration. These products are not intended to diagnose, treat, cure, or prevent any disease.
Shown in Product Identification Guide, page 503

PURE GARDENS CREAM®

Description: 100% natural, may help to improve dry skin, fine lines and age spots.

Ingredients: Apple oil, vitamin C, vitamin E, Aloe Vera Leaf, Almond Oil, Cold Press Virgin Olive Oil, Sesame Oil, Chamomile Flowers Oil, Calendula Officinalis Oil, Beeswax, Jojoba Oil, Linseed Oil.

Directions: Application for both face and body. External use only

How Supplied: 2 ounce jar, Clinically tested

PURETRIM™ CAPSULES

Description: Helps Control Appetite and Cravings Naturally*.

Ingredients: Mediterranean Proprietary Blend of Forskohlii root extract, guarana seed extract, green tea leaf extract, olive leaf extract, rosemary, mate leaf extract, cocoa bean, artichoke leaf extract, kelp, nigella, cinnamon twig extract, greater galangal extract, polygonatum, pepper (black) extract, grape leaf extract, an pomegranate fruit extract.

Directions: Take 1 capsule mid-morning & 1 capsule mid-afternoon with water.

Warnings: Do not use this product if you are pregnant or breastfeeding, or have hypertension. Consult your doctor prior to using this product if you are taking any prescription medication. Consult your physician before using if you are on a caffeine-restricted diet. Keep out of reach of children.

How Supplied: 60 Vegetarian capsules. Clinically Tested Ingredients

———
*These statements have not been evaluated by the Food and Drug Administration. These products are not intended to diagnose, treat, cure, or prevent any disease.
Shown in Product Identification Guide, page 503

PURETRIM™ WHOLEFOOD WELLNESS SHAKE

Description: Vegetarian Natural Wholefood High Protein Low Carb Energy Shake. No Dairy, No Soy

Ingredients: Vegetable Pea & Brown Rice Protein, Antioxidants, Prebiotics, Essential Fatty Acids & Enzyme Active Greens

Directions: Mix contents in 10 oz. of cold water.

Warnings: Not for use by pregnant or lactating women. Must be 18 years or older to use.

How Supplied: 10 Packets (Net Wt 500 g)
Shown in Product Identification Guide, page 503

SYNERGYDEFENSE® Capsules

Description: Maintain a healthy intestinal tract, boosts the immune system, & strengthens the body's natural defense.

Ingredients: Proprietary Blend of Enzymes, Probiotics, Antioxidants, Prebiotics

Directions: Take 1 capsule with a glass of water during or before your largest meal of the day. You may increase to 1 capsule twice a day, taken with your largest meals.

Warnings: Do not use if pregnant or lactating. If under 18, consult a physician before use.

How Supplied: 30 Vegetarian Capsules individually sealed

———
*These statements have not been evaluated by the Food and Drug Administration. These products are not intended to diagnose, treat, cure, or prevent any disease.
Shown in Product Identification Guide, page 503

**Bayer HealthCare LLC
Consumer Care
Division**

**36 Columbia Road
P.O. Box 1910
Morristown, NJ 07962-1910**

Direct Inquiries to:
Consumer Relations
(800) 331-4536
www.bayercare.com

For Medical Emergency Contact:
Bayer HealthCare LLC
Consumer Care Division
(800) 331-4536

FERGON®
**Ferrous Gluconate
Iron Supplement
High Potency**

Fergon Tablets are for use as a dietary iron supplement.

Directions: Adults: One tablet daily, with food.

Supplement Facts
Serving Size: One tablet

	Amount Per Serving	% Daily Value
Iron	27 mg	150%

Ingredients: Ferrous Gluconate Sucrose, Corn Starch, Hypromellose, Talc, Maltodextrin, Magnesium Stearate, Silicon Dioxide, Titanium Dioxide, Polyethylene Glycol, FD&C Yellow #5 (tartrazine) Aluminum Lake, FD&C Blue #1 Aluminum Lake, Polysorbate 80, Carnauba Wax.
AVOID EXCESSIVE HEAT
USP: Fergon meets the USP standards for strength, quality, and purity.

Warning: Accidental overdose of iron-containing products is a leading cause of fatal poisoning in children under 6. Keep this product out of reach of children. In case of accidental overdose, call a doctor or Poison Control Center immediately.

If pregnant or breast feeding, ask a health professional before use.
CHILD RESISTANT CAP
DO NOT USE IF SAFETY SEAL UNDER CAP WITH BLUE "Bayer Coporation" PRINT IS TORN OR MISSING.

How Supplied: Bottle of 100 Easy to Swallow Tablets
Questions? Comments?
Please call 1-800-331-4536.

Continued on next page

Fergon—Cont.

Visit our website at
www.bayercare.com
Bayer HealthCare LLC
Consumer Care Division
Morristown, NJ 07960 USA

Shown in Product Identification Guide, page 504

FLINTSTONES® COMPLETE
Children's Chewable Multivitamin/ Multimineral Supplement

Directions: 2 & 3 years of age —**Chew** one-half tablet daily. Adults and children 4 years of age and older—**Chew** one tablet daily.

Supplement Facts
Serving Size: $\frac{1}{2}$ tablet (2 & 3 years of age); 1 tablet (4 years of age and older)

Amount Per Tablet	% Daily Value for Children 2 & 3 Years of Age ($^1/_2$ Tablet)	% Daily Value for Adults and Children 4 Years of Age and older (1 Tablet)
Vitamin A		
3000 IU	60%	60%
Vitamin C 60 mg	75%	100%
Vitamin D 400 IU	50%	100%
Vitamin E 30 IU	150%	100%
Thiamin (B$_1$)		
1.5 mg	107%	100%
Riboflavin (B$_2$)		
1.7 mg	106%	100%
Niacin 15 mg	83%	75%
Vitamin B$_6$ 2 mg	143%	100%
Folic Acid		
400 mcg	100%	100%
Vitamin B$_{12}$		
6 mcg	100%	100%
Biotin 40 mcg	13%	13%
Pantothenic Acid		
10 mg	100%	100%
Calcium (elemental)		
100 mg	6%	10%
Iron		
18 mg	90%	100%
Phosphorus		
100 mg	6%	10%
Iodine 150 mcg	107%	100%
Magnesium		
20 mg	5%	5%
Zinc 12 mg	75%	80%
Copper 2 mg	100%	100%

Ingredients: Dicalcium Phosphate, Sorbitol, Magnesium Phosphate, Sodium Ascorbate, Ferrous Fumarate, Gelatin, Natural and Artificial Flavors (including fruit acids), Pregelatinized Starch, Vitamin E Acetate, Stearic Acid, Carrageenan, Hydrogenated Vegetable Oil, Magnesium Stearate, FD&C Red #40 Aluminum Lake, Zinc Oxide, Niacinamide, Calcium Pantothenate, FD&C Yellow #6 Aluminum Lake, Xylitol, Aspartame* (a sweetener), FD&C Blue #2 Aluminum Lake, Cupric Oxide, Pyridoxine Hydrochloride, Riboflavin, Thiamine Mononitrate, Monoammonium Glycyrrhizinate, Vitamin A Acetate, Beta Carotene, Folic Acid, Potassium Iodide, Vitamin D, Biotin, Magnesium Oxide, Vitamin B$_{12}$.

***PHENYLKETONURICS: CONTAINS PHENYLALANINE.**

Warning: Accidental overdose of iron-containing products is a leading cause of fatal poisoning in children under 6. Keep this product out of reach of children. In case of accidental overdose, call a doctor or Poison Control Center immediately.

KEEP OUT OF REACH OF CHILDREN.
CHILD RESISTANT CAP

How Supplied: Bottles of 60s, 150's 20's, 240's

THE FLINTSTONES and all related characters and elements are trademarks of Hanna-Barbera © 2000.

Questions or comments?
Please call 1-800-800-4793
Visit our website at www.bayercare.com
Bayer Healthcare
Consumer Care Division
P.O. Box 1910
Morristown, NJ 07962-1910 USA

Shown in Product Identification Guide, page 504

MY FIRST FLINTSTONES®
Children's Multivitamin Supplement

#1 Pediatricians' Choice

For children's chewable vitamins
• Specially formulated for children 2 and 3 years of age.
• Provides 10 essential vitamins, including A, D, and C, important for your child's healthy growth and development.
• Small, easy to chew tablets
• **GREAT TASTING** flavors
• **FUN CHARACTER SHAPES**
NUTRIENTS NEEDED TO GROW-UP STRONG AND HEALTHY.
B VITAMINS
Aid in the release of energy from food.*
VITAMIN C
Helps support the immune system.*

VITAMIN D
Helps absorption of calcium for strong bones and teeth.*

***These statements have not been evaluated by the FDA. This product is not intended to diagnose, treat, cure, or prevent any disease.**

Directions: Children 2 & 3 years of age – **Chew** one tablet daily. Tablet should be fully chewed or crushed for children who cannot chew.

Supplement Facts
Serving Size: One tablet

	Amount Per Tablet	% Daily Value for Children 2 & 3 Years of Age
Vitamin A	2500 IU	100%
Vitamin C	60 mg	150%
Vitamin D	400 IU	100%
Vitamin E	15 IU	150%
Thiamin (B$_1$)	1.05 mg	150%
Riboflavin (B$_2$)	1.2 mg	150%
Niacin	13.5 mg	150%
Vitamin B$_6$	1.05 mg	150%
Folic Acid	300 mcg	150%
Vitamin B$_{12}$	4.5 mcg	150%

Ingredients: Sucrose (a natural sweetener), Sodium Ascorbate, Stearic Acid, Invert Sugar, Artificial Flavors (including fruit acids), Gelatin, Vitamin E Acetate, Niacinamide, FD&C Red #40 Lake, FD&C Yellow #6 Lake, FD&C Blue #2 Lake, Pyridoxine Hydrochloride, Riboflavin, Thiamine Mononitrate, Vitamin A Acetate, Folic Acid, Beta Carotene, Vitamin D, Vitamin B$_{12}$.
USP: My First Flintstones formula meets the USP standards for strength, quality, and purity for Oil- and Water-soluble Vitamins Tablets. Complies with USP Method 2: Vitamins A, D, E, B12, Thiamin, Riboflavin, Niacin, and B6.
Keep out of reach of children.

How Supplied: bottles of 60's
THE FLINTSTONES and all related characters and elements are trademarks of and © Hanna-Barbera.
(s01)
CHILD RESISTANT CAP
Questions or comments?
Please call 1-800-800-4793.
Visit our website at
www.bayercare.com
Do not use this product if safety seal bearing "Bayer Corporation" under cap is torn or missing
Bayer HealthCare LLC
P.O. Box 1910
Morristown, NJ 07962-1910
Shown in Product Identification Guide, page 504

FLINTSTONES® BONE BUILDING CALCIUM CHEWS
Building a lifetime of Strong Bones*

Flintstones Bone-Building Calcium Chews are a tasty way to give your growing kids key nutrients they need to help build a lifetime of strong and healthy bones*.

Each delicious, chocolate creamy chew contains as much calcium as two 6 1/2 ounce glasses of milk plus Vitamin D to help absorb calcium.

Give your kids this calcium supplement in addition to a Flintstones multivitamin. Each chew is an excellent source of calcium for Moms and Dads too!

*These statements have not been evaluated by the Food and Drug Administration. This product is not intended to diagnose, treat, cure or prevent any disease.

Directions: Adults and children 4 years of age and older, chew one to two pieces daily with a meal.

Supplement Facts

Serving Size: One Piece

	Amount Per Serving	% Daily Value
Calories	20	
Total Carbohydrate	3 g	1%*
Sugars	2 g	**
Vitamin D	200 IU	50%
Calcium (elemental)	500 mg	50%
Sodium	10 mg	<1%

* Percent Daily Values are based on a 2,000 calorie diet.
** Daily Value not established.

Ingredients: Corn Syrup, Calcium Carbonate, Sugar, Partially Hydrogenated Coconut Oil, Dried Milk Solids, Cocoa. Contains less than 2% of the following: Acacia, Butylated Hydroxytoluene (BHT), Caramel Flavor, Coconut Oil, Corn Starch, Dicalcium Phosphate, Glycerin, Lactose, Lecithin, Salt, Silicon Dioxide, Sodium Benzoate, Sodium Prussiate Yellow, Sorbic Acid, Soybean Oil, Tricalcium Phosphate, Vanilla Flavor, Vitamin D3.

Keep out of reach of children.

"Do not use if plastic band around lid is torn or missing."

THE FLINTSTONES and all related characters and elements are trademarks of and © Hanna-Barbera.

(s02)

Questions or comments?
Please call 1-800-800-4793.
Visit our website at
www.bayercare.com
90000038-00
Made in U.S.A.
Distributed by:
Bayer HealthCare LLC
Consumer Care Division
P.O. Box 1910
Morristown, NJ 07962-1910 USA

Shown in Product Identification Guide, page 504

Amount Per Tablet	% Daily Value for Children 2 & 3 Years of Age (½ Tablet)	% Daily Value for Adults and Children 4 Years of Age and Older (1 Tablet)
Vitamin A 3000 IU	60%	60%
Vitamin C 60 mg	75%	100%
Vitamin D 400 IU	50%	100%
Vitamin E 30 IU	150%	100%
Thiamin (B₁) 1.5 mg	107%	100%
Riboflavin (B₂) 1.7 mg	106%	100%
Niacin 15 mg	83%	75%
Vitamin B₆ 2 mg	143%	100%
Folic Acid 400 mcg	100%	100%
Vitamin B₁₂ 6 mcg	100%	100%
Biotin 40 mcg	13%	13%
Pantothenic Acid 10 mg	100%	100%
Calcium (elemental) 100 mg	6%	10%
Iron 18 mg	90%	100%
Phosphorus 100 mg	6%	10%
Iodine 150 mcg	107%	100%
Magnesium 20 mg	5%	5%
Zinc 12 mg	75%	80%
Copper 2 mg	100%	100%

ONE-A-DAY® KIDS
BUGS BUNNY AND FRIENDS COMPLETE SUGAR FREE CHILDREN'S MULTIVITAMIN/ MULTIMINERAL SUPPLEMENT

Complete with 19 essential vitamins and minerals, including Vitamin C, Iron, and Calcium for your child's healthy growth and development.

Directions: 2 & 3 years of age—**Chew** one-half tablet daily. Adults and children 4 years of age and older—**Chew** one tablet daily.

Supplement Facts

Serving Size: ½ tablet – (2 & 3 years of age); 1 tablot   (4 years of age and older) [See table above]

Ingredients: Dicalcium Phosphate, Sorbitol, Magnesium Phosphate, Sodium Ascorbate, Gelatin, Ferrous Fumarate, Natural and Artificial Flavors (including fruit acids), Starch, Stearic Acid, FD&C Red #40 Lake, Vitamin E Acetate, Carrageenan, Niacinamide, Magnesium Stearate, Hydrogenated Vegetable Oil, Zinc Oxide, FD&C Yellow #6 Lake, FD&C Blue #2 Lake, Calcium Pantothenate, Aspartame* (a sweetener), Cupric Oxide, Pyridoxine Hydrochloride, Vitamin A Acetate, Riboflavin, Thiamine Mononitrate, Beta Carotene, Folic Acid, Potassium Iodide, Vitamin D, Biotin, Magnesium Oxide, Vitamin B₁₂.

* PHENYLKETONURICS: CONTAINS PHENYLALANINE

Keep out of reach of children

WARNING: Accidental overdose of iron-containing products is a leading cause of fatal poisoning in children under 6. Keep this product out of reach of children. In case of accidental overdose, call a doctor or Poison Control Center immediately.

USP: Bugs Bunny Complete formula meets the USP standards for strength,

quality, and purity for Oil- and Water-soluble Vitamins and Minerals Tablets.

How Supplied: Contains 60 chewable tablets

Cartoon Network and logo are trademarks of Cartoon Network ©2001
CHILD RESISTANT CAP
Do not use this product if safety seal bearing "Bayer Corporation" under cap is torn or missing
LOONEY TUNES, characters, names and all related indicia are trademarks of Warner Bros. ©2001
Questions or comments?
Please call 1-800-800-4793
Visit our website at www.oneaday.com
Bayer HealthCare LLC
Consumer Care Division
P.O. Box 1910
Morristown, NJ 07962-1910 USA

ONE-A-DAY® KIDS
SCOOBY-DOO!™ COMPLETE CHILDREN'S MULTIVITAMIN/ MULTIMINERAL SUPPLEMENT

Provides 19 essential vitamins and minerals, including Vitamin C, Iron, and Calcium for your child's healthy growth and development.

Directions: 2 & 3 years of age—**Chew** one-half tablet daily. Adults and children 4 years of age and older—**Chew** one tablet daily.

Supplement Facts

Serving Size: ½ tablet (2 & 3 years of age); 1 tablet (4 years of age and older) [See table at top of next page]

Ingredients: Dicalcium Phosphate, Sorbitol, Magnesium Phosphate, Sodium Ascorbate, Ferrous Fumarate, Gelatin, Natural and Artificial Flavors (including fruit acids), Pregelatinized Starch, Vita-

Continued on next page

Amount Per Tablet	% Daily Value for Children 2 & 3 Years of Age (½ Tablet)	% Daily Value for Adults and Children 4 Years of Age and older (1 Tablet)
Vitamin A 3000 IU	60%	60%
Vitamin C 60 mg	75%	100%
Vitamin D 400 IU	50%	100%
Vitamin E 30 IU	150%	100%
Thiamin (B_1) 1.5 mg	107%	100%
Riboflavin (B_2) 1.7 mg	106%	100%
Niacin 15 mg	83%	75%
Vitamin B_6 2 mg	143%	100%
Folic Acid 400 mcg	100%	100%
Vitamin B_{12} 6 mcg	100%	100%
Biotin 40 mcg	13%	13%
Pantothenic Acid 10 mg	100%	100%
Calcium (elemental) 100 mg	6%	10%
Iron 18 mg	90%	100%
Phosphorus 100 mg	6%	10%
Iodine 150 mcg	107%	100%
Magnesium 20 mg	5%	5%
Zinc 12 mg	75%	80%
Copper 2 mg	100%	100%

One-A-Day Kids Scooby—Cont.

min E Acetate, Stearic Acid, Carrageenan, Hydrogenated Vegetable Oil, Magnesium Stearate, FD&C Red #40 Aluminum Lake, Zinc Oxide, Niacinamide, Calcium Pantothenate, FD&C Yellow #6 Aluminum Lake, Xylitol, Aspartame* (a sweetener), FD&C Blue #2 Aluminum Lake, Cupric Oxide, Pyridoxine Hydrochloride, Riboflavin, Thiamine Mononitrate, Monoammonium Glycyrrhizinate, Vitamin A Acetate, Beta Carotene, Folic Acid, Potassium Iodide, Vitamin D, Biotin, Magnesium Oxide, Vitamin B_{12}.

*PHENYLKETONURICS: CONTAINS PHENYLALANINE

WARNING: Accidental overdose of iron-containing products is a leading cause of fatal poisoning in children under 6. Keep this product out of reach of children. In case of accidental overdose, call a doctor or Poison Control Center immediately.

Scooby-Doo Complete formula meets the **USP** standards for strength, quality, and purity for Oil- and Water-soluble Vitamins and Minerals Tablets.

**Keep out of reach of children
CHILD RESISTANT CAP**

Do not use this product if safety seal bearing "Bayer Corporation" under cap is torn or missing

How Supplied: ONE-A-DAY® KIDS SCOOBY-DOO COMPLETE bottles of 50's, 100's

SCOOBY-DOO, characters, names and all related indicia are trademarks of Hanna-Barbera © 2001.

CARTOON NETWORK and logo are trademarks of Cartoon Network © 2001

**Questions or comments?
Please call 1-800-800-4793.
Visit our website at www.oneaday.com**

Bayer HealthCare LLC
Consumer Care Division
P.O. Box 1910
Morristown, NJ 07962-1910 USA

ONE-A-DAY® KIDS SCOOBY-DOO™ PLUS CALCIUM
CHILDREN'S MULTIVITAMIN SUPPLEMENT

Provides 10 essential vitamins plus calcium for your child's healthy growth and development. Contains as much calcium as one 5 oz glass of milk.

Directions: Adults and children 2 years of age and older—**Chew** one tablet daily.

Supplement Facts
Serving Size: One tablet

Amount Per Tablet	% Daily Value for Children 2 & 3 Years of Age	% Daily Value for Adults and Children 4 Years of Age and older
Vitamin A 2500 IU	100%	50%
Vitamin C 60 mg	150%	100%
Vitamin D 400 IU	100%	100%
Vitamin E 15 IU	150%	50%
Thiamin (B_1) 1.05 mg	150%	70%
Riboflavin (B_2) 1.2 mg	150%	70%
Niacin 13.5 mg	150%	67%
Vitamin B_6 1.05 mg	150%	52%
Folic Acid 300 mcg	150%	75%
Vitamin B_{12} 4.5 mcg	150%	75%
Calcium (elemental) 200 mg	25%	20%

Ingredients: Calcium Carbonate, Sorbitol, Pregelatinized Starch, Sodium Ascorbate, Natural and Artificial Flavors (including fruit acids), Stearic Acid, Gelatin, Magnesium Stearate, Vitamin E Acetate, Niacinamide, FD&C Red #40 Lake, FD&C Yellow #6 Lake, Aspartame* (a sweetener), FD&C Blue #2 Lake, Pyridoxine Hydrochloride, Riboflavin, Thiamine Mononitrate, Vitamin A Acetate, Monoammonium Glycyrrhizinate, Folic Acid, Beta Carotene, Vitamin D, Vitamin B_{12}.

*** PHENYLKETONURICS: CONTAINS PHENYLALANINE
Keep out of reach of children**

USP: Scooby-Doo Plus Calcium formula meets the USP standards for strength, quality, and purity for Oil- and Water-soluble Vitamins and Minerals Tablets.

How Supplied: Contains 50 Chewable Tablets.

SCOOBY-DOO, characters, names and all related indicia are trademarks of Hanna-Barbera ©2001.
CARTOON NETWORK and logo are trademarks of Cartoon Network ©2001

**CHILD RESISTANT CAP
Do not use this product if safety seal bearing "Bayer Corporation" under cap is torn or missing**

Questions or comments?
**Please call 1-800-800-4793.
Visit our website at www.oneaday.com**
Made in U.S.A.
Bayer HealthCare LLC
Consumer Care Division
P.O. Box 1910
Morristown, NJ 07962-1910 USA

ONE-A-DAY® MEN'S HEALTH FORMULA
Dietary Supplement

Complete Multivitamin for Men Plus More† to support:*
- **HEALTHY PROSTATE**
- **HEALTHY HEART**

With 2 times the amount of **Lycopene** in Centrum® or Centrum® Silver®

---

†Refers to vitamins C, B_6, B_{12}, Calcium, Selenium, Chromium, Magnesium, Copper, Zinc compared to One-A-Day® essential.

---

*These statements have not been evaluated by the Food and Drug Administration. This product is not intended to diagnose, treat, cure, or prevent any disease.

Complete Multivitamin designed for Men to:
- Support Prostate Health with a unique combination of **Lycopene, Selenium, Vitamin E** and **Zinc.***
- Promote Healthy Homocysteine levels, an emerging measure of Heart Health, with **Vitamins B6, B12** and **Folic Acid.***
- Help Maintain Normal Blood Pressure†† with **Calcium, Magnesium, Potassium** and **Vitamin C.***

- **No Iron** – Research suggests excess iron may increase a man's risk of heart disease

††For people with blood pressure already within the normal range

Directions: Adults: One tablet daily, with food.

Supplement Facts
Serving Size: One Tablet

	AMOUNT PER SERVING		% DAILY VALUE
Vitamin A	3500	IU	70%
(14% as beta carotene)			
Vitamin C	90	mg	150%
Vitamin D	400	IU	100%
Vitamin E	45	IU	150%
Vitamin K	20	mcg	25%
Thiamin (B$_1$)	1.2	mg	80%
Riboflavin (B$_2$)	1.7	mg	100%
Niacin	16	mg	80%
Vitamin B$_6$	3	mg	150%
Folic Acid	400	mcg	100%
Vitamin B$_{12}$	18	mcg	300%
Biotin	30	mcg	10%
Pantothenic Acid	5	mg	50%
Calcium (elemental)	210	mg	21%
Magnesium	120	mg	30%
Zinc	15	mg	100%
Selenium	105	mcg	150%
Copper	2	mg	100%
Manganese	2	mg	100%
Chromium	120	mcg	100%
Potassium	100	mg	3%
Lycopene	600	mcg	*

*Daily value not established

Ingredients: Calcium Carbonate, Magnesium Oxide, Potassium Chloride, Cellulose, Ascorbic Acid, dl-Alpha Tocopheryl Acetate, Gelatin, Croscarmellose Sodium, Acacia, Dicalcium Phosphate, Zinc Oxide, Niacinamide, Stearic Acid, Silicon Dioxide, Dextrin, Magnesium Stearate, Corn Starch, d-Calcium Pantothenate, Manganese Sulfate, Calcium Silicate, Pyridoxine Hydrochloride, Sucrose, Mannitol, Hypromellose, Cupric Oxide, Resin, Riboflavin, Thiamine Mononitrate, Vitamin A Acetate, Dextrose, Lecithin, Chromium Chloride, Lycopene, Sodium Carboxymethylcellulose, Folic Acid, Ascorbyl Palmitate, Beta Carotene, Sodium Selenate, Sodium Ascorbate, Sodium Citrate, dl-Alpha Tocopherol, Biotin, Phytonadione, Cyanocobalamin, Ergocalciferol.

KEEP OUT OF REACH OF CHILDREN
CHILD RESISTANT CAP
Do not use this product if safety seal bearing "SEALED for YOUR PROTECTION" under cap is torn or missing

How Supplied: Bottles of 60's & 100's.

USP: One-A-Day Men's Health formula meets the USP standards of strength, quality, and purity for Oil- and Water-Soluble Vitamins with Minerals Tablets.

Questions or comments?
Please call 1-800-800-4793.
Visit our website at www.oneaday.com
Distributed by:
Bayer HealthCare LLC
Consumer Care Division
P.O. Box 1910
Morristown, NJ 07962-1910 USA
Shown in Product Identification Guide, page 505

ONE A DAY® WEIGHTSMART™
Dietary Supplement
With EGCG
Specially formulated to help you while you control your weight.

Complete Multivitamin Plus More†
to:
- **ENHANCE YOUR METABOLISM** WITH EGCG (GREEN TEA EXTRACT)*
- **CONVERT FOOD TO FUEL** WITH EXTRA† CHROMIUM AND KEY B VITAMINS*

Complete Multivitamin specially designed to help you while you're controlling your weight
- **100%** of key daily essential vitamins and minerals
- **EGCG, a natural green tea extract,** to enhance your metabolism*
- Extra† levels of **Chromium** and important **B Vitamins** to help convert food to fuel*
- **Vitamins C, E, B6** and **B12** to help support a healthy heart*
Ephedra Free

***These statements have not been evaluated by the Food and Drug Administration. This product is not intended to diagnose, treat, cure, or prevent any disease.**
† Refers to chromium, B$_1$, B$_2$, niacin, B$_6$, B$_{12}$, and pantothenic acid as compared to Centrum®

Directions: Adults: One tablet daily, with food.

Supplement Facts
Serving size: One tablet

	Amount Per Serving	% Daily Value
Vitamin A	2500 IU	50%
(100% as beta carotene)		
Vitamin C	60 mg	100%
Vitamin D	400 IU	100%
Vitamin E	30 IU	100%
Vitamin K	80 mcg	100%
Thiamin (B$_1$)	1.9 mg	127%
Riboflavin (B$_2$)	2.125 mg	125%
Niacin	25 mg	125%
Vitamin B$_6$	2.5 mg	125%
Folic Acid	400 mcg	100%
Vitamin B$_{12}$	7.5 mcg	125%
Pantothenic Acid	12.5 mg	125%
Calcium (elemental)	300 mg	30%
Iron	18 mg	100%
Magnesium	50 mg	12%
Zinc	15 mg	100%
Selenium	70 mcg	100%
Copper	2 mg	100%
Manganese	2 mg	100%
Chromium	200 mcg	167%
EGCG (from Green Tea Extract, *Camellia sinensis* leaf)	32 mg	*

* Daily Value not established

Ingredients: Calcium Carbonate, Cellulose, Green Tea Extract, Magnesium Oxide, Ascorbic Acid, Ferrous Fumarate, Acacia, dl-alpha Tocopheryl Acetate, Niacinamide, Croscarmellose Sodium, Zinc Oxide, Dicalcium Phosphate, Dextrin, d-Calcium Pantothenate, Silicon Dioxide, Caffeine Powder, Hypromellose, Magnesium Stearate, Titanium Dioxide, Gelatin, Corn Starch, Glucose, Crospovidone, Calcium Silicate, Manganese Sulfate, Cupric Sulfate, Polyethylene Glycol, Pyridoxine Hydrochloride, Riboflavin, Dextrose, Thiamine Mononitrate, Lecithin, Beta Carotene, Chromium Chloride, Resin, Folic Acid, FD&C Blue #1 Lake, Sodium Selenate, Phytonadione, Tricalcium Phosphate, Cholecalciferol, Cyanocobalamin.

> **Warning:** Accidental overdose of iron-containing products is a leading cause of fatal poisoning in children under 6. Keep this product out of reach of children. In case of accidental overdose, call a doctor or Poison Control Center immediately.

If pregnant or breast-feeding, ask a health professional before use.
KEEP OUT OF REACH OF CHILDREN
CHILD RESISTANT CAP
Do not use this product if safety seal bearing *"SEALED for YOUR PROTECTION"* under cap is torn or missing.

How Supplied: 100 Tablets
Questions or comments?
Please call 1-800-800-4793.
Visit our website at www.oneaday.com
USP One-A-Day WeightSmart meets the USP standards of strength, quality, and purity for Oil- and Water-Soluble Vitamins with Minerals Tablets. Complies with USP-Method 1: Vitamin A, D, E, B$_{12}$, Thiamin, Riboflavin, Niacin, B$_6$, Pantothenic Acid.
Made in the U.S.A.
Distributed by:
Bayer HealthCare LLC
Consumer Care Division
P.O. Box 1910
Morristown, NJ 07962-1910 USA
Shown in Product Identification Guide, page 505

ONE-A-DAY® WOMEN'S
Multivitamin/Multimineral
Supplement

Directions: Adults: One tablet daily with food.

Continued on next page

One-A-Day Women's—Cont.

Supplement Facts
Serving Size: One tablet

	AMOUNT PER SERVING		% DAILY VALUE
Vitamin A (20% as beta carotene)	2500	IU	50%
Vitamin C	60	mg	100%
Vitamin D	400	IU	100%
Vitamin E	30	IU	100%
Thiamine (B_1)	1.5	mg	100%
Riboflavin (B_2)	1.7	mg	100%
Niacin	10	mg	50%
Vitamin B_6	2	mg	100%
Folic Acid	400	mcg	100%
Vitamin B_{12}	6	mcg	100%
Pantothenic Acid	5	mg	50%
Calcium (elemental)	450	mg	45%
Iron	18	mg	100%
Magnesium	50	mg	12%
Zinc	15	mg	100%

Ingredients: Calcium Carbonate, Cellulose, Magnesium Oxide, Ascorbic Acid, Acacia, Ferrous Fumarate, dl-alpha Tocopheryl Acetate, Croscarmellose Sodium, Zinc Oxide, Magnesium Stearate, Titanium Dioxide, Dextrin, Hypromellose, Niacinamide, Gelatin, Starch, d-Calcium Pantothenate, Calcium Silicate, Polyethylene Glycol, Silicon Dioxide, Dextrose, Pyridoxine Hydrochloride, Lecithin, Riboflavin, Thiamine Mononitrate, Vitamin A Acetate, Resin, Folic Acid, Beta Carotene, FD&C Yellow #5 (tartrazine) Lake, FD&C Yellow #6 Lake, FD&C Blue #2 Lake, Cholecalciferol, Cyanocobalamin.

USP: One-A-Day Women's formula meets the USP standards of strength, quality, and purity for Oil- and Water-Soluble Vitamins with Minerals Tablets.

WARNING: Accidental overdose of iron-containing products is a leading cause of fatal poisoning in children under 6. Keep this product out of reach of children. In case of accidental overdose, call a doctor or Poison Control Center immediately.

KEEP OUT OF REACH OF CHILDREN CHILD RESISTANT CAP
Do not use this product if safety seal bearing *"SEALED for YOUR PROTECTION"* **under cap is torn or missing**

How Supplied: Bottles of 60 and 100.
Questions or comments?
Please call 1-800-800-4793.
Visit our website at www.oneaday.com
Distributed by:
Bayer HealthCare LLC
Consumer Care Division
P.O. Box 1910
Morristown, NJ 07962-1910 USA
Shown in Product Identification Guide, page 505

PHILLIPS'® SOFT CHEWS
[*fĭ-lĭps sŏft chews*]
laxative dietary supplement
Chocolate Creme Flavor

Comfortable Overnight Relief of Occasional Constipation* Cramp-free

* This statement has not been evaluated by the Food and Drug Administration. This product is not intended to diagnose, treat, cure, or prevent any disease.

Directions: For adults and children 12 years and older. Take 2 to 4 Chews daily, preferably all at bedtime, or individually throughout the day. Drink a full glass (8 oz.) of liquid with each serving. Do not exceed the recommended daily amount. Children under 12, ask a doctor before use.

Supplement Facts
Serving Size: 1 Chew

	Amount Per Serving	% Daily Value
Calories	20	
Total Carbohydrate	3 g	1%*
Sugars	2 g	†
Magnesium	500 mg	125%
Sodium	10 mg	<1%

*Percent Daily Values are based on a 2,000 calorie diet.
†Daily Value not established.

Ingredients: Corn Syrup, Sugar, Magnesium Hydroxide, Partially Hydrogenated Coconut Oil, Cocoa, Chocolate Powder, Natural and Artificial Flavors. Contains less than 2% of the following: Acesulfame Potassium, Corn Starch, Dextrose, Glycerin, Propylene Glycol, Salt, Sodium Prussiate, Soy Lecithin, Soybean Oil, Sucralose, Tricalcium Phosphate.

Warnings: Keep out of reach of children. If you are pregnant or breastfeeding, ask a health professional before use. Ask a doctor before use if you have kidney disease, stomach pain, nausea or vomiting, or a sudden change in bowel habits that lasts over 14 days. Ask your doctor or pharmacist before use if you are taking a prescription drug. This product may interact with certain prescription drugs. Stop use and talk to your doctor if you need to use a laxative for more than one week, or have rectal bleeding or no bowel movement after using this product. These could be signs of a serious condition.
Store at room temperature. Protect from excessive heat and humidity. **Do not use if foil pouch is torn or open.**

How Supplied: 18 chews
Made in U.S.A.

Distributed by:
Bayer HealthCare LLC
Consumer Care Division
P.O. Box 1910
Morristown, NJ 07962-1910 USA
Shown in Product Identification Guide, page 505

Beach Pharmaceuticals
Division of Beach Products, Inc.
5220 SOUTH MANHATTAN AVE.
TAMPA, FL 33611

Direct Inquiries to:
Richard Stephen Jenkins, Exec. V.P.:
(813) 839-6565

BEELITH Tablets
magnesium supplement with pyridoxine HCl

Description: Each tablet contains magnesium oxide 600 mg and pyridoxine hydrochloride (Vitamin B_6) 25 mg equivalent to Vitamin B_6 20 mg.

Supplement Facts
Serving Size: 1 Tablet

	Amount Per Tablet	% Daily Value
Magnesium	362 mg	90%
Vitamin B_6	20 mg	1000%

Inactive Ingredients: D&C Yellow No. 10, FD&C Yellow No. 6 (Sunset Yellow), hydroxypropylmethylcellulose, magnesium stearate, microcrystalline cellulose, polyethylene glycol, sodium starch glycolate, titanium dioxide, and water.

Indications: As a dietary supplement for patients with magnesium and/or Vitamin B_6 deficiencies resulting from malnutrition, alcoholism, magnesium depleting drugs, chemotherapy, and inadequate nutritional intake or absorption. Also, increases urinary magnesium levels.

Dosage: One tablet daily or as directed by a physician.

Warnings: Do not take this product if you are presently taking a prescription drug without consulting your physician or other health professional. If you have kidney disease, take only under the supervision of a physician. Excessive dosage may cause laxation. If pregnant or breast-feeding, ask a health professional before use. **KEEP OUT OF THE REACH OF CHILDREN.**

How Supplied: Golden yellow, film-coated tablet with the letters **BP** and the number **132** imprinted on each tablet. Packaged in bottles of 100 (Item No. 0486-1132-01) tablets.

Beutlich LP Pharmaceuticals
1541 SHIELDS DRIVE
WAUKEGAN, IL 60085-8304

Direct Inquiries to:
847-473-1100
800-238-8542 in US & Canada
FAX 847–473-1122
www.beutlich.com
e-mail beutlich@beutlich.com

PERIDIN-C®
Vitamin C Supplement

Dietary supplement helps alleviate hot flashes by improving capillary strength and maintaining vascular integrity, reducing the physiologic potential for flushing.

Suggested Use: As a Dietary Supplement - 1 tablet daily or as directed/For Hot Flashes - 2 tablets, 3 times per day after meals. Reduce servings gradually after one month until effective daily intake is determined.

Ingredients:
Ascorbic Acid (Vitamin C) 200 mg
Hesperidin Complex (Bioflavonoids) - 150 mg
Hesperidin Methyl Chalcone (Bioflavonoid) - 50 mg

Other Ingredients: hydroxypropyl methylcellulose, Microcrystalline cellulose, crospovidone, stearic acid, polydextrose, titanium dioxide, yellow 6 lake, polyethylene glycol, magnesium stearate, silicon dioxide, triacetin, carnauba wax and polysorbate 80.

How Supplied: In bottles of:
100 tablets NDC #0283-0597-01
500 tablets NDC #0283-0597-05

Earthspring, LLC
7620 E McKELLIPS RD
SUITE 4 PMB 86
SCOTTSDALE, ARIZONA USA 85257

Direct Inquiries to:
www.greencalcium.com
www.totalgreens.com
www.earthspring.com
888-841-7363

GREEN CALCIUM™

Description: Calcium From Vegetables & Green Plants
Ingredients: Vitamin B1, Vitamin D, Calcium, Magnesium from 43 plants & vegetables sources
Directions: Take 1 Tablespoon Daily

Warnings: Do not use this product if you are pregnant or breastfeeding.
How Supplied: 16 Oz Bottle

TOTAL GREENS™

Description: Daily Green Drink of Fruits, Vegetables, & Green Plants
Ingredients: Over 75 Green Plants, Fruits, Vegetables per serving
Directions: 1 Scoop in Water Daily
Warnings: Do not use this product if you are pregnant or breastfeeding.
How Supplied: Powder in 30 serving canister

Fleming & Company
1733 GILSINN LANE
FENTON, MO 63026

Direct Inquiries to:
Tom Johnson
636 343-5306
800-633-1886
FAX (636) 343-5322
www.flemingcompany.com

MAGONATE® Tablets
MAGONATE® Liquid
Magnesium Gluconate (Dihydrate), USP
(Dietary Supplement)

Description: Each 2 tablets contain magnesium 54 mg (from 1000 mg magnesium gluconate dihydrate) calcium 175 mg and phosphorous 182 mg (from 752 mgs dibasic calcium phosphate dihydrate). Each 5 mL of MAGONATE® liquid contains magnesium (elemental) 54 mg. (Each 5 mL contains the same amount of magnesium as contained in 1000 mg of magnesium gluconate dihydrate).

Suggested Uses: MAGONATE® Tablets and Liquid are indicated to maintain magnesium levels when the dietary intake of magnesium is inadequate or when excretion and loss are excessive. MAGONATE® is recommended during and for three weeks after a course in chemotherapy, then monitored regularly.

Precautions: Excessive dosage may cause loose stools.

Contraindications: Patients with kidney disease should not take magnesium supplements without the supervision of a physician.

Dosages and Administration: Two MAGONATE® tablets or 1 teaspoon MAGONATE® Liquid three times a day (mid-morning, mid-afternoon and bedtime) on an empty stomach with a glass of water.

How Supplied: MAGONATE® Tablets are orange scored, and supplied in bottles of 100 (0256-0172-01), and 1000 (0256-0172-02) tablets. MAGONATE® Liquid is supplied in pints, (0256-0184-01).

Rev. 7/00

4Life Research
9850 S 300 W
SANDY, UT 84070

Direct Inquiries to:
Ph: (801) 562-3600
Fax: (801) 562-3699
Email: productsupport@4life.com
Website: www.4life.com

4LIFE® TRANSFER FACTOR CARDIO™

Description: 4Life Transfer Factor Cardio combines Targeted Transfer Factor® derived from egg yolks, (U.S. patent 6,468,534) with scientifically validated nutrients that are designed to address (via immune system response) the pathogens that cause cardiovascular tissue damage and inflammation. 4Life Transfer Factor Cardio supports healthy cardiac function with Targeted Transfer Factor—immune system identification codes for specific cardio viruses and bacteria and suppressor cells that help the immune system control inflammation. Additional cardiovascular support ingredients protect the heart against cholesterol, homocysteine, oxidative damage, and unhealthy blood pressure levels include vitamins A, C, E, B6, B12 and phytochemicals from herbs such as garlic, red rice yeast, hawthorn, ginkgo biloba and butchers broom.

Summary of Research: Research indicates that elevated homocysteine levels and infections that cause inflammation are some of the most common causes of cardiovascular (atherosclerotic—arteria plaque collection) risk factors. Other risk factors for cardiovascular disease (CVD) include: unhealthy cholesterol levels, hardening of the arteries, blood vessel constriction, toxin and oxidative damage and inefficient pumping of the heart. 4Life Transfer Factor Cardio contains key ingredients to support the body's efforts to block oxidative damage, improve toxin clearance, maintain cholesterol balance, activate the immune response against inflammation, relax the blood vessels and support the pumping efficiency of the heart. 4Life Transfer Factor Cardio is formulated to support and strengthen these specific cardiovascular processes.

Directions for use: Take 4 capsules daily with 8 oz of fluid.

Shown in Product Identification Guide, page 507

Continued on next page

4LIFE® TRANSFER FACTOR PLUS®

Description: Transfer factors are small peptides of approximately 44 amino acids that "transfer" or have the ability to express cell-mediated immunity from immune donors to non-immune recipients. 4Life Transfer Factor™ Advanced Formula is derived from egg yolk and cow colostrum extracts containing antigens. The extraction of Transfer Factor is protected by US patents 6,468,534 and 4,816,563 with other patents pending.

4Life Transfer Factor Plus combines Transfer Factor Advanced Formula with a proprietary formulation of innate and adaptive immune system enhancers such as Inositol Hexaphosphate, Cordyceps, Beta Glucans, Maitake and Shiitake Mushrooms. These ingredients work together to trigger and enhance the various immune protective mechanisms of the body. Clinical studies show that 4Life Transfer Factor Plus can increase Natural Killer cell activity up to 437% above baseline.

Summary of Research: In 1949 transfer factors were discovered by Dr. HS Lawrence. Since that time hundreds of studies have been completed involving transfer factors' effect on various diseases. Transfer factors have been shown to be immune modulators effective in providing immune system support for people with cancer, immune disorders and infections. Recent studies completed:
Rak, AV et al. Effectiveness of Transfer Factor (TF) in the Treatment of Osteomyelitis Patients. International Symposium in Moscow 2002, Nov 5–7, 62–63.
Granitov, VM et al. Usage of Transfer Factor Plus in Treatment of HIV – Infected Patients. Russian Journal of HIV, AIDS and Related Problems 2002, 1, 79–80.
Karbysheva, NV et al. Enhanced Transfer Factor in the Complex Treatment of Patients with Opisthorchiasis. International Symposium in Moscow 2002, May, 104–105.
Luikova, SG et al. Transfer Factor in Dermatovenerology. Syberian Journal of Dermatology and Venerology 2002, 3, 34–35.

Directions for Use: Transfer Factor Plus – Take two (2) capsules daily with 8 oz. of fluid.
4Life Transfer Factor™ Products Include:
  4Life Transfer Factor Advanced Formula
  4Life Transfer Factor Chewable
  4Life Transfer Factor Plus with Advanced Formula
  4Life Transfer Factor ReCall®
  4Life Transfer Factor Classic™
  4Life Transfer Factor Immune Spray™
  4Life Transfer Factor RenewAll™
  4Life Transfer Factor Kids

Shown in Product Identification Guide, page 507

GlaxoSmithKline Consumer Healthcare, L.P.

P.O. BOX 1467
PITTSBURGH, PA 15230

Direct Inquiries to:
Consumer Affairs
1-800-245-1040
For Medical Emergencies Contact:
Consumer Affairs
1-800-245-1040

ALLUNA™ SLEEP
Herbal Supplement Tablet

Use: Alluna Sleep is an herbal supplement that can relieve occasional sleeplessness.* It works by helping you relax, so you can drift off to sleep naturally.*
Alluna Sleep has been clinically tested and shown to be effective in actually promoting your body's own natural sleep pattern – safely and gently.* This is a natural process. Depending upon your particular circumstances, benefits are typically seen within a few nights with more consistent results within two weeks.
Alluna Sleep is not habit forming and is safe to take over time. You can expect to wake up refreshed, with no groggy side effects, because you experience a natural, healthy sleep through the night.*

Supplement Facts:
Serving Size: 2 Tablets

	Amount Per 2 Tablets	% Daily Value
Calories	5	
Valerian Root Extract	500 mg	†
Hops Extract	120 mg	†

†Daily Value Not Established

Other Ingredients: microcrystalline cellulose, soy polysaccharide, hydrogenated castor oil, hypromellose. Contains less than 2% of titanium dioxide, propylene glycol, magnesium stearate, silica, polyethylene glycol (400, 6,000 and 20,000), blue 2 lake, artificial flavoring.

Directions: Take **two** (2) tablets one hour before bedtime with a glass of water.

Warning: As with all dietary supplements, contact your doctor before use if you are pregnant or lactating. Keep this and all dietary supplements out of the reach of children. Driving or operating machinery while using this product is not recommended. Chronic insomniacs should consult their doctor before using this product.

Please Note: The herbs in this product have a distinct natural aroma.
Store in a cool, dry place. Avoid temperatures above 86°F.

How Supplied: Packets of 28 and 56 Tablets

BEANO®
[bēan ō]
Food Enzyme Dietary Supplement

PRODUCT INFORMATION

Description:
Beano drops: each 5 drop dosage follows Food Chemical Codex (FCC) standards for activity and contains 150 GalU (galactosidase units) of alpha-D-galactosidase derived from *Aspergillus niger* mold. The enzyme is in a liquid carrier of water and xylitol. Add about 5 drops on the first bite of problem food serving, but remember a normal meal has 2-3 servings of the problem foods.
Beano tablets: each tablet follows Food Chemical Codex (FCC) standards for activity and contains 150 GalU (galactosidase units) of alpha-D-galactosidase derived from *Aspergillus niger* mold. The enzyme is in a carrier of cellulose gel, mannitol, invertase, potato starch, magnesium stearate, gelatin (fish), colloidal silica. 3 tablets swallowed, chewed, or crumbled onto food should be enough for a normal meal of 3 servings of problem foods (1 tablet per ½ cup serving). Beano® will hydrolyze complex sugars, raffinose, stachyose and verbascose, into the simple sugars - glucose, galactose and fructose, and the easily digestible disaccharide, sucrose. (Sucrose hydrolysis happens simultaneously with normal digestion.) In some cases, more enzyme than 5 drops or 3 tablets will be required, and this is a function of the quantity of food eaten, the levels of alpha-linked sugars in the food, and the gas-producing propensity of the person.

Use: Helps prevent flatulence and/or bloat from a variety of grains, cereals, nuts, seeds, and vegetables containing the sugars raffinose, stachyose and/or verbascose. This includes all or most legumes and all or most cruciferous vegetables. Examples of such foods are oats, wheat, beans of all kinds, chickpeas, peas, lentils, peanuts, soy-content foods, broccoli, brussel sprouts, cabbage, carrots, corn, leeks, onions, parsnips, squash. Note: Most vegetables and beans also contain fiber, which is gas productive in some people, but usually far less so than the alpha-linked sugars. Beano® has no effect on fiber.

Usage: About 5 drops per food serving or 3 tablets per meal (1 tablet per ½ cup serving) of 3 servings of problem foods; higher levels depending on symptoms.

Precautions: If you are pregnant or nursing, ask your doctor before product use. Beano is made from a safe, food-grade mold. However, if a rare sensitivity occurs, discontinue use. Galactosemics should not use without physician's advice, since one of the breakdown sugars is galactose.

How Supplied: Beano® is supplied in both a liquid form (30 and 75 serving sizes, at 5 drops per serving), and a tablet form (30, 60, and 100 tablet sizes as well as 24 tablets in packets of 3). These statements have not been evaluated by the Food and Drug Administration. This product is not intended to diagnose, treat, cure or prevent any disease.

For more information and free samples, please write or call toll-free 1-800-257-8650 or visit www.beano.net.

FEOSOL® Caplets
Hematinic
Iron Supplement

Description: FEOSOL Caplets contain pure iron micro particles called carbonyl iron. Replacing FEOSOL Capsules, this advanced formula is specially designed to be well absorbed, gentle on the stomach and offers enhanced safety in the event of an accidental overdose. Each FEOSOL carbonyl iron caplet delivers 45 mg of pure elemental iron, the same amount of elemental iron contained in the 225 mg ferrous sulfate capsule. At equivalent doses, carbonyl iron and ferrous sulfate were shown to be equally efficacious in correcting hemoglobin, hematocrit and serum iron levels in iron-deficient patients[1].

Safety: According to the American Association of Poison Control Centers, iron containing supplements are the leading cause of pediatric poisoning deaths for children under six in the United States[2]. Widely used as a food additive, carbonyl iron must be gastrically solubilized before it can be absorbed, giving it lower toxicity and enhancing its safety versus any of the ferrous salts[3]. As a result, carbonyl iron presents less chance of harm from accidental overdose. In addition, at equivalent doses, carbonyl iron side effects are no greater than those experienced with ferrous sulfate[4].

Warnings: Do not exceed recommended dosage. The treatment of any anemic condition should be under the advice and supervision of a physician. Since oral iron products interfere with absorption of oral tetracycline antibiotics, these products should not be taken within two hours of each other. Occasional gastrointestinal discomfort (such as nausea) may be minimized by taking with meals. Iron containing medication may occasionally cause constipation or diarrhea. If you are pregnant or nursing a baby, seek the advice of a health professional before using this product.
WARNING: **Accidental overdose of iron-containing products is a leading cause of fatal poisoning in children un-**

der 6. Keep this product out of reach of children. In case of accidental overdose, call a doctor or poison control center immediately.

SUPPLEMENT FACTS
Serving Size: 1 Caplet

Amount per Caplet	% Daily Value
Iron 45 mg	250%

Ingredients: Lactose, Sorbitol, Carbonyl Iron, Hypromellose. Contains 1% or less of the following ingredients: Carnauba Wax, Crospovidone, FD&C Blue #2 Al Lake, FD&C Red #40 Al Lake, FD&C Yellow #6 Al Lake, Magnesium Stearate, Polydextrose, Polyethylene Glycol, Polyethylene Glycol 8000 (Powder), Stearic Acid, Titanium Dioxide, Triacetin.

Directions: Adults—one caplet daily or as directed by a physician. Children under 12 years: Consult a physician.

Tamper-Evident Feature: Each caplet is encased in a plastic cell with a foil back; do not use if cell or foil is broken.

References: [1]Devasthali SD, Gordeuk VR, Brittenham GM, et al, "Bioavailability of Carbonyl Iron: A randomized, double-blind study." Eur J Haematology, 1991; 46:272–278.
[2]FDA Consumer; March 1996:7
[3]Heubers, JA, Brittenham GM, Csiba E and Finch CA. "Absorption of carbonyl iron." J Lab Clin Med 1986; 108:473–78.
[4]Devasthali SD, Gordeuk VR, Brittenham GM, et al, "Bioavailability of a Carbonyl Iron: A randomized, double-blind study." Eur J Haematology, 1991; 46:272–278.
Store at room temperature, avoid excessive heat (greater than 100°F) or humidity.

How Supplied: Boxes of 30 and 60 caplets in blisters. Also available in single unit packages of 100 caplets intended for institutional use
Also available: Feosol Tablets.
Comments or Questions? Call Toll-Free 1-800-245-1040 Weekdays.
GlaxoSmithKline Consumer Healthcare, L.P.
Moon Township, PA 15108

                Made in USA
Shown in Product Identification Guide, page 507

FEOSOL® TABLETS
Hematinic
Iron Supplement

Description: Feosol tablets provide the body with ferrous sulfate—an iron supplement for iron deficiency and iron deficiency anemia when the need for

such therapy has been determined by a physician.

SUPPLEMENT FACTS
Serving Size: 1 Tablet

Amount per Tablet	% Daily Value
Iron 65 mg	360%

Ingredients: Dried ferrous sulfate 200 mg (65 mg of elemental iron) equivalent to 325 mg of ferrous sulfate per tablet. Lactose, Sorbitol, Crospovidone, Magnesium Stearate, Carnauba Wax. Contains 2% or less of the following ingredients: FD&C Blue #1, FD&C Yellow #6, Hypromellose, Polydextrose, Polyethylene Glycol, Titanium Dioxide, Triacetin.

Directions: Adults and children 12 years and over—One tablet daily or as directed by a physician. Children under 12 years—Consult a physician.
Tamper-Evident Feature: Each tablet is encased in a plastic cell with a foil back; do not use if cell or foil is broken.

Warnings: **Do not exceed recommended dosage.** The treatment of any anemic condition should be under the advice and supervision of a physician. Since oral iron products interfere with absorption of oral tetracycline antibiotics, these products should not be taken within two hours of each other. Occasional gastrointestinal discomfort (such as nausea) may be minimized by taking with meals. Iron containing medication may occasionally cause constipation or diarrhea.
If you are pregnant or nursing a baby, seek the advice of a health professional before using this product.
WARNING: **Accidental overdose of iron-contraining products is a leading cause of fatal poisoning in children under 6. Keep this product out of reach of children. In case of accidental overdose, call a doctor, or poison control center immediately.**
Store at room temperature (59–86°F).
Not USP for dissolution.

How Supplied: Cartons of 100 tablets in child-resistant blisters.
Previously packaged in bottles.
Also available: Feosol caplets.
Comments or Questions?
Call toll-free 1-800-245-1040 weekdays.
GlaxoSmithKline Consumer Healthcare, L.P.
Moon Township, PA 15108

                Made in USA
Shown in Product Identification Guide, page 507

OS-CAL® CHEWABLE
Calcium Supplement

Description: Calcium supplement to help reduce the risk of osteoporosis. Osteoporosis affects middle-aged and older persons, especially Caucasian and

Continued on next page

Os-Cal Chewable—Cont.

Asian women, and those whose families tend to have fragile bones in later years. A lifetime of regular exercise and eating a healthful diet that includes enough calcium, especially during teen and early adult years, builds and maintains good bone health and may reduce the risk of osteoporosis in later life.

Adequate calcium intake is important, but daily intakes above 2000 mg are not likely to provide any additional benefit. [See first table at right]

Ingredients: Calcium carbonate, dextrose monohydrate, maltodextrin, microcrystalline cellulose, magnesium stearate, artificial flavors, sodium chloride. Each tablet provides 500 mg of elemental calcium

Directions: One tablet two to three times a day with meals, or as recommended by your physician.

How Supplied: Bottle of 60 tablets Store at room temperature. Keep out of reach of children.

Shown in Product Identification Guide, page 508

OS-CAL® 250 + D
Calcium with Vitamin D Supplement

Description: Calcium supplement to help reduce the risk of osteoporosis (see below*). Also contains Vitamin D.

Supplement Facts
Serving Size 1 Tablet
[See second table at right]

Ingredients: Oyster shell powder, corn syrup solids, talc, corn starch, hypromellose. Contains less than 1% of calcium stearate, polysorbate 80, titanium dioxide, polyethylene glycol, Vitamin D, propylparaben and methylparaben (preservative), simethicone, yellow 5 lake, blue 1 lake, carnauba wax, edetate sodium.

Directions: One tablet three times a day with meals, or as recommended by your physician.

How Supplied: Bottle of 100 and 240 tablets
Store at room temperature.
Keep out of reach of children.
*Osteoporosis affects middle-aged and older persons, especially Caucasian and Asian women, and those whose families tend to have fragile bones in later years. A lifetime of regular exercise and eating a healthful diet that includes enough calcium, especially during teen and early adult years, builds and maintains good bone health and may reduce the risk of osteoporosis in later life.

Adequate calcium intake is important, but daily intakes above 2000 mg are not likely to provide any additional benefit.

Shown in Product Identification Guide, page 508

Supplement Facts
Serving Size 1 Tablet

Amount Per Serving	% Daily Value for Pregnant or Lactating Women	% Daily Value for Adults and Children 4 or more years of age
Calories 5		
Calcium 500 mg	38%	50%

Amount Per Tablet	% Daily Value for Pregnant or Lactating Women	% Daily Value for Adults and Children 4 or More Years of Age
Vitamin D 125 IU	31%	31%
Calcium 250 mg	19%	25%

Amount Per Tablet	% Daily Value for Pregnant or Lactating Women	% Daily Value for Adults and children 4 or more years of age
Calcium 500 mg	38%	50%

Supplement Facts
Serving Size 1 Tablet

Amount Per Tablet	% Daily Value for Pregnant or Lactating Women	% Daily Value for Adults and Children 4 or more years of age
Vitamin D 200 IU	50%	50%
Calcium 500 mg	38%	50%

OS-CAL® 500
Calcium Supplement

Description: Calcium supplement to help reduce the risk of osteoporosis. Osteoporosis affects middle-aged and older persons, especially Caucasian and Asian women, and those whose families tend to have fragile bones in later years. A lifetime of regular exercise and eating a healthful diet that includes enough calcium, especially during teen and early adult years, builds and maintains good bone health and may reduce the risk of osteoporosis in later life.

Adequate calcium intake is important, but daily intakes above 2000 mg are not likely to provide any additional benefit.

Supplement Facts
Serving Size 1 Tablet
[See third table above]

Ingredients: Oyster shell powder, corn syrup solids, talc, corn starch. Contains less than 1% of sodium starch glycolate, calcium stearate, polysorbate 80, hypromellose, polydextrose, titanium dioxide, propylparaben and methylparaben (preservative), triacetin, yellow 5 lake, blue 1 lake, polyethylene glycol, carnauba wax.

Directions: One tablet two to three times a day with meals, or as recommended by your physician.

How Supplied: Bottles of 75 and 160 tablets
Store at room temperature.
Keep out of reach of children.

Shown in Product Identification Guide, page 508

OS-CAL® 500 + D
Calcium with Vitamin D Supplement

Description: Calcium supplement to help reduce the risk of osteoporosis (see below*). Also contains Vitamin D. [See fourth table above]

Ingredients: Oyster shell powder, corn syrup solids, talc, corn starch. Contains less than 1% of sodium starch glycolate, calcium stearate, polysorbate 80, hypromellose, polydextrose, titanium dioxide, Vitamin D, propylparaben and methylparaben (preservative), triacetin, yellow 5 lake, blue 1 lake, polyethylene glycol, carnauba wax.

Directions: One tablet two to three times a day with meals, or as recommended by your physician.

How Supplied: Bottle of 75 and 160 tablets
Store at room temperature.
Keep out of reach of children.
*Osteoporosis affects middle-aged and older persons, especially Caucasian and Asian women, and those whose families tend to have fragile bones in later years. A lifetime of regular exercise and eating a healthful diet that includes enough calcium, especially during teen and early adult years, builds and maintains good bone health and may reduce the risk of osteoporosis in later life.

Adequate calcium intake is important, but daily intakes above 2000 mg are not likely to provide any additional benefit.

Shown in Product Identification Guide, page 508

REMIFEMIN Menopause
Drug Free
Herbal Supplement
A safe, natural, effective way to help ease the physical and emotional symptoms of menopause*

Remifemin Menopause is a unique, natural formula. For over 40 years in Europe, it has helped reduce the unpleasant physical and emotional symptoms associated with menopause, such as hot flashes, night sweats and mood swings. Clinically shown to be safe and effective. Not a drug.
Remifemin Menopause helps you approach menopause with confidence – naturally.*

Supplement Facts
Serving Size 1 tablet

Ingredients:	Amount Per Tablet:	% Daily Value:
Black Cohosh Extract (Root and Rhizome) Equivalent to	20 mg	†

†Daily Value Not Established.

Other Ingredients: Lactose, Cellulose, Potato Starch, Magnesium Stearate, and Natural Peppermint Flavor. Standardized to be equivalent to 20 mg Black Cohosh (*Cimicifuga racemosa*) root and rhizome.
Contains no salt, yeast, wheat, gluten, corn, soy, coloring, or preservatives.

Directions: Take one tablet in the morning and one tablet in the evening, with water. You can expect to notice improvements within a few weeks with full benefits after using Remifemin twice a day for 4 to 12 weeks. This product is intended for use by women who are experiencing menopausal symptoms. Does not contain estrogen. Remifemin is not meant to replace any drug therapy.

Warnings: **This product should not be used by women who are pregnant or considering becoming pregnant or are nursing.** As with any dietary supplement, always keep out of reach of children. For a few consumers, gastric discomfort may occur but should not be persistent. If gastric discomfort persists, discontinue use and see your health care practitioner. As part of an overall good health care program, we encourage you to see your health care practitioner on a regular basis.

Making Sense Out of Menopause with Remifemin Menopause
Today, women are leading very dynamic and diverse lifestyles. Despite this diversity, there is one constant. They are all experiencing physiological changes. They will all experience menopause. The time when you have menopausal symptoms is a multiphasic period. Technically, the change or transitional process of menopause is known as the *"Climacteric"*. There are different phases of the climacteric that a woman experiences:

1. Perimenopause is the transitional phase when hormone levels begin to drop. This phase lasts typically 3 to 5 years but can last up to 10 years. This gradual decline in estrogen levels causes the troublesome effects of menopause.

2. Menopause is the permanent cessation of menstruation. The average age at menopause is 51, but there is considerable variation in this timing among women. Menopause is medically defined as one year without menstruation.

3. Postmenopause is the phase following menopause. During this phase, your body gets used to the loss of estrogen and eventually the symptoms such as hot flashes go away.

Some Commonly Asked Questions Regarding Remifemin Menopause
1. What is Remifemin Menopause? Remifemin Menopause is a uniquely formulated natural herbal supplement derived from the black cohosh plant. It is formulated to work with your body to promote physical and emotional balance during menopause. Over 40 years of clinical research has shown Remifemin Menopause helps reduce hot flashes, night sweats, related occasional sleeplessness, irritability and mood swings. In a recent clinical study, on average, women experienced the following overall improvements:

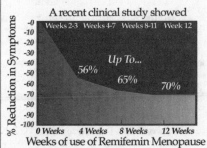

A recent clinical study showed

% Reduction in Symptoms

Weeks 2-3 Weeks 4-7 Weeks 8-11 Week 12

Up To...
56%   65%   70%

0 Weeks   4 Weeks   8 Weeks   12 Weeks
Weeks of use of Remifemin Menopause

2. What makes Remifemin Menopause so special? Remifemin Menopause contains an *exclusive* extract of black cohosh. Unlike many other black cohosh products, it is developed with specific modern analytical techniques which produce a standardized extract of the black cohosh root and rhizome. In addition, Remifemin is estrogen free and does not influence hormone levels, unlike estrogens and phytoestrogens such as soy.

3. With so many products out there claiming to be "natural," how can I be sure that this product is safe and effective? Remifemin Menopause's formulation is supported by over 40 years of clinical research, and millions of women in Europe have safely used it. Remifemin Menopause is drug free and estrogen free. And it is brought to you from a world-renowned health care company.

4. How does Remifemin Menopause work? Remifemin Menopause contains a proprietary standardized extract taken from the rootstock of the black cohosh plant. Studies have shown that the compounds found within this standardized herbal extract seem to interact with certain hormone receptors – without influencing hormone levels.*

5. How long does it take for Remifemin Menopause to work? Remifemin Menopause is a natural herbal supplement, not a drug. It will take time for your body's cycles to respond to its gentle onset. Personally, you may notice improvements within a few weeks. But for some women, it may take 4 to 12 weeks to benefit fully from Remifemin Menopause. Since the effects of Remifemin Menopause increase after extended twice daily use, we recommend that you take Remifemin Menopause for at least 12 weeks. If you do not find any difference in your well being after 12 weeks, please consult your physician to discuss other options.

6. Can I take it over a long period of time, since the menopausal period lasts for years? Every woman's menopause symptoms are different. Depending on your particular circumstances, you should expect that over time your body will be adjusted to its lower level of estrogen and you may find that you no longer need to take Remifemin. You should listen to your body. We recommend that you take Remifemin Menopause twice daily for up to 6 months continuously. If, after discontinuing use your symptoms return, you may start taking Remifemin Menopause again. Keep in mind that Remifemin Menopause is a natural herbal supplement that supports a natural change that may take you years to go through. As part of an overall good healthcare program, we encourage you to see your health care practitioner on a regular basis.

7. Are there any known side effects? When used properly following the package directions, Remifemin Menopause has few side effects, if any. In clinical research, there was a small percentage of gastric discomfort complaints. If you have been taking Remifemin Menopause and find that this or any other condition develops and persists, please discontinue use and see your physician.

8. Is there a certain time of the day when I should take this product? Do I need to take it with food? You can take Remifemin Menopause with or without food any time of the day. We recommend that you take one tablet in the morning with your breakfast and one tablet in the evening with water.

9. Can I take my herbal tea, vitamins, or other dietary supplements with Remifemin Menopause? Typically, dietary supplements can be taken with other dietary supplements. Always follow package directions. If you should notice any undesirable effects, discontinue taking them together.

Expiration and Storage Information
The expiration date of this package is printed on the side panel flap of the outer carton as well as on the blister packs. Do not use this product after this date.

Store this product in a cool, dry place. Keep out of the reach of children. Avoid storing at temperatures above 86°F.

***These statements have not been evaluated by the Food and Drug Administration. This product is not intended to diagnose, treat, cure, or prevent any disease.**

Continued on next page

Remifemin—Cont.

Questions or Comments? Call toll-free 1-800-965-8804 weekdays, or visit www.remifemin.com anytime.

Remifemin ® is a trademark of Schaper & Brümmer GmbH & Co. KG, licensed to GlaxoSmithKline.

Kyowa Engineering-Sundory

6-964 NAKAMOZU-CHO, SAKAI-CITY, OSAKA, JAPAN

Direct Inquiries to:
Consumer Relations
Tel: 81-722-57-8568
Osaka
Fax: 81-722-57-8655
URL: http://www.sundory.co.jp

SEN-SEI-RO LIQUID GOLD™
Kyowa's *Agaricus blazei Murill*
Mushroom Extract
100 ml liquid
Dietary Supplement

SEN-SEI-RO LIQUID ROYAL™
Kyowa's *Agaricus blazei Murill*
Mushroom Extract
50ml liquid (2 × Concentrate of Liquid Gold, v/v)
Dietary Supplement

Description: Sen-Sei-Ro Liquid Gold™, and Sen-Sei-Ro Liquid Royal™ a dietary supplement containing an exclusive all-natural, standardized extracts of the Kyowa's cultured *Agaricus blazei Murill* mushroom are primarily used to reduce symptoms of fatigue, to promote vitality, overall well-being, and to support immune functions.[†] Normal immune function can decline with age, and are necessary for maintenance of vitality, energy, good health, and quality of life. A few major biomarkers for decreased immune functions are decreased natural killer cell (NK) activity, and the number of lymphocytes and macrophage cells. These cells, primarily attack diseased cells and thereby, maintain body homeostasis, promote health and quality of life. For the past half a century in Brazil and other countries, *Agaricus blazei Murill* mushroom has been used to restore vitality, and energy, and to serve as a potent tonic conducive to general health and aging concerns.[†]

Clinical Trials: The effectiveness of ABMK22 in Sen-Sei-Ro Gold™, and Sen-Sei-Ro Liquid Royal™ for health benefits were tested in several controlled pre- and clinical trials in animals and in humans.[†] Recent studies in Japan led researchers to report that in humans, ABMK22 in Sen-Sei-Ro Gold™, and

Sen-Sei-Ro Liquid Royal™ enhanced NK cell activity, promoted maturation and activation of dendritic cells indicated by increased cell kill, elevated expression of CD80 and CD83 expressions (Biotherapy 15(4): 503–507, 2001), increased the number of macrophage (Anticancer Research 17(1A): 274–284, 1997; Japanese Association of Cancer Research, no. 2268, 1999) and tumor necrosis factor α (TNF-α)(Japanese Association of Cancer Research, no. 1406, 1999; Japanese J. Veterinary Clin. Medicine 17(2):31–42, 1998).[†] Further clinical studies with Sen-Sei-Ro Liquid Royal™ among 100 cervical cancer patients undergoing chemotherapy in Korea have shown that NK cell activity were significantly enhanced, while NK cell activity in the placebo group was markedly diminished. (International J. Gynecological Cancer, in press).[†] Earlier and recent both pre- and clinical studies in Japan, and Korea, led researchers to report that Kyowa's *Agaricus blazei Murill* mushroom extract can be part of an effective treatment for supporting the immune systems of cancer patients by stimulating host defense system (Biotherapy 15(4): 503–507, 2001; Carbohydrate Res. 186(2): 267–273, 1989; Japanese J. Pharmacology 662: 265–271, 1994; Agricultural and Biological Chemistry 54: 2889–2905, 1990).[†]

Ingredients: Each 100ml heat-treated high pressure pack of all natural Kyowa's *Agaricus blazei Murill* water extract is scientifically standardized to contain 300mg% carbohydrate, 700mg% protein, 0mg% fat,; 1.4mg% sodium, 0% food quality cellulose, and 4 Kcal energy. Molecular weights of polysaccharopeptides ranges between 600∼8,000. Water: 99.2g%,; includes a variety of amino acids and vitamins (arginine 12mg%, lysine 6mg%, histidine 2mg%, phenylalanine 4mg%, tyrosine 4mg%, leucine 5mg%, isoleucine 3mg%, methionine 1mg%, valine 5mg%, alanine 13mg%, glycine 7mg%, proline 13mg%, glutamic acid 53mg%, serine 6mg%, threonine 5mg%, and asparagine 10mg%.

Recommended Use: As a dietary supplement, take 1∼3 packs per day. Pour the liquid content into a cup or drink directly from the pack. Do not heat the pack either in a microwave oven or heating range or leave the pack open since the product does not contain any preservatives. If warming is necessary, place the pack in warm to mildly hot water for desired length of time. Once the pack is open, drink immediately.

Adverse Reactions: No subjects have reported any side effects since the dietary supplement was placed for consumers in Japan, and Korea for the past 9, and 4 years, respectively. The use of this dietary supplement is generally safe based on FDA's INDA required tripartite genotoxicities, and 28-day subacute toxicity tests involving a comprehensive microscopic pathology of rats and dogs. In addition, two-year chronic toxicity studies of the products carried out by the

Good Laboratory Practice (GLP) and American Association of Accreditation of Laboratory Animal Certification (AAA-LAC) certified Toxicology Research Center. Toxicity evaluation of general, CNS, reproductive and developmental, cardiovascular, immunology, and the two-year bioassay for carcinogenicity was negative. Recent clinical studies with 100 cancer patients undergoing chemotherapy in Korea have shown no known side effects or contraindications.[†]

Warnings: Sen-Sei-Ro Liquid Gold™, and Sen-Sei-Ro Liquid Royal™ have not been evaluated in pregnant and breast feeding mothers or children and should consult a physician prior to use. Also consult a physician prior to use if taking a prescription medication. **Keep this product out of the reach of children. Do not use if you are pregnant, can become pregnant or breast feeding.**

How Supplied: Sen-Sei-Ro Liquid Gold™ 100ml, and Sen-Sei-Ro Liquid Royal™ 50ml water extract are high pressure heat sealed. A box contains 30, 100, or 50 ml packs, respectively, and can be purchased directly from company representatives, health food stores, and independent pharmacies. Storage condition keep at room temperature and avoid any direct heat or sun light.

[†]These statements have not been evaluated by the Food and Drug Administration. These products are not intended to diagnose, treat, cure or prevent any disease.

Shown in Product Identification Guide, page 509

SEN-SEI-RO POWDER GOLD™
KYOWA'S *Agaricus blazei Murill*
Mushroom
1800mg standard granulated powder
Dietary Supplement

Description: Sen-Sei-Ro Powder Gold™ slim pack, a dietary supplement containing an exclusively all natural and prepared from Kyowa's *Agaricus blazei Murill* mushroom is primarily used to reduce symptoms of fatigue, to promote vitality, overall well-being, and to support immune functions.[†] Normal immune function can decline with age, and are necessary for maintenance of vitality, energy, good health, and quality of life. A few major biomarkers for decreased immune functions are decreased natural killer cell (NK) activity, and the number of lymphocytes and macrophage cells. These cells, primarily attack diseased cells and thereby, maintain body homeostasis, promote health and quality of life. For the past half a century in Brazil and other countries, *Agaricus blazei Murill* mushroom has been used to restore vitality, and energy, and to serve as a potent tonic conducive to general health and aging concerns.[†]

Clinical Trials: The effectiveness of Sen-Sei-Ro Powder Gold™ for health benefits were tested in several controlled pre- and clinical trials in animals and in humans.[†] Recent studies in Japan, and Korea led researcher to report that in humans, Sen-Sei-Ro Powder Gold™ enhanced NK cell activity, increased the number of macrophage cells (Anticancer Research 17 (1A): 274–284, 1997; Japanese Association of Cancer Research, no. 2268, 1999) and tumor necrosis factor α (TNF-α)(Japanese Association of Cancer Research, no. 1406, 1999).[†] Antitumor effects of Sen-Sei-Ro against various murine and dog tumors were thought to be mediated by stimulation of NK cell activity, increased number of macrophage cells, and increased activity of tumor necrosis factor α (TNF-α)(Japanese J. Veterinary Clin. Medicine 17(2):31–42, 1998).[†] Recent clinical studies in Japan, and Korea, led researchers to report that *Agaricus blazei Murill* mushroom extract can be part of an effective treatment for supporting the immune systems of cancer patients by stimulating host defense system (Biotherapy 15(4): 503–507, 2001; Carbohydrate Res. 186(2): 267–273, 1989; Japanese J. Pharmacology 662: 265–271, 1994; Agricultural and Biological Chemistry 54: 2889–2905, 1990).[†]

Ingredients: Each 1800mg granulated powder in a slim pack contains 488 mg protein, 820 mg carbohydrate, 47 mg fat, 0.19 mg Sodium; 284 mg food grade cellulose; 5.7 kcal energy.
Water: 68mg, includes 0.1 mg Fe, 0.24 mg Ca, 37 mg K, 0.01mg thiamine, 0.04mg ergosterol, 0.59mg niacin.

Recommended Use: As a dietary supplement, take 1~3 packs per day. Pour the content into a cup containing warm water or other desirable beverage and mix and drink. Do not heat the pack either in a microwave oven or heating range or leave the pack open since the product does not contain any preservatives. Once the pack is open, drink immediately.

Adverse Reactions: No subjects have reported any side effects since the dietary supplement was placed for consumers in Japan and Korea for the past 9, and 4 years, respectively. The use of this dietary supplement is generally safe based on two-year chronic toxicity studies of the product by the Good Laboratory Practice (GLP) and American Association of Accreditation of Laboratory Animal Certification (AAALAC) certified Toxicology Research Center. Toxicity evaluation of general, CNS, reproductive and developmental, cardiovascular, immunology, and the two-year bioassay for carcinogenicity was negative.[†]

Warnings: Sen-Sei-Ro Powder Gold™ has not been evaluated in pregnant and breast feeding mothers or children and should consult a physician prior to use. Also consult a physician prior to use if

taking a prescription medications. **Keep this product out of the reach of children. Do not use if you are pregnant, can become pregnant or breast feeding.** Quality of the dietary supplement is guaranteed for 2 years from the manufactured date, but for more information, please write or call 81-72-257-8568 or 81-3-3512-5032.

How Supplied: Sen-Sei-Ro Powder Gold™ is high pressure heat sealed. A box contains 30 slim packs of each with 1800mg per pack, and can be purchased directly from company representatives, health food stores, and independent pharmacies. Storage condition keep at room temperature and avoid any direct heat or sun light.

---

†**These statements have not been evaluated by the Food and Drug Administration. These products are not intended to diagnose, treat, cure or prevent any disease.**
Shown in Product Identification Guide, page 509

Legacy for Life, LLC
P.O. BOX 410376
MELBOURNE, FL 32941-0376

Direct Inquiries to:
(800) 557-8477
(321) 951-8815
www.legacyforlife.net

IMMUNE[26®]
IMMUNE [26®] COMPLETE SUPPORT

Description: These immune[26®] products contain hyperimmune egg powder, a pure all-natural egg powder derived from hens hyperimmunized with over 26 inactivated enteric pathogens of human origin.

Clinical Background: Upon oral administration, immune[26®] specific immunoglobulins and immunomodulatory factors are passively transferred. immune[26®] and immune[26®] COMPLETE Support modulate autoimmune responses, plus support and balance cardiovascular function, healthy cholesterol levels, a vital circulatory system, a fully functional digestive tract, flexible and healthy joints and energy levels.

How Supplied: immune[26®] is available as immune[26®], hyperimmune egg in powder and capsule form, wellness bars and chewable tablets, as immune[26®] Complete Support, hyperimmune egg enriched with protein, minerals and 100% of the daily value of more than 13 essential vitamins and as an ingredient in the Legacy BALANCE shake, a meal alternative product.

Precautions: Those with known allergies to eggs should consult with a health practitioner before consuming this product.
Note: immune[26®] is not intended to diagnose, treat, cure, or prevent any disease. These statements have not been evaluated by the Food and Drug Administration.

Mannatech, Inc.
600 S. ROYAL LANE
SUITE 200
COPPELL, TX 75019

For Medical Professional Inquiries Contact:
Kia Gary, RN LNCC
(972) 471-8189
Kgary@mannatech.com

Direct Inquiries to:
Customer Service
(972) 471-8111

Product Information:
www.mannatech.com

Ingredient Information:
www.glycoscience.com

AMBROTOSE®
A Glyconutritional Dietary Supplement

Supplement Facts:
Ambrotose® powder:
Serving Size 0.44 g (approx. ¼ teaspoon)
Powder canister: 100g or 50g

Amount Per Serving	% Daily Value
0.44g	*

* Daily Values not established.

Ambrotose® capsules:
Serving Size: two capsules
Capsules per container: 60

Amount Per Serving	% Daily Value
2 capsules	*

* Daily Values not established.

Ambrotose® with Lecithin capsules:
Ambrotose® with Lecithin
Supplement Facts:
Serving Size: two capsules
Capsules per container: 60

Amount Per Serving	% Daily Value
1–2 capsules	*

* Daily Values not established.

Continued on next page

Ambrotose—Cont.

Ingredients:
Ambrotose® Powder
(patent pending)
Arabinogalactan (Larix decidua) (gum), Rice starch, Aloe vera extract, (inner leaf gel)- Manapol® powder, Ghatti (Anogeissus latifolia)(gum), Glucosamine HCl, Tragacanth (Astragalus Gummifer) (gum).

Ambrotose® capsules
(patent pending)
Arabinogalactan (Larix decidua) (gum), Rice starch, Aloe vera extract, (inner leaf gel)- Manapol® powder, Ghatti (Anogeissus latifolia) (gum), Tragacanth (Astragalus gummifer) (gum).

Ambrotose® with Lecithin capsules
(patent pending)
Arabinogalactan (Larix decidua) (gum), Rice starch, Aloe vera extract, (inner leaf gel) - Manapol® powder, Ghatti (Anogeissus latifolia) (gum), Tragacanth (Astragalus gummifer) (gum).
Other ingredients: Calcium, lecithin powder
For additional information on ingredients, visit www.glycoscience.com

Use: Ambrotose complex is a proprietary formula designed to help provide saccharides used in glycoconjugate synthesis to promote cellular communication and immune support.** Consumers who are healthy may notice improved concentration, more energy, better sleep, improved athletic performance, and a greater sense of well-being.

Directions: The recommended intake of Ambrotose powder is ¼ teaspoon two times a day; the recommended intake of Ambrotose capsules or Ambrotose with Lecithin is one capsule two times daily. If desired, you may begin by taking less than the recommended intake. If well tolerated, you may gradually increase to the recommended intake. As a blend of plant saccharides, Ambrotose complex is safe in amounts well in excess of the label recommendations. Children between the ages of 12 and 48 months with growth/nutritional problems (failure to thrive) have been given 1 tablespoon a day of Ambrotose powder for 3 months with no adverse effects. Individuals have reported taking as much as 10 tablespoons of Ambrotose powder (approx. 50 grams) each day for several months with no adverse effects. The amount needed by each individual may vary with time, age, genetic makeup, metabolic rate, and activities, stress level, current dietary intake, and health challenges of the moment. A health care professional experienced with use of Ambrotose complex may be helpful.

Warning: Anyone who is taking medication may wish to advise his/her physician. One teaspoon of Ambrotose powder (equivalent to approximately 12 Ambrotose capsules) contains the amount of glucose equivalent to 1/25 teaspoon of sucrose (table sugar)

KEEP BOTTLE TIGHTLY CLOSED. STORE IN A COOL, DRY PLACE.

How Supplied: Bottle of 3.50 oz (100g) powder. Bottle of 1.75 oz (50g) powder. Bottle of 60 (150mg) capsules.

** This statement has not been evaluated by the Food and Drug Administration. This product is not intended to diagnose, treat, cure or prevent any disease.

Mannatech Inc.
600 S. Royal Lane, Suite 200
Coppell, Texas 75019
www.mannatech.com
Shown in Product Identification Guide, page 510

AMBROTOSE AO™
[ăm-brō-tōs]
Glyco-Antioxidant Supplement

[See table below]
For additional information on ingredients, Visit www.glycoscience.com

Use: Ambrotose AO™ capsules helps protect both water and fat soluble portions of cells from free radical attacks while supporting your immune system.** Defend your health by supporting overall immune function through the natural glyconutrients in Ambrotose® complex.** Protect against the daily onslaught of toxins, poor food, stress and the environment, all of which contribute to an increase in free radicals, accelerating the aging process. ** Help restore cellular damage and the overall balance your body may have lost due to the harmful effect of free radical damage that results from pollutants in the air we breathe, the water we drink and the lives we live.**

** **This statement has not been evaluated by the Food and Drug Administration. This product is not intended to diagnose, treat, cure or prevent any disease.**

Directions: The recommended intake of Ambrotose AO™ capsules is one capsule two times daily.

Oxygen Radical Absorption Capacity (ORAC) can be used to assess the antioxidant status of human blood and serum. One recent study reported that increasing fruit and vegetable consumption from the usual five to an experimental ten servings per day over two weeks can increase serum ORAC values by roughly 13%.[1] In an open-label pilot study of 12 healthy human volunteers, the antioxidant effects of increasing amounts of supplementation with Ambrotose AO™ were evaluated. A battery of tests was selected in order to assess both oxidative damage and protection. Independent companies were contracted to conduct blood and urine chemistry tests and statistical data analyses. An increase in $ORAC_{\beta-PE}$, a measure of oxidative protection, was found at all three doses: 19.1% at 500 mg per day, 37.4% at 1.0 g per day, and 14.3% at 1.5 g per day. A trend of decreased urinary lipid hydroperoxides/creatinine, a marker of oxidative damage, was observed as well. No significant trends were found in regard to urinary alkenal or 8-OHdG levels.[2] Thus, over the same time period, 1.0 g per day of Ambrotose AO™ provided over twice the antioxidant protection (37.4%) provided by 5 servings of fruits and vegetables (13%).

Supplement Facts:
Serving Size - 1 Capsule

	Amount Per Serving	% Daily Value
Vitamin E (as mixed d-alpha-, d-beta, d-delta and d-gamma tocopherols)	18 IU	60%
Mtech AO Blend™	113mg	
Quercetin dihydrate		*
Grape pomace extract		*
Green tea extract (leaves)		*
Australian Bush Plum (fruit) (Terminalia ferdinandiana)		*
Ambrotose® Phyto Formula	333mg	
Gum Arabic		*
Xanthan Gum		*
Gum Tragacanth		*
Gum Ghatti		*
Aloe vera gel extract (inner leaf gel)- Manapol® powder		*
Phyt-Aloe® complex (broccoli, Brussels sprout, cabbage, carrot, Cauliflower, garlic, kale, onion, Tomato, turnip, papaya, pineapple)		*

Other Ingredients: Vegetable-based cellulose capsules

---

*Daily value not established.

1. Cao G;Booth SL;Sadowski JA;Prior RL;. Increases in human plasma antioxidant capacity after consumption of controlled diets high in fruit and vegetables. *Am J Clin Nutr.* 1998 Nov; 68: 1081-1087.
2. Boyd S, Gary K, Koepke CM, et al. An open-label pilot study of the antioxidant activity in humans of Ambrotose AO™: Results. *GlycoScience & Nutrition (Official Publication of Glyco-Science com: The Nutrition Science Site).* 2003;4(6).

Shown in Product Identification Guide, page 510

PLUS with AMBROTOSE® Complex
Dietary Supplement Caplets

Supplement Facts:
Serving Size - 1 Caplet

	Amount Per Serving	% Daily Value
Iron	1mg	5
Wild Yam (root) Standardized for	200mg	*
Phytosterols	25mg	
L-Glutamic acid	200mg	*
L-Glycine	200mg	*
L-Lysine	200mg	*
L-Arginine	100mg	*
Beta Sitosterol	25mg	*
Ambrotose® Complex (patent pending)	2.5mg	*

Naturally occurring plant polysaccharides including freeze-dried Aloe vera inner gel extract-Manapol® powder.

Other Ingredients: Microcrystalline cellulose, silicon dioxide, croscarmellose sodium, magnesium stearate, titanium dioxide coating.

*Daily value not established.

For additional information on ingredients, visit www.glycoscience.com

Use: PLUS caplets provide nutrients to help support the endocrine system's production and balance of hormones.** A well-functioning endocrine system works in harmony with the body's immune system, helps support the efficient metabolism of fat, and supports natural recovery from physical or emotional stress.** The functional components of PLUS caplets are wild yam extract, amino acids, and beta sitosterol. PLUS caplets contain no hormones.

Directions: The recommended intake of PLUS caplets is two caplets per day.

Warning: After an extensive review of the literature, no documented evidence was found linking the ingredients in PLUS caplets with any form of human cancer or with any problems associated with pregnancy. However, as with all supplements, you should consult your health care professional if you are pregnant.

KEEP BOTTLE TIGHTLY CLOSED. STORE IN A COOL, DRY PLACE.

How Supplied: Bottle of 90 caplets.

** This statement has not been evaluated by the Food and Drug Administration. This product is not intended to diagnose, treat, cure or prevent any disease.

Shown in Product Identification Guide, page 510

Matol Botanical International Ltd.

290 LABROSSE AVENUE
MONTREAL, QUEBEC
CANADA, H9R 6R6

Direct Inquiries to:
Ph: (800) 363-1890
website: www.matol.com

BIOMUNE OSF™ PLUS

Description: Biomune OSF™ Plus is an immune system support product for all ages.

Biomune OSF™ Plus is a combination of a special extract of antigen infused colostrum and whey with the herb Astragalus.

Indications: Biomune OSF Plus™ is a unique combination.

Astragalus has a synergistic effect when used with Ai/E10®. It accelerates and optimizes immune system function.

Ai/E10®: The exclusive colostrum/whey extract named Ai/E10® is prepared using a patented and proprietary process. It supports healthy immune cell communication by providing a concentrate of immune system messengers, including interleukins, interferon, and other memory transfer factors. Ai/E10® also provides additional low molecular weight molecules including macrophages, lactoferrin, lysozymes, and polysaccharides.

ASTRAGALUS: Astragalus is a traditional Chinese herb that is known over the years for its proven immune enhancing properties. The "stem cells" in bone marrow are increased and their development is stimulated into active immune cells that are then released into the body. Essentially, every phase of immune system activity is affected by Astragalus including increased interferon production and resistance to viral conditions while enhancing NK and T cell function. It has also been shown to support the body in peripheral vascular disease, peripheral circulation and aids adrenal gland function that often needs support in chronic and degenerative health states.

Clinical studies show that Biomune OSF™ Plus is effective in consistently and dramatically increasing Natural Killer cell activity. Medical research has shown that low NK cell activity is present in most illness. A double blind study with antigen infused dialyzable bovine colostrum/whey shows its effectiveness as an immune system modulator.

Summary of clinical studies:
The Use of Dialyzable Bovine Colostrum/Whey Extract in Conjunction with a Holistic Treatment Model for Natural Killer Cell Stimulation in Chronic Illness by Jesse A. Stoff, MD.
This clinical study consists of 107 patients with an average treatment time of 13.2 months. The average initial Natural Killer (NK) cell activity was 18 Lytic Units (LU) and the average final NK cell was 246 LU. All patients in this study improved, went into remission or recovered. Conclusions: The Study Group demonstrated that increased NK activity paralleled restored resistance to illness and recovery from illness.
An Examination of Immune Response Modulation in Humans by Antigen Infused Dialyzable Bovine Colostrum/Whey Extract Utilizing a Double Blind Study by Jesse A. Stoff, MD.
This study provides double blind evidence that the cytokines, peptide neuro-hormones and other informational molecules in Antigen Infused Dialyzable Bovine Colostrum/Whey Extract modulate and normalize immune function. Further, Antigen Infused Dialyzable Bovine Colostrum/Whey Extract demonstrates its effectiveness as a Biological Immune Response Modulator for increasing the protective functions of the immune system. Both studies are available from Matol Botanical International Ltd. upon request.

Directions for Use: One (1) or two (2) capsules every 2–3 hours when additional immune support is needed. Take one (1) capsule daily for maintenance. **Since human immune cell development is continuous, it is recommended that the product be taken daily and consistently to optimize immune system support.**

How Supplied: One bottle contains 30 capsules – also available in an economical family 3 pack (90 capsules).
Ai/E10® is a registered trademark of Quantum Research, Inc.
These statements have not been evaluated by the FDA. The product is not intended to diagnose, cure, prevent or treat any disease.

Shown in Product Identification Guide, page 510

Continued on next page

Supplement Facts

Serving Size one (1) tablespoon (15 ml)
Servings Per Container 63

Amount Per Serving		**% Daily Value**
Calcium (glycerophosphate)	30.5 mg	3%
Iron (ferric glycerophosphate)	1.4 mg	8%
Iodine (potassium iodide)	22.5 mcg	15%
Potassium (citrate and glycerophosphate)	350 mg	10%
Proprietary herbal extract blend:	108 mg	*

Camomile (herb) 4.1; Sarsaparilla (root) 4:1;
Dandelion (root) 3:1; Horehound (herb) 4:1;
Licorice (root) 3:1; Senega (root) 4:1;
Passion flower (herb) 4:1; Thyme (herb) 4:1;
Gentian (root) 2:1; Saw palmetto (berry) 4:1;
Alfalfa (herb) 4:1; Angelica (root) 3:1;
Celery (seed) 4:1; Cascara sagrada (bark) 3:1

*Daily Value not established

KM® – POTASSIUM MINERAL SUPPLEMENT

Description: With over 28 million bottles sold in 20 years, the Original Km® Formula is the highest selling potassium mineral supplement available on the market.

Indications: The Original Km® Formula has shown the ability to help eliminate toxins due to antioxidant properties in the herbal blend, while acting as a blood stream catalyst which activates the oxygenation process.

It stimulates oxygenation of the blood system and helps keep cells healthy by maintaining the body's pH balance.

The Km® formula combines active botanical ingredients and minerals to form a unique and beneficial blend that works in concert with the human body for optimal health.

Km® is recommended for all ages.

Active Ingredients: Km® is a natural phytonutrient-rich potassium mineral formulation, using a proprietary process, from a synergistic combination of minerals and extracts of 14 traditional botanicals.

Km® is an excellent source of recommended daily minerals in particular: potassium, iron and iodine. Potassium is one of the minerals vital to human cells' permeability and their inherent ability to absorb nutrients from foods.

The formula includes a proprietary herbal extract blend of foliage, roots, flowers, barks and fruits selected for their purity and active ingredients by means of stringent quality control procedures. Most of the herbs are an antioxidant which detoxifies and prevents the production of free radicals.

The properties of the carefully selected 14 botanicals that make up the Km® formula have been joined together at the molecular level creating a microscopic bonding. This specific process encourages each component to propel the other to work at its optimum level.

Km® gives the body the ability to respond with renewed levels of vital force, energy and most of all, profound well-being.

Directions: Daily use or as recommended by physicians.
Liquid: One (1) tablespoon (15 ml) in the morning and one (1) tablespoon at night mixed with your choice of cold beverage or on its own.
Capsules: Two (2) capsules twice daily with water.
[See table above]

How Supplied: Available in 32 fl. oz. bottles - also available in convenient travel formats: 8 fl. oz. bottles and capsule form of 120 capsules per bottle.

These statements have not been evaluated by the FDA. The product is not intended to diagnose, cure, prevent or treat any disease.

Shown in Product Identification Guide, page 510

Maxorb Health Products A Div. of Pharmco Int'l

670 INTERNATIONAL PKWY, STE. 130 RICHARDSON, TEXAS 75081

Direct Product Inquiries to:
Toll Free: (866) 886-6668
Fax: (972) 699-0495

OSTEOFORM

[ŏ-stē-ō-fŏrm]

Enhanced Calcium absorption dietary supplement

Supplement Facts

Serving size: 1 capsule
Each Osteoform capsule contains the following vitamin and minerals:

Calcium	250.00mg
Magnesium	30.00mg
Phosphorus	25.00mg
Zinc	8.00mg
Manganese	2.10mg
Copper	0.20mg
Vanadium	10mcg
Silicon	0.70mg
Boron	0.20mg
Vitamin D3	200.0 IU

Ingredients: Calcium Amino Acid Chelate, Calcium Ascorbate, Dicalcium Phosphate, Magnesium Amino Acid Chelate, Zinc Amino Acid Chelate, Manganese Amino Acid Chelate, Vanadium Amino Acid Complex, Silicon Amino Acid Complex, Boron Amino Acid complex.

Other Ingredients: Gelatin (capsule) and Magnesium Stearate

Advantages: Each capsule contains a blend of a unique form of chelated Calcium, vitamin D_3 and eight minerals required for bone development, bone remodeling and skeletal health. This non-prescription product meets USP guidelines for potency (as applicable), uniformity and disintegration, and is manufactured according to pharmaceutical cGMP standards.

Recommended Use: Take 1 to 2 capsules twice daily or as recommended by a physician, pharmacist or health professional.

How Supplied: Supplied as 00 size white gelatin capsules with Osteoform® imprint. Available in bottles of 60 UPC682297-00201, and bottles of 120 UPC682297-00204.

Storage: Store at room temperature 15°C–30°C (59°F–86°F). Store away from heat, light and moisture.

Mayor Pharmaceutical Laboratories

2401 S. 24TH ST. PHOENIX, AZ 85034

Direct Inquiries to:
Medical Director
(602) 244-8899

www.vitamist.com

VITAMIST® Intra-Oral Spray

[vĭt '-ə-mĭst]

Nutraceuticals/Dietary Supplements

Description: VitaMist® products are patented, intra-oral sprays for the delivery of vitamins, minerals, and other nutritional supplements, directly into the oral cavity. A 55 microliter spray delivers high concentrations of nutrients directly onto the mouth's sensitive tissue. The buccal mucosa transfers the nutrients into the bloodstream. (U.S. Patent 4,525,341—Foreign patents issued and pending.)

[See figure at top of next column]

Benefits:
• Spray supplementation provides an absorption rate approximately nine times greater than that of pills.
• Once the formula is sprayed into the mouth and swallowed, the nutrients reach the bloodstream within minutes.

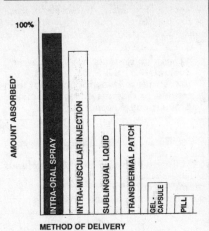

METHOD OF DELIVERY

*Representative of the product class.

- No fillers or binders are added; the body receives only pure ingredients.
- An alternative method of supplementation for those that cannot take pills, or simply do not enjoy swallowing pills.
- Convenient administration; no water needed.

Product Overview: Multi-Vitamin Formulations: VitaMist is available in four unique multivitamin formulations, each designed for the needs of a specific population grouping – Pre-Natal, for pregnant and lactating mothers and for anyone considering pregnancy, Children's Multiple, for children aged 4 – 12, Women's Health and Men's Formula, for women and men of all ages.

Anti-Oxidant: a unique blend of vitamins A, C and E with grape seed extract, lycopene and lutein, to fight the damaging effects of free-radicals.

ArthriFlex: a powerful combination of glucosamine sulfate and MSM, together with vitamins C and D, calcium, manganese and boron.

Cold Weather Formula: formulation containing vitamins C and E and the amino acid lysine. Ideal for cold weather use.

D-Stress: herbal formula with added B-complex vitamins.

Heart Healthy: with folic acid, vitamin B6 and vitamin B12 – a combination proven to reduce blood levels of homocysteine, an indicator of coronary artery disease.

Immune: with extracts of both echinacea and goldenseal, two herbs that have been used extensively to enhance the immune system. This powerful blend also contains vitamin E, honey, lemon and garlic extract.

ReVitalizer®: enhanced multi-vitamin formulation with B-complex vitamins, vitamins A, C and E, and a proprietary herbal extract. ReVitalizer may assist in providing an energy boost when you need it most.

Sleep: melatonin, 5-HTP and amino acids blended with herbal extracts designed for use in re-establishing normal sleep patterns.

B12: contains 1000% of the US RDI of vitamin B12.

St. John's Wort: St. John's wort extract with vitamin B12, ginkgo biloba, kava kava and folic acid.

E+Selenium: contains vitamin E and selenomethionine.

VitaSight®: with vitamins A, C and E, beta-carotene, zinc, selenium, bilberry, lutein, and ginkgo biloba.

Colloidal Minerals: more than 70 trace and essential minerals from natural sources.

Smoke-Less™: herbal combination with additional nutrients designed to reduce cravings.

PMS and LadyMate: supplementation for the nutritional needs of pre-menstrual syndrome.

Slender-Mist®: dietary snack supplements containing a combination of B vitamins, hydroxy-citric acid, L-carnitine and chromium. Four different flavors.

Blue-Green Sea Spray: spirulina extract, additional omega 3 fatty acids from flaxseed oil, and vitamin E.

Re-Leaf: a blend of more than 10 herbs that are recommended for minor discomfort, anxiety, and stress.

Osteo-CalMag: herbal supplement with additional vitamin D, calcium and magnesium.

Pine Bark and Grape Seed: powerful proanthocyanidins (anti-oxidants) from natural sources, with additional B vitamins.

1-Before, 2-During, 3-After: three performance sprays designed for the needs of physical activity.

CardioCare™: with vitamins C and E, the amino acids L-lysine and L-proline, coenzyme Q10 and additional herbal extracts.

DHEA: dehydroepiandrosterone in both men's and women's formulations.

GinkgoMist™: with ginkgo biloba, vitamin B12, acetyl-L-carnitine, choline, inositol, phosphatidylserine and niacin.

Ex. O: powerful blend of cayenne and peppermint with additional herbs recommended for allergy control.

How Supplied: VitaMist dietary supplements are supplied in sealed containers fitted with a natural pump. Each container provides a 30-day supply.

Recommended Dosage: Two sprays, four times per day, for a total dosage of eight sprays per day.

UNKNOWN DRUG?
Consult the
Product Identification Guide
(Gray Pages)
for full-color photos of
leading over-the-counter
medications

McNeil Consumer & Specialty Pharmaceuticals

**Division of McNeil-PPC, Inc.
FORT WASHINGTON, PA 19034**

Direct Inquiries to:
Consumer Relationship Center
Fort Washington, PA 19034
(800) 962-5357

LACTAID® ORIGINAL STRENGTH CAPLETS
(lactase enzyme)

LACTAID® EXTRA STRENGTH CAPLETS
(lactase enzyme)

LACTAID® ULTRA CAPLETS AND CHEWABLE TABLETS
(lactase enzyme)

Description: Each serving size (3 caplets) of *LACTAID® Original Strength* contains 9000 FCC (Food Chemical Codex) units of lactase enzyme (derived from *Aspergillus oryzae*).
Each serving size (2 caplets) of *LACTAID® Extra Strength* contains 9000 FCC units of lactase enzyme (derived from *Aspergillus oryzae*).
Each serving size (1 caplet) of *LACTAID® Ultra Caplet* contains 9000 FCC units of lactase enzyme (derived from *Aspergillus oryzae*).
Each serving size (1 tablet) of *LACTAID® Ultra Chewable Tablet* contains 9000 FCC units of lactase enzyme (derived from *Aspergillus oryzae*).
LACTAID® is the original lactase dietary supplement that makes milk and dairy foods more digestible for individuals with lactose intolerance. *LACTAID®* lactase enzyme hydrolyzes lactose into two digestible simple sugars: glucose and galactose. *LACTAID® Caplets/Chewable Tablets* are taken orally for *in vivo* hydrolysis of lactose.

Actions: *LACTAID® Caplets/Chewable Tablets* work by providing the enzyme that hydrolyzes the milk sugar lactose (disaccharide) into the two monosaccharides, glucose and galactose.

Uses: LACTAID contains a natural enzyme that helps your body break down lactose, the complex sugar found in dairy foods. If not properly digested, lactose can cause flatulence, bloating, cramps or diarrhea.*

*This statement has not been evaluated by the Food and Drug Administration. This product is not intended to diagnose, treat, cure, or prevent any disease.

Directions: Original Strength: Swallow 3 caplets with the first bite of dairy food. For best results, you may have to adjust the number of caplets up

Continued on next page

Lactaid—Cont.

or down. **Extra Strength:** Swallow 2 caplets with first bite of dairy food. For best results, you may have to adjust the number of caplets up or down. **Ultra Caplets:** Swallow 1 caplet with the first bite of dairy food. If you suffer from severe digestive discomfort, you may have to take more than one caplet, but no more than two at a time. **Ultra Chewables:** Chew and swallow 1 chewable tablet with your first bite of dairy food. If you suffer from severe digestive discomfort, you may have to take more than one tablet but no more than two at a time. Don't be discouraged if at first LACTAID does not work to your satisfaction. Because the degree of enzyme deficiency naturally varies from person to person and the amount of lactose varies from food to food, you may have to adjust the number of caplets/chewable tablets up or down to find your own level of comfort. Since LACTAID Caplets/Chewable Tablets work only on the food as you eat it, use them every time you consume dairy foods.

Warnings: *Consult your doctor if* your symptoms continue after using the product or if your symptoms are unusual or seem unrelated to eating dairy. Keep out of reach of children. **Do not use if carton is open or if printed plastic neckwrap is broken or if single serve packet is open.**
LACTAID® Ultra Chewable Tablets:
Phenylketonurics: Contains Phenylalanine.

Ingredients: *LACTAID® Original Strength Caplets:* Lactase Enzyme (9000 FCC Lactase units/3 caplets), Mannitol, Cellulose, Sodium Citrate, Magnesium Stearate.
LACTAID® Extra Strength Caplets: Lactase Enzyme (9000 FCC Lactase units/2 caplets), Mannitol, Cellulose, Sodium Citrate, Magnesium Stearate.
LACTAID® Ultra Caplets: Lactase Enzyme (9000 FCC Lactase units/Caplet), Cellulose, Sodium Citrate, Magnesium Stearate, Colloidal Silicon Dioxide.
LACTAID® Ultra Chewable Tablets: Lactase Enzyme (9000 FCC Lactase units/tablet), Mannitol, Cellulose, Sodium Citrate, Magnesium Stearate, Flavor, Citric Acid, Acesulfame K, Aspartame.

How Supplied: *LACTAID® Original Strength Caplets* are available in bottles of 120 count. Store at or below room temperature (below 77°F) but do not refrigerate. Keep away from heat. *LACTAID® Extra Strength Caplets* are available in bottles of 50 count. Store at or below room temperature (below 77°F) but do not refrigerate. Keep away from heat. *LACTAID® Ultra Caplets* are available in single serve packets in 12, 32, 60 and 90 count packages. Store at or below 86°F. Keep away from heat. *LACTAID® Ultra Chewable Tablets* are available in single serve packets of 32 and 60 counts.

Store at or below room temperature (below 77°F), but do not refrigerate. Keep away from heat and moisture.
LACTAID® Caplets and *LACTAID® Ultra Chewable Tablets* are certified kosher from the Orthodox Union.
Also available: 70% lactose-reduced Lactaid Milk and 100% lactose-free Lactaid Milk.
Shown in Product Identification Guide, page 511

Memory Secret
1221 BRICKELL AVENUE
SUITE 1000
MIAMI FL 33131 USA

For Direct Inquiries Contact:
(866) 673 2738
fax 1-305-675-2279
e-mail intelectol@memorysecret.net

INTELECTOL® MEMORY ENHANCER
VINPOCETINE TABLETS MEMORY SECRET

Description: **INTELECTOL®** is the purest form of Vinpocetine available. Vinpocetine is a derivative of Vincamine, which is extracted from the Periwinkle plant (*Vinca Minor, Vinca Pervinca*). Research suggests that Vinpocetine helps to maintain healthy blood circulation in the brain and supports certain neurotransmitters in the memory process.* Vinpocetine supports and protects brain blood vessel health and aids mental function.*

Directions: As a dietary supplement, take 2 tablets twice daily with meals. Vinpocetine should be taken as part of an on-going regimen with exercise, a healthy diet and keeping active the mind. Do not use if tamper-evident seal is broken.

Cautions: Take product with food to avoid stomach upset. Not recommended for use by pregnant women, nursing mothers or anyone under 18 years old. Consult a doctor or health care professional before use if you have any medical condition or if taking any medication. Not recommended for use by anyone with hemophilia, heart problems or low blood pressure. **Keep out of reach of children.**
Store in a cool, dry place.

Supplement Facts
Serving Size 2 tablets
Servings Per Container: 25

	Amount Per Serving	% DV
Vinpocetine	10 mg	*
(from Periwinkle seed extract)		

*Daily Value not established.

Other Ingredients: Lactose, hydroxypropylcellulose, magnesium stearate and talc.

> ***These statements have not been evaluated by the Food & Drug Administration. This product is not intended to diagnose, treat, cure, or prevent any disease.**

Distributed by: The Memory Secret, Inc.
1221 Brickell Ave., Suite 1000, Miami, FL 33131/USA
memorysecret™
www.memorysecret.net
Shown in Product Identification Guide, page 515

Mission Pharmacal Company
10999 IH 10 WEST
SUITE 1000
SAN ANTONIO, TX 78230-1355

Direct Inquiries to:
PO Box 786099
San Antonio, TX 78278-6099
TOLL FREE: (800) 292-7364
(210) 696-8400
FAX: (210) 696-6010
For Medical Information Contact:
In Emergencies:
Mary Ann Walter

CITRACAL®Ⓤ
[*sit'ra-cal*]
Ultradense® calcium citrate dietary supplement

Ingredients: Each tablet contains calcium (as Ultradense® calcium citrate) 200 mg, polyethylene glycol, croscarmellose sodium, hydroxypropyl methylcellulose, color added, magnesium silicate, magnesium stearate.

Sensitive Patients: CITRACAL® contains no wheat, barley, yeast or rye; is sugar, dairy and gluten free and contains no artificial colors.
One Tablet Provides:
200 mg. calcium (elemental), equaling 20% of the U.S. recommended daily allowance for adults and children 4 or more years of age.

Directions: Take 1 to 2 tablets two times daily or as recommended by a physician, pharmacist or health professional. Store at room temperature.

How Supplied: Supplied as white, barrel shaped, coated tablets in bottles of 100, UPC 0178-0800-01, and bottles of 200, UPC 0178-0800-20.
Ⓤ=Kosher Parvae approved by Orthodox Union.

CITRACAL® 250 MG + D

[sit 'ra-cal]

Ultradense® calcium citrate-Vitamin D dietary supplement

Ingredients: Each tablet contains: calcium (as Ultradense® calcium citrate) 250 mg., polyethylene glycol, citric acid, microcrystalline cellulose, hydroxypropyl methylcellulose, croscarmellose sodium, color added, magnesium silicate, magnesium stearate, vitamin D_3 (62.5 IU).

How Supplied: Supplied as white, modified rectangle shaped, coated tablets in bottles of 150, UPC 0178-0837-15.

CITRACAL® Caplets + D

[sit ' ra-cal]

Ultradense® calcium citrate-Vitamin D dietary supplement

Ingredients: Each caplet contains calcium (as Ultradense® calcium citrate) 315 mg., polyethylene glycol, croscarmellose sodium, hydroxypropyl methylcellulose, color added, magnesium silicate, magnesium stearate, vitamin D_3 (200 IU).

How Supplied: Supplied as white, arc rectangle shaped, coated tablets in bottles of 60 UPC 0178-0815-60, and bottles of 120 UPC 0178-0815-12, and bottles of 180 UPC 0178-0815-18.

CITRACAL® PLUS

[sit 'ra-cal]

Ultradense® calcium citrate-Vitamin D-multimineral dietary supplement

Ingredients: Each tablet contains calcium (as Ultradense® calcium citrate) 250 mg., polyethylene glycol, magnesium oxide, hydroxypropyl methylcellulose, povidone, croscarmellose sodium, color added, pyridoxine hydrochloride, zinc oxide, sodium borate, manganese gluconate, magnesium silicate, copper gluconate, maltodextrin, magnesium stearate, vitamin D_3 (125 IU).

How Supplied: Supplied as white, arc rectangle, coated tablets in bottles of 150 tablets, UPC 0178-0825-15.

Novartis Consumer Health, Inc.

**200 KIMBALL DRIVE
PARSIPPANY, NJ 07054-0622**

Direct Product Inquiries to:
Consumer & Professional Affairs
(800) 452-0051
Fax: (800) 635-2801
Or write to above address.

BENEFIBER® Fiber Supplement

Description: Benefiber® is a 100% natural fiber, that can be mixed with almost anything. It's taste free, grit-free, and will never thicken. So it won't alter the taste or texture of foods or non-carbonated beverages. It can be used in coffee, pudding, soup, or whatever is desired.

Supplement Facts:
**Serving Size: 1 tbsp (4g)
(makes 4 fl oz prepared)**

Amount Per Serving	%DV
Calories 20	
Total Carbohydrate 4g	**1%***
Dietary Fiber 3g	12%*
Soluble Fiber 3g	†
Sodium 20mg	**1%**

*Percent Daily Values (DV) are based on a 2,000 calorie diet.
†Daily Value not established.

Ingredients: Partially Hydrolyzed Guar Gum (A 100% natural fiber). Guar Gum is derived from the seed of the cluster bean.
Ⓤ 100% Natural Fiber–Sugar Free

Directions for use: Stir 1 tablespoon (tbsp) of Benefiber into at least 4 oz. of any beverage or soft food (hot or cold). Use 8 oz. if using 2 tbsp. Stir until dissolved.††

Age	Dosage
12 yrs. to adult	1–2 tbsp up to 3 times daily*
7 to 11 yrs.	1/2–1 tbsp up to 3 times daily**
Under 6 yrs.	Ask your doctor

tbsp=tablespoon
* Not to exceed 5 tbsp per day.

**Not to exceed 2.5 tbsp per day.
††Not recommended for carbonated beverages.

Store at controlled room temperature 20–25°C (68–77°F). Protect from moisture.
Use within 6 months of opening.
Keep out of reach of children.
If you are pregnant or nursing a baby, ask a health professional before use.
Tamper Evident Feature: Do not use if printed bottle inner seal is broken or missing or if sealed packet is broken or torn.

How Supplied:
• 24 serving cannister = 3.4 oz/96 g
• 42 serving cannister = 6 oz/168 g
• 80 serving cannister = 11.3 oz/320 g
• Box of 14 ct. individual packets = 2 oz/56 g
Packaged by weight, not volume. Contents may settle during shipping and handling.
Benefiber® guarantees your satisfaction or your money back.
Questions? Call **1-800-452-0051** 24 hours a day, 7 days a week or visit us at **www.benefiber.com** for recipe ideas and additional information.
Novartis Consumer Health, Inc.
Parsippany, NJ 07054-0622 ©2003
Shown in Product Identification Guide, page 515

BENEFIBER®
**Fiber Supplement
Chewable Tablets Orange Creme Flavored**

Benefiber Chewable Tablets are an easy way to add fiber to your diet. These great tasting tablets provide as much fiber per dose as the leading bulk fiber powder, but because there's no need for water or mixing, you can take them virtually anywhere, anytime.

Supplement Facts:
Serving Size: 3 Tablets
Servings Per Container: Varies

Amount Per Serving	%DV*
Calories 35	
Total Carbohydrate 8g	**3%***
Dietary Fiber 3g	12%*
Soluble Fiber 3g	†
Sugars 3g	
Sodium 10mg	**<1%**

*Percent Daily Values (DV) are based on a 2,000 calorie diet.
†Daily Value (DV) not established.

Ingredients: partially hydrolyzed guar gum, sorbitol, maltodextrin, confection-

Continued on next page

Information on Novartis Consumer Health, Inc. products appearing on these pages is effective as of November 2003.

Benefiber Chewable—Cont.

er's sugar, dextrates, citric acid, magnesium stearate, sucralose, sucrose, natural and artificial flavors, modified food starch, acacia, FD&C yellow 6 aluminum lake, silicon dioxide, lecithin, tocopherols, soybean oil

Directions for use: Adults: Chew 1 to 3 tablets up to 5 times daily to supplement the fiber content of your diet. Do not take more than 15 tablets in a 24 hour period.

Age	Dosage
12 yrs. to adult	1–3 tablets up to 5 times daily*
7 to 11 yrs.	1/2–1 1/2 tablets up to 5 times daily**
Under 6 yrs.	ask your doctor

* Not to exceed 15 tablets per day.
**Not to exceed 7 1/2 tablets per day.

Other Information: Store at controlled room temperature 20–25°C (68–77°F). Protect from excessive heat and moisture.
Keep out of reach of children.
If you are pregnant or nursing a baby, ask a health professional before use.
Tamper Evident Feature: Notice Protective printed inner seal beneath cap. If missing or damaged, do not use contents.

> Product may contain dark specks due to the processing of natural ingredients.

Questions? call **1-800-452-0051** 24 hours a day, 7 days a week.
www.benefiber.com
for additional information.
Benefiber guarantees your satisfaction or your money back.
Manufactured for and Distributed by:
Novartis Consumer Health, Inc.
Parsippany, NJ 07054-0622
©2004

How Supplied: Available in bottles of 36 ct. and 100 ct. tablets.
Shown in Product Identification Guide, page 515

SLOW FE®
Slow Release Iron Tablets

Drug Facts:
Active Ingredient
(in each tablet):   **Purpose:**
160 mg dried ferrous sulfate, USP (equivalent to 50 mg elemental iron) .... Iron deficiency

Uses: For use in the prevention of iron deficiency when the need for such therapy has been determined by a doctor.

Warnings:
- The treatment of any anemic condition should be under the advice and supervision of a doctor.
- As oral iron products interfere with absorption of oral tetracycline antibiotics, these products should not be taken within two hours of each other.
- **If pregnant or breast-feeding,** ask a health professional before use.

> **Warning:** Accidental overdose of iron-containing products is a leading cause of fatal poisoning in children under 6. Keep this product out of reach of children. In case of accidental overdose, call a doctor or poison control center immediately.

Directions:
- Tablets must be swallowed whole.
- ADULTS: One or two tablets daily or as recommended by a doctor. A maximum of four tablets daily may be taken.
- CHILDREN UNDER 12: consult a doctor

Other Information:
- store at controlled room temperature 20–25°C (68–77°F)
- protect from moisture

Inactive Ingredients: cetostearyl alcohol, FD&C blue #2 aluminum lake, hypromellose, lactose, magnesium stearate, polysorbate 80, talc, titanium dioxide, yellow iron oxide

Questions? call **1-800-452-0051** 24 hours a day, 7 days a week.

How Supplied: Child-resistant blister packages of 30 ct., 60 ct. and 90 ct. NDC 0067-0125-47.

Child Resistant

Blister packaged for your protection.
Do not use if individual seals are broken.
Tablets non-USP (disintegration, content uniformity)
Tablets made in Great Britain
Distributed by:
Novartis Consumer Health, Inc.
Parsippany, NJ 07054-0622 © 2003
Shown in Product Identification Guide, page 517

SLOW FE® WITH FOLIC ACID
(Slow Release Iron, Folic Acid)
Dietary Supplement

Description: Slow Fe + Folic Acid delivers 47.5 mg elemental iron as ferrous sulfate plus 350 mcg folic acid using the unique wax matrix delivery system described above (for SLOW FE® Slow Release Iron Tablets).

Provides women of childbearing potential with folic acid to help reduce the risk of neural tube birth defects. These birth defects are rare, but serious, and occur within 28 days of conception, often before a woman knows she's pregnant.

Formula: Each tablet contains: 47.5 mg elemental iron as ferrous sulfate and 350 mcg folic acid.
Other Ingredients: lactose, hypromellose, talc, magnesium stearate, cetostearyl alcohol, polysorbate 80, titanium dioxide, yellow iron oxide.

Dosage: ADULTS—One or two tablets once a day or as recommended by a physician. A maximum of two tablets daily may be taken. CHILDREN UNDER 12—Consult a physician. Tablets must be swallowed whole.

Warning: The treatment of any anemic condition should be under the advice and supervision of a physician. As oral iron products interfere with absorption of oral tetracycline antibiotics, these products should not be taken within two hours of each other. Intake of folic acid from all sources should be limited to 1000 mcg per day to prevent the masking of Vitamin B_{12} deficiencies. Should you become pregnant while using this product, consult a physician as soon as possible about good prenatal care and the continued use of this product. If you are already pregnant or nursing a baby, seek the advice of a health care professional before using this product.

> **Warning:** Accidental overdose of iron-containing products is a leading cause of fatal poisoning in children under 6. Keep this product out of reach of children. In case of accidental overdose, call a doctor or poison control center immediately.

How Supplied: Blister packages of 20 supplied in Child-Resistant packaging. Store at controlled room temperature 20–25°C (68°–77°F). Protect from moisture.
Tablets made in Great Britain
Novartis Consumer Health, Inc.
Parsippany, NJ 07054-0622 © 2003
Shown in Product Identification Guide, page 517

UNKNOWN DRUG?
Consult the
Product Identification Guide
(Gray Pages)
for full-color photos of
leading over-the-counter
medications

OBIKEN
JAPAN APPLIED MICROBIOLOGY RESEARCH INSTITUTE LTD.

326 Otoguro, Tamaho-cho,
Nakakoma-gun,
Yamanashi, 409-3812 JAPAN

For Direct Inquiries contact:
1) Tel: 81-55-240-3511
2) Fax: 81-55-240-3512
3) E-mail: sales@oubiken.co.jp
4) website: httn://www.oubiken.co.jp

ABPC® (Agaricus Blazei Practical Compound)

ABPC® is the processed food, which is mycelia of Agaricus blazei mushroom treated by digestive enzyme and is applied as dietary supplement.

*Product Description: Agaricus blazei Murrill H-1, which we have originally isolated from wild Agaricus blazei mushroom, is used to produce ABPC® (Enzyme digested Agaricus blazei mushroom mycelium processed food).
ABPC® is prepared from mycelium of Agaricus blazei mushroom cultured in the fermentor that we have originally designed. Mycelia processed by enzyme. After completion of enzyme treatment, the product are freeze-dried and powdered.
It is essential for keeping the quality of product consistently from lots to lots that mycelium is cultured by fermentor. The amount of β-D-glucan of the mycellia by this method (ca 30% (wt/wt)) is more than that of Agaricus blazei fruit body (ca 8% (wt/wt)).
Agaricus blazei mushroom has been used habitually in Brazil and other South American countries for the sake of health.
ABPC® is one of the best processed foods for the sake of health, because it protects us from physiological imbalance due to irregular habits and aging, or enhances immune system.
We, OBIKEN has obtained the U. S. patent concerning with the mycelium culturing method. U. S. patent number: USP6465218 registered October 15, 2002 and have been assessed, registered ISO9001:2000 for design/development and manufacturing ABPC® in March 14, 2003.

Clinical Data: The first publication as regarding clinical test of ABPC® was the treatment report at 35th Conference of Japan Society of Clinical Oncology in 1997, where Dr. Yukie NIWA (Tosashimizu Hospital, Tosashimizu-city, Kochi), Dr. Jiro ITAMI (Shibata Hospital) presented the cases of high survival rate of breast cancer, stomach cancer and spleen cancer among 1,260 patients. The test have been conducted at the hospitals including Kanazawa Medical University, University of Yamanashi Faculity of Medical, Juntendo University School of Medicine, Akiyama Neurosurgery Hospital and Sano Surgical Hospital.

*Recommended Dosage: ABPC® is the dietary supplement which is produced by culturing mycelium of Agaricus blazei mushroom in fermentor.
It enhances immune system and one of the best processed food for keeping good health.
As a dietary supplement, ABPC® should be taken 1 to 2 sticks per day, usually with water or lukewarm water, or could be taken by chewing. It may be used before or after meal. Store at room temperature in the dark.

Ingredients: The content of ABPC® per stick (contain 1.00 gr) is as followings.
1) ABPC powder freeze-dried:
   :68% (Wt/Wt)
2) Lactose
   :20% (Wt/Wt)
3) Calcium from egg shell
   :10% (Wt/Wt)
4) Lipid
   :2% (Wt/Wt)
5) Energy : 345Kcal/100gr

Adverse Reactions: Since we have released ABPC® in Japan 7 years ago, no adverse reaction have been reported. The acute toxicity test with mice[1],[2],[3] proved safety of ABPC®.
References;
1) Test report dated December 4, 1997 conducted by The Japan Food Analysis Center
2) Test report dated June 14, 2002 conducted by Japan Applied Microbiology Research Institute Ltd.
3) Test report dated June 26, 2002 conducted by The Japan Food Analysis Center

Warning: Women who are pregnant or in a period of lactation and infant should better avoid to take. Although no sign of adverse reaction observed in taking a large amount, it is better not to exceed 5 times of daily dosage.

How to Supplied: The box contains 90 sticks (Total amount 90 gr). Each stick contains 1.0 gr granule of ABPC®.
However, We can also supply in the shape of tablet.

---

*These statements have not been evaluated by the Food And Drug Administration. This products are not intended to diagnose, treat, cure OR prevent any disease.

Shown in Product Identification Guide, page 518

**IF YOU SUSPECT
AN INTERACTION. . .**
The 1,800-page
PDR Companion Guide™ can help.
Use the order form
in the front of this book.

The Procter & Gamble Company

P. O. BOX 599
CINCINNATI, OH 45201

Direct Inquiries to:
Consumer Relations
(800) 832–3064

METAMUCIL®
DIETARY FIBER SUPPLEMENT
[met uh-mū sil]
(psyllium husk)
*Also see **Metamucil Fiber Laxative** in Nonprescription Drugs section*

Description: Metamucil contains psyllium husk (from the plant *Plantago ovata*), a concentrated source of soluble fiber which can be used to increase one's dietary fiber intake. When used as part of a diet low in saturated fat and cholesterol, 7g per day of soluble fiber from psyllium husk (the amount in 3 doses of Metamucil) may reduce the risk of heart disease by lowering cholesterol. Each dose of Metamucil powder and Metamucil Fiber Wafers contains approximately 3.4 grams of psyllium husk (or 2.4 grams of soluble fiber). A listing of ingredients and nutrition information is available in the listing of Metamucil Fiber Laxative in the Nonprescription Drug section. Metamucil Smooth Texture Sugar-Free Regular Flavor and Metamucil capsules contains no sugar and no artificial sweeteners. Metamucil Smooth Texture Sugar-Free Orange Flavor contains aspartame (phenylalanine content of 25 mg per dose). Metamucil powdered products are gluten-free.

Uses: Metamucil Dietary Fiber Supplement can be used as a concentrated source of soluble fiber to increase the dietary intake of fiber. Diets low in saturated fat and cholesterol that include 7 grams of soluble fiber per day from psyllium husk, as in Metamucil, may reduce the risk of heart disease by lowering cholesterol. One adult dose of Metamucil has 2.4 grams of this soluble fiber. Consult a doctor if you are considering use of this product as part of a cholesterol-lowering program.

Warnings: Read entire Drug Facts section in listing for Metamucil Fiber Laxative in the Nonprescription Drug section.

Directions: Adults 12 yrs. & older: 1 dose in 8 oz of liquid *3 times daily*. Capsules: 2–6 capsules for increasing daily fiber intake; 6 capsules for cholesterol lowering use. Up to three times daily. Under 12 yrs.: Consult a doctor. See mixing directions in Drug Facts in listing for Metamucil Fiber Laxative in the Nonprescription Drug section.

Continued on next page

Metamucil—Cont.

NOTICE: Mix this product with at least 8 oz (a full glass) of liquid. Taking without enough liquid may cause choking. Do not take if you have difficulty swallowing.

For listing of ingredients and nutritional information for Metamucil Dietary Fiber Supplement, and for laxative indications and directions for use, see Metamucil Fiber Laxative in the Nonprescription Drug section.

Notice to Health Care Professionals: To minimize the potential for allergic reaction, health care professionals who frequently dispense powdered psyllium products should avoid inhaling airborne dust while dispensing these products.

Handling and Dispensing: To minimize generating airborne dust, spoon product from the canister into a glass according to label directions.

How Supplied: Powder: canisters and cartons of single-dose packets. Capsules: 100 and 160 count bottles. For complete ingredients and sizes for each version, see Metamucil Table 1, page 740, Nonprescription Drug section.

Questions? 1-800-983-4237

Wellness International Network, Ltd.

**5800 DEMOCRACY DRIVE
PLANO, TX 75024**

Direct Inquiries to:
Product Coordinator
(972) 312-1100
FAX: (972) 943-5250

BIOLEAN II®

[bī-ō-lēn]
Herbal & Amino Acid Dietary Supplement

Uses: BIOLEAN II® contains a rich supply of natural herbal extracts and pharmaceutical grade amino acids that, when used as a daily nutritional supplement, helps stimulate thermogenesis, reduce weight and increase lean muscle mass to total body mass.

One of the key ingredients in BIOLEAN II is Advantra Z®, a unique extract of the Chinese herb zhi shi, also commonly referred to as citrus aurantium or bitter orange. Advantra Z, as the only patented citrus aurantium extract for weight loss and physical performance on the market today, contains alkaloids which are related to the ephedrine alkaloids and have similar effects on metabolism and breakdown of stored fat. As a result, they increase the metabolic rate and increase the rate of breakdown of stored fat (lipol-

ysis) in the body (Jones, 1998). The alkaloids present in Advantra Z include synephrine, N-methyltyramine, hordenine, octopamine, and tyramine.

Advantra Z is distinguished from generic extracts of citrus aurantium due to its specific standarization of the five adrenergic amines: synephrine, hordenine, octopamine, tyramine and N-methyltyramine. It contains higher levels of these than are normally found in other products (6.6%). Also, the amounts are fixed in relationship to each other with synephrine at 4.6%, N-methyltyramine at 1.04%, tyramine at 0.32%, hordenine at 0.33% and octopamine at 0.35%. Thus, BIOLEAN II ensures a high potency of a fixed formula extraction.

The main adrenergic amines (alkaloids) of the citrus extract Advantra Z are synephrine and N-methyltyramine, which act almost wholly independently and are active by mouth. In classical tests, these citrus alkaloids show properties similar to ephedrine (Goodman and Gilamn, 1941), with activation of B-receptors (Munson, 1995). More recently, studies have shown that both octopamine and synephrine appear particularly effective in stimulating lipolysis (Carpene et al., 1999; Fontana et al., 2000), by a postulated B3-receptor effect (Dulloo, 1993). Wenke et al. (1967) had previously revealed that synephrine was about 3.5 times as effective in stimulating lipolysis as octopamine. There are thus indications that the alkaloid mixture in Advantra Z is superior to the mixture of ephedrine alkaloids in Ma-huang (Ephedra sinica) in terms of effects on B receptors in general.

However, this theoretical superiority does not extend to side effects. Initial studies in lean volunteers (Hedrei & Gougeon, 1997) and obese volunteers (Pathak & Gougeon, 1998), while showing excellent thermogenic responses, failed to reveal any evidence of increased heart rate, blood pressure or central nervous system stimulation. A clinical study reported by Coker et al. (1999) also demonstrated excellent effects on weight loss with an absence of side effects.

Thus, though the citrus alkaloids appear to be at least as thermogenic as the ephedrine alkaloids, they do not cause the minor side effects associated with use of Ma-huang (nervousness, agitation, palpitations, increases in blood pressure). The lack of central nervous system side effects can be attributed to the relatively low lipophilicity of the citrus alkaloids, which will slow their passage across the blood-brain barrier. However, the absence of cardiovascular activity implies that Advantra Z alkaloids have little effect on alpha-, beta-1, and beta-2 receptors, while the thermogenic effect confirms that they do activate the peripheral beta-3 receptors, targeting fat cells rather more specifically. While the actions of adrenergic agents that demonstrate thermogenesis without significant cardiovascular and central nervous system effects make them

ideal adjuncts for regulating and controlling weight problems, they can also be used as erogenic aids to improve physical performance (Yang & Elligott, 1989). The acute action is to increase energy availability and, thus, increase the capacity for physical exertion, while longer-term actions result in an increase in muscle mass, particularly when combined with appropriate diet programs and training (Jones 1998).

Advantra Z's actions are boosted when combined with the synergistic grouping of three caffeine-containing herbs—guarana, green tea and yerba mate. In terms of safety and efficacy, these botanicals are preferable caffeine sources, as they do not elicit an adrenal response. Some studies have shown that the lipolytic effect of caffeine may be less in leaner individuals. (Braceo, 1995). Caffeine has been in at least four studies to stimulate the metabolic rate for up to 24 hours after ingesting (Bracco, 1995; Astrup, 1990; Horton, 1996; Graham, 1994). It has also been shown to decrease the perception of work effort (Cole, 1996).

The herbal extracts and amino acids in BIOLEAN II are known to cause fat loss through thermogenic activity and altered fuel metabolism resulting from sympathomimetic response to stimulation of beta receptors in adipose and muscle cells. The positive immune response, though not completely understood, is at least partially attributable to beta stimulation in adipocytes and the adaptogenic and tonifying action of certain of the herbal extracts. The extremely potent antioxidant properties found in some of the component plants, most notably in the Green Tea and Schizandrea extracts, work together with the amino acids to extend the adaptogenic, thermogenic, and restorative effects of BIOLEAN II.

Guarana is an herb long recognized for increasing mental alertness, fighting fatigue, and increasing stamina and physical endurance. Active compounds in guarana have an effect on increasing metabolism by suppressing appetite by aiding in a temporary, natural increase in body temperature and metabolic thermogensis. Guarana does this through stimulation of the body's B receptor pathway. It can induce the breakdown and release of stored body fat, thereby allowing stored fats to be turned into energy. Active compounds in guarana called xanthines suppress appetite and enhance both physical and mental performance. The caffeine present in guarana is known as guaranine and its effect on the body is without the side effects commonly associated with caffeine. This is because the herb contains other key components along with the caffeine that modify the activity of this substance.

Green tea is a natural herbal stimulant shown to significantly increase energy levels and to have a significant effect on fat metabolism (Amer J Clin Nut, 1999).

Green tea extract has potent pharmacologically active compounds, bioflavonoids and polyphenols, that oppose free radicals in the body. There are four primary polyphenols in green tea. While all four appear to have protective value, epigallocatechin-3-gallate (EGCG) occurs in the greater amounts and has the strongest benefit. EGCG enhances mental drive and energy, stimulates thermogenesis to provide major fat burning, and helps to control overeating by significantly reducing food intake Ahmed, 1997). EGCG is an antioxidant that is several times more potent than Vitamin E; it also prolongs the MIF life of noradrenaline, which triggers thermogenesis. Methylxanthines in green tea increase cAMP levels by inhibiting the enzyme phosphodiesterace. These compounds have also been shown to increase mental alertness, improve vitality, decrease the appetite, and increase energy. Green tea provides steady energy without eliciting an adrenal response.

Yerba mate is a plant long known for its ability to energize the body, stimulate the mind, relieve stress and aid in weight loss (Martinet, 1999); (Anderson et al. 2001). One study (Pasteur Institute, 1995) found yerba mate to be a more potent antioxidant than Vitamin C and an invitro study (University of Montreal, 1995) showed it can inhibit the oxidation of low-density lipoprotein. Although yerba mate has a chemical structure similar to caffeine, it stimulates the body without the CNS side effects. Acting as a tonic, yerba mate may provide energy through nutrition, rather than through stimulant properties, and actively works as a tonic for the central nervous system. Clinical studies show that caffeine-sensitive individuals can consume yerba mate without adverse reactions. (Keats, 1993).

L-carnitine aids in the transport of fatty acids into the mitochondria for thermogenesisis (Lurz, 1998). Other studies have shown it to increase the body's resistance to stress, lower cholesterol, improve heart, liver, and kidney functions, and increase endurance during physical exercise (Cacciatore, 1991; Kobayashi, 1992; Giamberadino, 1996). The amino acids, L-tyrosine and L-phenylalanine, inhibit appetite and promote satiety through hypothalamic release of cholycystokinin (CCK) and catecholamines. Catecholamines, like epinephrine, elevate mood and reduce the desire to eat, causing an increase in lipolysis coinciding with an inhibition of glycogen synthesis (Wingard et al., 1991), while L-tyrosine helps your body stay at its desired weight once you reach it (Wingard et al. 1991).

BIOLEAN II's herbal extracts are produced in a unique and exclusive process which is proprietary to this product. Instead of creating extracts based on a set quantity of one particular active within many which may be present in any particular plant, BIOLEAN II components are concentrated to maintain the natural and complete spectrum of biologically active factors, in the same ratio presented by the unprocessed plant.

Directions: Recommended Use: AM Serving - Adults take one white tablet and two green tablets with low calorie food. PM Serving - Adults may take one green tablet with low calorie food. If using BioLean II for the first time, limit daily intake to one white tablet and one green tablet on days one and two and one white tablet and two green tablets on day three. Needs vary with each individual.

Warnings: Not for use by children under the age of 18. If you are pregnant or nursing, if you have heart disease, thyroid disease, diabetes, high blood pressure, depression or other psychiatric condition, glaucoma, difficulty urinating, prostate enlargement, or seizure disorder, if you are using a monoamine oxidase inhibitor (MAOI), consult a health professional before using this product. Exceeding recommended serving may cause serious adverse effects. Discontinue use and consult your health professional if dizziness, sleeplessness, severe headache, heart palpitations or other similar symptoms occur. The recommended dose of this product contains about as much caffeine as a cup of coffee. Limit the use of caffeine-containing medications, food, or beverages while taking this product because too much caffeine may cause nervousness, irritability, sleeplessness, and occasionally, rapid heart beat. Phenylketonurics: Contains phenylalanine 196 mg per AM serving.

Ingredients: Calcium (as calcium carbonate, calcium phosphate dibasic), Proprietary Blend: [Caffeine(as Guarana Seed 50% Extract, Yerba Mate Leaf 10% Extract, Green Tea Leaf 40% Extract), Citrus Aurantium Fruit 30% Extract (Advantra Z®), Schizandra Berry, Gymnema Sylvestre Leaf 25% Extract, Rehmannia Root, Hawthorne Root, Jujube Seed, Alisma Root, Angelicae dahuricae Radix, Epemidium grandiflorum Radix, Poria Cocos Mushroom, Rhubarb Root, Angelicae sinensis Radix, Codonopsis Root, Eucommia Bark, Panax notoginseng Radi], L-Tyrosine, L-Phenylalanine, L-Carnitine (as L-Carnitine Bitartrate), Calcium Carbonate, Starch, Stearic Acid, Cellulose, Hydroxypropylcellulose, Croscarmelose Sodium, Magnesium Stearate, Silicon Dioxide, Calcium Phosphate Dibasic, Stearic acid, Silicon Dioxide, Croscarmelose Sodium, Hydroxypropylcellulose, Magnesium Stearate, Ethylcellulose.

Advantra Z® - registered trademark of Nutratech, Inc./Zhishin, LLC licensor of U.S. Patents.

How Supplied: One box contains 112 tablets (28 daily servings), with one white tablet and three green tablets per packet. Store at controlled temperature between 59° F and 86° F to maintain freshness.

BIOLEAN Accelerator™
Herbal & Amino Acid Formulation

Uses: BIOLEAN Accelerator™ is a unique combination of Chinese herbal extracts and pharmaceutical grade amino acids specifically designed to complement both BIOLEAN® and BIOLEAN Free® by extending and accelerating their actions. BIOLEAN and BIOLEAN Free are, in the traditional view of Chinese herbal medicine, strong Yang blends. This means that they are energy or heat-producing at their core. The addition of the amino acids and certain of the herbal components lends a very definite restorative or Yin element, as well. BIOLEAN Accelerator is a strong Yin herbal formula, intended to augment the lesser replenishing Yin elements of the other two herbal and amino acid supplements. Though the physiological actions of many herbs are complex and not totally understood, the formula in BIOLEAN Accelerator extends the adaptogenic, thermogenic, restorative and detoxifying results experienced with BIOLEAN and BIOLEAN Free, with an emphasis on the restorative and adaptogenic effects. The herbal formula is a combination of tonifiers traditionally used in China for the lungs, liver and kidneys.

Directions: For maximum effectiveness, use in conjunction with original BIOLEAN or BIOLEAN Free. (Do not consume BIOLEAN and BIOLEAN Free on the same day.) Take one tablet in the morning with original BIOLEAN or BIOLEAN Free. BIOLEAN Accelerator™ may also be taken in the afternoon with or without additional BIOLEAN or BIOLEAN Free if desired. Maximum absorption will be attained if taken with low-calorie food.

Warnings: Phenylketonurics: Contains 200 mg phenylalanine per serving. Not for use by children. Consult your physician before using this product if you are taking appetite suppressing drugs or antidepressants, or if you are pregnant or lactating. If symptoms of allergy develop, discontinue use.

Ingredients: Proprietary herbal extract (Cuscula Seed, Black Sesame Seed, Rehmannia Root, Achyranthes Root, Cornus Fruit, Chinese Yam, Eclipta Herb, Rose Hips, Ligustrum Fruit, Mulberry Fruit, Polygonati Rhizome, Foti Poria Cocos, Euryale Seed, Alisma Rhizome, Moutan Bark, Phellodendron Bark, Anemarrhena Rhizome, Schisandra Berry, Royal Jelly), L-Phenylalanine, L-Tyrosine, Calcium Carbonate, Calcium Phosphate Dibasic, Partially Hydrogenated Vegetable Oil, Hydroxypropyl Cellulose, Croscarmelose Sodium, Magnesium Stearate, Silicon Dioxide and Sodium Lauryl Sulfate.

How Supplied: One bottle contains 56 tablets.

Continued on next page

BIOLEAN Free®
Herbal & Amino Acid Dietary Supplement

Uses: BIOLEAN Free® is a strategic blend of herbs, spices, vitamins, minerals and amino acids specifically formulated to enhance fat utilization and energy production through various metabolic pathways. It has been shown to reduce body fat through its thermogenic effects and to enhance both physical and mental performance.

Thermogenesis refers to the body's ability to convert substrates such as proteins, fats and carbohydrates into heat energy. This is carried out most efficiently in the Brown Adipose Tissue of our body which uses fatty acids as its preferred fuel. Other fat cells, namely White Adipose Tissue, are concerned primarily with the storage of fat rather than its conversion to energy. The thermogenic pathway is complex and relies upon a series of reactions to occur. BIOLEAN Free utilizes many compounds which act at various locations in this pathway to ensure the maximum efficiency of the thermogenic process. Quebracho is one of these very special compounds. This South American plant contains quebrachine, aspidiospermine and other alkaloids that possess the ability to block alpha-2 adrenergic receptors in the body. This produces an enhanced sympathetic nervous system effect which, in turn, increases lipolysis (fat breakdown) within fat cells. The fatty acids released by this process can then be transported into the mitochondria to be used as a fuel. Ginger, cinnamon, horseradish, turmeric, cayenne and mustard are spices that stimulate thermogenesis in different ways. Some stimulate lipid mobilization in adipose tissue; others raise the resting metabolic rate; and some increase cAMP levels by inducing more beta receptors on fat cells and by increasing the concentration of adenylate cyclase. cAMP increases the breakdown of triglycerides to free fatty acids which are later used as fuel by the mitochondria in the cell. Methylxanthines (such as those found in green tea and yerba maté) also increase cAMP levels, but do this by inhibiting the enzyme, phosphodiesterase. These compounds have been noted to increase mental alertness, improve vitality, satisfy the appetite and increase energy. In addition to its methylxanthine content, green tea has recently been shown to possess strong antioxidant properties. Yerba maté is a plant that has been shown to produce the positive effects above without causing the insomnia seen with other methylxanthine-containing plants (such as coffee and kola nut). BIOLEAN Free also contains vitamin B-3 (niacin), vitamin B-6 (pyridoxine) and chromium and vanadium, which aid in the proper metabolism of fats, proteins and carbohydrates. L-tyrosine also aids in metabolism and promotes satiety through hypothalamic release of CCK. Methio-

nine is a precursor of L-carnitine which aids in the transport of fatty acids into the mitochondria for thermogenesis. Other herbs have been utilized in BIOLEAN Free. Ginseng and ho shou wu possess adaptogenic properties. Adaptogens help the body adapt to physiological and environmental stresses. Ginseng accomplishes this through its stabilizing effect on the hypothalamic-pituitary-adrenal-sympathetic nervous system. It can mediate an increased adrenal response to stress.

Ho shou wu has a stabilizing effect on the endocrine system and has restorative properties. It is also an antioxidant with a high flavonoid content. *Centella asiatica* contains asiaticoside and has been shown to increase activity levels and ease the body's ability to overcome fatigue when taken with ginseng and cayenne. Individually, *centella* has been shown to increase memory and mental acuity in studies abroad. Uva ursi contains the glycoside arbutin and promotes urinary health and body strength through its purifying effects. Ginkgo biloba is a tree whose leaves have been used for centuries as an herbal medicine. It contains flavonoids and is therefore a strong antioxidant. It reduces the tendency of platelets to stick together by inhibiting Platelet Activating Factor. It has been shown to increase blood flow to the heart, brain and other organs.

Directions: Adults (18 years and older) may take 4 tablets in the mid to late morning with a low-calorie food. Needs may vary with each individual. Some persons may require less than 4 caplets, or may prefer taking 3 tablets mid morning and 1 additional tablet mid afternoon to achieve optimum results. Do not exceed recommended daily amounts. It is recommended that you drink at least eight glasses of water daily.

Warnings: Not for use by children, pregnant women or lactating women. Consult your physician before using this product if you are taking appetite suppressing drugs or cardiovascular medication. Consult your physician if you have hypertension, heart disease, arrhythmias, prostatic hypertrophy, glaucoma, liver disease, renal disease or diabetes. Do not use if you have hyperthyroidism, psychosis, Parkinson's Disease, or are taking Monoamine oxidase inhibitors. BIOLEAN Free should not be taken on the same day as original BIOLEAN®. It is recommended that you minimize your caffeine intake while consuming this product. If allergic symptoms develop, discontinue use. Store in a cool, dry place. Keep out of reach of children.

Ingredients: Niacin (as niacinamide), Vitamin B6 (as pyridoxine HCl), Chromium (as chromium Chelavite® chloride), Potassium (as potassium citrate), Green tea leaf extract (10% methylxanthines), Yerba mate leaf extract (10% methylxanthines), Korean ginseng root extract (4% ginsenosides), Uva ursi leaf (20% arbutin), Guarana seed (22% meth-

ylxanthines), Quebracho bark extract (10% quebrachine), Gotu kola leaf (Centella asiatica), Ceylon cinnamon bark, Chinese horseradish root, Jamaican ginger root, Turmeric rhizome, Nigerian cayenne pepper (fruit), English mustard seed, Ho shou wu root, Ginkgo biloba leaf (24% ginkgoflavoneslycosides and 6% bilobalides), L-Tyrosine, L-Methionine, Vanadium (as BMOV), Dicalcium phosphate, Cellulose, Cellulose gum, Vegetable stearic acid, Silica, Vegetable magnesium stearate and Vegetable resin glaze.

How Supplied: One box contains 28 packets, four tablets per packet.

BIOLEAN LipoTrim™
All-Natural Dietary Supplement

Uses: LipoTrim™ is a highly active, synergistic combination of garcinia cambogia extract and chromium polynicotinate specifically created for use with the other products in the BIOLEAN® System. The method of action is by inhibition of lipogenesis and regulation of blood glucose levels. Serum glucose derived from dietary carbohydrates and not immediately converted to energy or glycogen tends to be converted into fat stores and cholesterol. In individuals with excess body fat stores or slow basal metabolism, this tendency is thought to be higher. The garcinia cambogia extract present in LipoTrim is verified by HPLC analysis to be no less than 50%(-) hydroxycitrate (HCA). HCA inhibits ATP-citrate lyase which retards Acetyl CoA synthesis, severely restricting conversion of excess glucose into fatty acids and cholesterol. Animal studies have shown a post-meal fatty acid synthesis reduction of 40–80% for an 8–12 hour period. When glucose to fat/cholesterol conversion is retarded, glycogen conversion continues, increasing liver stores and causing satiety signals to be sent to the brain resulting in appetite suppression. In situations of intense physical exercise, increased glycogen stores have been shown to result in enhanced endurance and recovery.

Directions: As a dietary supplement, take one capsule three times daily, 30 minutes before each meal. LipoTrim should be used in conjunction with a healthy diet and exercise plan.

Warnings: Do not consume if you are pregnant or lactating. Not for use by young children. Consult your physician before using this product if your diet consists of less than 1,000 calories per day.

Ingredients: Chromium as chromium polynicotinate, Garcinia Cambogia Fruit Extract, Hydroxypropylmethylcellulose, calcium sulfate, starch, and silicone dioxide.

How Supplied: One bottle contains 84 easy-to-swallow capsules.

*CitriMax™ is a trademark of Inter-Health.
ChromeMate® is a registered trademark of InterHealth.

FOOD FOR THOUGHT™
Choline-Enriched Supplement

Uses: By utilizing scientifically established "smart nutrients," Food For Thought™ is ideal for work, school or anytime peak mental performance is desired.

Choline, a member of the B-complex family, is determined to be one of the few substances that possesses the ability to penetrate the blood-brain barrier—a protectant of the brain from the onslaught of chemicals taken into the body each day—and go directly into the brain cells to produce acetylcholine.

The most abundant neurotransmitter in the body, acetylcholine is the primary neurotransmitter between neurons and muscles. It is vital because of its role in motor behavior (muscular movement) and memory. Acetylcholine helps control muscle tone, learning, and primitive drives and emotions, while also controlling the release of the pituitary hormone vasopressin—which is involved in learning and in the regulation of urine output. Studies show that low levels of acetylcholine can contribute to lack of concentration and forgetfulness, and may interfere with sleep patterns.

Food For Thought further enhances its effectiveness through the utilization of essential vitamins—required for promoting the synthesis of brain neurotransmitters—with a unique blend of minerals. The brain uses vitamins B3 (niacin) and B6 (pyridoxine), to convert the amino acid L-tryptophan into the mood- and sleep-regulating neurotransmitter serotonin, while vitamins B1 (thiamin), B5 (pantothenic acid), B6 (pyridoxine), and C and the minerals zinc and calcium are required for the production of acetylcholine.

Directions: Add 3/4 cup of chilled water or fruit juice to one packet of mix. Stir briskly. Consume 1–2 times per day. Keep in a cool, dry place. For maximum results, combine this product with one serving of Winrgy™.

Warnings: Not for use by children, pregnant or lactating women. Persons taking medications should seek medical advice before taking this product. Persons with ulcers or a history of ulcers should consult their physician before using a choline supplement. Do not consume more than four servings per day. Avoid the use of antacids containing aluminum with this product.

Ingredients: Carbohydrates, Sugars, Vitamin C (as ascorbic acid), Vitamin E (as dl-alpha tocopheryl acetate), Thiamin (as thiamin mononitrate), Riboflavin, Niacin (as niacinamide niacin), Vitamin B6 (as pyridoxine hydrochloride), Vitamin B12 (as cyanocobalamin), Pantothenic Acid (as calcium pantothenate), Calcium (as calcium pantothenate), Zinc (as zinc gluconate), Copper (as copper gluconate), Chromium (as chromium aspartate), Choline (as choline bitartrate), Glycine, Lysine (as L-lysine hydrochloride), Fructose, Natural Flavors, Silicon Dioxide and Magnesium Gluconate.

How Supplied: One box contains 28 packets Food For Thought. Serving size equals one packet.

DHEA Plus™
Pharmaceutical-Grade Formulation

Uses: By utilizing the latest and most advanced breakthrough applications in age management, DHEA Plus™ uniquely combines dihydroxyepiandrosterone (DHEA), Bioperine® and ginkgo biloba leaf to safely and effectively aid the body.

These age management factors are mainly attributed to the properties of DHEA, a natural substance obtained from the barbasco root, also known as Mexican Wild Yam, which is synthesized in a pharmaceutical laboratory to be utilized for specific health applications. Once supplemental DHEA is orally consumed, it is quickly absorbed into the bloodstream through the intestines and binds to a sulfate compound which creates DHEA-S. DHEA-S is the ultimate substance for which the body uses to manufacture hormones. Natural DHEA levels, abundant in the bloodstream and present at an even higher level in the tissues of the brain, are known to decline with age in both sexes. Scientific research proves that adequate levels of DHEA in the body can actually slow the aging process.

Bioperine, a pure piperine extract, enhances the body's natural thermogenic activity and is another important ingredient in DHEA Plus. Thermogenesis is the metabolic process that generates energy at the cellular level. While thermogenesis plays an integral role in our body's ability to properly utilize daily foods and nutrients in the body, it also sets in motion the mechanisms that lead to digestion and subsequent gastrointestinal absorption.

Known for possessing antioxidant activity, or flavonoid effects, ginkgo biloba proves to decrease platelet aggregation and increase vasodilation which appears to extend blood flow to the peripheral arteries and the brain. Some improvement in cognitive abilities has been noted as well as inhibition of lipid peroxidation, thereby stabilizing the cell wall against free-radical attack.

Directions: Adults take one capsule daily with food.

Warnings: This product should only be consumed by adults and is not intended for use by children. Do not consume if you are pregnant or lactating. Consult your physician before using this product if you are taking prescription medications. Persons with a history of prostate cancer should seek medical advice before using this product.

Ingredients: Dihydroxyepiandrosterone (DHEA), Ginkgo Biloba leaf, Bioperine* (Piper nigrum L.), Calcium Phosphate Dibasic, Partially Hydrogenated Vegetable Oil, Starch, Magnesium Stearate, Silicon Dioxide and Croscarmellose Sodium.

How Supplied: One bottle contains 60 enteric-coated tablets.

---

*Bioperine is a registered trademark of Sabinsa Corporation.

MASS APPEAL™
Amino Acid & Mineral Workout Supplement

Uses: Utilizing natural compounds which mimic the beneficial effects of anabolic steroids, Mass Appeal™ is specifically formulated to enhance athletic performance without the harmful side effects of steroids.

Among Mass Appeal's scientifically researched and proven ingredients is creatine, a naturally occurring substance which functions as a storage molecule for high-energy phosphate – the ultimate source of muscular energy known as adenosine triphosphate, or ATP. More than 95 percent of the body's total amount of creatine is contained within the muscles, with type II muscle fibers (fibers that generate large amounts of force) possessing greater initial levels and higher rates of utilization. Unlike other artificial aids used to enhance performance, creatine monohydrate saturates the muscle cells and causes a muscle "cell volumizing" effect by beneficially forcing water molecules inside the muscle cell. This promotes an increase in muscle growth by helping muscles form new proteins faster while slowing down the destructive breakdown of muscle cells during exercise. Studies show that creatine loading not only improves performance during short-duration, high intensity and intermittent exercises, but it accelerates energy recovery and reduces muscle fatigue by reducing lactic acid build-up as well.

Found in high concentrations within muscle cells and proteins throughout the body, the branched chain amino acids (BCAAs) L-leucine, L-valine and L-isoleucine are also incorporated into Mass Appeal's scientifically engineered formulation. BCAAs increase protein synthesis and can be oxidized inside muscle cells as ATP, a protein-sparing effect which indirectly increases anabolism by reducing the muscle's need to burn its own proteins during bodybuilding or strenuous exercise. When dietary intake of these amino acids is inadequate, muscle protein is broken down into its individual amino acid constituents and utilized in other essential metabolic reactions within the body. Through supplementation, the catabolic breakdown of muscle can be minimized and the muscle tissue preserved.

Continued on next page

Mass Appeal—Cont.

Alpha-ketoglutaric acid and the amino acid L-glutamine also protect against muscle catabolism by assisting muscle protein synthesis and preserving the body's natural stores of glutamine in the muscle.

Another major contributor to the Mass Appeal™ formulation is the amino acid inosine. By increasing hemoglobin's affinity for binding oxygen within red blood cells, inosine supplementation enables red blood cells to carry more oxygen as they travel from the lungs to the muscles.

Vanadyl sulfate, known for its vasodilator effects, has been shown to markedly increase the blood flow to muscle cells. Researchers also believe that this mineral not only contributes to increased efficiency in the metabolic pathways controlled by the body's insulin, but also triggers certain glucose transporters much in the same way insulin does. This results in increased glucose transport into the muscle tissue, increased glycogen storage, and decreases the breakdown of muscle protein as an energy source.

Directions: Adults (18 years and older) may take a loading dose of 3 packets in the morning and 2 packets in the late afternoon for one week. This dose may be repeated every three months. Following one week of the loading dose, begin the maintenance dose of 1 packet daily two hours after exercise. Needs may vary with each individual.

For individuals desiring enhanced effects, increase the loading dose to 3 to 4 packets, three times per day (morning, afternoon and evening). Following one week of this enhanced loading dose, begin the enhanced maintenance dose of 2 packets in the morning and 2 packets in the late afternoon. It is recommended that one maintain a low-fat, high-protein diet; drink at least eight glasses of water per day; and engage in 30 to 60 minutes of aerobic and anaerobic exercise three to four times per week. For optimal effects, take in conjunction with Phyto-Vite®, Pro-Xtreme™ and Sure2Endure™.

Warnings: Not for use by children, pregnant women or lactating women. Consult your physician before using this product if you have any medical conditions. Do not take if you have kidney disease, muscle disease or are on a protein-restricted diet. Discontinue immediately if allergic symptoms develop. Keep out of the reach of children. Store in a cool, dry place.

Ingredients: Creatine Monohydrate, Inosine (phosphate-bonded), L-leucine, L-valine, L-isoleucine, Alpha-Ketoglutaric acid, KIC (calcium keto-isocaproate), L-glutamine, Vanadyl Sulfate, Dicalcium phosphate, Microcrystalline Cellulose, Stearic Acid, Croscarmellose Sodium, Silica, Magnesium Stearate and film coating (hydroxypropyl methylcellulose, hydroxypropyl cellulose, polyethylene glycol, titanium dioxide and propylene glycol).

How Supplied: One box contains 28 packets, four tablets per packet.

PRO-XTREME™
Protein-Enriched Dietary Supplement

Uses: The need for protein in the human diet has been increasingly studied, especially in the last decade. As a result of this research, several factors regarding the optimal daily requirements and sources of protein have become very clear. Even the current government published RDIs, which are based solely on minimal needs for survival, have increased to .6–.8 grams per kilogram of body weight per day.

Current clinical findings however indicate that an RDI necessary to maintain optimum health for even a sedentary adult are closer to double that. Circumstances including illness, fat-loss diets, regular exercise, accelerated adolescent growth, or chronic mental or emotional stress indicate requirements 2–3 times that. Competitive or strength athletes, post surgical patients or any situation causing wasting disease such as chemotherapy, HIV, burn trauma or radiation therapy can increase the metabolic need for protein by a factor of up to 6 times the official government RDIs.

Furthermore, these figures represent protein which has been absorbed and made available to the tissues of the body and *not* merely that which has been consumed. This is a distinction current clinical research has recognized as *critical* to proper understanding of the need for protein in the human diet.

Before protein can be absorbed and utilized it must first be digested. Following digestion the free amino acids and di and tripeptides that result from protein breakdown are absorbed at the surface of the small intestine. The process of digestion and absorption requires several steps and is most efficient in the upper portion or proximal section of the jejunum (small intestine). In order for absorption of dietary protein to occur, it must first be reduced from larger oligo and polypeptides to di and tripeptides, the smallest protein fragments consisting of only two or three peptide-bonded amino acids, and free amino acids. Di and tripeptides have been clearly shown to be preferential over free forms. This process must occur fast enough and at a rate high enough to take advantage of the proximal transporters, those that specialize in di and tripeptides and which are in abundance only in this short section of upper intestinal bowel. Once protein has passed this lumenal area, relatively no further protein breakdown or absorption occurs. The balance moves on relatively unchanged into the colon, where it is definitely a negative health factor causing minimal gas and gastrointestinal distress, and when experienced chronically, can lead to colon disease and malignancy. It is now generally believed to be the number one factor responsible for the world's highest rate of colon cancer experienced in the U.S.

Pro-Xtreme™ is specifically engineered based on a new profile for protein in optimum human metabolism arising from these new clinical findings. With an exceptionally high di and tripeptide content of 40 percent, Pro-Xtreme™ not only promotes increased nitrogen retention—thereby minimizing the negative effects of increased protein intake or reduced caloric intake—but it works in harmony with natural gastrointestinal activity to produce maximum absorption as well.

Because of the fat content and the density of the bolus, meals containing tissue-source protein are released from the stomach and travel through the intestines at a rate which is naturally slower and more conducive to efficient digestion and absorption. The problems begin when too much tissue protein is consumed or the process of digestion and absorption is incomplete. It is estimated that at best only 30–35% of the protein consumed in an average protein-containing meal is absorbed allowing the balance of now detrimental undigested protein to pass into the colon.

In the case of liquid protein supplements, the problem is one not only of excessive amounts of protein being consumed but also the speed at which the bolus travels throughout the jejunum. Consequently, even in individuals with normal gastrointestinal function, liquid forms of whole proteins generally result in equally incomplete and oftentimes less absorption than their tissue food counterparts.

Pro-Xtreme™ utilizes sequentially hydrolyzed whey protein isolates of the highest quality to insure complete and rapid absorption of the highest levels of essential and branched-chain amino acids (BCAAs) in the preferred smallest peptide bonded form. These features, coupled with its industry-leading lowest average molecular weight, and soluble-fiber content, offer a primary source of protein that may be used any time a protein supplement is desired.

The combination and sequencing of amino acids in whey protein also results in increased tissue storage of glutathione, a stable tripeptide whose antioxidant activity is known to improve immune function. And, although whey protein naturally contains 5 to 7 percent of glutamine, the formula for Pro-Xtreme™ incorporates additional gram amounts of L-glutamine to its list of highly evolved ingredients as well. This extra step is designed to promote anti-catabolic effects in skeletal muscle while focusing on gastrointestinal and immune function improvement. Glutamine and the critical BCAA leucine are deemed indispensable for the healthy functioning of other tissues and metabolic processes. By maintaining a rich supply of BCAAs, Pro-Xtreme™ proves protein sparing within muscle and offers the highest biological value possible. Pro-Xtreme™ is formulated specifically for use with the other products in the BIOLEAN® System.

Directions: Add 1 packet (36 grams) Pro-Xtreme™ to 1 cup (8 ounces) cold water and stir. There is no need for blending or shaking. Pro-Xtreme™ may also be mixed with lowfat or nonfat milk, milk substitutes or blended with ice.

Warnings: Accidental overdose of iron-containing products is a leading cause of fatal poisoning in children under 6. Keep this product out of reach of children. In case of accidental overdose, call a doctor or poison control center immediately.

Ingredients: Carbohydrates, Dietary fiber, Sugars, Calcium, Iron, Magnesium, Chloride, Sodium, Potassium, Glutamic acid (as Whey Protein Hydrolysate & L-glutamine), The following ingredients as Whey Protein Hydrolysate (Leucine, Aspartic Acid, Lysine, Threonine, Isoleucine, Proline, Valine, Alanine, Serine, Cysteine, Phenylalanine, Tyrosine, Arginine, Methionine, Glycine, Histidine, Tryptophan), Maltodextrin, Natural and Artificial Flavorings (vanilla cappuccino flavoring), Fructose, Cocoa, Salt and Sucralose.

How Supplied: One box contains 14 packets. Serving size equals one packet.

SATIETE®
Herbal and Amino Acid Supplement

Uses: With its synergistic blend of herbs and amino acids, Satiete® addresses many of today's health concerns by ensuring maximum nutritional support.

One such ingredient is 5-HTP (5-Hydroxytryptophan). 5-HTP is an amino acid derivative and the immediate precursor to serotonin, a neurotransmitter involved in regulating mood, sleep, appetite, energy level and sensitivity to pain. Like drugs known as selective serotonin reuptake inhibitors (SSRI's), 5-HTP enhances the activity of serotonin, a hormone produced by the brain that is involved in mood, sleep, and appetite. Low levels of serotonin are associated with depression, anxiety, and sleep disorders. SSRI's prevent the brain cells from using up serotonin too quickly, thereby causing a deficiency. 5-HTP increases the cell's production of serotonin, which boosts serotonin levels.

L-5-HTP is a standardized extract of Griffonia simplicifolia (containing greater than 95% anhydrous 5-HTP). The diverse physiological functions of serotonin in the body include actions as a neurotransmitter, a regulator of

smooth muscle function in the cardiovascular and gastrointestinal system, and a regulator of platelet function. Serotonin is involved in numerous central nervous system actions such as regulating mood, sleep and appetite. In the gastrointestinal system, serotonin stimulates gastric motility. Serotonin also stimulates platelet aggregation.

As a precursor to serotonin, 5-HTP helps to normalize serotonin activity in the body. Considerable research has been conducted regarding the activity of 5-HTP. Some of the clinical studies are summarized below:

Mood—Dysregulation of serotonin metabolism in the central nervous system has been shown to affect mood. 5-HTP helps to normalize serotonin levels and, thereby, positively affect mood. In a double-blind study using objective assessments of mood, researchers in Zurich reported significant improvements in mood with 5-HTP. Likewise, in a double-blind, multi-center study in Germany, researchers reported significant improvements in both objective and self-assessment indices of mood.

Sleep—Many studies have shown that depletion of serotonin results in insomnia, which is reversed by administration of 5-HTP. Likewise, Soulairac and Lambinet reported that 100 mg of 5-HTP resulted in significant improvement for people who complained of trouble sleeping. Futhermore, serotonin is metabolized to the hormone melatonin, which is known to help regulate the sleep cycle; by increasing serotonin levels with 5-HTP, melatonin levels are also increased.

Appetite—Food intake is thought to suppress appetite through the production of serotonin from the amino acid tryptophan. Because it is an intermediary in the conversion process of tryptophan to serotonin, 5-HTP may reduce appetite in a similar manner as food intake, but without the calories. In a recent double-blind placebo-controlled study, subjects taking 5-HTP lost significant weight compared to control subjects. A reduction in carbohydrate intake and early satiety were seen in the 5-HTP group.

Another key ingredient in the Satiete formulation is Gymnema sylvestre, whose active ingredient "gymnemic acid" affects the taste buds in the oral cavity as the acid prevents the taste buds from being activated by any sugar molecules in the food; and the absorptive surface of the intestines where the acid prevents the intestine from absorbing sugar molecules. Practically speaking, this creates a reduced appetite for sweet tasting food, as well as reducing the metabolic effect of sugar by reducing its digestion in the intestines thus reducing the blood sugar level. In experimental and clinical trials, Gymnema sylvestre has been successful in treating both insulin-dependent and non-insulin dependent diabetics without reducing the blood sugar level to below

the normal blood sugar levels, an effect seen with the use of insulin oral hypoglycemic sulphony lurea compounds. Studies show that vanadyl sulfate is very effective in normalizing blood sugar levels and controlling conditions such as insulin resistance, or Type II diabetes.

Magnesium, malic acid and St. John's Wort are also combined in Satiete's proven formulation. Magnesium is a key mineral cofactor for many anaerobic as well as aerobic reactions that generate energy, and has an oxygen-sparing effect. It is essential for the cell's mitochondria "powerhouses" to function normally, being involved in both the production and utilization of ATP.

Malic Acid has an oxygen-sparing effect and there are a number of indications that malic acid is a very critical molecule in controlling mitochondrial function. Malate is a source of energy from the Krebs cycle and is the only metabolite of the cycle which falls in concentration during exhaustive physical activity. Depletion of malate has also been linked to physical exhaustion. By giving malic acid and magnesium as dietary supplements, flexibility to use aerobic and anaerobic energy sources can be enhanced and energy production can be boosted. Lab studies show that many patients with fibromyalgia (or with chronic fatigue) have low magnesium levels. Magnesium supplementation enhances the treatment of both conditions. Its benefits appear to result, at least in part, from its positive impact on serotonin function.

Combining 5-HTP with St. John's Wort Extract (0.3% hypericin context), malic acid, and magnesium, is part of an overall fibromyalgia treatment plan providing excellent results, due in large measure to its improvement of sleep quality and mood.

Directions: Start by taking one hypoallergenic tablet three times per day 30 to 60 minutes before meals. If needed after two weeks of use, increase the dosage to two tablets three times per day. Do not exceed nine tablets daily without medical supervision.

Warning: If you are taking MAO inhibitor drugs, tricyclic antidepressants, SSRI antidepressants (Prozac, Paxil, Zoloft) or prescription diet drugs, do not take this product without medical supervision. If you suffer from liver or kidney diseases, serious gastrointestinal disorders or carcinoid syndrome, do not take this product without medical supervision. If gastrointestinal upset develops and persists, reduce dosage, take only with large meals or discontinue use.

Ingredients: Three enteric-coated Satieté tablets contain: Griffonia Seed Extract (Supplying 95% min. naturally occurring L-5htp), Gymnema Sylvestre, Vanadyl Sulfate, Vitamin B-2, Niacinamide, Magnesium (Oxide), Vitamin B-1, Vitamin B-6, Malic Acid, St. John's Wort

Continued on next page

Satiete—Cont.

Extract, Ginkgo Biloba Extract, Vitamin B-12, Folic Acid, Microcrystalline Cellulose, Stearic Acid, Croscarmelose Sodium, Magnesium Stearate, Silicon Dioxide, Ethylcellulose and Hydroxypropylcellulose.

How Supplied: One bottle contains 84 tablets.

STEPHAN Clarity™
Nutritional Supplement

Uses: STEPHAN Clarity™, designed for use by both men and women, contains selected tissue proteins in the form of nutrients important to memory and concentration.

This is achieved by utilizing such ingredients as lecithin and glutamic acid. Lecithin is a popular supplement widely embraced for memory health, while glutamic acid is an amino acid which influences the body by serving as brain fuel, and has been scientifically proven to increase the firing of neurons in the nervous system. It also metabolizes sugars and fats, as well as detoxifies.

Ginkgo biloba, a third primary ingredient in STEPHAN Clarity™, is a special additive which increases the flow of blood to the brain and is noted for improving concentration and learning ability. A study published in the *Journal of the American Medical Association* demonstrated ginkgo biloba's effects on individuals with Alzheimer's disease and multi-infarct dementia. It was reported to stabilize and – in 20% of the cases – improve the subjects' functioning for periods of six months to a year.

Together with the support of carefully selected vitamins, minerals, amino acids, and herbs, STEPHAN Clarity™ is a natural and effective way to better one's health.

Directions: As a dietary supplement, take one capsule daily.

Warnings: Contains 9.2 mg phenylalanine per serving.

Ingredients: Proprietary blend (Lecithin, Bee Pollen, L-Glutamic Acid, Ribonucleic Acid Yeast, L-Aspartic Acid, L-Arginine HCI, L-Leucine, L-Lysine HCI, L-Phenylalanine, L-Serine, L-Proline, L-Valine, L-Isoleucine, L-Alanine, L-Glycine, L-Threonine, L-Tyrosine, L-Histidine, L-Cysteine HCI, L-Methionine, Adenosine Triphosphate, Ginkgo Biloba 50:1 Extract), Hydroxypropylmethylcellulose, Dl-Alpha Tocopheryl Acetate, Ascorbic Acid, Niacinamide, Stearic Acid, Ethylcellulose, Vitamin A Acetate, D-Calcium Pantothenate, Thiamine HCI, Silicon Dioxide, Dicalcium Phosphate, Pyridoxine HCI, Riboflavin, Folic Acid, Cholecalciferol, Biotin, Cyancobalamin.

How Supplied: One bottle contains 60 easy-to-swallow capsules.

STEPHAN™ Elasticity®
Nutritional Supplement

Uses: A dietary supplement for men and women, STEPHAN™ Elasticity® contains a scientifically balanced mixture of specific tissue proteins established as important for skin tone and texture.

Utilizing such scientifically respected ingredients as vitamin A and selenium, STEPHAN Elasticity is also supported by various other vitamins, minerals and amino acids dedicated to epidermal appearance.

Due to its antioxidant properties, vitamin A has been dubbed the "skin vitamin." It is commonly used as a means of preventing premature aging of the skin. In addition, synthetic derivatives of vitamin A are often used to treat acne and psoriasis.

Selenium is also considered beneficial to the skin. It was recently reported that low blood selenium in the context of low blood vitamin A increases the risk for certain types of skin cancer.

Directions: As a dietary supplement, take one capsule daily.

Warnings: Accidental overdose of iron-containing products is a leading cause of fatal poisoning in children under 6. Keep this product out of the reach of children. In case of accidental overdose, call a doctor or poison control center immediately.

Ingredients: Proprietary Blend (Shavegrass Herb, L-Glutamic Acid, Bladderwrack Extract, Ribonucleic Acid Yeast, L-Aspartic Acid, L-Arginine HCI, L-Leucine, L-Lysine HCI, L-Phenylalanine, L-Serine, L-Proline, L-Valine, L-Isoleucine, L-Alanine, L-Glycine, L-Threonine, L-Tyrosine, L-Histidine, L-Cysteine HCI, L-Methionine, Adenosine Triphosphate), Hydroxypropylmethylcellulose, DL-Alpha Tocopheryl Acetate, Ascorbic Acid, Ethylcellulose, Stearic Acid, Silicon Dioxide, Calcium Amino Acid Chelate, Manganese Amino Acid Chelate, Iron Amino Acid Chelate, Magnesium Amino Acid Chelate, Zinc Amino Acid Chelate, Vitamin A Acetate, Selenium Amino Acid Chelate, Chromium Amino Acid Chelate.

How Supplied: One bottle contains 60 easy-to-swallow capsules.

STEPHAN Elixir®
Nutritional Supplement

Uses: Formulated with an exclusive blend of specific proteins, STEPHAN Elixir® is ideal for both men and women. These tissue proteins are supported by vitamins, minerals, amino acids and herbs recognized as important for general health and well-being.

Among the scientifically researched and proven ingredients utilized in STEPHAN Elixir are vitamin E and cysteine. Vitamin E protects against the ravages of aging in several ways. It is essential for the normal functioning of the body and is especially important for normal neurological functions in humans. It also serves as a potent antioxidant and has been dubbed the body's "first line of defense" against free-radical attack by helping to guard against free radicals. Cysteine has also been found to inactivate free radicals and thus protect and preserve the cells. This sulfur-containing amino acid is a precursor of glutathione, a tripeptide that is claimed to safeguard the body against various toxins and pollutants.

Directions: As a dietary supplement, take one (1) capsule daily.

Warnings: Accidental overdose of iron-containing products is a leading cause of fatal poisoning in children under 6. Keep this product out of the reach of children. In case of accidental overdose, call a doctor or poison control center immediately. CAUTION PHENYLKETONURICS: Contains 6.9 mg phenylalanine per serving.

Ingredients: Proprietary Blend (Isolated Soy Protein, Bee Pollen, Citric Acid, Malic Acid, Ribonucleic Acid Yeast, Ginkgo Biloba Leaf Extract, Adenosine Triphosphate), Hydroxypropylmethylcellulose, Zinc Amino Acid Chelate, Iron Amino Acid Chelate, Dl–alpha tocopheryl Acetate, Starch, Ascorbic Acid, Calcium Carbonate, Niacinamide, D-calcium Pantothenate, Vitamin A Acetate, Silicon Dioxide, Thiamine HCl, dicalcium Phosphate, Pyridoxine HCl, Riboflavin, Folic Acid, Selenium Amino Acid Chelate, Cholecalciferol, Biotin, Cyano-cobalamin.

How Supplied: One bottle contains 60 easy-to-swallow capsules.

STEPHAN Essential®
Nutritional Supplement

Uses: STEPHAN Essential® is a nutritional supplement which contains specific tissue proteins supported by vitamins, minerals, herbs and amino acids that are proactive to cardiovascular and circulatory management. L-carnitine, vitamin E and linoleic acid are only some of these very important components.

Scientifically researched and a major contributor to the effects of STEPHAN Essential, L-carnitine is necessary for the transport of long-chain fatty acids into the mitochondria, the metabolic furnaces of the cells. These fatty acids prove a major source for the production of energy in the heart and skeletal muscles, structures that are particularly vulnerable to L-carnitine deficiency.

While vitamin E has proven beneficial in serving to boost the immune system and protect against cardiovascular disease, it has also been established as an important therapy for disorders related to neurologic symptoms. Omega 3–Oil, another important addition to STEPHAN Essential, can lower serum cholesterol levels and decrease platelet stickiness, proving beneficial in the prevention of coronary heart disease.

STEPHAN Essential may be consumed by both men and women.

Directions: As a dietary supplement, take one (1) capsule daily.

Warnings: Contains 6.9 mg phenylalanine per serving.

Ingredients: Proprietary Blend (Isolated Soy Protein, L-carnitine Bitartrate, Bee Pollen, Marine Lipid Concentrate, Ribonucleic Acid Yeast, Adenosine Triphosphate), Hydroxypropylmethylcellulose, Magnesium Amino Acid Chelate, Starch, D-alpha Tocopheryl Succinate, Selenium Amino Acid Chelate, Silicon Dioxide.

How Supplied: One bottle contains 60 easy-to-swallow capsules.

STEPHAN Feminine®
Nutritional Supplement

Uses: Specifically designed for women, STEPHAN Feminine® contains selected tissue proteins supported by vitamins, minerals and amino acids regarded as important to the ever-changing female body. This is achieved through such scientifically researched ingredients as magnesium and boron.

STEPHAN Feminine utilizes magnesium as an important ingredient responsible for regulating the flow of calcium between cells. Studies reveal that women with high-calcium diets report fewer PMS symptoms including less irritability and depression, as well as fewer headaches, backaches and cramps. Magnesium allows for maximum benefits from calcium intake.

Researchers also report many promising results on the effects of dietary boron. Conclusions show that supplementary boron markedly reduces the excretion of both calcium and magnesium while increasing production of an active form of estrogen and testosterone.

Directions: As a dietary supplement, take one (1) capsule daily.

Warnings: Contains 9.2 mg phenylalanine per serving.

Ingredients: Proprietary blend (isolated soy protein, magnesium oxide, boron aspartate, ribonucelic acid yeast, adenosine triphosphate), hydroxypropyl-methylcellulose, dl-alpha tocopheryl acetate, starch, silicon dioxide, selenium amino acid chelate.

How Supplied: One bottle contains 60 easy-to-swallow capsules.

STEPHAN™ Flexibility®
Nutritional Supplement

Uses: A nutritional supplement for both men and women, STEPHAN™ Flexibility® is rich with exclusive proteins which are supported by vitamins, minerals and amino acids recognized as beneficial to the health of joint and soft tissues.

Glycine, an amino acid, is one very significant ingredient utilized in STEPHAN Flexibility. In a pilot study investigating the possibility of glycine's effect on spastic control, a 25% improvement was noted on subjects with chronic multiple sclerosis. Furthermore, all patients benefited to some degree, and no toxicity or other adverse side effects were noted.

Another important amino acid in STEPHAN Flexibility is L-histidine. Reports suggest that supplementary L-histidine may actually boost the activity of suppressor T cells. Because rheumatoid arthritis is one of the many autoimmune diseases in which T-cell activity is subnormal, these conclusions lend further support that normal levels of L-histidine are beneficial to joint health.

Vitamin E can also be found in STEPHAN Flexibility because of its ability to relieve muscular cramps. According to one popular study, supplemental vitamin E caused remarkable relief from nocturnal leg and foot cramps in 82% of the 125 patients tested.

Directions: As a dietary supplement, take one capsule daily.

Warnings: Contains 9.2 mg phenylalanine per serving.

Ingredients: Proprietary Blend (Boron Gluconate, L-Glutamic Acid, Ribonucleic Acid Yeast, L-Aspartic Acid, L-Arginine HCl, L-Leucine, L-Lysine HCl, Bee Pollen, L-Phenylalanine, L-Serine, L-Proline, L-Valine, L-Isoleucine, L-Alanine, L-Glycine, L-Threonine, L-Tyrosine, L-Histidine, L-Cysteine HCl, L-Methionine, Adenosine Triphosphate), Hydroxypropylmethylcellulose, Zinc Amino Acid Chelate, Calcium Amino Acid Chelate, Stearic Acid, Ascorbic Acid, Whey, D-Alpha Tocopheryl Succinate, Magnesium Stearate, Niacinamide, Silicon Dioxide, Cellulose, Vitamin A Palmitate, D-Calcium Pantothenate, Thiamine HCl, Dicalcium Phosphate, Pyridoxine HCl, Riboflavin, Folic Acid, Selenomethionine, Cholecalciferol, Biotin, Cyanocobalamin.

How Supplied: One bottle contains 60 easy-to-swallow capsules.

STEPHAN Lovpil™
Nutritional Supplement

Uses: STEPHAN Lovpil™ is a nutritional supplement for men and women of all ages that is formulated with vitamins, minerals, herbs, amino acids and selected proteins recognized as important for general health and sexual vitality. Damiana, typically thought of as an aphrodisiac by those who are familiar with its effects, is an important ingredient utilized in STEPHAN Lovpil. A major herbal remedy in Mexican medical folklore, damiana is proven for its stimulating properties of male virility and libido. A number of scientific studies have shown a direct relationship between low sperm count and diets deficient in arginine.

Scientific studies on Vitamin C have uncovered that ascorbic acid may actually protect human sperm from oxidative DNA damage.

Directions: As a dietary supplement, take one (1) capsule daily.

Ingredients: Proprietary blend (damiana leaf, isolated soy protein, ribonucleic acid yeast, adenosine triphosphate), calcium carbonate, hydroxypropylmethylcellulose, ascorbic acid, stearic acid, zinc amino acid chelate, magnesium stearate, manganese amino acid chelate, silicon dioxide, vitamin A acetate, dicalcium phosphate, cholecalciferol, folic acid, selenomethionine, cyanocobalamin.

How Supplied: One bottle contains 60 easy-to-swallow capsules.

STEPHAN Masculine®
Nutritional Supplement

Uses: A nutritional supplement formulated for the adult male, STEPHAN Masculine® contains a special blend of nutrients with vitamins, minerals, herbs and amino acids.

Scientifically researched ingredients have been carefully selected to help ensure STEPHAN Masculine's effectiveness. Zinc is one such ingredient. Proven to be closely interrelated with the male sex hormone, testosterone, zinc deficiency often results in regression of the male sex glands, decreased sexual interest, mental lethargy, emotional problems and even poor appetite. It has been found that in males with only a mild zinc deficiency, zinc supplementation was accompanied by increased sperm count and plasma testosterone.

Directions: As a dietary supplement, take one capsule daily.

Ingredients: Proprietary Blend (L-Histidine, Bee Pollen, Parsley Leaf, Ribonucleic Acid, Adenosine Triphosphate), Calcium Carbonate, Zinc Amino Acid Chelate, Hydroxypropylmethylcellulose, Magnesium Amino Acid Chelate, Stearic Acid, Magnesium Stearate.

How Supplied: One bottle contains 60 easy-to-swallow capsules.

PHYTO-VITE®
Advanced Antioxidant, Vitamin and Mineral Supplement

Uses: Phyto-Vite® is a state-of-the-art nutritional supplement providing chelated minerals, vitamins and a diverse

Continued on next page

Phyto-Vite—Cont.

group of antioxidants. It was formulated to meet the nutritional needs of our society where studies estimate only 9% consume foods in the quantities necessary to protect against the oxidative damage caused by free radicals.

The antioxidant coverage provided by Phyto-Vite is both comprehensive and diverse. First, it includes optimal amounts of vitamins A, C, and E as well as the pro-vitamins alpha and beta carotene. Vitamin A, in addition to its antioxidant capabilities, is also felt to improve immune function, protein synthesis, RNA synthesis and steroid hormone synthesis. In this product, vitamin A is derived from two sources: retinyl palmitate and lemongrass. Additional vitamin A activity is provided by the alpha and beta carotene found in *Dunaliella salina*. These carotenoids are strong antioxidants in their own right; however, they can also be converted to vitamin A. This occurs only when the body is deficient in this vitamin. Consequently, vitamin A toxicity cannot be caused by alpha or beta carotene. Vitamin C has long been associated with wound healing, collagen formation, and maintaining the structural integrity of capillaries, cartilage, dentine and bone. Phyto-Vite utilizes esterified vitamin C which has been shown to provide a quicker uptake and a decreased rate of excretion when compared with conventional vitamin C. This allows for higher, more sustained levels of this vitamin in the body. Phyto-Vite also contains 400 I.U. of vitamin E, from natural sources. The antioxidant effects of vitamin E have been shown to stabilize cell membranes, increase HDL cholesterol, and decrease platelet aggregation.

Many flavonoids are incorporated into Phyto-Vite. These substances possess antioxidant activity themselves and also potentiate the effects of vitamins C and E. This later effect is produced by decreasing the degradation of vitamin C and E into inactive metabolites. Ginkgo biloba has flavonoid activity as well as other significant effects. Among these are a decrease in platelet aggregation and an increase in vasodilation which appears to increase blood flow to the peripheral arteries and the brain. Some improvement in cognitive abilities has been noted. It also helps to inhibit lipid peroxidation, thereby stabilizing the cell wall against free radical attack.

A phytonutrient blend has been incorporated into Phyto-Vite to further enhance its antioxidant effects. Phytonutrient is a term given to the thousands of chemical compounds found in fruits and vegetables. Some of these compounds have shown great promise in aiding the cardiovascular system. Currently, much research is ongoing to isolate and identify more of these compounds, but it has already been clearly established that phytonutrients work best when the entire plant source is used rather than just the isolated compound. The phytonutrients found in Phyto-Vite are obtained from alfalfa (lutein), broccoli (indoles), cabbage (isothiocyanates), cayenne (capsanthin and capsorubin), green onion (thioallyl compounds), parsley (chlorophyll), spirulina (gamma linolenic acid), tomato (lycopene), soy isoflavones (genistein, lecithin and daidzein), aged garlic concentrate, and Pure-Gar-A-8000™ (allicin).

The antioxidant minerals copper, zinc, manganese and selenium have also been incorporated into Phyto-Vite. These minerals have been chelated via a patented process in which the mineral is wrapped within an amino acid. Once inside the body, the minerals can then be utilized in the millions of metabolic reactions that take place in the body. With this process, overall mineral absorption can approach 95% instead of the 5 to 10% absorption seen with other mineral supplements.

Phyto-Vite also provides two antioxidant enzymes (catalase and peroxidase). These help to reduce the body's free radical burden by neutralizing free radicals in the pharynx or stomach.

There are three other features that make Phyto-Vite unique among supplements. First, a small amount of canola oil was included to aid in the proper absorption of fat soluble vitamins, even on an empty stomach. Canola oil also provides essential fatty acids. Second, the product is formed into prolonged-release tablets which allow flexibility in dosing frequency. It can be taken all at once or staggered throughout the day. Dissolution testing has been performed to insure that the product will dissolve properly. Lastly, Phyto-Vite tablets are covered with a Betacoat™. This is a beta carotene coating that is designed to provide antioxidant coverage to the tablet itself. This helps to protect the integrity and activity of the product.

Directions: As a dietary supplement take six tablets per day with eight ounces of liquid. Tablets may be taken all at once or staggered throughout the day.

Warnings: If pregnant or lactating, consult physician before using. Accidental overdose of iron-containing products is a leading cause of fatal poisoning in children under 6. Keep this product out of reach of children. In case of accidental overdose, call a doctor or poison control center immediately. This hypoallergenic formula is free of dairy, yeast, wheat, sugar, starch, animal products, dyes, preservatives, artificial flavors and pesticide residues.

Ingredients: Vitamin A, Vitamin C, Vitamin D, Vitamin E, Vitamin K, Thiamin, Riboflavin, Niacin, Vitamin B6, Folate, Vitamin B12, Biotin, Pantothenic Acid, Calcium, Iron, Phosphorus, Iodine, Magnesium, Zinc, Selenium, Copper, Manganese, Chromium, Potassium, Phytonutrient Blend (alfalfa leaf, aged garlic bulb concentrate, Pur-Gar® A-10,000 [garlic bulb], soy protein isolate, broccoli floret, cabbage leaf, cayenne pepper fruit, green onion bulb, parsley leaf, tomato, spirulina), canola oil concentrate, citrus bioflavonoid complex, rutin, quercetin dehydrate, choline, Inositol, PABA, ginkgo biloba leaf standardized extract, bilberry fruit standardized extract, catalase enzymes, grape seed proanthocyanidins, red grape skin extract, boron, dicalcium phosphate, magnesium oxide, calcium carbonate, calcium ascorbate, microcrystalline cellulose, d-alpha-tocopheryl succinate, croscarmellose sodium, stearic acid, potassium citrate, choline bitartrate, beta-carotene, niacinamide, silica, d-calcium pantothenate, magnesium stearate, copper Chelazome® glycinate, zinc Chelazome® glycinate, calcium citrate, calcium lactate, magnesium amino acid chelate, inositol, L-selenomethionine, kelp, manganese Chelazome® glycinate, biotin, pyridoxine HCl, Ferrochel® iron bisglycinate, boron chelate, riboflavin, magnesium citrate, thiamin mononitrate, retinyl palmitate, chromium Chelavite® glycinate, phylloquinone, cyanocobalamin, vanillin, cholecalciferol, folic acid.

How Supplied: One bottle contains 180 Betacoat™ tablets.

STEPHAN Protector® Nutritional Supplement

Uses: STEPHAN Protector® is a nutritional supplement that combines specific proteins, vitamins, minerals and amino acids recognized as important for the health of areas associated with the human immune system.

Among these specially selected and scientifically researched ingredients are astragalus and kelp. Known for its strengthening effects of both the immune and digestive systems, astragalus can be combined with other herbs to increase phagocytosis, interferon production and the number of macrophages. It, in combination, enhances T-cell transformation and functions as an adaptogen to relieve stress-induced immune system suppression.

Research clearly indicates that kelp supplies dozens of important nutrients for improved cardiovascular health and function.

Directions: As a dietary supplement, take one (1) capsule daily.

Warnings: Contains 9.2 mg phenylalanine per serving.

Ingredients: Proprietary blend (isolated soy protein, astragalus root, bee pollen, kelp, ribonucleic acid yeast, adenosine triphosphate), hydroxypropylmethylcellulose, cellulose, stearic acid, magnesium stearate, silicon dioxide.

How Supplied: One bottle contains 60 easy-to-swallow capsules.

STEPHAN Relief® Nutritional Supplement

Uses: Designed for both men and women, STEPHAN Relief® has been formulated with a special combination of nutrients, vitamins, minerals, amino acids and herbs which are recognized as important to the digestive and excretory systems.

Parsley, a member of the carrot family, can be used as a carminative and an aid to digestion. While the root has a mild diuretic property, parsley has also been reported, in large doses, to affect blood pressure.

Psyllium is a gel-forming fiber used in many bulk laxatives to promote bowel regularity. In recent years, because of its affects on healthy cholesterol levels, psyllium has gained wide-spread popularity and can be found in some ready-to-eat cereals.

Directions: As a dietary supplement, take one (1) capsule daily.

Ingredients: Proprietary blend (Psyllium Seed Powder, L-isoleucine, L-leucine, L-valine, Bee Pollen, Bladderwrack Herb 5:1 Extract, Parsley Leaf 4:1 extract, Ribonucleic Acid Yeast, Adenosine Triphosphate), Hydroxypropylmethylcellulose, Starch, D-calcium Pantothenate, Silicon Dioxide.

How Supplied: One bottle contains 60 easy-to-swallow capsules.

SLEEP-TITE™ Herbal Sleep Aid

Uses: Sleep-Tite™ is a non-addicting herbal sleep aid formulated to promote a deeper, more restorative sleep without the use of pharmaceutically synthesized hormones. With the body's overall health, and proper functioning, dependent upon efficient sleep patterns in order to achieve cellular, organ, tissue and emotional repair, this powerful tool's primary function is to rejuvenate and restore by assisting the body in initiating and maintaining sleep.

Sleep-Tite is a blend of 10 highly effective, all-natural herbs. California poppy, passion flower, valerian, kava kava and skullcap have been used for centuries as a remedy for insomnia because of their calming effects and ability to relieve muscle tension. Hops and celery seed produce a generalized calming effect and are especially helpful for indigestion, gastrointestinal and smooth muscle relaxation. Chamomile also has a relaxing effect on the body and the gastrointestinal tract, but with the added benefit of producing anti-inflammatory effects on joints. Feverfew has been used as a treatment for fever, migraines and arthritic complaints dating back to ancient Greece. A study published in *Lancet* demonstrated that feverfew inhibited the body's production of prostaglandin and serotonin. These biochemicals can cause inflammation, fever and the vasoactive response that triggers migraine headaches.

By utilizing this unique blend of herbs to aid in the effective initiation and maintenance of sleep patterns, Sleep-Tite can be consumed by adults, thereby promoting physical and emotional well-being in a safe, active manner.

Directions: Adults (18 years and older) may take two Sleep-Tite caplets approximately 30 to 60 minutes prior to bedtime. Needs may vary with each individual. Some persons may require less than two caplets to achieve optimum results. Do not exceed recommended nightly amounts.

Warnings: Not for use by children, pregnant women or lactating women. Consult your physician before using this product if you have any medical condition or are taking antidepressant, sedative or hypnotic medications. Do not take this product if using Monoamine Oxidase Inhibitors (MAOI). This product may cause drowsiness and should not be taken with alcohol or while operating a vehicle or other machinery. If allergic symptoms develop, discontinue use. Store in a cool, dry place. Keep out of reach of children.

Ingredients: European Valerian Root 4:1 extract, Celery Seed 4:1 extract, Hops Strobile 4:1 extract, Passion Flower 4:1 extract (whole plant), California Poppy 5:1 extract (aerial parts), Chamomile Flower 5:1 extract, Chinese Fu Ling 5:1 extract (Poria Cocos), Kava Kava Root 5:1 extract, Feverfew 5:1 extract (aerial parts), Skullcap (aerial parts), Dicalcium Phosphate, Microcrystalline Cellulose, Croscarmellose Sodium, Stearic Acid, Silica, Magnesium Stearate and Sugar Coat (calcium sulfate, sucrose, kaolin, talc, gelatin, shellac, titanium dioxide, anise oil, beeswax and carnauba wax).

How Supplied: One box contains 28 packets. Two caplets per packet.

STEPHAN Tranquility™ Nutritional Supplement

Uses: Designed for both men and women, STEPHAN Tranquility™ is a nutritional supplement which contains a blend of vitamins, minerals and amino acids recognized as important to areas involved in stress management.

Myo-Inositol is among these specially researched ingredients. It has long been claimed to lower blood concentrations of triglycerides and cholesterol, as well as to generally protect against cardiovascular disease. In addition, Myo-Inositol intake can influence the phosphatidylinositol levels in the membranes of brain cells. Compounds derived from this process could conceivably have some beneficial effect on insomnia and anxiety.

Valerian root contains valepotriates which are said to be the source of its sedative effects. Studies reveal that valeranon, an essential oil component of this herb, produces a pronounced smooth-muscle effect on the intestine.

Directions: As a dietary supplement, take one (1) capsule daily.

Warnings: Contains 9.2 mg phenylalanine per serving.

Ingredients: Proprietary blend (isolated soy protein, choline bitartrate, inositol, lecithin, ribonucelic acid yeast, valerian root extract, adenosine triphosphate), hydroxypropylmethylcellulose, dl-alpha tocopheryl acetate, calcium aspartate, silicon dioxide, ascorbic acid, stearic acid, niacinamide, magnesium amino acid chelate, vitamin A palmitate, hydroxypropylcellulose, d-calcium pantothenate, thiamine HCl, dicalcium phosphate, pyridoxine HCl, riboflavin, folic acid, cholecalciferol, biotin, cyanocobalamin.

How Supplied: One bottle contains 60 easy-to-swallow capsules.

SURE2ENDURE™ Herbal, Vitamin & Mineral Workout Supplement

Uses: Attaining peak physical and athletic performance can be an elusive and time-consuming endeavor. It requires a conditioning process whereby the body's endurance, stamina and ability to recover are enhanced. Sure2Endure™ is formulated to aid in this process through an innovative blend of herbs, vitamins and minerals.

Among these specially selected ingredients is ciwujia (*Radix Acanthopanax senticosus*). Used in traditional Chinese medicine for almost 1,700 years to treat fatigue and boost the immune system, ciwujia has been shown to improve overall performance in aerobic exercise, endurance activities and weight lifting without any stimulant effects. According to a recent study, ciwujia increases fat metabolism during exercise by shifting toward the use of fat as an energy source instead of carbohydrates. In addition, the caffeine-free herb improves endurance by reducing lactic acid build-up in the muscles. This process delays the muscle fatigue which often leads to muscle pain and cramps.

Sure2Endure™ also provides antioxidant coverage and enzyme cofactors. Vitamins C and E address the otherwise high levels of free radicals generated from the oxidation of fuel substrates during exercise, while vitamins B1 (thiamin), B2 (riboflavin), B6 (pyridoxine), and B12 (cyanocobalamin) aid in proper carbohydrate metabolism and serve as cofactors in numerous biochemical reactions in the body. Ciwujia has been credited with antioxidant properties as well. Since tissue stress and damage are often the result of strenuous exercise, it is im-

Continued on next page

Sure2Endure—Cont.

portant to maintain proper integrity and recovery of connective tissue. Glucosamine, one of the basic constituents making up joint cartilage, is another special additive to Sure2Endure™. This substance enhances the synthesis of cartilage cells and protects against destructive enzymes. It stabilizes cell membranes and intercellular collagen thereby protecting cartilage during rest, exercise and recovery.

The anti-inflammatory activities of bromelain and boswellia further prove beneficial to the health of joint and soft tissues.

Directions: Adults (18 years and older) take 3 tablets one hour prior to exercise. Needs may vary with each individual. For optimum performance, use in conjunction with BIOLEAN® or BIOLEAN Free® one hour before exercise. Phyto-Vite® may be taken with this product to maximize the antioxidant effect necessary with exercise. Pro-Xtreme™ and Mass Appeal™ may also be consumed for maximum effectiveness.

Warnings: Not for use by children, pregnant women or lactating women. Consult your physician before using this product if you have any medical conditions. Discontinue immediately if allergic symptoms develop. Keep out of the reach of children. Store in a cool, dry place.

Ingredients: Vitamin C (as ascorbic acid), Vitamin E (as d-alpha tocopheryl succinate), Thiamin (as thiamin mononitrate), Riboflavin, Vitamin B6 (as pyridoxine hydrochloride), Vitamin B12 (as cyanocobalamin), Chromium (as patented Chelavite® chromium dinicotinate glycinate), Ciwujia root standardized extract (0.8% eleutherosides) (Acanthopanax senticosus), Magnesium L-aspartate, Potassium L-aspartate, Boswellia Serrata standardized extract (40% boswellic acids (as gum resins), Bromelain (600 GDU/g), Glucosamine hydrochloride, Dicalcium Phosphate, Microcrystalline Cellulose, Croscarmellose Sodium, Stearic Acid, Silica, Magnesium Stearate and Sugar Coat (calcium sulfate, sucrose, kaolin, talc, gelatin, shellac, titanium dioxide, wintergreen oil, FD&C yellow #5, FD&C blue #1, beeswax and carnauba wax).

How Supplied: One box contains 28 packets, three tablets per packet.

WINRGY™
Nutritional Supplement with Vitamin C

Uses: Through nutrients in the diet, nerves are able to send signals throughout the body called neurotransmitters. One such neurotransmitter, noradrenaline, provides individuals with the necessary alertness and energy required in day-to-day activity. A unique blend of vitamins and minerals important to the creation of noradrenaline has been incorporated into Winrgy™.

Studies reveal that vitamin B2 (riboflavin) helps the body release energy from protein, carbohydrates and fat, while vitamin B12 (cobalamin) is given to combat fatigue and alleviate neurological problems, including weakness and memory loss. Another important component of Winrgy, vitamin B3 (niacin), works with both thiamin and riboflavin in the metabolism of carbohydrates and is essential for providing energy for cell tissue growth. Niacin has also proven to dilate blood vessels and thereby increase the blood flow to various organs of the body, sometimes resulting in a blush of the skin and a healthy sense of warmth. Unlike caffeine, Winrgy offers the raw materials necessary to continue the production of noradrenaline and is ideal for anytime performance is required.

Directions: Add 3/4 cup of chilled water or fruit juice to one packet of mix. Stir briskly. Consume 1–2 times per day. Keep in a cool, dry place. For maximum results, combine this product with one serving size of Food For Thought.™

Warnings: Phenylketonurics: Contains Phenylalanine. Not for use by children, pregnant or lactating women. Persons taking medications should seek medical advice before taking this product. Do not consume more than four servings per day. Avoid the use of antacids containing aluminum with this product.

Ingredients: Vitamin C (as ascorbic acid), Vitamin E (as dl-alpha tocopheryl acetate), Thiamin (as thiamin mononitrate), Riboflavin, Niacin (as niacinamide), Vitamin B6 (as pyridoxine hydrochloride), Folate (as folic acid), Vitamin B12 (as cyanocobalamin), Pantothenic Acid (as calcium pantothenate), Zinc (as zinc gluconate), Copper (as copper gluconate), Manganese (as manganese aspartate), Chromium (as chromium aspartate), Potassium (as potassium aspartate), Phenylalanine (as L-phenylalanine), Taurine, Glycine, Caffeine, Fructose, Natural Flavor, Citric Acid and Silicon Dioxide.

How Supplied: One box contains 28 packets. Serving size equals one packet.

FACED WITH AN Rx SIDE EFFECT?
Turn to the Companion Drug Index for products that provide symptomatic relief.

Wyeth Consumer Healthcare
Wyeth
FIVE GIRALDA FARMS MADISON, NJ 07940

Direct Inquiries to:
Wyeth Consumer Healthcare Product Information 800-322-3129

CALTRATE® 600 + D
CALTRATE® 600 + SOY

Description: CALCIUM SUPPLEMENT WITH VITAMIN D, NATURE'S MOST CONCENTRATED FORM OF CALCIUM®; TABLET SHAPE SPECIALLY DESIGNED FOR EASIER SWALLOWING
CALTRATE 600 + SOY CONTAINS SOY ISOFLAVONES

SUPPLEMENT FACTS
Serving Size 1 Tablet

AMOUNT PER SERVING		% DAILY VALUE
CALTRATE® 600 + D	Vitamin D 200 IU	50%
	Calcium 600 mg	60%
CALTRATE® 600 + SOY	Vitamin D 200 IU	50%
	Calcium 600 mg	60%
	Soy Isoflavones 25 mg	*

*Daily Value Not Established

CALTRATE® 600 + D: Calcium Carbonate, Starch. **Contains less than 2% of the following:** cholecalciferol, Croscarmellose Sodium, dl-Alpha Tocopherol, FD&C Yellow No. 6 Aluminum Lake, Gelatin, Magnesium Stearate, Partially Hydrogenated Soybean Oil, Sucrose, Titanium Dioxide. **May contain less than 2% of the following:** Glycerin, Hypromellose, Polydextrose, Polyethylene Glycol, Polyvinyl Alcohol, Talc. ***CALTRATE® 600 + SOY:*** Calcium Carbonate, Maltodextrin, Soy Isoflavones Extract, Cellulose, Mineral Oil, Soy Polysaccharides, Hydroxypropyl Methylcellulose, Gelatin, Sucrose, Corn Starch, Polyethylene Glycol, Canola Oil, Carnauba Wax, Crospovidone, Magnesium Stearate, Stearic Acid, Cholecalciferol (Vit. D), dl-Alpha Tocopherol.

Caltrate® 600 + D
As with any supplement, if you are pregnant or nursing a baby, contact your healthcare professional. **Keep out of reach of children.**

Caltrate® 600 + Soy

Precaution: Use only as directed. Do not exceed recommended dosage. As with any supplement, if you are taking a prescription medication, or if you are pregnant or nursing a baby, contact your physician before using this product. **Keep out of reach of children.**

This is not a substitute for a prescription therapy. Ask your doctor about the approach to menopause that's best for you.

Suggested Use: Take one tablet twice daily with food or as directed by your physician. Not formulated for use in children.
Bottle sealed with printed foil under cap. Do not use if foil is torn.

Storage: Store at Room temperature. Keep bottle tightly closed.

How Supplied:
Caltrate 600 + D, Bottles of 60, 120 tablets
Caltrate 600 + SOY, Bottle of 60 tablets

CALTRATE® 600 PLUS™ Tablets
Calcium Carbonate

Calcium Supplement With Vitamin D & Minerals

Supplement Facts
Serving Size 1 Tablet
AMOUNT PER
SERVING   % Daily Value

Vitamin D 200 IU	50%
Calcium 600 mg	60%
Magnesium 45 mg	11%
Zinc 7.5 mg	50%
Copper 1 mg	50%
Manganese 1.8 mg	90%
Boron 250 mcg	*

* Daily Value not established.
† Percent daily value based on a 2000 calorie diet.

Ingredients: Calcium Carbonate, Starch, Microcrystalline Cellulose, Magnesium oxide.
Contains <2% of: Cholecalciferol (Vit. D), Croscarmellose Sodium, Cupric Sulfate, dl-Alpha Tocopherol (Vit. E), FD&C Blue #1 Aluminum Lake, FD&C Red #40 Aluminum Lake, FD&C Yellow #6 Aluminum Lake, Gelatin, Hypromellose, Magnesium Stearate, Manganese Sulfate, Partially Hydrogenated Soybean Oil, Polysorbate 80, Sodium Borate, Sucrose, Titanium Dioxide, Triacetin, Zinc Oxide.

Suggested Use: Take one tablet twice daily with food or as directed by your physician. Not formulated for use in children.
As with any supplement, if you are pregnant or nursing a baby, contact your healthcare professional.
Keep out of reach of children.
Bottle sealed with printed foil under cap. Do not use if foil is torn.
Store at room temperature. Keep bottle tightly closed.
© 1999

How Supplied: Bottles of 60 & 120 tablets.

CALTRATE COLON HEALTH
Calcium Supplement with Vitamin D

Supplement Facts
Serving Size 1 Tablet

Amount Per Serving	% Daily Value
Vitamin D 200 IU	50%
Calcium 600 mg	60%

Ingredients: Calcium Carbonate, Starch. **Contains less than 2% of the following:** Cholecalciferol, croscarmellose sodium, dl-Alpha Tocopherol, FD&C Yellow No. 6 Aluminum Lake, Gelatin, Magnesium Stearate, Partially Hydrogenated Soybean Oil, Sucrose, Titanium Dioxide. **May contain <2% of:** Glycerin, Hypromellose, Polydextrose, Polyethylene Glycol, Polyvinyl Alcohol, Talc.

Suggested Use: Take one tablet twice daily with food or as directed by your physician. Replaces your daily calcium supplement.
Not formulated for use in children.
As with any supplement, if you are pregnant or nursing a baby, contact your healthcare professional.
Store at room temperature. Keep bottle tightly closed.
Keep out of reach of children.
Bottle sealed with printed foil under cap. Do not use if foil is torn.

How Supplied: Bottles of 60 tablets

CENTRUM®
High Potency
Multivitamin-Multimineral
Supplement, Advanced Formula
From A to Zinc®

Supplement Facts:
Serving Size 1 Tablet

Each Tablet Contains	% DV
Vitamin A 3500 IU	70%
(29% as Beta Carotene)	
Vitamin C 60 mg	100%
Vitamin D 400 IU	100%
Vitamin E 30 IU	100%
Vitamin K 25 mcg	31%
Thiamin 1.5 mg	100%
Riboflavin 1.7 mg	100%
Niacin 20 mg	100%
Vitamin B₆ 2 mg	100%
Folic Acid 400 mcg	100%
Vitamin B₁₂ 6 mcg	100%
Biotin 30 mcg	10%
Pantothenic Acid 10 mg	100%
Calcium 162 mg	16%
Iron 18 mg	100%
Phosphorus 109 mg	11%
Iodine 150 mcg	100%
Magnesium 100 mg	25%
Zinc 15 mg	100%
Selenium 20 mcg	29%
Copper 2 mg	100%
Manganese 2 mg	100%
Chromium 120 mcg	100%
Molybdenum 75 mcg	100%
Chloride 72 mg	2%
Potassium 80 mg	2%
Boron 150 mcg	*
Nickel 5 mcg	*
Silicon 2 mg	*
Tin 10 mcg	*
Vanadium 10 mcg	*
Lutein 250 mcg	*
Lycopene 300 mcg	*

*Daily Value (%DV) not established.

Ingredients: Dibasic Calcium Phosphate, Magnesium Oxide, Potassium Chloride, Microcrystalline Cellulose, Ascorbic Acid (Vit. C), Ferrous Fumarate, Calcium Carbonate, Gelatin, dl-Alpha Tocopheryl Acetate (Vit. E). **Contains less than 2% of the following:** Acacia Senegal Gum, Ascorbyl Palmitate, Beta Carotene, Biotin, Boron, Butylated Hydroxytoluene, Calcium Pantothenate, Chromic Chloride, Citric Acid, Colloidal Silicon Dioxide, Crospovidone, Cupric Acid, Cyanocobalamin (Vit. B₁₂), Ergocalciferol (Vit. D), FD&C Yellow No. 6 Aluminum Lake, Folic Acid, Hypromellose, Lutein, Lycopene, Magnesium Stearate, Manganese Sulfate, Niacinamide, Nickelous Sulfate, Phytonadione (Vit. K), Polysorbate 80, Potassium Iodide, Potassium Sorbate, Pregelatinized Starch, Purified Water, Pyridoxine Hydrochloride (Vit. B₆), Riboflavin (Vit. B₂), Silicon Dioxide, Sodium Ascorbate, Sodium Benzoate, Sodium Citrate, Sodium Metavanadate, Sodium Molybdate, Sodium Selenate, Sodium Silicoaluminate, Sorbic Acid, Stannous Chloride, Starch, Sucrose, Thiamine Mononitrate (Vit. B₁), Titanium Dioxide, Tocopherol, Tribasic Calcium Phosphate, Triethyl Citrate, Vitamin A Acetate (Vit. A), Zinc Oxide. **May also contain:** Calcium Stearate, Glucose, Lactose Monohydrate.

Suggested Use:
One tablet daily with food. Not formulated for use in children.

Warnings: Accidental overdose of iron-containing products is a leading cause of fatal poisoning in children under 6. Keep this product out of reach of children. In case of accidental overdose, call a doctor or poison control center immediately.
As with any supplement, if you are pregnant or nursing a baby, contact your healthcare professional.
IMPORTANT INFORMATION: Long-term intake of high levels of vitamin A (excluding that sourced from beta-carotene) may increase the risk of osteoporosis in postmenopausal women. Do not take this product if taking other vitamin A supplements.

How Supplied: Light peach, engraved CENTRUM C1.
Bottles of 15, 50, 130, 180, 250 tablets
Storage: Store at room temperature. Keep bottle tightly closed.
Bottle sealed with printed foil under cap. Do not use if foil is torn.

Continued on next page

CENTRUM KIDS COMPLETE
Rugrats®
Chewable Multivitamin Supplement
(Orange, Cherry, Fruit Punch)

Supplement Facts:
[See table below]

Ingredients: Sucrose, Dibasic Calcium Phosphate, Mannitol, Calcium Carbonate, Stearic Acid, Magnesium Oxide, Ascorbic Acid (Vit. C), Pregelatinized Starch, Microcrystalline Cellulose, dl-Alpha Tocopheryl Acetate (Vit. E). **Contains less than 2% of the following:** Acacia, Aspartame**, Beta Carotene, Biotin, Butylated Hydroxytoluene (BHT), Calcium Pantothenate, Carbonyl Iron, Carrageenan, Chromic Chloride, Citric Acid, Cupric Oxide, Cyanocobalamin (Vit. B_{12}), Dextrose, Ergocalciferol (Vit. D), FD&C Blue 2 Aluminum Lake, FD&C Red 40 Aluminum Lake, FD&C Yellow 6 Aluminum Lake, Folic Acid, Gelatin, Glucose, Guar Gum, Lactose, Magnesium Stearate, Malic Acid, Manganese Sulfate, Mono and Diglycerides, Natural and Artificial Flavors, Niacinamide, Phytonadione (Vit. K), Potassium Iodide, Potassium Sorbate, Purified Water, Pyridoxine Hydrochloride (Vit. B_6), Riboflavin (Vit. B_2), Silicon Dioxide, Sodium Ascorbate, Sodium Benzoate, Sodium Citrate, Sodium Molybdate, Sodium Silicoaluminate, Sorbic Acid, Starch, Thiamine Mononitrate (Vit. B_1), Tocopherol, Tribasic Calcium Phosphate, Vanillin, Vitamin A Acetate (Vit. A), Zinc Oxide. **May also contain:** Fructose, Maltodextrin.

Suggested Use: Children 2 and 3 years of age, chew approximately ½ tablet daily with food. Adults and children 4 years of age and older, chew 1 tablet daily with food. Not formulated for use in children less than 2 years of age.

Warnings: Accidental overdose of iron-containing products is a leading cause of fatal poisoning in children under 6. Keep this product out of reach of children. In case of accidental overdose, call a doctor or poison control center immediately. **CONTAINS ASPARTAME.**
** PHENYLKETONURICS: CONTAINS PHENYLALANINE.

Storage: Store at room temperature. Keep bottle tightly closed.
Bottle sealed with printed foil under cap. Do not use if foil is torn.

How Supplied: Assorted Flavors— Uncoated Tablet—Bottles of 60, 100 tablets

Also available as: Centrum® Kids™ + Extra C (250 mg); and as: **Centrum® Kids™ + Extra Calcium** (200 mg).

Marketed by: Wyeth Consumer Healthcare, Madison, NJ 07940

CENTRUM® PERFORMANCE COMPLETE MULTIVITAMIN SUPPLEMENT Tablets

Supplement Facts
Serving Size 1 Tablet

Each Tablet Contains	%DV
Vitamin A 3500 IU (29% as Beta Carotene)	70%
Vitamin C 120 mg	200%
Vitamin D 400 IU	100%
Vitamin E 60 IU	200%
Vitamin K 25 mcg	31%
Thiamin 4.5 mg	300%
Riboflavin 5.1 mg	300%
Niacin 40 mg	200%
Vitamin B_6 6 mg	300%
Folic Acid 400 mcg	100%
Vitamin B_{12} 18 mcg	300%
Biotin 40 mcg	13%
Pantothenic Acid 10 mg	100%
Calcium 100 mg	10%
Iron 18 mg	100%
Phosphorus 48 mg	5%
Iodine 150 mcg	100%
Magnesium 40 mg	10%
Zinc 15 mg	100%
Selenium 70 mcg	100%
Copper 2 mg	100%
Manganese 4 mg	200%
Chromium 120 mcg	100%
Molybdenum 75 mcg	100%
Chloride 72 mg	2%
Potassium 80 mg	2%
Ginseng Root (*Panax ginseng*) 50 mg Standardized Extract	*
Ginkgo Biloba Leaf (*Ginkgo biloba*) 60 mg Standardized Extract	*
Boron 60 mcg	*
Nickel 5 mcg	*
Silicon 4 mg	*
Tin 10 mcg	*
Vanadium 10 mcg	*

*Daily Value (%DV) not established.

Ingredients: Dibasic Calcium Phosphate, Potassium Chloride, Ascorbic Acid (Vit. C), Microcrystalline Cellulose, Calcium Carbonate, dl-Alpha Tocopheryl Acetate (Vit. E), Magnesium Oxide, Ginkgo Biloba Leaf (*Ginkgo biloba*) Standardized Extract, Gelatin, Ginseng Root (*Panax ginseng*) Standardized Extract, Ferrous Fumarate, Niacinamide, Crospovidone, Starch. **Contains less than 2% of the following:** Acacia Senegal Gum, Beta Carotene, Biotin, Butyl-

Serving Size:	½ Tablet	1 Tablet
Amount Per Serving:	% DV for Children 2 and 3 Years (1/2 Tablet)	% DV for Adults and Children 4 Years and Older (1 Tablet)
Total Carbohydrate <1g	*	<1%+
Vitamin A 3500 IU (29% as Beta Carotene)	70%	70%
Vitamin C 60 mg	75%	100%
Vitamin D 400 IU	50%	100%
Vitamin E 30 IU	150%	100%
Vitamin K 10 mcg	*	13%
Thiamin 1.5 mg	107%	100%
Riboflavin 1.7 mg	106%	100%
Niacin 20 mg	111%	100%
Vitamin B_6 2 mg	143%	100%
Folic Acid 400 mcg	100%	100%
Vitamin B_{12} 6 mcg	100%	100%
Biotin 45 mcg	15%	15%
Pantothenic Acid 10 mg	100%	100%
Calcium 108 mg	7%	11%
Iron 18 mg	90%	100%
Phosphorus 50 mg	3%	5%
Iodine 150 mcg	107%	100%
Magnesium 40 mg	10%	10%
Zinc 15 mg	94%	100%
Copper 2 mg	100%	100%
Manganese 1 mg	*	50%
Chromium 20 mcg	*	17%
Molybdenum 20 mcg	*	27%

*Daily Value (%DV) not established.
+Percent Daily Values based on a 2,000 calorie diet.

ated Hydroxytoluene, Calcium Pantothenate, Chromic Chloride, Citric Acid, Cupric Oxide, Cyanocobalamin (Vit. B_{12}), Ergocalciferol (Vit. D), FD&C Red No. 40 Aluminum Lake, FD&C Yellow No. 6 Aluminum Lake, Folic Acid, Glucose, Hypromellose, Lactose Monohydrate, Magnesium Borate, Magnesium Stearate, Manganese Sulfate, Nickelous Sulfate, Phytonadione (Vit.K), Polyethylene Glycol, Polysorbate 80, Potassium Iodide, Potassium Sorbate, Purified Water, Pyridoxine Hydrochloride (Vit. B_6), Riboflavin (Vit. B_2), Silicon Dioxide, Sodium Ascorbate, Sodium Benzoate, Sodium Borate, Sodium Citrate, Sodium Metavanadate, Sodium Molybdate, Sodium Selenate, Sodium Silicoaluminate, Sorbic Acid, Stannous Chloride, Sucrose, Thiamin Mononitrate (Vit. B_1), Titanium Dioxide, Tocopherol, Tribasic Calcium Phosphate, Vitamin A Acetate (Vit. A), Zinc Oxide. **May also contain:** Maltodextrin.

Suggested Use: Adults—One tablet daily with food. Not formulated for use in children.

Warning: Accidental overdose of iron-containing products is a leading cause of fatal poisoning in children under 6. Keep this product out of reach of children. In case of accidental overdose, call a doctor or poison control center immediately.

Precaution: As with any supplement, if you are taking a prescription medication, or if you are pregnant or nursing a baby, contact your physician before using this product.

Important Information: Long-term intake of high levels of vitamin A (excluding that sourced from beta-carotene) may increase the risk of osteoporosis in postmenopausal women. Do not take this product if taking other vitamin A supplements.

Store at room temperature. Keep bottle tightly closed. Bottle sealed with printed foil under cap. Do not use if foil is torn.

How Supplied: Bottles of 45, 75 and 120 Tablets.

CENTRUM® SILVER®
Multivitamin/Multimineral Dietary Supplement for Adults 50+ From A to Zinc®

Supplement Facts
Serving Size 1 Tablet

Each Tablet Contains	% DV
Vitamin A 3500 IU (29% as Beta Carotene)	70%
Vitamin C 60 mg	100%
Vitamin D 400 IU	100%
Vitamin E 45 IU	150%
Vitamin K 10 mcg	13%
Thiamin 1.5 mg	100%
Riboflavin 1.7 mg	100%
Niacin 20 mg	100%
Vitamin B_6 3 mg	150%
Folic Acid 400 mcg	100%
Vitamin B_{12} 25 mcg	417%
Biotin 30 mcg	10%
Pantothenic Acid 10 mg	100%
Calcium 200 mg	20%
Phosphorus 48 mg	5%
Iodine 150 mcg	100%
Magnesium 100 mg	25%
Zinc 15 mg	100%
Selenium 20 mcg	29%
Copper 2 mg	100%
Manganese 2 mg	100%
Chromium 150 mcg	125%
Molybdenum 75 mcg	100%
Chloride 72 mg	2%
Potassium 80 mg	2%
Boron 150 mcg	*
Nickel 5 mcg	*
Silicon 2 mg	*
Vanadium 10 mcg	*
Lutein 250 mcg	*
Lycopene 300 mcg	*

*Daily Value (%DV) not established.

Ingredients: Calcium Carbonate, Dibasic Calcium Phosphate, Magnesium Oxide, Potassium Chloride, Microcrystalline Cellulose, Ascorbic Acid (Vit. C), dl-Alpha Tocopheryl Acetate (Vit. E), Gelatin, Pregelatinized Starch, Crospovidone. **Contains less than 2% of the following:** Acacia Senegal Gum, Ascorbyl Palmitate, Beta Carotene, Biotin, Boron, Butylated Hydroxytoluene, Calcium Pantothenate, Chromic Chloride, Citric Acid, Colloidal Silicon Dioxide, Cupric Oxide, Cyanocobalamin (Vit. B_{12}), Ergocalciferol (Vit. D), FD&C Blue No. 2 Aluminum Lake, FD&C Red No. 40 Aluminum Lake, FD&C Yellow No. 6 Aluminum Lake, Folic Acid, Hypromellose, Lutein, Lycopene, Magnesium Stearate, Manganese Sulfate, Niacinamide, Nickelous Sulfate, Phytonadione (Vit. K), Polysorbate 80, Potassium Iodide, Potassium Sorbate, Purified Water, Pyridoxine Hydrochloride (Vit. B_6), Riboflavin (Vit. B_2), Silicon Dioxide, Sodium Ascorbate, Sodium Benzoate, Sodium Citrate, Sodium Metavanadate, Sodium Molybdate, Sodium Selenate, Sodium Silicoaluminate, Sorbic Acid, Starch, Sucrose, Thiamine Mononitrate (Vit. B_1), Titanium Dioxide, Tocopherol, Tribasic Calcium Phosphate, Triethyl Citrate, Vitamin A Acetate (Vit. A), Zinc Oxide. **May also contain:** Calcium Stearate, Glucose, Lactose Monohydrate.

Recommended Intake: Adults, 1 tablet daily with food. Not formulated for use in children.

Warnings: Keep out of the reach of children. As with any supplement, if you are pregnant or nursing a baby, contact your healthcare professional.

Important Information: Long-term intake of high levels of vitamin A (excluding that sourced from beta-carotene) may increase the risk of osteoporosis in postmenopausal women. Do not take this product if taking other vitamin A supplements.

How Supplied: Bottles of 60, 100, 150, and 220 tablets.

Storage: Store at Room Temperature. Keep bottle tightly closed. Bottle is sealed with printed foil under cap. Do not use if foil is torn.

Earthspring, LLC
7620 E McKELLIPS RD.,
SUITE 4 PMB 86
SCOTTSDALE, ARIZONA USA
85257

Direct Inquiries to:
www.greencalcium.com
www.totalgreens.com
www.earthspring.com
888-841-7363

PHARMABETIC™

Description: A 100% natural dietary supplement.

Ingredients: proprietary blend Sage Leaves, Horsetail, Mullein, Coriander Seed, Black Seed, Cornsilk, Neem Leaves, Gymnema Sylvestre, Bitter Melon, Fenugreek, Guava Leaves, Bilberry, Mulberry Leaves, Olive Leaves

Directions: Only take this product with water. Take 1 capsules in the morning and 1 capsules before bedtime. Contact your healthcare practitioner for further advice.

Warning: Do not use if pregnant or breast-feeding. Consult your doctor prior to using this product if you are taking any prescription medication.

How Supplied: 30 Capsules (Vegetarian) per Bottle